R. Steffen, H.O. Lobel, J. Haworth, D.J. Bradley (Eds.)

# Travel Medicine

Proceedings of the First Conference on International Travel Medicine, Zürich, Switzerland, 5-8 April 1988

With 83 Figures and 138 Tables

Springer-Verlag Berlin Heidelberg New York
London Paris Tokyo Hong Kong

PD Dr. med. Robert Steffen
Institut für Sozial- und Präventivmedizin
der Universität Zürich, Sumatrastraße 30,
CH-8006 Zürich, Switzerland

Dr. Hans Lobel
Malaria Branch, Centers for Disease Control
Atlanta, GA 30333, United States of America

Dr. James Haworth
Chemin Roitelet 5,
CH-1292 Chambèsy, Switzerland

Professor David J. Bradley
MA, DM, FRCPath, FFCM, FRCP, FIBiol, Hon. FIPHE
London School of Hygiene and Tropical Medicine
Keppel Street, London WCLE 7HT, England

ISBN 3-540-19356-1 Springer-Verlag Berlin Heidelberg New York
ISBN 0-387-19356-1 Springer-Verlag New York Berlin Heidelberg

Library of Congress Cataloging-in-Publication Data
Conference on International Travel Medicine (1st: 1988: Zurich, Switzerland) Travel medicine. proceedings of the First Conference on International Travel Medicine, Zurich, Switzerland, 5–8 April 1988 / R. Steffen ... [et al.] (eds.).
ISBN 0-387-19356-1 (U.S.: alk. paper)
1. Travel – Health aspects – Congresses. 2. Travel – congresses. I. Steffen, Robert. II. Title [DNLM: 1. Preventive Medicine – congresses. WA 110 C7485t 1988] RA783.5.C66 1988 613.6'8 – dc20
DNLM/DLC 89-10114



Typesetting: Brühlsche Universitätsdruckerei, Giessen
Offsetprinting: Zach, Berlin. Bookbinding: Lüderitz & Bauer, Berlin
2119/3020-543210 – Printed on acid-free paper

# Preface

The interest in health problems of travelers has grown as transportation has become faster and many distant places have become accessible for millions of travelers (Fig. 1). This interest was evidenced by the attendance at the First Conference on International Travel Medicine in Zurich, Switzerland, 4–8 April 1988. The conference was cosponsored by the World Health Organization, the World Tourism Organization, the US Centers for Disease Control, the London School of Hygiene and Tropical Medicine, the UK Public Health Laboratory Service, the Swiss Federal Office of Public Health, and the University of Zurich.

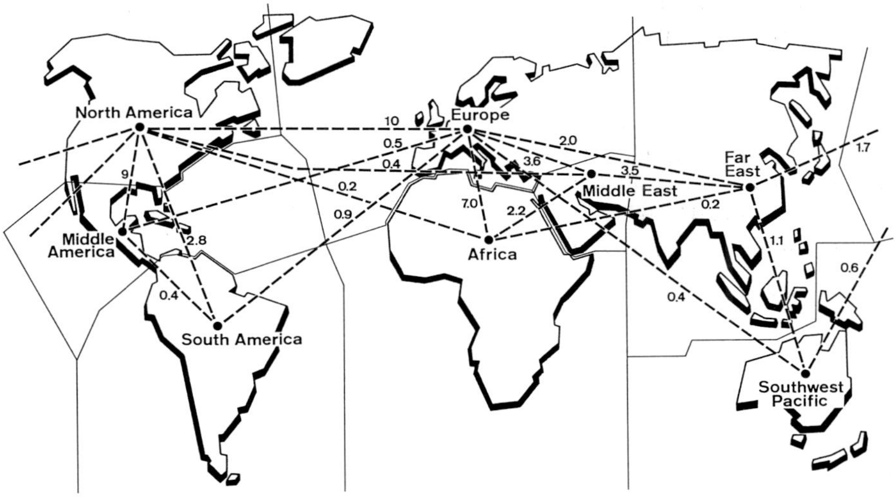


**Fig. 1.** Passengers (millions return flights on interregional scheduled and charter services, 1985. The total of 46.5 million return flights is based on interregional scheduled and charter services 1985, including passengers of companies who are not members of the International Air Transport Association. From the total number, 13.5 million interregional return flights between industrialized countries (taking into account subregions, e.g., Japan), 6 million between developing countries were subtracted. From the remaining 27 million, 25%–30% were deducted as allowance to persons originating their flights in the Third World, leaving 20 million travelers originating in industrialized countries for a visit in developing countries.

The conference brought together 413 participants from 43 countries. They represented many different disciplines and included clinicians, epidemiologists, health administrators, policy makers, medical advisors to airlines and industrial enterprises and to relief and volunteer agencies, and representatives of the travel and pharmaceutical industries.

The aim of the conference was to improve the protection of the traveler by developing more effective recommendations for the prevention of illness in travelers, to promote uniformity of the advice given to travelers, and to exchange information on the health aspects associated with intercontinental travel.

The diversity of the presentations reflected the wide range of issues which confront short-term and long-term travelers. They included pre-travel health information, immunizations and other preventive measures, aspects of travel itself such as kinetosis, jet lag, and high altitude sickness, psychological adaptation to foreign environments, and the risks of death or health impairment in various population groups and at diverse destinations. Round table discussions were held on malaria, diarrheal diseases, AIDS, immunizations, and health information.

Several presentations and discussions concentrated on the responsibility to inform travelers about health issues. Although some representatives of travel agents and the airline industry indicated that it was neither in their interest nor their responsibility to let their customers know of potential health hazards, evidence was presented that several large tour operators take a more sensible attitude and recognize their responsibility to safeguard the health of their clients.

The conference demonstrated a need for improved communication and a more frequent exchange of views and information between experts in travel medicine, the travel industry, and the media.

We are indebted to the publishers for their patience and assistence in the preparation of these proceedings.

June 15, 1988

Robert Steffen
Hans O. Lobel
James Haworth
David J. Bradley

# List of Contributors

Abos, R.
Unidad de Medicina Tropical, Hospital Clinico, Provincial de Barcelona, Carrer Monges 28, E-08030 Barcelona, Spain

Abounaja, S.S., Dr.
Department of Microbiology & Community Medicine, Great Al-Fateh University, Tripoli, Libya

Adamowicz, L.
Pasteur Vaccins, 3, Avenue Pasteur, BP 10, F-92430 Marnes-La-Coquette, France

Albuquerque, J.
Algarve Health Department, Faro, Portugal

Alisjahbana, A.
Faculty of Medicine, Padjadjaran University, Bandung, Indonesia

Alonge, D.O.
Department of Veterinary Public Health, and Preventive Medicine, University of Ibadan, Ibadan, Nigeria

Ambrosch, F.
Institute for Specific Prophylaxis and Tropical Medicine, University of Vienna, Kinderspitalgasse 15, A-1095 Vienna, Austria

Amsallem, D.
Service des Maladies Infectieuses et Tropicales, C.H.U. "St.-Jacques", F-25030 Besançon Cedex, France

Añaños, G.
Unidad de Medicina Tropical, Hospital Clinic Provincial de Barcelona, Via Augusta 128, E-08006 Barcelona, Spain

Andersen, P.
Department of Infectious Diseases, University Hospital, Marselisborg Hospital, P.P. Orumsgade 11, DK-8000 Aarhus, Denmark

Andersson, Y.
National Bacteriological Laboratory, S-10521 Stockholm, Sweden

Andremont, A.
Institut G. Roussy, Villejuif, France

André, F.E.
Smith Kline Biologicals, 89 Rue de l'Institut, B-1330 Rixensart, Belgium

Bailey, T.
Centers for Disease Control, Parasitic Disease Branch, Atlanta, GA 30333, USA

Baker, T.
Johns Hopkins School of Public Health, International Health Department, Baltimore, MD 21205, USA

Balvay, P.
Service des Maladies Infectieuses et Tropicales, C.H.U. "St-Jacques", F-25030 Besançon Cedex, France

Bandet, R.
Institut Mérieux, 56 Avenue Leclerc, F-69348 Lyon Cedex 07, France

Babalola, R.O.
University College Hospital, School of Midwifery, Ibadan, Nigeria

Barbarini, G.
Institute of Infectious Diseases, IRCCS Policlinico S. Matteo, University of Pavia, Via Taramelli, I-27100 Pavia, Italy

Barnas, G.P.
Department of Internal Medicine, Box 135, Milwaukee County Medical Complex, 8700 West Wisconsin Avenue, Milwaukee, WI 53226, USA

Beales, P.F.
Chief Medical Officer, Programming and Training, Malaria Action Programme, WHO Headquarters, CH-1211 Geneva 27, Switzerland

Begg, N.T.
PHLS Communicable Diseases Surveillance Centre, 61 Colindale Avenue, London NW9 5EQ, England

Bell, E.J.
Communicable Diseases (Scotland) Unit, Ruchill Hospital, Glasgow G20 9NB, Scotland

Berger, R.
University Children's Hospital, Römergasse 8, CH-4058 Basel, Switzerland

Bern, K.
University of Pennsylvania Medical School, Philadelphia, PA, USA

Bernard, K.W.
International Health Program Office, Centers for Disease Control, 1600 Clifton Road, Atlanta, GA 30333, USA

Bertolaso, G.
Ministry of Foreign Affairs, Directorate General for Development Cooperation, Via Contarini 25, I-00194 Rome, Italy

Binder, M.
Medical Counsellor, Club Méditerranée, 25, rue Vivienne, F-75002 Paris, France

Black, F.T.
Department of Infectious Diseases, University Hospital, Marseliborg Hospital, Aarhus, Denmark

Blanche, X.
Hospital Clinic Provincial de Barcelona, Carrer Monges 28, E-08030 Barcelona, Spain

Bock, H.L.
Behringwerke AG, P.O.B. 1140, D-3550 Marburg, Federal Republic of Germany

Boettiger, M.
National Bacteriological Laboratory, S-10521 Stockholm, Sweden

Borbély, A.A.
Institute of Pharmacology, University of Zurich, CH-8006 Zurich, Switzerland

Bouvet, E.
Direction Générale de la Santé, Paris, France

Bovet, P.
Medical Policlinic, Division of Immunology and Allergology, University of Lausanne, Rue César Roux 19, CH-1005 Lausanne, Switzerland

Bowker, L.
Department of Pediatrics, University of Ottawa, Infectious Diseases Service, Children's Hospital of Eastern Ontario, 401 Smyth Rd., Ottawa, Ontario, K1H 8L1, Canada

Bradley, D.J.
P.H.L.S. Malaria Reference Laboratory and Ross Institute, London School of Hygiene and Tropical Medicine, Keppel Street, London WC1E7HT, England

Bradley, S.G.
Department of Microbiology and Immunology, Virginia Commonwealth University, Box 678, Richmond, VA 23298-0678, USA

Brink, E.W.
Surveillance, Investigations, and Research Branch, Division of Immunization, Center for Prevention Services, Centers of Disease Control, 1600 Clifton Road NE, Atlanta, GA 30333, USA

Brockmeyer, N.
Dermatological Clinic, University of Essen Medical School, Hufelandstr. 55, D-4300 Essen 1, Federal Republic of Germany

Bruce-Chwatt, L.J. †
Wellcome Tropical Institute, 200 Euston Road, London NW1, England

Bryan, R.T.
Centers of Disease Control, Parasitic Diseases, Atlanta, GA 30333, USA

Buck, A.
Institute of Pharmacology, University of Zurich, CH-8006 Zurich, Switzerland

Burchard, G.D.
Bernhard-Nocht Institute for Tropical Medicine, Clinical Department, Bernhard-Nocht-Str. 74, D-2000 Hamburg 4, Federal Republic of Germany

Burnier, E.
St. Francis District Designated Hospital, Box 73, Ifakara, Tanzania

Bwibo, N.O.
College of Health Sciences, University of Nairobi, Kenyatta National Hospital, P.O. Box 30588, Nairobi, Kenya

Calderon, W.
Institute of Infectious Diseases, IRCCS Policlinico S. Matteo, University of Pavia, Via Taramelli, I-27100 Pavia, Italy

Cartwright, R.Y.
Public Health Laboratory, St. Luke's Hospital, Warren Road, Guildford, Surrey GU1 3NT, England

Chambers, R.
Emergency Medicine, Regional Hospital, C.H.R., Vesoul, France

Chan-Kam, C.
Aids Prevention and Control Unit, Civil Hopsital, Port Louis, Mauritius

Char, D.F.B.
Director of Student Health, Professor of Pediatrics, University of Hawaii, 1710 East West Road, Honolulu, HI 96822, USA

Chiesa, A.
Institute of Infectious Diseases, IRCCS Policlinico S. Matteo, University of Pavia, Via Taramelli, I-27100 Pavia, Italy

Clarke, P.D.
London School of Hygiene and Tropical Medicine, Keppel Street, London WC1E 7HT, England

Clemens, R.
Behringwerke AG, P.O.B. 1140, D-3550 Marburg, Federal Republic of Germany

Conant-Sloane, B.
Dartmouth Medical School, Hanover, NH, USA

Corachan, M.
University of Barcelona, Hospital Clinic, Villaroel 170, E-08036 Barcelona, Spain

Cossar, J.H.
Principal in General Practice and Research Associate, Communicable Diseases (Scotland) Unit, Ruchill Hospital, Glasgow G20 9NB, Scotland

Crawford, C.M.
General Practitioner Ruchill Hospital, Glasgow G20 9NB, Scotland

D'Agata, E.
Tropical Disease Unit, Toronto General Hospital, Toronto M5G 2C4, Canada

Danielides, B.
Laboratory of Bacteriology, Infectious Diseases Hospital, P.O.B. 11191, GR-54110 Thessaloniki, Greece

Darioli, R.
Medical Policlinic, Division of Immunology and Allergology, University of Lausanne, Rue César Roux 19, CH-1005 Lausanne, Switzerland

Dawson, D.G.
International Medicine, Unocal UK Limited, 32 Cadburg Road, Sunbury-on-Thames Middx. FW 167 LU OAG, England

Dax, E.M.
Department of Medicine, Johns Hopkins Medical Institutions, Medical Advisor's Office, Hampton B-139, Baltimore, MD 21205, USA

Deuber, H.J.
III. Med. Klinik, Klinikum Bamberg, Buger Straße 80, D-8600 Bamberg, Federal Republic of Germany

Deville, W.
Epidemiology and Community Medicine, University of Antwerp, Antwerp, Belgium

Dewar, R.D.
Communicable Diseases Scotland Unit, Ruchill Hospital, Glasgow G20 9NB, Scotland

Dietrich, M.
Bernhard-Nocht Institute for Tropical Medicine, Bernhard-Nocht-Straße 74, D-2000 Hamburg 4, Federal Republic of Germany

Djakovic, N.
Clinical Hospital "Dr. M. Stojanovic", Zagreb, Yugoslavia

Djeddah, C.
Documentation Center, Italian Society of Tropical Medicine, P. le Ponte Milvio n. 20, Rome, Italy

Dos Dantos, J.
Medical College of Virginia, Department of Pathology, Box 597, MCV Station, Richtmond, VA 23298-0597, USA

DuPont, H.L.
Department of Medicine, The University of Texas Medical School, 6431 Fannin, 1728 Freeman Bldg., Houston, TX 77030, USA

Ebisawa, I.
Department of Public Health, Toho University School of Medicine,
5-21-16 Omori-nishi, Otaku, Tokyo 143, Japan

Echeverria, P.
Department of Bacteriology, A.F.R.I.M.S., Bangkok 10400, Thailand

Edwards, B.
Division of Infectious Diseases, Long Island Jewish Medical Center,
New Hyde Park, NY 11042, USA

Ericsson, C.
The University of Texas Health, Science Center at Houston, 1150 MSB,
P.O. Box 20708, Houston, TX 77225, USA

Estavoyer, J.M.
Service des Maladies Infectieuses et Tropicales, C.H.U. "St-Jacques",
F-25030 Besançon Cedex, France

Fidler, A.
Arbeitskreis für Vorsorge- und Sozialmedizin, Lindauerstraße 58,
A-6912 Hoerbranz, Austria

Fallon, R.J.
Communicable Diseases (Scotland) Unit, Ruchill Hospital, Glasgow G20 9NB, Scotland

Fouant, M.M.
School of Basic Health Sciences, Virginia Commonwealth University
Richmond, VA 23298, USA

Foyle, M.F.
Missionary and Volunteers Health Service to Inter Health,
Mildmay Mission Hospital, Hackney Road, London E2 7NA, England

Frei, P.
Medical Policlinic, Division of Immunology and Allergology, University of
Lausanne, Rue César Roux 19, CH-1005 Lausanne, Switzerland

Fritzell, B.
Pasteur Vaccins, 1 Bd Raymond Poincaré, F-92430 Marnes-La-Coquette,
France

Gamble, K.L.
Missionary Health Institute, 4800 Leslie St., Willowdale, Ontario M2K 2R9,
Canada

Gatzoflia, B.
Laboratory of Bacteriology, Infectious Diseases Hospital, P.O.B. 11191, GR-54110 Thessaloniki, Greece

Gennaro, M. di
Ministery of Foreign Affairs, Directorate General for Development Cooperation, Via Contarini 25, I-00194 Rome, Italy

Gesemann, M.
Institute for Medical Virology and Immunology, University of Essen Medical School, Hufelandstr. 55, D-4300 Essen 1, Federal Republic of Germany

Gobert, P., Institut Mérieux, 58 Avenue Leclerc, BP 7046, F-69348 Lyon Cedex 07, France

Goilav, C.
Institute of Tropical Medicine, 155 Nationalestraat, B-2000 Antwerp, Belgium

Gola, T.
Institute of Infectious Diseases, IRCCS Polioclinico S. Matteo, University of Pavia, Via Taramelli, I-27100 Pavia, Italy

Goldsmid, J.M.
Department of Pathology, University of Tasmania, GPO, Box 252C, 7001 Hobart, Australia

Gordon, M.E.
Yale School of Medicine, 111 Sherman Avenue, New Haven, CT 06511, USA

Goujon, C.
Institut Pasteur, 211 rue de Vaugirard, F-75015 Paris, France

Grimes, P.
Condé Nast's Traveler's Magazine, 360 Madison Avenue, New York, NY 10017, USA

Guerra, R.
Ministry of Foreign Affairs, Directorate General for Development Cooperation, Via Contarini 25, I-00194 Rome, Italy

Gunn, A.D.G.
University of Reading, University Health Centre, Northcourt Avenue, Reading RG2 7HE, England

Guptill, K.
Johns Hopkins School of Public Health, International Health Department, Baltimore, MD 21205, USA

Gurung, K.
University Hosptial Travel Clinic, Dept. Medicine RC-02, Seattle, WA 98195, USA

Gyr, K.
Innere Medizin, Kantonsspital, CH-4410 Liestal, Switzerland

Hargarten, S.W.
Medical College of Wisconsin, Emergency Medicine, 8700 W. Wisconsin Avenue, Box 204, Milwaukee, WI 53226

Hatz, C.
Swiss Tropical Institute, Field Laboratory, Box 53, Ifakara, Tanzania

Heber, L.
College of Nursing, University of Saskatchewan, Saskatoon, Saskatchewan S7N OWO, Canada

Heizmann, W.
Hygiene-Institut der Universität Tübingen, Wilhelmstraße 31, D-7400 Tübingen, Federal Republic of Germany

Heusser, R.
Institute for Social and Preventive Medicine of the University, Sumatrastr. 30, CH-8006 Zurich, Switzerland

Hill, D.R.
Division of Infectious Diseases, Room L-3108, University of Connecticut Health Center, Farmington, CT 06032, USA

Hilton, E.
Division of Infectious Diseases, Long Island Jewish Medical Center, New Hyde Park, NY 11042, USA

Hirschl, A.
Institute of Hygiene, University of Vienna, Kinderspitalgasse 15, A-1095 Vienna, Austria

Hitze, K.L.
W.H.O. Communicable Disease Control, Am Halbenstein 5, A-6912 Hoerbranz, Austria

Höfler, W.
Tropenmedizinisches Institut, Universität Tübingen, Wilhelmstraße 31,
D-7400 Tübingen, Federal Republic of Germany

Höring, E.
Krankenhaus Bad Cannstatt, Stuttgart, Federal Republic of Germany

Houston, R.
Peace Corps Medical Clinic, Kathmandu, Nepal

Jardel, J.P.
Assistant Director-General, World Health Organization,
CH-1211 Geneva 27, Switzerland

Jansen-Rossek, R.
Landesinstitut für Tropenmedizin, Königin-Elisabeth Str. 32,
D-1000 B 19 Berlin (West), Germany

Jedlička, J.
Research Laboratory of Tropical Health, Institute of Hygiene and
Epidemiology, Ruska 85, CS-10005 Prague 10, Czechoslovakia

Jong, E.C.
University Hospital Travel Clinic, Department of Medicine RC-02,
University of Washington School of Medicine, Seattle, WA 98195, USA

Junga, C.
Krankenhaus Bad Cannstatt, Stuttgart, Federal Republic of Germany

Juranek, D.
Centers for Disease Control, Parasitic Disease Branch, Division of Parasitic
Disease, Atlanta, GA 30333, USA

Just, M.
Department of Microbiology, University Childrens Hospital, Römergasse,
CH-4058 Basel, Switzerland

Kaay van der, H.J.
Laboratory of Parasitology/Institute of Tropical Medicine,
Faculty of Medicine, University of Leiden, The Netherlands

Kanzouzidou, A.
Laboratory of Bacteriology, Infectious Diseases Hospital, P.O.B. 11191,
54110 Thessaloniki, USA

Karpilow, C.
International Professional Association, Queen Anne Medical Center,
1902 Victoria Ave SW, Seattle, WA 98126, England

Keefe, D.M.K.
Royal Cornwall Hospital, Treliske, Truro TR1 3LJ, UK

Keene, W.
University of California, San Francisco, CA 94611, USA

Keller, P.
Tourism Department Swiss Federal Office of Labour and Industry,
Bundesgasse 8, CH-3003 Berne, Switzerland

Kermorvant, M.
DRASS D'lle de France, Paris, France

Keystone, J.S.
Tropical Disease Unit, Toronto General Hospital, Toronto M5G 2C4,
Canada

Kiosses, V.G.
Laboratory of Bacteriology, Infectious Diseases Hospital, P.O.B. 11191,
GR-54110 Thessaloniki, Greece

Klerk de, L.
Central Development and Support Group Hospital Information Systems
BAZIS, Rijnsburgerweg 10, Leiden, The Netherlands

Klugman, K.P.
Department of Bacteriology and Immunology, The Rockefeller University,
1230 York Avenue, New York, NY 10021, USA

Knaus, L.
Division of Infectious Diseases, Departement of International Medicine,
University of Ulm, Steinhövelstraße 9, D-7900 Ulm,
Federal Republic of Germany

Koch, K.
Tourism Department, Swiss Federal Office of Labour and Industry,
Bundesgasse 8, CH-3003 Berne, Switzerland

Kollaritsch, H.
Institute for Specific Prophylaxis and Tropical Medicine,
Kinderspitalgasse 15, A-1095 Vienna, Austria

Kollaritsch, R.
Institute for Specific Prophylaxis and Tropical Medicine,
Kinderspitalgasse 15, A-1095 Vienna, Austria

Korger, G.
Behringwerke AG, P.O. Box 1140, D-3550 Marburg,
Federal Republic of Germany

Kouznetsov, R.L.
Programming and Training, Malaria Action Programme, World Health Organization, CH-1211 Geneva 27, Switzerland

Kreider, S.D.
Department of Medicine, Johns Hopkins Medical Institutions, Medical Advisors's Office, Hampton, B-139, Baltimore, MD 21205, USA

Kremsner, P.
Institute for Specific Prophylaxis and Tropical Medicine, University of Vienna, Kinderspitalgasse 15, A-1095 Vienna, Austria

Kreuzfelder, E.
Institute for Medical Virology and Immunology, Hufelandstr. 55, D-4300 Essen 1, Federal Republic of Germany

Krishna, V.R.
University of Washington, Department of Medicine RC-02, University Hospital Travel Clinic, Seattle, WA 98195, USA

Kusch, G.
Medizinische Universitätsklinik, Tübingen, D-7400 Tübingen, Federal Republic of Germany

Kyrönseppä, H.
Clinic for Tropical Diseases, Aurora Hospital, Nordenskiöldinkatu 20, SF-00250 Helsinki, Finland

Lange, W.R.
Department of Medicine, Johns Hopkins Medical Institutions, Medical Advisor's Office, Hampton, B-139, Baltimore, MD 21205, USA

Lapresle, C.
Hopital de l'Institute Pasteur, Centre de Vaccination, Paris, France

Laulund, S.
Chr. Hansesn's Bio Systems, Copenhagen, Denmark

Lapropoulou, M.
Laboratory of Bacteriology, Infectious Diseases Hospital, P.O.B. 11191, GR-54110 Thessaloniki, Greece

Lavanchy, D.
Medical Policlinic, Division of Immunology and Allergology, University of Lausanne, Rue César Roux 19, CH-1005 Lausanne, Switzerland

Lawee, D.
Department of Family and Community Medicine, University of Toronto and Toronto General Hospital, 200 Elizabeth Street, Toronto, Ontario M5G 2C4, Canada

Le Mouel, A.
Service de Radiologie, C.H.U. "St-Jacques", F-25030 Besançon Cedex, France

Lea, G.
British Airways Medical Centre, 75 Regent Street, London W1R 7HG, England

Lee, R.V.
Department of Medicine, Children's Hospital of Buffalo, 219 Bryant Street, Buffalo, NY 14222, USA

Lefur, M.
Pasteur Vaccins 1, Bd Raymond Poincaré, F-92430 Marnes-La-Coquette, France

Leimer, R.
F. Hoffmann-La Roche Ltd., CH-4002 Basel, Switzerland

Leroy, J.
Service des Maladies Infectieuses et Tropicales, C.H.U. "St.-Jacques", F-25030 Besançon Cedex, France

Lhuillier, M.
Institut Pasteur, Paris, France

Lobel, H.O.
Malaria Branch, DPD, CID, Centers for Disease Control, 1600 Clifton Rd, C-22, Atlanta, Georgia 30333, USA

Maccabruni, A.
Institute of Infectious Diseases, IRCCS Policlinico S. Matteo, University of Pavia, Via Taramelli, I-27100 Pavia, Italy

Mailer, R.
F. Hoffmann-La Roche Ltd., CH-4002 Basel, Switzerland

Mann, J.M.
Special Programme on AIDS, World Health Organization, CH-1211 Geneva 27, Switzerland

Mas, J.
Seccion de Parasitologia, Hospital Clinic Provincial de Barcelona, Via Augusta 128, E-08006 Barcelona, Spain

McCann, J.P.
Corporate Medical Director, Pan American World Airways, John F. Kennedy International Airport, Jamaica, NY 11430, USA

McKinney, W.P., M.D.
Department of Internal Medicine, Box 135, Milwaukee County Medical Complex, 8700 West Wisconsin Avenue, Milwaukee, WI 53226, USA

McMullen, R.
University Hospital Travel Clinic RC-02, Department of Medicine, University of Washington School of Medicine, Seattle, WA 98195, USA

Meade, J.
Department of Veterinary Science, University of Arizona, Tucson, AZ 85721, USA

Meer van der, J.W.M.
Department of Infectious Diseases, University Hospital, Leiden, The Netherlands

Meheus, A.
Epidemiology and Community Medicine, University of Antwerp, Antwerp, Belgium

Meier, R.
Innere Medizin, Kantonsspital, CH-4410 Liestal, Switzerland

Mercer, N.
Dartmouth Medical School, Hanover, NH, USA

Mirelman, D.
Department of Biophysics, Weizman Institute, Rehovot, Israel

Missoni, E.
Health Division, General Direction of Cooporation Development, Ministry of Foreign Affairs, Directorate General for Development Cooperation, Via Contarini 25, I-00194 Rome, Italy

Mitchell, S.
Scottish Health Education Group, Caanan Lane, Edinburgh, Scotland

Moran, J.S.
Peace Corps, Office of Medical Service, 806 Connecticut Ave NW, Washington, DC 20526, USA

Motamedi, M.
DIWEC Clinic, P.O. Box 1340, Kathmandu, Nepal

Müller, C.
University Children's Hospital, Römergasse 8, CH-4058 Basel, Switzerland

Naef, U.
F. Hoffmann-La Roche & Co., CH-4002 Basel, Switzerland

Navarro, P.
Departamento Bioestadistica, School of Medicine, University of Barcelona, Barcelona, Spain

Nereli, B.
Pasteur Vaccins, 1, Bd Raymond Poincaré, F-92430 Marnes-La-Coquette, France

Neto, J.G. dos Santos
Department of Pathology, Box 597 – MCV Station, Medical College of Virginia, Richmond, VA 23298-0597, USA

Ngantung, W.
Faculty of Medicine, Padjadjaran University, Bandung, Indonesia

Nicholson, A.N.
Royal Air Force Institute of Aviation Medicine, Farnborough, Hampshire GU146SZ, England

Nutini, M.T.
Pasteur Vaccins, Direction Medical, F-92430 Marnes-La-Coquette, France

Obrecht, O.
Assistance Publique de Paris, Direction du Plan, 3, Avenue Victoria, F-75004 Paris, France

Oelz, O.
Medical Clinic, University Hospital, CH-8091 Zurich, Switzerland

Ohara, H.
Department of Public Health, Toho University School of Medicine, 5-21-16 Omori-nishi, Otaku, Tokyo 143, Japan

Orenstein, W.
Surveillance, Investigations and Research Branch, Division of Immunizations, Centers for Disease Control, United States Public Health and Human Services, 1600 Clifton Road NE, Atlanta, GA 30333, USA

Orskov, F.
Statens Seruminstitut, Copenhagen, Denmark

Overbosch, D.
Red Cross Hospital, The Hague, The Netherlands

Paixao, M.T.
Instituto Nacional de Saude, Lisbon, Portugal

Pasini, W.
Italian Association for Touristic Medicine, Via Dardanelli 64, I-47037 Rimini, Italy

Peltola, H.
Clinic for Tropical Diseases, Aurora Hospital, Nordenskiöldinkatu 20, SF-00250 Helsinki, Finland

Perrin, J.
Direction Générale de la Santé, Paris, France

Phillips-Howard, P.
P.H.L.S. Malaria Reference Laboratory and Ross Institute, London School of Hygiene and Tropical Medicine, Keppel Street, London WC1E 7HT, England

Pichard, E.
Institut Mérieux, 58 Avenue Leclerc, F-69348 Lyon Cedex 07, France

Piot, P.
Institut de Médecine Tropicale, Prince Leopold, Nationalestraat 155, B-2000 Antwerp, Belgium

Plentz, K.
Public Health Services, Waldhausenstr. 11, D-3000 Hannover 81, Federal Republic of Germany

Preblud, S.W.†
Surveillance, Investigation and Research Branch, Division of Immunization, Center for Prevention Services, Centers for Disease Control, 1600 Clifton Road NE, Atlanta, GA 30333, USA

Prinsen, H.
Institute for Tropical Medicine, 155 Nationalestraat, B-2000 Antwerp, Belgium

Prokopec, J.
Research Laboratory of Tropical Health, Institute of Hygiene and Epidemiology, Ruska 85, CS-10005 Prague 10, Czechoslovakia

Quast, U.
Behringwerke AG, P.O.B. 1140, D-3550 Marburg, Federal Republic of Germany

Raeber, P.A.
Medical Policlinic, Division of Immunology and Allergology, University of Lausanne, Rue César Roux 19, CH-1005 Lausanne, Switzerland

Rappold, E.
Institute for Specific Prophylaxis and Tropical Medicine, University of Vienna, Kinderspitalgasse 15, A-1095 Vienna, Austria

Raymond, M., Dr.
Scottish Health Education Group, Caanan Lane, Edinburgh, Scotland

Reid, D.
Communicable Diseases (Scotland) Unit, Ruchill Hospital, Glasgow G20 9NB, Scotland

Reid, T.M.S.
Regional Laboratory, City Hospital, Aberdeen AB9 8AU, Scotland

Richards, F.
Centers for Disease Control, Parasitic Disease Branch, Division of Parasitic Diseases, Atlanta, GA 30333, USA

Riding, M.H.
Communicable Diseases (Scotland) Unit, Ruchill Hospital, Glasgow G20 9NB, Scotland

Rigamer, E.F.
U.S. State Department, Medical Division, Washington, CD 20520, USA

Ritchie, L.D.
Community Medicine Specialist, Grampian Health Board, Aberdeen, Scotland

Roldan, M.L.
Servicio de Pediatria, Hospital Clinic Provincial de Barcelona,
Via Augusta 128, E-08006 Barcelona, Spain

Sabate, F.
C.A.P. "Can Rull" Sabadell, Institut Catala de la Salut, Bailen 165,
E-08037 Barcelona, Spain

Safary, A.
Smith Kline Biological, 89 Rue de l'Institut, B-1330 Rixensart, Belgium

Saliou, P.
3, Avenue Pasteur, BP 10, F-92430 Marnes-La-Coquette, France

Saout, C., Dr.
DRASS D'lle de France, Paris, France

Sawyer, L.
Tropical Disease Unit, Toronto General Hospital, Toronto M5G 2C4,
Canada

Scappatura, F.P.
Department of Family and Community Medicine, University of Toronto and
Toronto General Hospital, 200 Elizabeth Street, Totonto, Ontario,
M5G 2C4, Canada

Scevola, D.
Institute of Infectious Diseases IRCCS Polioclinio S. Matteo,
University of Pavia, Via Taramelli, I-27100 Pavia, Italy

Schär, M.
Institute of Social and Preventive Medicine of the University,
Sumatrastr. 30, CH-8006 Zurich, Switzerland

Scheiermann, N.
University of Essen Medical School, Institute for Laboratory Medicine,
Municipal Hospital Heilbronn, Heilbronn, Federal Republic of Germany

Schultz, M.
Division of Quarantine, Center for Prevention Services, Centers for
Disease Control, 1600 Clifton Road NE, Atlanta, GA 30333, USA

Shlim, D.R.
The CIWEC Clinic, P.O. Box 1340, Kathmandu, Nepal

Sinclair, R.
International Health Center for the Volvo Group, Carlanderika Hospital,
S-41255 Gothenburg, Sweden

Singer, C.
Division of Infectious Diseases, Long Island Jewish Medical Center,
New Hyde Park, NY 11042, USA

Sinigaglia, F.
F. Hoffmann-La Roche & Co., CH-4002 Basel, Switzerland

Smith, C.R.
Missionary Health Institute, 4800 Leslie St., Willowdale, Ontario M2K 2R9,
Canada

Smith, D.
University of Pennsylvania Medical School, Philadelphia, PA, USA

Smith, R.P.
Department of Medicine, Maine Medical Center, Portland, Maine, USA

Sofianidou, A.
Laboratory of Bacteriology, Infectious Diseases Hospital, P.O.B. 11191,
GR-54110 Thessaloniki, Greece

Somaini, B.
Federal Office of Public Health, P.O. Box 2644, CH-3001 Berne, Switzerland

Soula, G.
Ecole national de Médecine et de Pharmacie, Bamako, Mali

Spence, L.
Toronto General Hospital, Toronto M5G 2C4, Canada

Steffen, R.
Division of Epidemiology and Prevention of Communicable Diseases,
Institute of Social and Preventive Medicine of the University,
Sumatrastr. 30, CH-8006 Zurich, Switzerland

Steiger, E.
Institute of Social and Preventive Medicine of the University,
Sumatrastr. 30, CH-8006 Zurich, Switzerland

Stemberger, H., Dr. med.
Institute of Specific Prophylaxis and Tropical Medicine, University of Vienna,
Kinderspitalgasse 15, A-1095 Vienna, Austria

Sterling, C.
Department of Veterinary Science, University of Arizona, Tucson, AZ 85721, USA

Strasser, T.
International Green Cross, 20 Ave du Bouchet, CH-1209 Geneva, Switzerland

Stuiver, P.C.
Department of Tropical Medicine, Havenziekenhuis, Haringvliet 2, NL-3011 TD Rotterdam, The Netherlands

Stürchler, D.
Roche Clinical Research, F. Hoffmann La Roche & Co. Ltd., P.O. Box, CH-4002 Basel, Switzerland

Sukadi, A.
Faculty of Medicine, Padjadjaran University, Bandung, Indonesia

Sugita, E.
Faculty of Medicine, Padjadjaran University, Bandung, Indonesia

Švandovà, E.
Research Laboratory of Tropical Health, Institute of Hygiene and Epidemiology, Ruska 85, CS-10005 Prague 10, Czechoslovakia

Takayanagi, M.
Department of Public Health, Toho University School of Medicine, 5-21-16 Omori-nishi, Otaku, Tokyo 143, Japan

Taylor, D.N.
Department of Bacteriology, A.F.R.I.M.S., Rajvithi Road, 10400 Bangkok, Thailand

Tobler, I.
Institute of Pharmacology, University of Zurich, CH-8006 Zurich, Switzerland

Tolarovà, V.
Research Laboratory of Tropical Health, Institute of Hygiene and Epidemiology, Ruska 85, CS-10005 Prague 10, Czechoslovakia

Tomaszunas, S.
Institute of Maritime and Tropical Medicine, Powstania Stycznniowego 9B, PL-81-519 Gdynia, Poland

Trespi, G.
Institute of Infectious Diseases, IRCCS Polioclinico S. Matteo, University of Pavia, Via Taramelli, I-27100 Pavia, Italy

Tschopp, A.
Institute of Social and Preventive Medicine of the University, Sumatrastr. 30 CH-8006 Zurich, Switzerland

Turner, A.
Sayers Cottage, Hoyle Lane, Heyshott, Midhurst, West Sussex, England

Urner, C.J.
Medical Director, Lykes Bros. Steamship Co. Inc., 300 Poydras Street, New Orleans, LA 70130, USA

Urwin, G.
Ruchill Hospital, Glasgow G20 9NB, Scotland

Valls, M.E.
Seccion de Parasitologia, Hospital Clinic I Provincial de Barcelona, Via Augusta 128, E-08006 Barcelona, Spain

Usman, A.
Faculty of Medicine Padjadjaran University, Bandung, Indonesia

Van der Reis, L.
Medical Director, KLM Royal Dutch Airlines, 1800 Sullivan Avenue, Daly City, CA 94015, USA

Vanek, E.
Division of Infectious Diseases, Dept. of International Medicine, University of Ulm, Steinhövelstraße 9, D-7900 Ulm, Federal Republic of Germany

Vichi, F.
Documentation Centre, Italian Society of Tropical Medicine, P. le Ponte Milvio n. 20, Rome, Italy

Vodopija, I.
Zagreb Institute of Public Health, Mirogojska 16, YU-41000 Zagreb, Yugoslavia

Vosloo, H.
National Institute for Tropical Diseases, Tzaneen, Republic of South Africa

Vranckx, R.
National Centre for Viral Hepatitis, Institute of Hygiene and Epidemiology, J. Wytsmanstraat 14, B-1050 Brussels, Belgium

Waclawski, E.R.
Occupational Health Service, Greater Glasgow Health Board,
Southern General Hospital, 1345 Govan Road, Glasgow G5I 4TF, Scotland

Walker, E.
University Department of Infectious Diseases, Ruchill Hospital,
Glasgow G20 9NB, Scotland

Waskin, H.
Centers for Disease Control, Parasitic Disease Branch, Division of Parasitic
Diseases, Atlanta, GA 30333, USA

Waterman, S.
Los Angeles County Department of Health Services, 313 N. Figueroa,
Room 231, Los Angeles, CA 90012, USA

Wegmann, W.
Pathologie, Kantonsspital, CH-4410 Liestal, Switzerland

Weidner, F.
Krankenhaus Bad Cannstatt, Stuttgart, Federal Republic of Germany

Wheal, R.
Thompson Holidays Ltd., Greater London House, Hapipstread Rd,
London, NW1, England

Wiedermann, W.
Institute for Specific Prophylaxis and Tropical Medicine, University of
Vienna, Kinderspitalgasse 15, A-1095 Vienna, Austria

Wilson, M.E.
Division of Infectious Diseases, Mt. Auburn Hospital, Cambridge,
02238, USA

Wolfe, M.S.
Office of Medical Services, Department of State, Washington,
DC 20520, USA

Wyss, R.
Medical Service, Swissair, P.O. Box, CH-8058 Zurich Airport, Switzerland

Young, E.J.
Baylor College of Medicine, V.A. Medical Center, 2002 Holcombe Blvd.,
Houston, TX 77030, USA

Zürrer, G.
Institute of Social and Preventive Medicine of the University,
Sumatrastr. 30, CH-8006 Zurich, Switzerland

# Table of Contents

# The Scope of Travel Medicine: An Introduction to the Conference on International Travel Medicine

D. J. Bradley

It is a great pleasure to welcome so many people of diverse disciplinary, occupational and national backgrounds to this Conference on International Travel Medicine, the first of its type. One has only to look at the programme to see the varied groups of problems which concern travel medicine and the many aspects of medicine involved. The focus is on travellers of all sorts – and the variety of travel patterns will be addressed below. There is however a common general theme which particularly arises in travel medicine, which is to be aware of the possibilities – once we perceive the possible hazards to which a traveller may be or has been exposed then much of the rest of the problem is relatively straightforward. There is more diversity, whether of travellers or of hazards, than we tend to perceive or accept. Hence the importance of this conference: it will surely broaden our perceptions and increase our awareness of the issues involved.

The programme for the conference and the contents page of the proceedings tell their own story about the scope of the subject and it is not my intention to repeat that. Rather, I would seek to draw the attention of participants, and of the press and our visitors, to the great changes that have occurred over the last century in the range and patterns of travel.

## Range of Travel

Zoologists have a nice term and a useful concept: the *life-time track*, which is a record, on a suitable map, of the entire movements of an animal from birth to its death. We may usefully apply it to people, though it is of course difficult to trace in detail for long-lived animals such as man. We usually only know it for very sedentary people or those with fixed and unvarying habits, or for close relations. It can be illustrated for four generations of my own family, for example.

My great-grandfather was born and died in Northamptonshire. His whole life took place in a square of only 40 km side. He was born in one village, worked for most of his life in a small market and manufacturing town nearby, and travelled to some of the neighbouring great houses and villages as postillion on the coach that operated from the main hotel in Kettering (Fig. 1). He lived a long and, to the best of my knowledge, happy life but it was geographically very circumscribed.

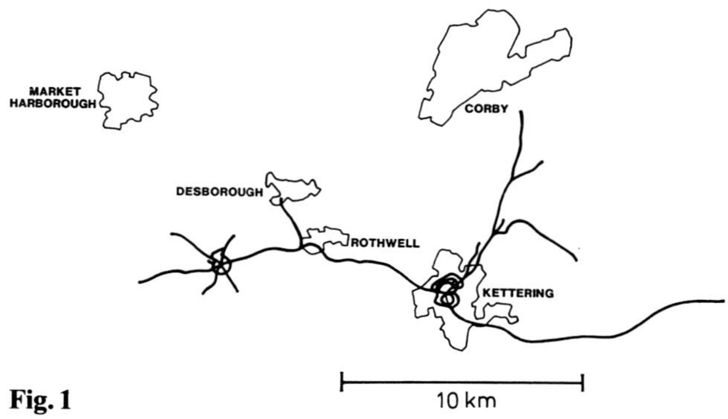


**Fig. 1**

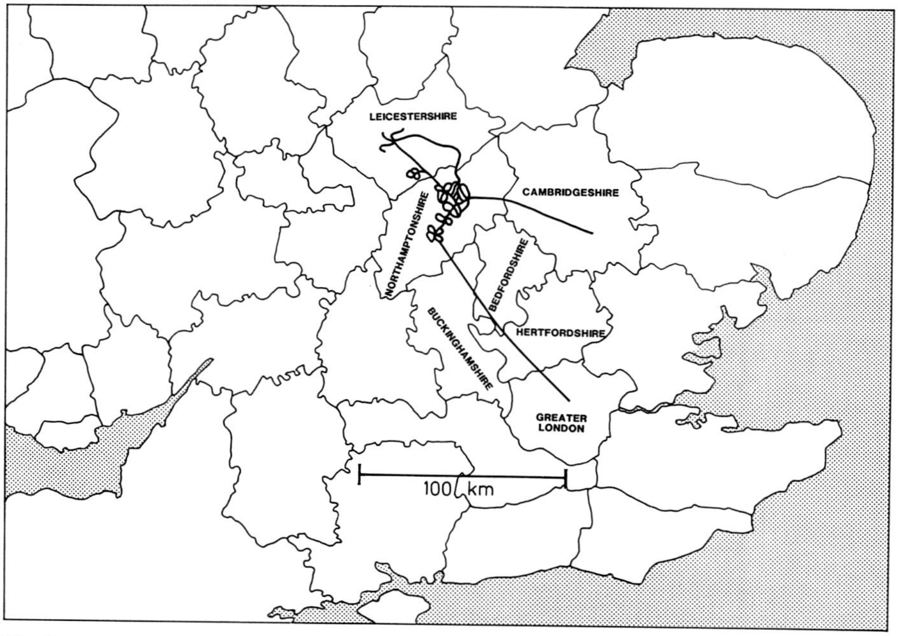


**Fig. 2**

**Figs. 1–4.** Maps of the life-time track of four generations of the same family. The linear scale increases by a factor of 10 and the map area by a factor of 100 between each pair of adjacent figures. Figure 1 represents the track of the authors' great-grandparent, Fig. 2 that of the grandparent, Fig. 3 the parent, and Fig. 4 the author's own movements

My grandfather lived in Northampton and Kettering. He was not a great traveller but he often went to nearby cities to see my parents and other relations, so he had visited Leicester and Cambridge, and at least once he went to London. His life-time track can be enclosed in a square of 400 km side, that

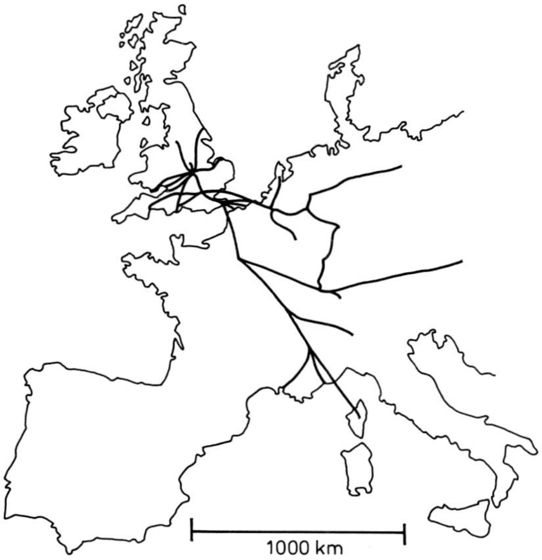


**Fig. 3**

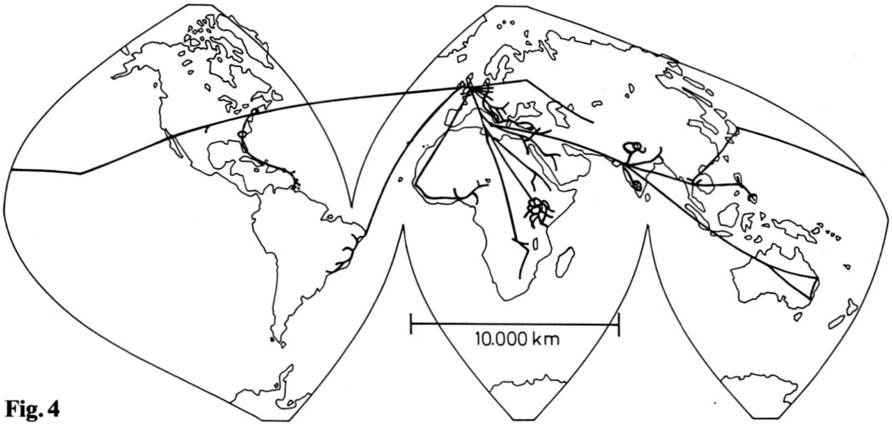


**Fig. 4**

is, ten times greater in length and a hundredfold in area as compared with his father's (Fig. 2).

My father travelled on the European continent in his youth, and probably knew Europe better than I, who grew up during the war. He visited many parts of England and continued to travel to Europe for business meetings about shoe design and manufacture, and for occasional holidays (Fig. 3). His lifetime track fits into a 4000-km square, again up tenfold linearly and a hundredfold in area from *his* father.

My own early life centred on Leicester and Northamptonshire, and subsequent visits covered a wide area. By the nature of my work, travel to the tropics is a major activity, but my occupation probably increases my frequency and diversity of travel more than the maximum distance travelled (Fig. 4), which now covers the globe, fitting into a 40 000-km square.

Thus in four generations the range of linear travelling has increased by a factor of 1000 and the area within which movement takes place has increased by a factor of one million. The experience described here is not atypical. Certainly some of those present at the conference have great-grandparents who sailed around the globe or migrated to another hemisphere. But in general the range and frequency of travel for inhabitants of developed countries and for the better educated members of third world nations has increased dramatically. The scope for travel medicine has greatly increased in quantitative terms.

But people have always travelled, since the time of Abraham and before. While travel has increased, the duration of the actual journey has fallen, for many people. The movements of the children of Israel or of the Greek army described by Xenophon in the Anabasis or of the Pilgrim Fathers have a completely different time scale from "jet clipper 101". The problems that once faced the ships' doctor have now become problems of imported disease. It is not accidental that, for example, the Hamburg School was founded for Tropical Diseases and Ships' Medicine, as the 6-week journey from many parts of the tropics to Europe ensured that the incubation period of most tropical diseases would be completed before the ship docked. There was time for contagious diseases to spread on board ship, and to be manifest. The ship's doctor was the travel medicine specialist.

By contrast, air travel restricts the time available for disease transmission on the voyage, but it makes the potential hazards of direct transmission greater, especially as the capacity of aircraft increases. Thus if a person is in the infectious stage of a virus fever before the rash appears, fellow-passengers are all potentially exposed but may disperse without being aware of this. With small, medium and large aeroplanes, corresponding to a quarter and a half century ago as well as today, if 1 person in 10 000 has a particular communicable disease problem then the chance of such a person being on the plane, and the number of contacts, are given in Table 1. There is a sense in which the scale of problem increases as the square of the passenger capacity, if considered on a per-flight basis.

**Table 1.** Risks and contacts for a communicable disease problem of prevalence 1:10 000 and varying aeroplane sizes

| Capacity of aeroplane: passengers *A* | Probability of having infected person on board *B* | Number of contacts *C* | Scale of problem per flight $B \times C$ |
|---|---|---|---|
| 4 | 1:2500 or 0.04% | 3 | 0.12 |
| 40 | 1:250 or 0.4% | 39 | 15.96 |
| 400 | 1:25 or 4% | 399 | 1596.00 |

However we choose to view the problem, it is clear that now the problems that were faced by the ships' doctor are substantially transferred to the GP, to the travel medicine specialist and more generally to the medical staff of the country from which the traveller came.

We may now usefully consider the migratory patterns followed by modern travellers. It is convenient to represent them schematically on a simple map-diagram (Fig. 5). The left side represents the home (h) country for the physician. The right-hand side represents the overseas (o/s) country or countries visited, viewed from the deliberately subjective point of view of the developed country traveller. Up to three overseas countries are available in the diagram. The journey falls in the centre of the diagram and may be by land, sea, or air. The three diamonds in the diagram represent stopover sites for the air traveller and ports of call for those travelling by sea. The traditional journey of the past, prior to regular air travel, is represented in Fig. 6. If it was to the tropics or other substantial distance, the voyages out and back would be measured in weeks and, because it took so long to make the journey, the overseas stay would often be for over a month, to make the whole effort worthwhile. Stops in port on the journey were usual.

The most common journeys of today are the package holiday, and many other visits abroad for business reasons resemble it (Fig. 7). The journey is measured in hours, is effectively non-stop in an aeroplane, and the time spent abroad is also short, generally 2 weeks or even less. The journey itself is negligible, except as a source of motion sickness (and possibly a hangover!) and exposure to respiratory infection. This is the archetypal modern traveller, but we need to bear in mind their diversity as shown in Figs. 8–14.

The first complicating factor is a possible stopover (Fig. 8), whose main importance for the travel physician is that it may escape unnoticed. The visitor to Australia, presenting with a fever to a clinician in Europe on his return, may fail to mention that his ticket allowed a 2-day stopover in a Southeast Asian country. This may provide the explanation of his fever. The practitioner whose

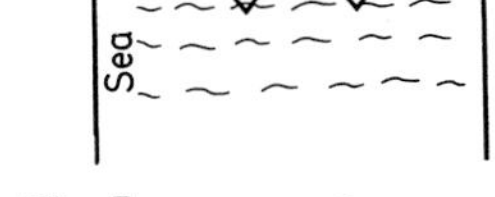


**Fig. 5**

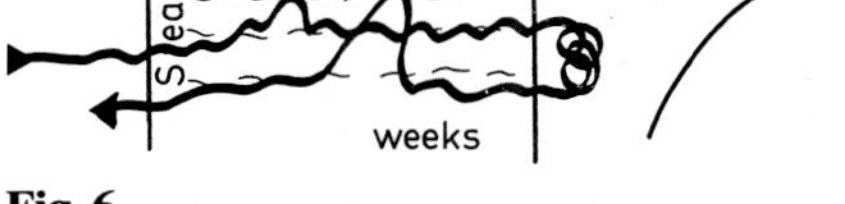


**Fig. 6**

**Figs. 5, 6.** Figure 5 represents the home, journey and destinations for the traveller (explanation in text) and Fig. 6 a typical journey to the tropics prior to availability of air travel

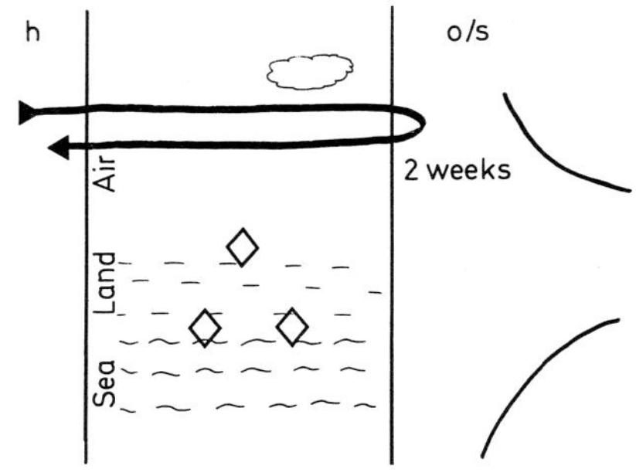


**Fig. 7**

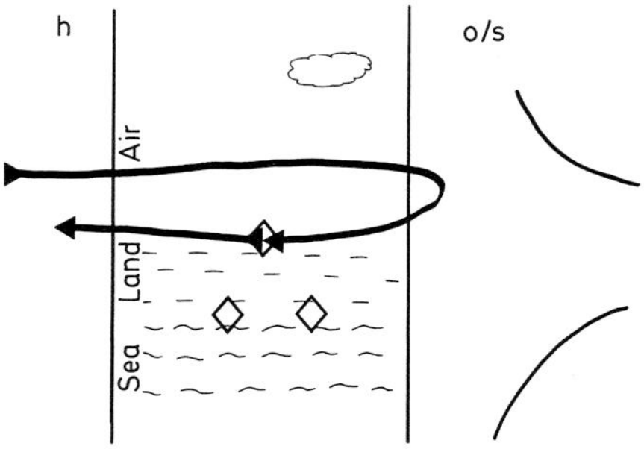


**Fig. 8**

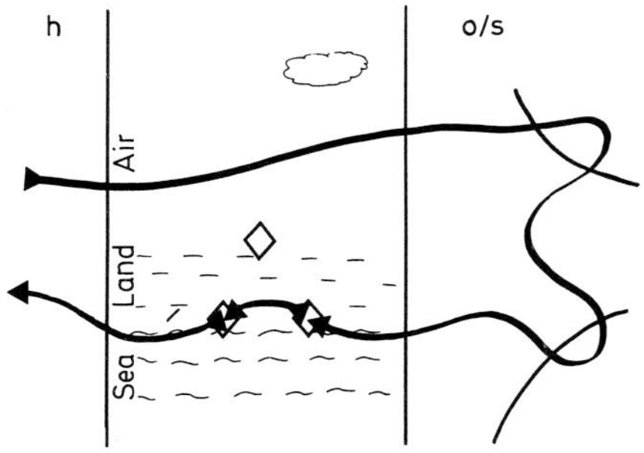


**Fig. 9**

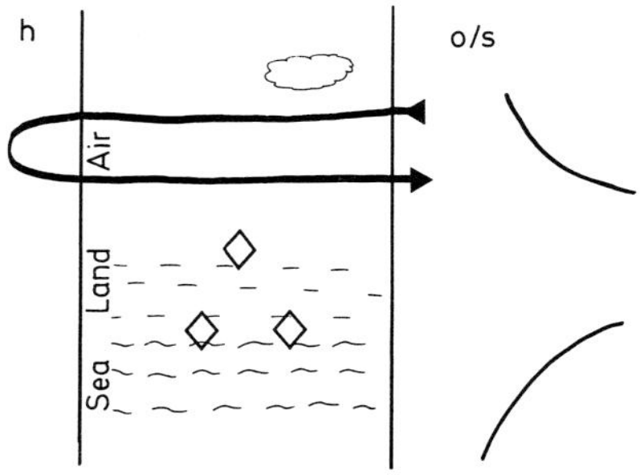


**Fig. 10**

**Figs. 7–10.** More complex but common modern journeys. Figure 7 fits the package tourist to the tropics, Fig. 8 the tourist with a stopover, Fig. 9 the "overlander" tourist who visits three overseas countries and has two stopovers on the way home, and Fig. 10 reminds us of the "reverse" tourist from overseas

main interest lies well outside travel medicine is most likely to miss this. An obvious elaboration of this problem is seen in Fig. 9, where the traveller visits three different overseas countries overtly, as well as having two short stops on his return route. The main problems here are working out the optimal immunization and malaria chemoprophylaxis regimes for the combined countries, and also ascertaining the journey rather than assuming that the first country mentioned is the only one to be visited.

Of increasing importance to all concerned with imported disease and travel medicine are the "mirror image" travellers; nationals of the third world and other overseas countries paying short visits for business or holiday to the "home" country (Fig. 10). Such visitors are medically important: they account for a substantial proportion of falciparum malaria seen in the United Kingdom, they may present with symptoms of infection modified by immunity acquired from previous attacks whilst in their own country, and so be difficult to diagnose, and they may be unfamiliar with the health care system of the country they are visiting and present late with disease. They also comprise a completely different group so far as effective health education is concerned.

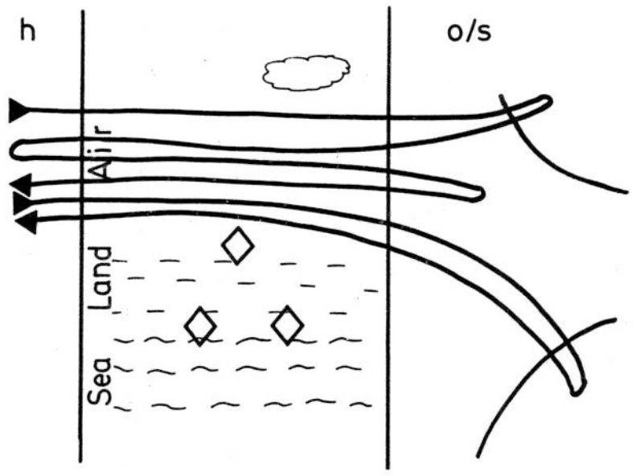


**Fig. 11**

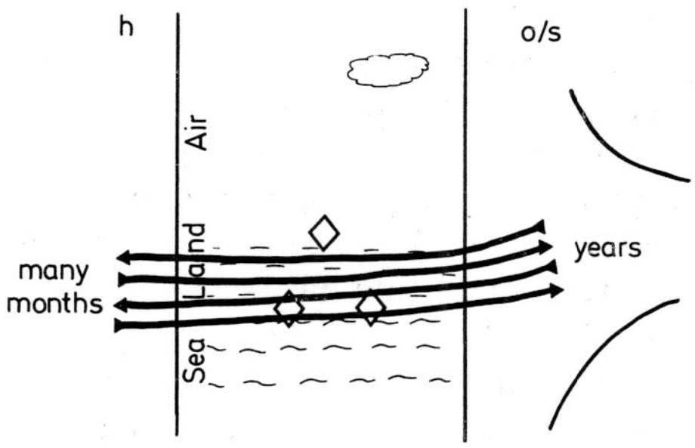


**Fig. 12**

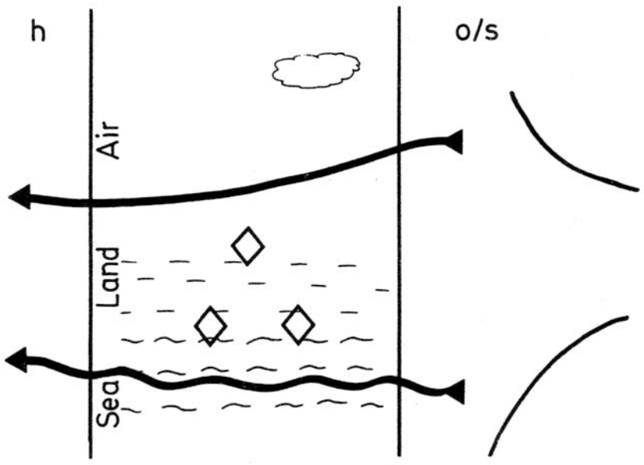


**Fig. 13**

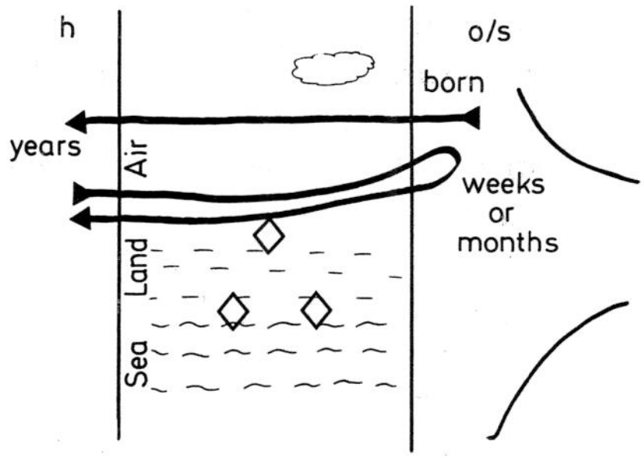


**Fig. 14**

**Figs. 11–14.** Special migratory patterns: Fig. 11 shows the high-speed business man, Fig. 12 the guest worker or seasonal migrant for work from a less-developed country, Fig. 13 the immigrant to an industrial country, and Fig. 14 the settled immigrant returning to his or her country of origin for a prolonged holiday to visit friends and relations. All are discussed in the text

Figure 11 draws attention to a relatively recent phenomenon, the jet-setting businessman (or academic or rock-star!) who may get ill on returning from New York, but as a result of visiting Lagos or Karachi two trips further back, but still all within 2 weeks. The immunization and prophylactic advisory needs of such travellers are complex, and may often best be handled from sophisticated computer-based material.

A much slower-motion similar type of migratory activity (Fig. 12) is seen in guest workers who may come from their homes in less prosperous countries to spend many months in more developed countries, and they may maintain this migratory pattern over years or even decades. They are exposed to various health risks, often have or seek little access to the health care system of the host country, and have a difficult time in many ways. The problems are more social than medical, and may go beyond the large-scale individual problems of migrants from Turkey to West Germany to having a major demographic effect in such countries as Lesotho where a large proportion of adult males may be away working as miners in South Africa. These "guest workers" are not the traditional concern of travel clinics, but it may well be that travel physicians should take an interest in them – the problems are partly those of travel medicine and the patients may otherwise simply get neglected.

There is much greater organized awareness of the health problems of immigrants (Fig. 13). The influx of nationals of their former colonies to European countries has been large and politically as well as medically apparent. Where immigration has been illicit, health problems have been less addressed directly, but attention has been given to health problems of, for example, Indonesian immigrants to the Netherlands and South Asians to the United Kingdom. Where the immigrants have been also refugees, as in the case of the Vietnamese "boat people", organized medical screening and care have been provided. Once they have settled, such immigrants become part of the ethnic minority groups of their host countries and often have health problems related to that status. Health educational materials need to be in appropriate languages.

A specific travel medicine problem is raised by the return of ethnic minority immigrants, or of their children born in the host country, to the lands of their fathers (Fig. 14), often for relatively long visits. Such visitors have usually lost any acquired immunity to infections prevalent in the overseas country, and they may be unaware of the risks, partly because of language difficulties, and so take inadequate preventive measures. A specific problem is faced by South Asians settled in the United Kingdom and returning to Asia. Many left there at the peak of malaria eradication efforts and do not realize that they are returning to a now highly malarious area.

There are many further ways in which the totality of travellers can be subdivided. Among those following the simple return journey of Fig. 6 there will be tourists who go to a single resort, businessmen who may go to several places, mainly urban, within their country of visit, and backpackers who live much closer to the land in rural areas. There are also special categories – babies and young children, pregnant women, the very aged or infirm, and so on. There are those whose actual journey is kept as short as possible as their goal is the destination, and those for whom the journey itself is the main aim – mountaineers, trekkers and those on a "bus" tour. The relative likelihood of injury, infection, or other health problem will vary between these.

The aggregate problems have been well set out by Dr. Steffen in a later paper and elaborated by other contributors. He points out that of 100 000 travellers on average half will have some health problem, 20 000 will feel ill and 8000 will consult a doctor; 6000 will be sufficiently ill that they go to bed and 400 will be hospitalized overseas, while 500 will have an accident of some sort and 8 of the 100 000 will not return alive. So with hundreds of millions of tourists, the health problems will be substantial.

In view of the scale of travel today and the health hazards associated with this, the diversity of travel and travellers described above can be used in subdividing those who travel and getting a more precise definition of the levels of risk and how to reduce them. The epidemiology of the health problems can be used to provide focussed advice on prevention and on coping with the health hazards.

It is clear that they key questions in travel medicine concern the journey in detail. Maegraith's original emphasis on *"unde venis"* remains the key to travel medicine. The aim of this conference will be to view this question in context: to specify the travellers, the risks, the preventive and management measures and, if necessary, rapid diagnosis and sound management for travel-related disease. The problems are becoming increasingly complex. More thought is needed on how to solve them and this conference marks significant progress in tackling them.

# World Tourism: Facts and Figures

P. Keller and K. Koch

## Summary

The World Tourism Organization aims to elaborate policies to enhance the harmonious development of tourism at national and international levels. Emphasis is given to assisting developing countries. Under its current programme, priority is given to facilitation, liberalization of trade, education and training and security and protection of tourists and tourist facilities. The latter involves, *inter alia*, sanitary and safety standards in tourist facilities and destinations, traveller health awareness, medical care and tourism insurance. WTO is keen to cooperate with the WHO and health experts to defend tourists against health problems and to see that such problems are not detrimental to the travel industry nor promoted by international tourism itself. Health problems may increase with the ever-larger number of travellers: tourism, measured in terms of tourist arrivals, hotel nights and receipts, is the fastest growing service industry, which continues to expand even in periods of economic slowdown. At world level, in 1987, 61% of all tourists came from Europe and 16% from North America. International tourist flows may be indicative of transmission of infections and diseases.

## Tourism as a Means of Development

Travelling provides many people with some of the happiest moments of their lives. But tourist needs can only be satisfied if a country's economy provides the necessary equipment and services. In addition, the state contributes in considerable measure to tourism. It guarantees freedom of travel, provides the necessary infrastructure and ensures that the landscape remains such that the tourist can relax in it.

Regions and business centres which are attractive because of their landscapes and their cultural monuments attract travellers who are no longer held back by national frontiers. With the jet age, travel has become a worldwide phenomenon. In order to further tourism as a contribution to peace and development, the world community in 1975 founded the World Tourism Organization (WTO), with headquarters in Madrid.

As a traditional tourist country, Switzerland was one of the founder members of the WTO. The WTO not only provides worldwide statistical data for the use of its 113 member states and 140 affiliated organizations, but its work is also organized with a view to creating conditions favourable to tourism in every possible sphere. In so doing, it aims always to think in terms of the tourist as an individual and to consider both his physical and his psychological needs.

## Explosive Growth in the Post-War Period

International – or cross-frontier – tourism has grown at an explosive rate in the post-war period. Up to 1980, we faced double-digit growth rates. In 1950, 25 million arrivals were registered in the various tourist countries, and this resulted in a turnover of 2.1 billion US dollars. In 1987, the WTO registered 355 million arrivals, with a turnover of US $150 billion. During this period – from 1950 to 1987 – growth in tourism exceeded growth in the national incomes of the respective countries 15-fold (Table 1).

These impressive economic statistics are in fact carefully worked-out aggregates, for the methods of collecting statistics are different in the various countries. Overseas, islands and third-world states count their tourists as they enter the country. States which are closely interrelated economically and have relatively open frontiers count arrivals as overnight stays in hotels and other types of accomodation. The statistics on currency turnover are in most countries collected by the central bank. Where data are missing, turnover is estimated by multiplying the number of overnight stays by the estimated average daily expenditure of the tourist.

International tourism counts as part of the "invisible" sector of exports or imports. Tourists travel in and out of a country. They thus bring about an exchange of payments and goods. A comparison with general international trade must be made in order to comprehend the economic importance of cross-frontier tourism. Its proportion of world trade in goods is still relatively small – at 5.25%.

International tourism also tends to promote the growth of domestic tourism. With respect to tourism within countries, some household surveys have been carried out in a number of states, but there are no worldwide statistics on this subject which can be regarded as definitive. The WTO estimates, however, that domestic tourism is about two to three times more important than international tourism in terms of overnight stays.

**Table 1.** Explosive growth of international tourism. (WTO)

| Year | Tourist arrivals (millions) | Tourism receipts (US$ million) |
|---|---|---|
| 1950 | 25 | 2100 |
| 1973 | 190 | 31054 |
| 1980 | 284 | 102363 |
| 1986 | 340 | 127828 |
| 1987[a] | 355 | 150000 |
| | 13 times more than 1950 | 70 times more than 1950 |

[a] Estimate

## Tourism in the Various Continents and Tourist Trends Within Regions

In the last 40 years, tourism in the various continents has not been distributed at all regularly (Fig. 1). During this period, Europe was able to maintain its very high proportion of 66% of all arrivals registered throughout the world. From 1950 to 1987, tourism in Europe increased from 16.8 million arrivals to 234.5 million. Europe has this leading position mainly because of the large number of relatively small states which coexist in a small areas – which naturally affects the statistics regarding frontier crossings. North America holds second place; but in spite of a growth from 6.1 million to 41 million arrivals the proportion of this half-continent in worldwide tourism has gone down from 24% to 12%.

The Asian and Pacific tourist market has grown at a remarkable speed in the period being considered – from 237 000 to 32.5 million arrivals. Tourism in Central and South America remained at about the same proportion throughout the period. In spite of a very rapid rate of growth from 524 000 to 8.8 million arrivals, Africa's proportion does not yet exceed 2%.

Much more significant than the distribution by continents is an analysis of the tourist streams between sending and receiving countries. The most important tourist movements in both Europe and America are between north and south. In Europe the Mediterranean and Alpine regions, in America Mexico and the island countries of the Caribbean area profit from these tourist streams. In the Asiatic-Pacific region, the main direction of international tourism is from Japan and Australia to the island states of Southeast Asia and the Pacific.

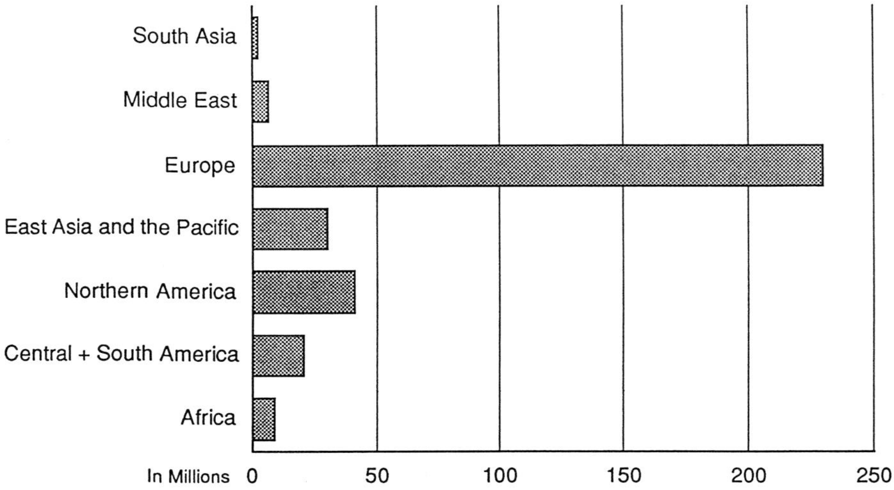


**Fig. 1.** International tourist arrivals (1986)

## Industrial States as the Most Important Tourist Markets

The Western industrial states receive 70% of arrivals and three quarters of the income from international tourism. Important intercontinental travel streams exist between the most important economic regions of the world – Western Europe, North America and Japan/Australasia. Thus, most international tourism takes place in the industrial states of the West.

Although 24 Western industrial states are the main providers of tourists to the rest of the world, these same states show only very small deficits in the balance of payments due to tourism (in 1986, US $4 billion; in 1987, US $12 billion). The reason for this is that there also exists a steady stream of travellers from the developing and partly developed countries to the industrialized countries, the latter being bound together in the framework of the Organization for Economic Cooperation and Development (OECD). This approximate balance in the tourist situation which has been achieved by the Western industrial states is due to the surplus of US $11 billion achieved by Western Europe in tourism's record year.

## The Situation of the Developing Countries

The developing countries which are most important for tourists have been integrated into a relatively free world tourism market. At present, they receive about one-quarter of all the revenue generated by international tourism. In contrast, the proportion of global currency exchange due to tourism in and out of the socialist countries – those with centralized economies – is small. In this sector, most tourism takes place among the countries of the socialist system and currency accounts are offset administratively against other goods and services.

The remarkable commercial success of the developing countries in terms of tourism so far gives some indication of the potential which still remains untapped. For the moment this success is mostly limited to certain countries which lie fairly near to the Western industrial states – some few island para-

**Table 2.** The most important tourism countries in the third world. (WTO)

| Thousands of arrivals 1986 | | | |
|---|---|---|---|
| 1. China | 9000 | 11. Argentina | 1600 |
| 2. Mexico | 4625 | 12. Porto Rico | 1573 |
| 3. Hong Kong | 3723 | 13. Tunesia | 1542 |
| 4. Bahamas | 3002 | 14. Virgin Islands | 1522 |
| 5. Singapore | 2905 | 15. India | 1462 |
| 6. Thailand | 2818 | 16. Egypt | 1311 |
| 7. Morocco | 2186 | 17. Uruguay | 1168 |
| 8. Brazil | 1934 | 18. Iraq | 1004 |
| 9. Jordan | 1900 | 19. Indonesia | 825 |
| 10. Republic of Korea | 1659 | 20. Phillippines | 604 |

dises and city states. Throughout the world, only 25 countries have accomodation capacities of more than 100 000 beds. The leading 20 countries are given in Table 2. In all other countries, toursim for the moment has only marginal economic significance.

If we take the income per head obtained from international tourism, it may be surprising to note that, apart from Austria and Switzerland, only tropical island states (Barbados, Fiji), small oil-producing countries (Bahrein, Kuwait) and city states (Singapore) reach a figure of more than US $ 300/head.

## Prosperity and Travel Intensity

The richer a country is, the more of its citizens travel abroad for their holidays. In a number of countries, household surveys have been made in order to discover the ratio of net travel intensity, defined as a least one journey abroad for private reasons per year comprising at least four nights. In the most prosperous countries, the proportion is around 80%. In the developing countries, it is usually under 10%. Already today there exists a travel stream between the countries of the third world which has been considerably underestimated. Out of 8.8 million arrivals in African countries in 1986, 3,9 million were travellers from other developing countries.

In the wake of the rapid increase in the immediate postwar period, opportunities for growth in tourism today are directly connected with general economic growth. When we take into account the fact that, even in the highly developed region of the European Community, only 20% of tourists cross their own frontier into another EC country, only 10% visit non-EC countries in Europe and only 3% travel to another continent, we can measure the enormous growth potential which is still available for international tourism.

## Health Strategies of the World Tourist Organization

This growth potential can only be exploited if the general framework of international travel is further improved. The WTO not only works in favour of cheaper flights to states which are handicapped in the field of tourism, but it is also trying to make travel all over the world freer and more secure. In this effort, the health of the tourist plays a primordial role. The main purpose of

**Table 3.** Tourism motivations. (WTO)

| Arrivals of tourists from abroad by purpose of visit (1985) | | | |
|---|---|---|---|
| | Recreation | Business | Visit friends |
| Brazil | 86.3% | 3.6% | 10.1% |
| Greece | 83.0% | 9.0% | 8.0% |
| Morocco | 60.0% | 9.0% | 31.0% |
| Sri Lanka | 90.9% | 7.1% | 2.0% |
| United States | 78.3% | 21.7% | – |

most tourism is relaxation and rest (see Table 3) leave the following retence is the most important preoccupation of most travellers. It is because of this that the risks to health involved in tourism should be kept as low as possible. You cannot relax if you fall ill.

The WTO is concerned with improving medical prophylaxis and care for tourists worldwide. At the present time a convention on new travel facilities is under preparation and it will include free first aid, mutual recognition of sickness insurance schemes between tourist-sending and -receiving countries and the creation of a minimum international travel insurance scheme.

If one out of every thousand tourists were to fall ill, this would mean that there would be at least 355 000 medical cases amongst the estimated 355 million tourists/year. This is approximately the population of the city of Geneva, where the headquarters of the World Health Organization is located – a body which maintains excellent contacts with the WTO. This goes to show that it is well worthwhile elaborating as rapidly as possible effective health strategies in the field of tourism.

# Medical Impact of Intercontinental Travel to Developing Countries

N. O. Bwibo


## Summary

Rapid air travel makes it possible for people to travel from temperate countries to developing countries, which are by and large tropical, and back to temperate within a very short time. While in the tropical countries, the traveller is exposed to the risks of tropical diseases, the majority of which are parasitic diseases such as malaria, intestinal parasites, gastrointestinal infections, chest infections as well as skin infections. The disease may manifest itself while the traveller is still in the tropics, where it may be diagnosed easily by health workers who are familiar with such diseases. It is increasingly becoming possible for the traveller to return to his country of origin before the disease shows its symptoms. Such imported diseases cause difficulties in diagnoses leading to delayed diagnosis. Travellers may get tropical diseases when they travel from one tropical country to another if such diseases do not normally occur in their own countries.

Travellers and physicians should be aware of such risks and be prepared for questions like. "Where are you from?" or "Where have you been recently?" or "Have you been abroad?" The information helps in making a quick differential diagnosis so that effective treatment can be given without undue delay.

Travellers should take precautions before they start their journeys. Their physicians should be able to guide them in preventive methods. Tropical diseases are discussed here, with emphasis on methods of prevention.


The health of travellers continues to receive much attention in both their host and home countries. This is more so for travellers to the developing countries which are also tropical. In these tropical countries, travellers encounter tropical diseases, the scourging heat of the tropical sun, high humidity, tropical insects and dangerous terrain, which may interfere with the intended reasons for travel; hence the risks need to be minimized or removed. There has been much written about the health risks for travellers to tropical countries [1–3]. The WHO and the World Tourism Organization have joined in providing the needed health information and have recently provided guidelines on AIDS [4] and also on health formalities and facilities for their member countries [5]. Adequate warning against malaria as the single most serious tropical disease has been sounded by all the concerned parties [6, 7].

Though the immediate medical impact of the health hazards is on the traveller, the home country and the host tropical country have concerns and hence a responsibility to minimize or prevent such hazards. For the host countries tourism is a welcome foreign currency earner and so the tourists need to remain safe and healthy. For the home countries the tourists may be a danger in importing tropical diseases [8–10] which pose health problems and which may fail to be diagnosed or be diagnosed late because of their unfamiliarity to the doctors, with sad consequences. The two countries therefore have a role to play in this matter but this paper discusses more the implications of preventive measures recommended for travellers on the public health policy in tourist target or host countries in the tropics, as well as the need for provision and utilization of health services for such foreign visitors while in the tropical countries.

Thousands of travellers visit tropical countries annually to see the fascinating natural sights and wildlife, so what we are dealing with are large numbers. With rapid air travel, these travellers may return home before the diseases acquired in the tropics have manifested themselves. Any policy or guidelines to the travellers should be stressed in their own country as well as in the host country. Apart from the tourists, there are large numbers of travellers to the tropics attending conferences in the capital cities in the new sophisticated international conference centres whose medical and health needs are quite different from those of the tourists who travel to remote parts of the countries. The medical advice and health guidelines should be tailored to the travellers depending upon where they are going and what they are going to do.

The host countries have ample opportunities to provide health information, health policy and guidelines on health matters to travellers. They can do so before the travellers leave their own home countries, at the ports of entry, and during the stay in the host countries and at the port of departure from the host countries. The information needed is on required immunization, patterns of tropical diseases, geographical and climatic environment and the types of protective measures.

Before travellers leave their countries, they are required to get visas from the High Commissions, Embassies and consulates of the host countries. It is at this stage that the health information and health policies should be made available to travellers. By that time travellers have had opportunities to read about the target countries, talk to friends who have already visited such countries and talk to their own physicians and may now countercheck and confirm the information and remove conflicts or incorrect information with the experts of the target host countries. Some developing countries have pamphlets on tourism with sections on health which travellers can collect at the time they obtain their visas. Otherwise this information is given verbally. Written information would be better since the traveller can refer to it and thus refresh the mind. Written information has the added advantages in that it is prepared by authorities and hence reduces uncertainities.

The policies on the required vaccinations for international travellers are uniform, with slight local variations. Most tropical countries require that travellers should have had valid vaccination against yellow fever; others require cholera as well. Due to differences in local occurrences of diseases, travellers may need to be advised about the need to get additional vaccinations such as TAB (typhoid and paratyphoid A and B), viral hepatitis A, poliomyelitis and rabies. Travellers going for a conference in the capital city would not require vaccination for scrab typhus and rabies as there is not likely be the risk of such diseases unless after the conference they wish to go on safari. So the scope of immunization is tailored to travellers' needs. It would be advisable to get vaccinated before departure for the host countries in case the vaccines are unavailable on arrival.

Before departure, travellers may wish to check with their physicians which medicines to take and which remedies they should carry for protection against the sun's rays and heat and insects. Lists of drugs and chemicals to be carried have been the subject of concern and guidelines are available [11]. Caution should be taken regarding these medicines as most countries are worried about drugs of addiction and drug peddling and their medical implications, which would make immigration officials need to know what medicines travellers have in their possession.

Travellers should be given adequate information on diseases acquired from swimming such as schistomiasis, diseases acquired from food, and the nuisance of insect bites.

At the port of entry, the host countries have facilities to check and inspect for internationally required vaccination and administer them if travellers still do not have them. Usually there are manned dispensaries at such ports of entry. In one country I know of, travellers are given a mandatory dose of chloroquine tablets to swallow at the port of entry. Further information on health can be obtained at such ports of entry together with checking of any queries.

Needless to say, countries with developed tourism have internationally reputable hotels and resorts with licensed restaurants where food and drink is of high quality. But the problem of traveller's diarrhoea, which commonly occurs the world over, is much more likely to occur in the humid tropical countries especially in those areas where sanitation and water supply are still poor. Travellers are given health information in such hotels. In addition each hotel has listings of private docotors who can be consulted by travellers in case of need. But the traveller should take precautions with foods which are particularly known to be notorious for food poisoning, especially in small cheap restaurants, and drink boiled water.

Travellers going for a conference and staying in the country's Hilton Hotel in the capital city would be unlikely to get schistosomiasis by swimming in the hotel swimming pool. This problem is of considerable importance for travellers swimming in a river. The former need not take precautions for schistosomiasis while the latter group of travellers must take all the precautions especially if they have been advised that the lake or river is infected. Situations arise where travellers are given adequate information about malaria or schistosomiasis but because they feel secure after their initial stay fail to continue observing the precautions. An example of this type occurred in American rafters on the Omo river in Ethiopia where 5 out of 11 developed acute schistosomiasis on returning home [12]. Travellers from one tropical country to another may encounter tropical diseases which are absent in their own countries; hence they should take same precautions as travellers from temperate countries.

Every country has a system for provision of health care and travellers may utilize it when in need. All developing countries have national hospitals and private hospitals. There are also private clinics and these are listed in the telephone directory, making them available to travellers in case of need. Hotels can provide information as well. Further information on medical matters can be obtained from professional medical associations and societies and are listed in the telephone directory. There are mission-run hospitals in some remote areas which can serve travellers visiting those remote parts. In case of a disaster, the national health service naturally participates with the assistance of the Red Cross and any charitable organizations. Travellers should be aware that the national health systems may not be in a position to provide the care equivalent to what is expected in their developed countries but the service is available with a built-in referral system which the patient can utilize.

In some countries like Kenya, there is a flying doctor scheme and this is very valuable in assisting tourists who fall sick or have accidents in remote parts of the country, referring them to the well-equipped city hospitals for medical treatment.

In international conference situations, there are usually manned dispensaries which provide health care and direct delegates to health institutions according to their special needs.

Finally, may I now give examples related to Kenya. Kenya's tourism industry is very advanced, hence the Ministry of Tourism and Ministry of Health have had workshops dealing with the health of tourists. In the recently organized workshop, a paper titled "Measures taken by the Ministry of Health on diseases affecting the tourist trade in Kenya, namely AIDS and malaria" was presented [13]. In the paper, the policy regarding vaccination requirements for entry into Kenya is stated; that yellow fever is the only vaccine required for people coming from endemic areas with this disease such as tropical African countries and South America excluding visitors from Europe, North America and Asia. The paper also highlighted the need to print an information card with information both for the traveller and for his personal physician. The information for the patient stresses that Kenya is a malarial country and hence prophylaxis should be taken during one's stay and continued for 4 weeks on return home and that on return home the card should be shown to the physician if the traveller feels unwell. The information for the physician states that the traveller has been to a malarial area and that appropriate tests for malaria should be taken.

If travellers adhered to this precaution and also sprayed his hotel room each night he would be protected from malaria and hence importation of malaria to his country would be prevented. But do all travellers do this? Personal behaviour and habits as well as misadventure lands some of them in trouble; it is not that there are not sufficient precautions.

One problem that immediately arises from an imported disease like malaria is the unfamiliar symptoms, delay in diagnosis and the unavailability of the required drug in the traveller's country of origin.

Precautions for AIDS are also stressed in Kenya's workshop, augumenting the guidelines of the WHO, which were endorsed by the World Tourism Organization [5].

It should be mentioned here that the World Tourism Organization, to which Kenya is a member, has discussed the issues of health for travellers and in the meeting held in Madrid it provided guidelines on recommendations for health formalities and facilities for travellers which the member states are expected to adhere to [5].

## References

1. Mann JM (1983) Commentary emporiatrics: policy and practice protecting the health of Americans abroad. JAMA 249:3323
2. Jensen B (1978) African travel. Br Med J 2:829
3. Schultz MG (1982) Emporiatrics: traveller's health. Br Med J 285:582
4. World Health Organization (1987) AIDS information for travellers (WHO special programme on AIDS). Geneva
5. World Tourism Organization. Health formalities and facilities and facilitation of travel and tourist stays for the disabled. FAL/6/5, Annex 11 a
6. World Health Organization (1978) Imported diseases – the epidemiological challenge. WHO Chron 32:355
7. Bruce-Chwatt LJ (1982) Imported malaria – an invited guest. Br Med Bull 38:179
8. Kendrick MA (1972) CDC study of illness among Americans returning from international travel (preliminary data). J Infect Dis 126:684
9. Woodruff AW, Bowes ETN, Platt GS (1978) Viral infections in travellers from tropical Africa. Br Med J 1:956
10. Helliwell CJ, Turner AC (1980) Imported disease at point of entry. Practitioner 224:793
11. Barber SG (1978) Drugs and doctoring for trans-Saharan travellers. Br Med J 2:404
12. Istre GR, Fontaine RE, Terr J, Hopkins RS (1984) Acute schistosomiasis among Americans rafting the Omo River Ethiopia. JAMA 251:508
13. Mueke F (1987) Measures taken by the Ministry of Health on diseases affecting tourist trade in Kenya, namely AIDS and malaria. DTC Workshop, Mombasa 1987

# Travel-Related Health Risks: A Question of Communication

J.-P. Jardel

## Summary

Communication between people through international tourism, labour migration and other types of travel has increased tremendously in the past decades, both in volume and in speed, at the same time increasing opportunities for the communication of disease, from minor ailments afflicting the traveller himself to major infectious diseases threatening public health.

The International Health Regulations adopted by the 166 Member States of the World Health Organization aim at protecting individuals and preventing the international spread of disease, with minimum interference with world traffic. However, regulations and preventive and protective measures can only be effective if supported by an adequate system for the communication of information. It is the responsibility of national health administrations to establish communicable disease surveillance and control programmes, to inform the international community, the health professionals and the general public of health risks associated with travel to given places and to advise on the general and specific preventive measures to be applied. The World Health Organization plays a major coordinating role in this communication chain, but the value of the information the Organization can provide depends on the timeliness and quality of the information received from countries.

In our world of increasing communication facilities, more and more people are travelling greater distances. International tourism has increased from 130 million to 350 million tourist arrivals in the last 2 decades. The majority travel to European countries but the rate of increase in travellers to Africa, Asia and the Pacific is impressive. Developing countries are now receiving about 20% of international tourists. The development of air transport has resulted in speedier travel, making it more possible than ever for the traveller to return to his point of departure within the incubation period of a disease contracted abroad. To travel related to international tourism must be added international migration due to pilgrimages, search for employment, and travel within national boundaries, which is difficult to assess.

Tourism is about to become the world's largest single industry and its economic impact is considerable. It offers ample opportunities for social and cultural exchange. It is also expected to be a health promotion activity. Unfortunately, travellers are exposed to health risks and they may become vectors of health risks to others.

The protection of public health against the risks from international travel was in fact at the very origin of international cooperation in the field of health. In 1851, the first international health conference ever convened dealt with the problem of harmonizing preventive measures against the spread of communicable diseases through maritime traffic in the Mediterranean, and particularly considered quarantine measurs applied to cholera, plague and yellow fever. The following 100 years witnessed a series of conventions and arrangements relating to health control measures at frontiers. International health cooperation developed on this basis and progressively entered other fields of interest. The present World Health Organization (WHO) may be seen as the distant relative of this first health conference.

## Communication of Diseases

### Health Risks to the Traveller

International travellers are subject to stresses that may lower their resistance to diseases. Changes in diet and lifestyle, jet lag, crowding, are likely to increase the risk of illness. Certain climatic conditions may be directly or indirectly responsible for physical aggression (sunburn, hypothermia, frostbite, etc.). Road traffic and sport accidents are among the most common causes of death or serious impairment to tourists, the issue being often aggravated by the lack of appropriate care facilities.

The list of communicable diseases a traveller may be exposed to is very long, and it is not my intention to mention them all here; a number of presentations during this conference will cover this subject. I would like only to mention some of the most frequent causes of illness. The most common health risk to the traveller comes from contaminated water and food. Twenty to 50% of international travellers suffer from diarrhoea due to a range of bacteria, viruses and protozoa. The majority of reported cases of food-borne illnesses are a result of food which has been mishandled at some stage in the food chain. The incidence of such illnesses could be greatly reduced through the correct application of food safety principles properly monitored by health authorities, and through adequate information to the traveller. Food and drink may also cause more serious diseases, including amoebiasis, helminthic infections, and above all viral hepatitis A and enterically transmitted hepatitis non-A and non-B, which are present worldwide with higher incidence in areas of poor sanitation. Cholera is still reported by about 40 countries in the world and some countries fail to timely notify outbreaks to WHO. However, given the relatively low risk to international travellers, and the fact that cholera vaccination cannot prevent the introduction of the disease into any country, vaccination should not be required.

In tropical areas, many communicable diseases are transmitted by insect vectors. The major risks for travellers in this regard are yellow fever and malaria. Yellow fever is endemic in Africa and South America and travellers entering infected areas must be vaccinated prior to arrival. Unvaccinated persons coming from an area where cases are occurring should be maintained under close surveillance for their own protection and the protection of the countries visited. Malaria is one of the more common and more serious of the tropical diseases and travellers to malarious areas are at high risk of acquiring

the infection. Chloroquine was until relatively recently a safe and effective chemoprophylactic agent. The situation is now far more complex, given the increase in chloroquine resistance, and the occurrence of severe adverse reaction to alternative drugs. The traveller and the physician should thus be better informed of other components of protection and of the fact that a fever may be due to malaria, even under chemoprophylaxis, and even if the symptoms are not typical. Many other tropical diseases are likely to be difficult to identify once the tourist has returned to his home country.

The increased risk of sexually transmitted diseases and the associated risk of AIDS and HIV infections justify better information to the traveller as well as a reasonable approach to the protection of public health. Extreme measures, such as the screening of international travellers for HIV infection, would have very little effect on the international spreading of AIDS, and would justify neither the tremendous social and legal implications, nor the expense.

Cerebrospinal meningitis is also worth mentioning in relation to international travel, being endemic throughout the world. Epidemic waves occur at intervals of several years, not only in countries of the so-called "cerebrospinal meningitis belt" in Africa, but also in other geographical areas. Polysaccharide vaccines may be of benefit to travellers planning to visit areas where the disease is epidemic.

## Public Health Risks

More important than the individual risks are the risks to public health from international travel. The risks from communicable diseases are increased during mass seasonal travel for vacations: tourism creates an influx of people during short periods of the year. This influx overloads essential basic services such as water supply and sanitation, food catering facilities and the health care services. It is at such sensitive periods that outbreaks of diseases are most likely to occur, affecting both indigenous populations and tourists. The development of tourism implies that such basic services are properly planned for and maintained. Failure to do so is likely to result in the medium term in the discouragement of tourists.

International travel also brings risks of transmission of diseases to populations in the country of destination and in the home country of the traveller. The speed of air travel is such that many diseases would occur only when the traveller is far away from the place of infection. There is a major risk, therefore, of an exotic disease not being recognized before it can spread. Besides the communication of diseases by the traveller himself, there is a non-negligible risk of transmission through the transportation of vectors and contaminated products.

International health regulations have been established in order to ensure the maximum security against the international spread of diseases, with a minimum interference in world traffic. The regulations are intended to strengthen the use of epidemiological principles to detect, reduce or eliminate the sources from which infection spreads; to improve sanitation in and around ports and airports; to prevent the dissemination of vectors; and, in general, to encourage epidemiological activities at the national level. Notification of diseases received by WHO according to the regulations are made available on the automatic telex reply service and published in the *Weekly Epidemiological Record.*

## Communication of Information

Information on the existing risks in a given country is a prerequisite to the adequacy of preventive and protective measures. It is essential, therefore, that epidemiological surveillance be properly organized in all countries. The development of epidemiological services in the developing world is one of the major concerns of WHO, within the general approach of primary health care and through specific programmes such as the Expanded Programme on Immunization and Diarrhoeal Diseases Control.

Even with the best epidemiological services, the information cannot be made useful to the international community if it is not notified to other countries through the global surveillance system of WHO. Unfortunately, there have been many instances of hesitation to disseminate the results of surveillance for fear of frightening away tourists in case of detection of important hazards. It must be made clear that this attitude is likely to be detrimental in the long term, as it is conducive to suspicion and lack of confidence. The existence of outbreaks of major diseases will eventually be reported and possibly amplified by the media, with the risk of generating excessive protective measures in some countries. WHO is able to report accurately only what has been properly and timely notified, not to confirm or deny rumours in the international press.

Information and education of the public, the health profession, travel agents and national authorities are finally the best way of reducing health risks from international travel, by improving the understanding of these risks and the knowledge of protective measures, thus promoting more responsible attitudes.

The World Health Organization has issued several guides related to hygiene and sanitation in aircrafts and ships and to vector control. WHO issues annually a publication on vaccination certificate requirements and health advice for international travel, and ensures the international transfer of information on international health risks through its *Weekly Epidemiological Record.*

The World Health Organization is of course not alone in this effort to inform and educate: national administrations, medical associations and individual experts are issuing excellent material for the information of travellers, travel agents, physicians, and people in all sectors of society who have some responsibility for international travel. What is required is an effort by all those concerned to make this information readily and easily accessible to those who need it. Again a question of communication.

# Health Risks for Short Term Travelers and Temporary Residents

# Health Risks for Short-Term Travelers

R. Steffen

## Summary

Epidemiologic data show that relatively minor ailments affect more than half of the travelers during a brief stay in the tropics. Diarrhea and upper respiratory tract infections are the most frequent problems. In contrast, infectious hepatitis affects only 1 in 500, typhoid fever 1 in 30000, cholera 1 in 500000 travelers to the tropics. The risk of malaria and of poliomyelitis is usually underestimated.

When tourists and foreign aid volunteers started to travel in greater number to developing countries, hardly any data were available about their health risks. Consequently, medical recommendations were vague and even more contradictory than nowadays. This prompted us among many others to conduct initially retrospective [1–4], later follow-up studies [5, 6]. Additionally, various case history studies were conducted, primarily to find the attack rates in illlnesses and accidents which rarely affect travelers.

## Health Impairments Abroad

The incidence rate of health impairments was astonishingly high (Fig. 1). During a stay of 1 week more than half of the travelers (mainly vacationers) who

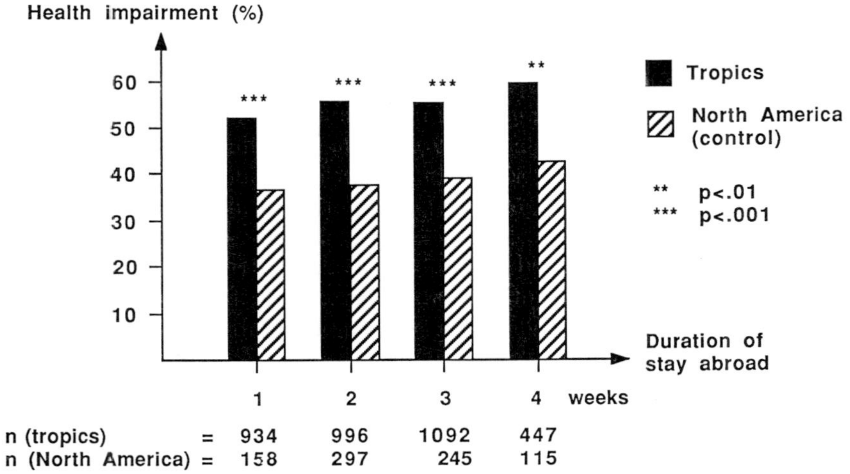


**Fig. 1.** Incidence of health impairments in intercontinental travelers 1976/1977. [3]

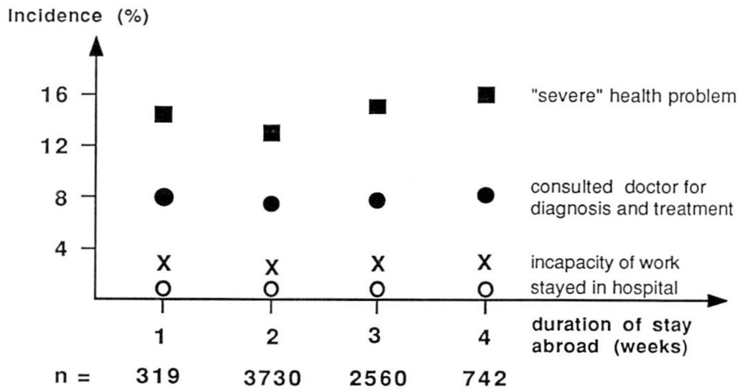


**Fig. 2.** Incidence of relevant health impairments in travelers to the tropics: problems abroad and upon return. [6]

had visited Africa, Asia or Latin America reported some trouble, and also more than one-third of travelers to North America were affected. These health impairments were defined as any subjective complaint, unaccustomed drug ingestion (except, of course, prophylactic drugs), or consultation with a doctor or a nurse. Also 43%–48% of Scottish [7] and Finnish [8] travelers staying mainly in Spain and North Africa experienced health problems. According to a more recent follow-up study [6], the majority of these health problems were not severe; less than 10% of the travelers needed medical attention, and less than 0.5% had to stay in hospital, usually for a few days only (Fig. 2). Surprisingly, the duration of stay abroad had very little influence. Those aged 30 years or less reported significantly more health impairments than those over 60, partly because they took greater risks. Women reported more ailments than men.

By far the predominant health problem in travelers to the tropics was diarrhea [2, 3, 6]. In contrast, travelers to North America experienced mainly constipation [3]. Respiratory infections also occurred frequently, but in less than 2% of all travelers it was accompanied by fever.

## Travelers' Diarrhea

The incidence of travelers' diarrhea depends not only on its definition, but on many variables, the most important of which is the destination of the traveler. We can distinguish three levels of risk for travelers' diarrhea in short-term travelers from highly industrialized countries (Fig. 3). Travelers to the United States, Canada, northern and central Europe, Australia and New Zealand are at low risk, that is at the most 8%. Intermediate risk (8%–20%) is found in travelers to most islands of the Caribbean, the major resorts on the northern Mediterranean, in the Pacific and, on the basis of limited data in our studies, presumably Israel, Japan and South Africa. Travelers to the developing countries in Africa, Asia and Latin America are at high risk, with incidence rates of 20% to over 50%.

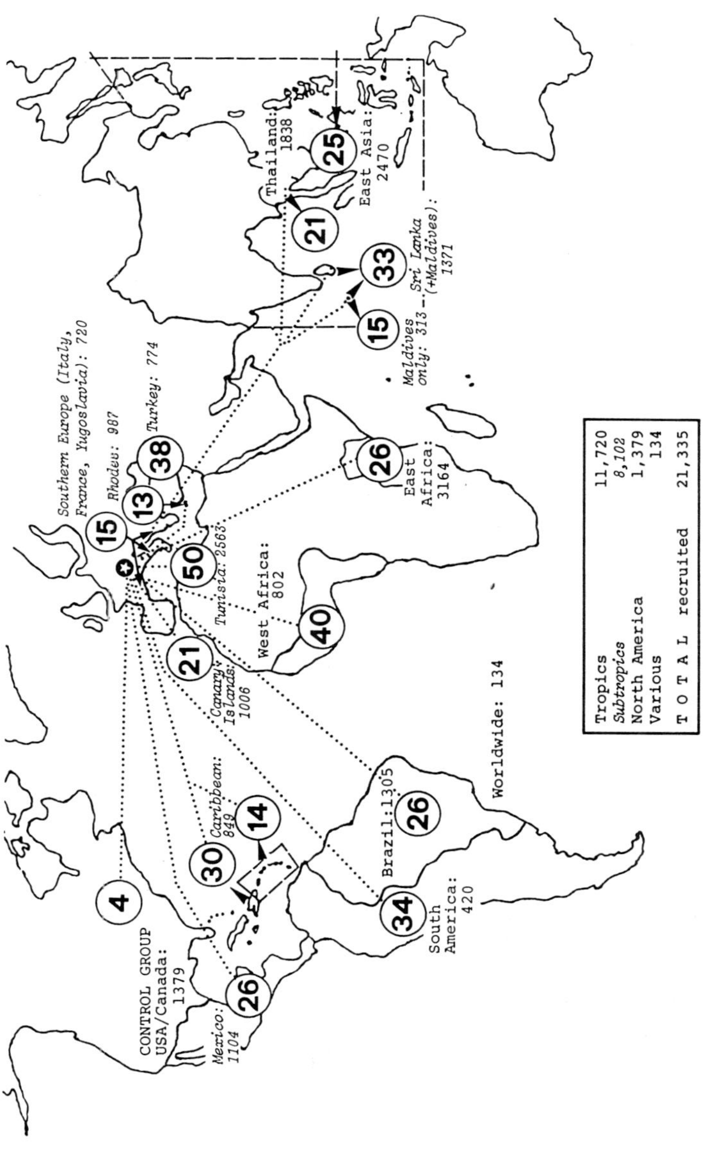


**Fig. 3.** Incidence (%) of traveler's diarrhea among 19 234 tourists during a stay of 14 days at various locations: 2101 travelers who stayed less than 13 days and those who manifested diarrhea after the 14th day were excluded

The situation in Tunisia deserves special attention, as the highest incidence rates of 46%–50% were found in travelers to this country in 1980, 1982 and 1986. In contrast, a decrease of the incidence from 28% in 1976–1977 to 19% in 1986 has been observed in travelers to Kenya.

Various host factors may play a role in the risk of acquiring travelers' diarrhea. The origin of the traveler is important, as has been demonstrated in several studies of convention participants, students or troops in Mexico, Iran and Lebanon [cited in 9]. Lower attack rates were observed among residents from developing countries. Further evidence that previous exposure to pathogenic agents results in subsequent partial immunity of short duration may be derived from the observation of DuPont and coworkers that United States students newly arrived in Mexico got travelers' diarrhea at an attack rate of 40%, whereas their colleagues who had studied there a year or more showed a rate of only 20% [10].

The incidence of travelers' diarrhea does not vary significantly in men and women, but age is an import risk factor. The 20- to 29-year-old age groups are the most often affected [3]. The reason for the increased risk is unknown: a larger appetite of the younger generation and hence the ingestion of larger numbers of pathogenic agents has been postulated, but a less-developed immunological defense mechanism must also be considered.

Some individuals seem to be particularly susceptible to travelers' diarrhea, possibly because of a lack of nonspecific gastrointestinal defense factors, such as antacids or gastrectomy. There are only anecdotal reports about this problem.

Travelers who risk more and care less are at greater risk. Recently, Kozicki and colleagues confirmed the role of food that is raw, or not freshly cooked, in causing diarrhea [11]. They asked 688 visitors to Kenya or Sri Lanka to record what they ate and drank during the first 3 days abroad and to note whether diarrhea occurred. Two results contradict older, retrospective studies: first, only 13 travelers (2%) committed no dietary mistakes. Seventy-one percent consumed salads or uncooked vegetables, 70% ate fruit which could not be peeled, and 53% did not refuse ice cubes. Second, the incidence of diarrhea depended on the number of dietary mistakes. In univariate analysis, diarrhea was associated with the consumption of raw oysters, steak tartare, bottled water, ice cubes, cold milk, puddings and sandwiches with mixed fillings. Those who brushed their teeth using tap water had marginally more diarrhea.

Most surveys show that diarrhea in travelers usually begins within the first few days of the stay abroad [3]. In various studies the highest proportion of new patients was recorded on the 3rd day. This was the case in each investigated region, including North America. Subgroups with symptoms, such as fever, vomiting, abdominal cramps and/or blood in the stool, showed no significantly different pattern of onset. A minority of travelers will experience a second attack of diarrhea abroad during a 2-week stay [9]. Untreated, this ailment has a mean duration of 4 days. In approximately 1% chronic diarrhea results of at least a month's duration. No fatalities have been recorded.

**Table 1.** Etiology of traveler's diarrhea. Range of isolation rates (%) in various studies. [12–14]

| | Asia | Central America | North or East Africa | West Africa |
|---|---|---|---|---|
| ETEC | 20–34 | 28–72 | 31–75 | 42 |
| *Salmonella* | 11–15 | 0–16 | 0 | 4 |
| *Shigella* | 4– 7 | 0–30 | 0–15 | 7 |
| *Campylobacter* | 2–11 | Few | Few | 1 |
| *Aeromonas hydrophila* | 1–57 | N/A | N/A | 0 |
| *Vibrio parahaemolyticus* | 1–16 | Few | Few | N/A |
| *Giardia lamblia* | < 5 | 0– 9 | N/A | 0 |
| *Entamoeba histolytica* | < 5 | 0– 9 | N/A | 2 |
| Rotavirus | N/A | ?–36 | 0 | N/A |
| Various | 0–10 | 0– 5 | 0– 8 | 14 |
| Multiple | 9–22 | N/A | N/A | 10 |
| No pathogen | 33–53 | 15–30 | 15–55 | 40 |
| Number of studies | 8 | 15 | 3 | 1 |

N/A, no data available

The attacks of diarrhea recorded in tourists usually take a mild course. More than 25% of the cases do not meet the classic criteria of an increase of the number of stools and they report only one to two daily bowel movements, but by definition used in the respective studies these patients with mild disease also noted concomitant symptoms. Even in the tropics, 77% of the patients did not suffer from more than five bowel movements per day [3].

In travelers to almost all regions, more than 50% of the patients with diarrhea reported having also had abdominal cramps, approximately 20% had observed mucus in their stools, and 15% had noted blood in the stools. The mean rate of fever and vomiting was slightly less than 15%. A minority of patients, who have dysenteric symptoms (roughly one in four of all patients), are of importance with respect to therapeutic considerations [9].

What is the route of transmission of traveler's diarrhea? It is usually acquired by the ingestion of food or beverages contaminated with infectious agents transmitted by those preparing them, by waste water or by flies. There is no evidence of person-to-person transmission. Numerous studies have assessed the many bacterial, parasitic and viral enteric pathogens [12–14]. In most studies, enterotoxigenic *Escherichia coli* (ETEC) was the most commonly isolated pathogen, followed by *Salmonella, Shigella*, other bacteria, parasites and viruses (Table 1). The same distribution has recently been observed in tourists staying in two hotels in the Gambia and Togo.

## Severe Gastrointestinal Infections

More severe infections due to typhoid fever and cholera deserve particular comment. To our knowledge four surveys [15–18] have documented the risk of typhoid fever per journey of undetermined duration (Table 2). All showed

**Table 2.** Risk of imported typhoid fever after a stay abroad. [15–18]

| Imported | Attack rate per 100000 travelers | | |
|---|---|---|---|
| To<br>From | Switzerland<br>$n=227$<br>1974–1981 | United States<br>$n=561$<br>1977–1979 | United Kingdom<br>$n=939$<br>1978–1982 |
| Northern Europe | 0.02 | 0.02 | N/A |
| Southern Europe | 0.5[a] | 0.25 | 0.33 |
| Developing country | 4 | 2.5 | N/A |
| India | 33[a] | N/A | 29[a] |

[a] Often after a stay in country of origin

similar results, that is a risk of 1 in 30000 for travelers to most developing countries except India, where a tenfold higher risk was found [17]. In none of the studies did the case fatality rate of imported typhoid fever exceed 1%. No data are available about typhoid treated abroad. Even less frequent is imported cholera. Only 129 cases were reported to the World Health Organization between 1975 and 1981 [19]. Detailed data were obtained on 117 of these patients: 56% were immigrants or refugees from endemic areas, or foreign workers returning from leave in their native countries. Only 51 (44%) were citizens of countries in Europe or North America. Considering that 40–50 million travelers visited Africa or Asia the risk was 1 in 500000. Snyder and Blake calculated the same risk estimate [20]. Stay in hospital was always short, and fewer than 2% of patients died.

Wheras the risks of cholera and typhoid fever are overestimated, the risks of acquiring hepatitis, malaria and poliomyelitis are underestimated by many travelers and their doctors.

## Infectious Hepatitis

According to retrospective surveys [21–24], hepatitis affected between 1 and 10/1000 travelers who were not protected by immune globulin (Table 3). Our follow-up study confirmed an incidence rate per month of 3.8/1000 for the sum of all serotypes [6]. The mean duration of inability to work was 33 days. Usually, 60% of the infections are due to hepatitis A, and 15% each to non-A, non-B hepatitis or hepatitis B, while 10% remain unclassified.

Hepatitis B is only exceptionally a risk for vacationers; it affects mainly persons working in developing countries. In French medical staff, 10% developed a symptomatic infection within 18–30 months according to Mercier (personal communication); 9% of men working for Unocal UK Ltd in southeast Asia seroconverted (Dawson, this volume). The excessive risk of Swiss male flight attendants of acquiring hepatitis B may be attributable to promiscuous homosexuality, as neither cockpit crews nor their female colleagues showed similar rates [25].

**Table 3.** Risk of traveler's hepatitis per journey abroad. [21–24]

| Imported | Risk per 100000 travelers Retrospective studies (only imported cases) | | | | Incidence/month Follow-up study |
|---|---|---|---|---|---|
| To / From | Zurich $n=221$ 1971–1976 | Copenhagen $n=105$ 1976–1978 | Zurich $n=137$ 1977–1981 | Göteborg $n=80$ 1980 | Zurich $n=23$ (+4) 1981–1984 |
| Northern Europe | 0.6 | 0.5 | 1.4 | N/A | N/A |
| Southern Europe | 11.1 | 3.1 | 4.3 | 16.6 | 0 (pop. 2296) |
| North Africa | 100.0 | 55.5 | 62.5 | 142.8 | N/A |
| Developing countries, other | 63–285 | 83.3 | 111.1 | 1000.0 | 291 (–342) (pop. 7886) |

## Malaria

The risk of malaria has so far mainly been estimated on the basis of surveillance data. however, we found that even in vacationers staying for less than 4 weeks in Africa, 22% of the cases were treated abroad. Our follow-up study, the details of which are presented elsewhere in this volume, showed that travelers to West Africa who took no chemoprophylaxis had a monthly incidence of 19/1000, while this incidence in travelers to East Africa was 12/1000. *Plasmodium falciparum* caused some 80% of these cases. Surveillance data suggest that travelers visiting endemic areas in Asia and Latin America have a much smaller risk. Far more details on the epidemiology of imported malaria are given elsewhere in the Proceedings.

## Poliomyelitis

Recently we have reviewed WHO and public health statistics. They showed that 175 cases of paralytic poliomyelitis were imported into industrialized countries between 1975 and 1984 [26]. Of particular interest were 47 cases in nationals traveling on holiday business, often for no longer than a week. Of these 16 were over 40 years of age, and in this age group the mortality was particularly high, with a rate of 47%.

Asymptomatic infections, however, are much more frequent than paralytic ones. Considering that only between 1 in 22 and 1 in 1000 infected people develop paralytic poliomyelitis, we can estimate that within the 10-year period up to 47000 travelers returning to industrialized countries imported the infection and may have excreted the virus for several weeks. The incidence of infection per journey to developing countries is estimated to be 0.7–33.6/100000 travelers. The lower incidence estimate is more realistic because a higher proportion of adults tend to have paralytic infections. Surprisingly, only 18 patients were reported among contacts of the cases. This, however, may be due to artifacts in reporting, and possibly some health authorities fail to conduct thorough case investigations.

## Conclusions

In conclusion, many data have been generated in the field of travel medicine in the past 15 years and we need no longer rely on vague experience. Are these data accurate? Often this is not the case, especially because subclinical infections or infections with spontaneous remission would only be identified by screening. These mild or asymptomatic cases, however, are clinically less important. Further, the incidence per month often had to be extrapolated. Despite these and other known biases, we believe that the order of magnitude of the documented relevant illnesses is adequate.

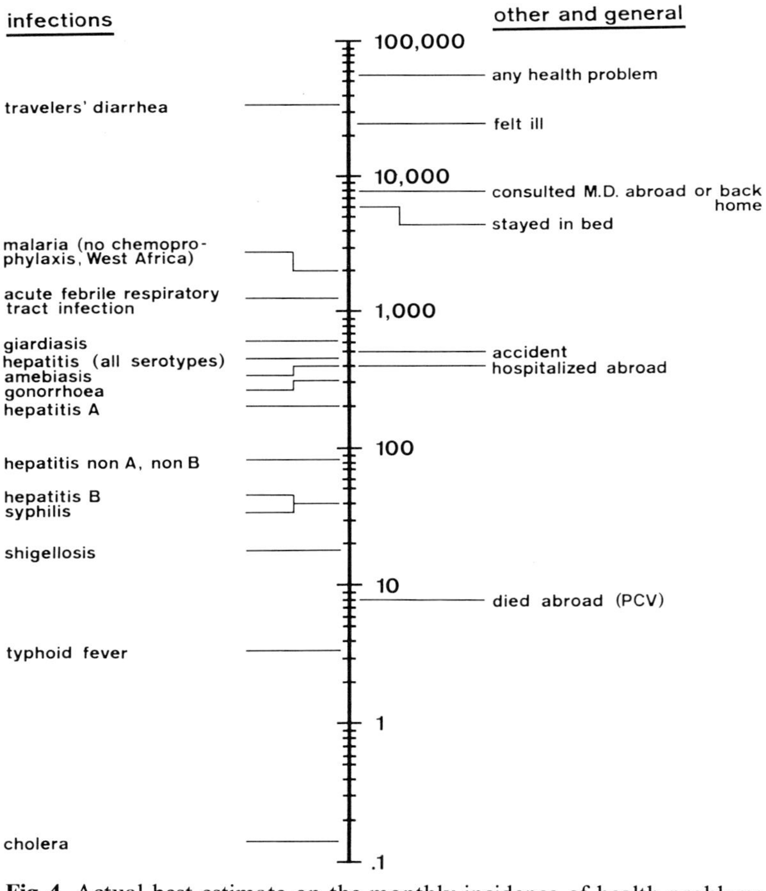


**Fig. 4.** Actual best estimate on the monthly incidence of health problems per 100 000 travelers to the tropics

In this brief review we have focused on those illnesses against which immunization or drug prophylaxis is possible. However, as Fig. 4 shows, data are available also about sexually transmitted diseases, parasitoses and accidents, which the smart traveler can avoid by reducing exposure to the various dangers. Accidents are particularly important, as they were the most frequent cause of death in Peace Corps Volunteers (Hargarten, this volume). Similarly, in the 90 Swiss citizens who died abroad in 1987, traffic and aircraft accidents and drowning were the most frequent known causes of death.

## References

1. Steffen R, Van der Linde F (1981) Intercontinental travel and its effect on pre-existing illnesses. Aviat Space Environ Med 52(1):57–58
2. Steffen R, Van der Linde F, Gyr K, Schär M (1983) Epidemiology of diarrhea in travelers. JAMA 249:1176–1180
3. Steffen R (1985) Epidemiology of health impairments during intercontinental travel. Travel Med Int 3:76–79
4. Kendrick MA (1972) Study of illness among Americans returning from international travel, Juli 11 – August 24, 1971 (preliminary data). J Infect Dis 126:684–685
5. Steffen R, Heusser R (1986) Zuverlässigkeit und Nebenwirkungen der Malariachemoprophylaxe. Schweiz Rundsch Med Prax 16:446–448
6. Steffen R, Rickenbach M, Wilhelm U, Helminger A, Schär M (1987) Health problems after travel to developing countries. J Infect Dis 156:84–91
7. Reid D, Dewar RD, Fallon RJ, Cossar JH, Grist NR (1980) Infection and travel: the experience of package tourists and other travellers. J Infect Dis 2:365–370
8. Peltola H, Kyrönseppä H, Hölsä P (1983) Trips to the South – a health hazard. Scand J Infect Dis 15:375–381
9. Steffen R, Boppart I (1987) Travellers' diarrhoea. Baillière's Clin Gastroenterol 2:361–376
10. DuPont HL, Haynes GA, Pickering LK, Tjoa W, Sullivan P, Olarte J (1977) Diarrhea of travelers to Mexico: relative susceptibility of United States' and Latin American students attending a Mexican university. Am J Epidemiol 105:37–41
11. Kozicki M, Steffen R, Schär M (1985) "Boil it, cook it, peel it, or forget it": does this rule prevent travellers' diarrhoea? Int J Epidemiol 14:169–172
12. Black RE (1986) Pathogens that cause travelers' diarrhea in Latin America and Africa. Rev Infect Dis 8:S131–S135
13. Taylor DN, Echeverria P (1986) Etiology and epidemiology of travelers' diarrhea in Asia. Rev Infect Dis 8:S136–S141
14. Steffen R, Mathewson JJ, Ericsson CD, DuPont HL, Helminger A, Balm TK, Wolff K, Witassek F (1988) Travelers' diarrhea in West Africa and in Mexico: fecal transport systems and liquid bismuth subsalicylate for self-therapy. J Infect Dis 157:1008–1013
15. Steffen R (1982) Typhoid vaccine, for whom? Lancet II:615–616
16. Taylor DN, Pollard RA, Blake PA (1983) Typhoid in the United States and the risk to international traveler. J Infect Dis 148:599–602
17. Anonymous (1984) Communicable disease report. Community Med 6:72–75
18. Wüthrich RP, Somaini B, Steffen R, Hirschel B (1985) Typhusepidemiologie in der Schweiz 1980–1983. Schweiz Med Wochenschr 115:1714–1720
19. Morger H, Steffen R, Schär M (1983) Epidemiology of cholera in travellers, and conclusions for vaccination recommendations. Br Med J 286:184–186
20. Snyder JD, Blake PA (1982) Is cholera a problem for US travelers? JAMA 247:2268–2269

21. Steffen R, Regli P, Grob PJ (1977) Wie groß ist das Risiko einer Reisehepatitis? Schweiz Med Wochenschr 107:1300–1307
22. Skinhøj P, Gluud C, Ramsøe K (1981) Traveller's hepatitis. Origin and characteristics of cases in Copenhagen 1976–1978. Scand J Infect Dis 13:1–4
23. Apothéloz M, Grob PJ, Steffen R, Schär M (1982) Welchen Auslandsreisenden ist ein Impfschutz gegen Heptatitis zu empfehlen? Soz Praventivmed 27:264–265
24. Iwarson S, Wahl M (1983) Hepatitis A in Swedish foreign travellers. Dev Biol Stand 54:419–422
25. Holdener F, Grob PJ, Joller-Jemelka HI (1982) Hepatitis virus infection in flying airline personnel. Aviat Space Environ Med 53(6):587–590
26. Kubli D, Steffen R, Schär M (1987) Importation of poliomyelitis to industrialised nations between 1975 and 1984: evaluation and conclusions for vaccination recommendations. Br Med J 295:169–171

# Health Risks for Temporary Residents of Developing Countries: The U.S. Peace Corps as an Epidemiologic Model

K. W. Bernard

## Summary

Health risks for temporary residents of developing countries may differ markedly from those in the vacation traveler. While some expatriates may live in protected communities in capital cities, many live in the rural towns and villages where they work. The United States Peace Corps is an international volunteer organization which supports over 5500 volunteers working in development projects in 62 countries worldwide. Peace Corps uses a computerized epidemiologic surveillance system to monitor trends in 31 health conditions and events. Data are collected monthly from each country and quarterly and annual incidence rates are calculated. In 1987, the most commonly reported health problems were diarrhea (unclassified), 48 cases/100 yolunteers/year; amebiasis, 24 cases/100 volunteers/year; injuries, 20 cases/100 volunteers/year; dental problems 19 cases/100 volunteers/year; and bacterial skin infections, 19 cases/100 volunteers/year. Based on these data, specific studies and disease control efforts have been initiated. Health problems with very low rates (less than 0.1/100 volunteers/year) include hepatitis, schistosomiasis, non-falciparum malaria, and filariasis. The epidemiologic surveillance system provides the health data needed to plan, implement, and evaluate health programs for Peace Corps Volunteers, and provides a model for surveillance in other groups of temporary and permanent residents of developing countries.

## Introduction

Although much has been written on the health problems of short-term visitors to developing countries, there is relatively little comprehensive information on health risks for long-term but still temporary residents of developing nations. These groups include diplomatic communities, personnel from international business and industrial organizations, and military personnel, in addition to over 200 000 missionaries, and 100 000 government and nongovernmental volunteers [1, 3]. Although having in common a prolonged length of stay (usually counted in months to years rather than weeks), temporary residents of developing countries are a heterogeneous population. Living conditions can range from the most basic and isolated, such as teachers working in rural Zaire, to truly elegant as in the case of high-level diplomatic and business personnel living in New Dehli or Abidjan. Nevertheless, epidemiologic and health data from these groups can provide useful information needed for triggering disease control and prevention efforts for their own communities, for short-term travelers, and perhaps for national populations in the host country.

Epidemiologic surveillance is the ongoing, systematic collection, and analysis and interpretation of health data needed to plan, implement, and evaluate public health programs. It is well recognized that acquisition of health-related data is necessary as a first step to provide rational recommendations intended to maximize health and safety. However, the difficulty in defining at-risk populations, limited health reporting infrastructure, and cost have limited the establishment of epidemiologic surveillance in many developing countries.

This report provides a description of the implementation of a comprehensive, active surveillance system designed to monitor health and morbidity trends in United States Peace Corps Volunteers (PCVs), a large group of volunteers serving in developing countries around the world. In addition to providing interesting new information on health of temporary residents of developing countries, it may serve as a model for epidemiologic surveillance in other expatriate organizations.

## Background

In 1987 Peace Corps supported approximately 5500 development volunteers located in 62 countries worldwide. The average age of the volunteers was 30.6 years with a range of 20–85 years; 50% were male. An increasing percentage of PCVs (12% in 1987) are 50 years of age or older. Because they often live in isolated rural locations and are exposed to diseases that are uncommon in the United States, PCVs must receive medical clearance and complete all needed dental work in the United States prior to placement in their assigned countries. A full-time Peace Corps Medical officer (PCMO), usually a registered nurse, is assigned in each country to provide physical examinations, disease diagnosis and treatment, and necessary health education for PCVs. If specific health care services are not available in-country, these services are obtained from other countries or after medical evacuation of the volunteer to the United States.

The surveillance system was instituted in October 1985. Each PCMO completes a monthly report form detailing the number of cases of 29 health conditions, the number of hospitalizations and medical evacuations, and the number of volunteers (total at-risk population) in each country (Table 1). Totals do not distinguish between multiple new cases of a disease in a single volunteer and single cases in multiple volunteers; the system counts cases, not patients. These data are cabled each month to Peace Corps/Washington and country-specific data are tabulated using a data entry program written in BASIC and resident on a small microcomputer. Data are then automatically analyzed using a commercially available spreadsheet program. Through the use of internal programming language, the resulting program is simple to use, and data can be entered and analyzed by personnel without extensive computer training.

Because the number of volunteers in a country ranges from as few as 4 to as many as 300, the program combines monthly data into quarterly and yearly figures. Raw numbers are converted to incidence rates as "cases/100 volunteers/month" over the quarterly time period. Yearly rates (cases/100 volunteers/year) are similarly computed. In this way, incidence rates of specific

**Table 1.** Health conditions and diseases monitored by the Peace Corps epidemiologic surveillance system[a]

| Health condition | Health condition |
|---|---|
| Assault | Malaria |
| Cardiovascular diseases | Falciparum malaria |
| Dental problems | Non-*falciparum* malaria |
| Diarrheal diseases | Presumptive malaria |
| Amebiasis | Pulmonary diseases |
| Giardiasis | Schistosomiasis |
| Intestinal helminths | Sexually transmitted diseases |
| Diarrheal diseases (other causes) | Genital herpes |
| Counseling | Gonorrhea |
| Febrile illnesses (other causes) | Syphilis |
| Filariasis | Sexually transmitted diseases (other) |
| Hepatitis | Skin diseases |
| Hepatitis A | Allergic dermatitis |
| Hepatitis B | Bacterial skin infections |
| Hepatitis (unspecified) | Fungal skin infections |
| Injuries | Urinary tract infections |
| Motorcycle injuries | Hospitalizations |
| Motor vehicle injuries (not motorcycle) | Medical evacuations |
| Physical trauma (not motorcycle or motor vehicle related) | |

[a] Data, including the number of volunteers in the country, are collected on a monthly basis

health conditions can be compared among countries and regions regardless of the number of volunteers. Quarterly and annual reports, including tables and graphs, are returned to the country and to Peace Corps, Washington DC administrative and policy-making staff.

## Results

Figure 1 compares the incidence of eight selected diseases and health conditions in PCVs for 1986 and 1987. Unspecified diarrheal disease (excluding amebiasis, giardiasis and helminths) had the highest annual incidence among PCVs in 1987, with 48 reports/100 volunteers/year. Combined with rates for laboratory-confirmed amebiasis, giardiasis, and intestinal helminths, the overall rate of reported diarrheal disease is over 95/100 volunteers/year. It should be emphasized that this is a very conservative figure in that diarrheal disease of a mild or moderate nature might never be reported to the medical officer – the data represent illnesses serious enough for volunteers to request treatment. Marked variation occurs in disease rates from country to country. For example. Nepal, Guatemala, and the Central African Republic had high rates of diarrheal disease, while Kenya, Lesotho, and Tonga report substantially lower rates – most likely due to variable country-specific rates of exposure to enteric pathogens. In Guatemala, the rates of diarrheal diseases, including

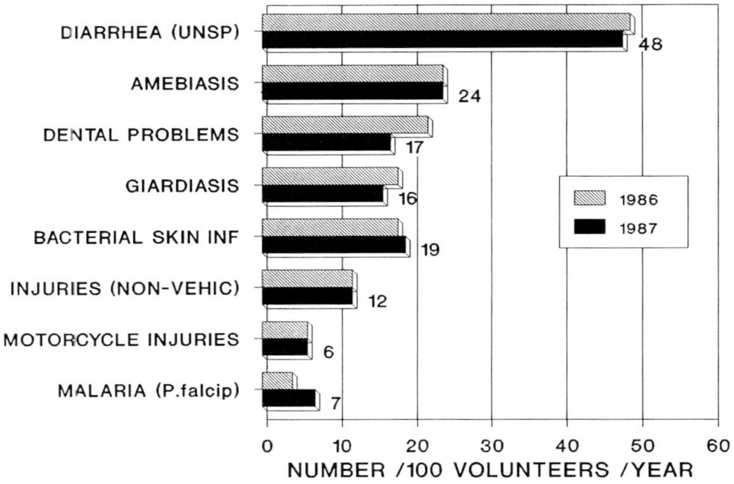


**Fig. 1.** Peace Corps health condition rates, 1986–1987

**Table 2.** Selected Peace Corps health condition rates, Guatemala, 1987[a]

| Health condition | Number/ year Guatemala | Rate (Number/100 volunteers/year) Guatemala | Rate (Number/100 volunteers/year) Inter-America Region |
|---|---|---|---|
| Diarrhea (unspecified) | 225 | 96.5 | 44.4 |
| Amebiasis | 99 | 42.5 | 27.7 |
| Injuries (total) | 43 | 18.4 | 24.9 |
| Febrile illneses | 9 | 3.9 | 9.6 |
| Bacterial skin infection | 46 | 19.7 | 12.3 |
| Dental problems | 37 | 15.9 | 21.4 |
| Giardiasis | 43 | 18.4 | 10.7 |
| Motorcycle injuries | 8 | 3.4 | 6.3 |
| Helminths | 38 | 16.3 | 9.7 |
| Cardiovascular disease | 3 | 1.3 | 1.4 |

[a] Mean monthly number of volunteers = 133

amebiasis and giardiasis, and bacterial skin infections are higher than the regional average, while the rates of dental problems and injuries are lower (Table 2).

There have been a number of unexpected results. Dental problems have consistently remained the third or fourth most frequently reported health problem overall (17/100 volunteers/year, 1987). Specific tropical disease such as schistosomiasis and filariasis are very uncommon among volunteers (less than 1.0/100 volunteers/year) except in highly localized areas. The rate of "all" hepatitis is also unexpectedly low at 0.7/100 volunteers/year, with hepatitis B reported in 0.2/100 volunteers/year.

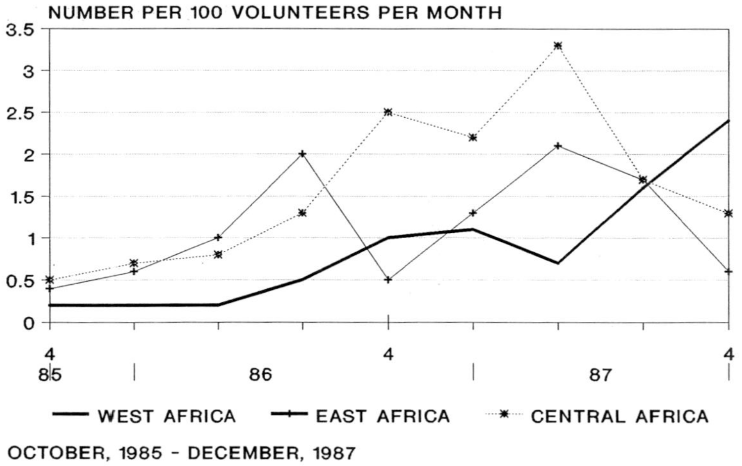


**Fig. 2.** Incidence of *P. falciparum* in Peace Corps volunteers in Africa by quarter, October 1985 – December 1987

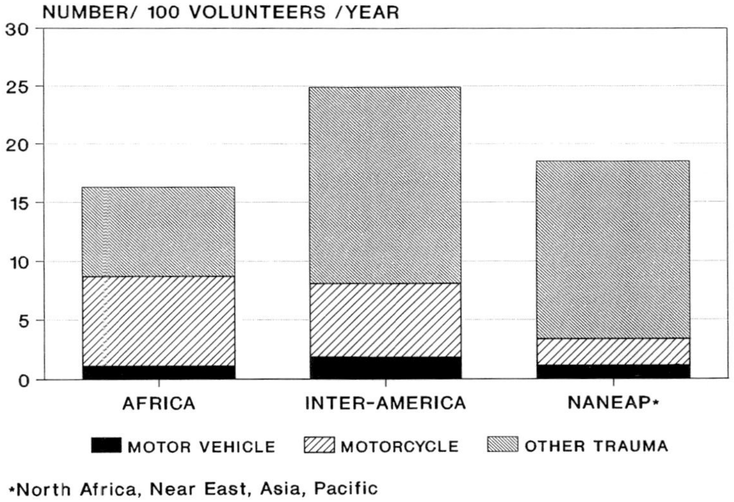


**Fig. 3.** Incidence of injuries in Peace Corps volunteers by region. 1987

Of the 62 countries in which PCVs are assigned, malaria is endemic in 47 (76%) and is therefore a health risk to volunteers. *Plasmoidum falciparum* resistant to chloroquine – the drug most commonly used for malaria prophylaxis and treatment – is rapidly spreading throughout the world. Using data obtained from the surveillance system, the Peace Corps is able to monitor the change in incidence of malaria in volunteers on a month-to-month basis. Figure 2 shows *P. falciparum* malaria rates in West, Central, and East Africa for 1986–1987. Of particular note is the overall increase in malaria in PCVs in West Africa beginning in the third quarter of 1986, when an explosive outbreak of resistant malaria occurred among Peace Corps Volunteers in Benin. Successive outbreaks of chloroquine-resistant malaria have subsequently occurred in PCVs in Togo [6] Ghana, Liberia, and Niger.

The occurrence of a number of diseases and health conditions of noninfectious etiology (including motor vehicle injuries, motorcycle injuries, and other trauma) are also monitored by the surveillance system. In 1987 Peace Corps reported 304 motorcycle injuries, 68 other motor vehicle injuries, and 645 cases of injuries from other causes, resulting in an overall injury rate of 20/100 volunteers/year (Fig. 3).

## Discussion

The comprehensive, computer-based, continuous monitoring of health conditions in a large expatriate community living and working in developing countries has not been heretofore reported. Diseases reported most frequently overall are generally those that would be expected in a group of volunteers in nontourist living situations.

The rates of diarrheal diseases may appear high; however, substantially higher rates have been observed in short-term travelers to developing countries. The rate of severe diarrhea in Swiss short-term travelers to developing countries was recently reported to be 15/100 travelers/month [9] compared with approximately 4.0/100 Peace Corps Volunteers/month for serious unspecified diarrheal illness. The rate of amebiasis in Swiss short-term travelers was 0.4/100 travelers/month compared with 2.0/100 PCVs/month. Diarrhea rates in other reports on short-term travelers to developing countries have exceeded 50% [8]. It has been speculated that the higher rates of parasitic diarrheal diseases in the volunteer population are due to increased exposure risk over time in volunteers living in rural locations. Because of these data, the Peace Corps has increased and emphasized its diarrheal prevention and education programs and embarked on two prospective studies, one in Nepal and one in Africa, to guide intervention strategies.

The incidence of hepatitis in Peace Corps Volunteers is 0.7/100 volunteers/year and has remained at a low level since 1964. The low rate is likely due to the standard Peace Corps policy of administering immune globulin to volunteers every 4 months during their service [10]. The incidence of hepatitis in other expatriates and short-term travelers, most of whom have not received immunoglobulin, has been reported to be over five times higher (primarily due to an increased rate of hepatitis A). It is apparent that routine use of immune globulin in nonimmune expatriates in rural living situations is indicated to reduce the substantial morbidity resulting from hepatitis A [4, 7].

Although it was initially surprising that dental problems were common in volunters, analysis revealed that the incidence may be similar to an age- and race-stratified group in the United States [5]. An evaluation prompted by these surveillance data demonstrated that the majority of dental problems occurred during the volunteer's 2nd year of service and resulted from dental caries and trauma secondary to hard objects such as stones in local foodstuffs.

The majority of Peace Corps deaths (over 70%) are secondary to injuries [2]; a study designed prospectively to evaluate the factors contributing to non-fatal injuries was instituted in five African countries with high injury rates. Of the 64 injuries occurring in a 6-month period, 58% resulted from motorcycle accidents. Of these motorcycle accidents, 62% involved loss of control with no other vehicle involved, 19% involved collision with an animal, and 19% involved collision with another vehicle. Clearly, driving motorcycles at speeds unsafe for prevailing conditions is a major factor leading to high rates of Peace Corps injuries. Specific injury reduction strategies have been implemented, and the surveillance system will allow immediate evaluation of the effectiveness of these interventions.

The surveillance system generally is quite sensitive, especially for the more serious illnesses and injuries. For problems in which the volunteer can easily obtain medical services outside the Peace Corps medical system, the sensitivity may be somewhat less; illnesses such as fungal skin infections may be reported at a much lower level than they actually occur. Other imperfections in the system include: (1) common diseases such as upper respiratory infections are not included; (2) case reporting biases occur resulting from factors such as the diligence of the medical officer, volunteer access to the medical office and physician, laboratory support; and (3), it is difficult to calculate statistical significance of disease rate differences because of wide confidence intervals around point estimates of the rates.

## Conclusions

Epidemiologic surveillance is being used by Peace Corps to: (1) provide quantitative estimates of morbidity and mortality; (2) detect epidemics; (3) identify factors affecting disease occurrence; (4) stimulate research to determine the specific focus for control or prevention; and (5) determine the effectiveness of previously implemented control measures. Surveillance data have traditionally been underutilized by expatriate organizations in developing countries. However, with the advent of sophisticated international telecommunications and the availability of portable computers, other groups could also monitor diseases and health conditions among their members. These data would not only be useful to persons with the responsibility of insuring the health and wellbeing of expatriate communities, but could also be used by persons advising short-term travelers and, potentially, those involved with making health policy decisions for permanent residents of host counties.

## References


1. Hamilton GR (1986) Health of the overseas volunteer. Travel Med Int 4:184–188
2. Hargarten SW, Baker SP (1985) Fatalities in Peace Corps, a retrospective study: 1962 through 1983. JAMA 254:1326–1329
3. Lange WR, Kreider SD, Kaczaniuk MA, Snyder FR (1987) Missionary health: the great omission. Am J Prevent Med 3:332–338
4. Larouze B, Gaudebout C, Mercier E et al. (1987) Infection with hepatitis A and B viruses in French volunteers working in tropical Africa. Am J Epidemiol 126:31–37
5. Miller AJ, Brunelle JP, Carlos JP, Brown LJ, Loe H (1985) Oral health of United States adults. National Institute of Dental Health, National Institutes of Health, U.S. Public Health Service, Bethesda MD
6. Moran JS, Bernard KW, Greenberg AW, Patchen L, Waterman S, Bennett HS (1987) Failure of chloroquine treatment to prevent malaria in Americans in West Africa. JAMA 258:2376–2377
7. Sleggs JH, Murray R (1986) Decline in hepatitis attack rate over two decades and effectiveness of immunoglobulin prophylaxis. Trop Doct 16:54–56
8. Steffen R, van der Linde F, Gyre K, Schar M (1983) Epidemiology of diarrhea in travelers. JAMA 249:1176–1180
9. Steffen R, Rickenbach M, Wilhelm U, Helminger A, Schar M (1987) Health problems after travel to developing countries. J Infect Dis 156:84–91
10. Woodson RD, Clinton JJ (1969) Hepatitis prophylaxis abroad: effectiveness of immune serum globulin in protecting Peace Corps Volunteers. JAMA 209:1053–1058

# Imported Disease in Australia: An Ongoing Problem

J. M. Goldsmid

Australia was for centuries isolated from outside influences, including infectious disease, by its geographical position and its surrounding sea barriers. The year 1988 marks the bicentenary of one of the most significant events in the history of the continent – its settlement in 1788 by Europeans – an event which marked the start of a long history of disease importation.

Prior to the coming of the whites, Australia was in all probability relatively free from infectious disease. The small numbers and nomadic habits of the indigenous Aboriginal people would have proved unsuitable for the persistence *in continuo* of acute infectious diseases (Cockburn 1977; Goldsmid 1984, 1988). Infectious diseases which do, however, seem to have been endemic at this time included yaws, treponarid (Sandison 1980) and, less certainly, trachoma (Goldsmid 1988) and perhaps benign tertian malaria (Black 1956). Also probably present were zoonotic infections harboured by native animals (Iveson 1977).

During this period, there seems to have been little contact with the outside world for the majority of the Aboriginal tribes, but occasional visits by traders and fishermen from Indonesia and Southeast Asia may at times have resulted in the introduction of epidemic diseases (Blainey 1975). Again, it would seem unlikely that these diseases could survive due to the low population density of the Aborigines (Goldsmid 1988).

Then, in 1788, the first permanent settlers from Europe arrived in New South Wales. These people brought with them all the infectious diseases common in Europe at that time, including measles, influenza, smallpox, diphtheria, pertussis, typhoid, syphilis, gonorrhoea and tuberculosis (Gandevia 1978; Curson 1985).

The result of this was disastrous for the highly susceptible Aboriginal people of Australia, with many tribes being decimated by these newly introduced diseases.

As the population of the new colonies increased and stabilized, so more and more of these diseases became endemic.

In 1856 gold was discovered in Australia and this resulted in a further influx of new settlers, including Europeans, Asians and Pacific Islanders into the country. Many of these migrants came from tropical destinations and this resulted in the importation of a whole new range of tropical diseases which spread into the interior and north of the continent with the explorers and expanding population. Diseases which became established at this time included dengue, leprosy, malaria, amoebiasis, Bancroftian filariasis and hookworm (Cilento 1942; Goldsmid 1984, 1988).

Then in 1901, the various colonies were united into the present Commonwealth of Australia, a union which brought improvements in living conditions, hygiene and sanitation as well as a uniform and efficient immunization policy. All of these developments resulted in a steady decline in the prevalence, morbidity and mortality from infection (Feery 1981; Goldsmid 1988).

Despite these improvements in the health of the nation, sporadic outbreaks of disease similar to the pre-Federation epidemics of diphtheria, scarlet fever and smallpox continued to occur. The most notable of these epidemics were the Bubonic Plague outbreak of 1900–1909, the Spanish influenza pandemic of 1918 and the tragic epidemic of poliomyelitis in 1937 (Goldsmid 1988).

Overall, as the country developed, most of these infectious diseases were successfully controlled or even eradicated (e.g. malaria, Bancroftian filariasis). The decline has, however, been notably slower amongst the Aboriginal people than amongst the other sectors of the population but this situation is undoubtedly improving albeit slowly (Moodie 1977; Hollows 1986; O'Dea 1986; Goldsmid 1988).

Australia is thus a classic example of the importation of disease introduced by international travel and migration.

This threat of imported disease associated with international travel does, however, remain. These imported diseases have, in fact, increased as a threat

**Table 1.** Visitor arrivals in Australia

| | |
|---|---|
| 1956 | 66018 |
| 1966 | 215071 |
| 1976 | 450217 |
| 1986 | 1467530 |

**Table 2.** Percentage of international arrivals cleared/state (1986)

| State | NSW | Vic | Q | WA | SA | NT | Tas | ACT | Total |
|---|---|---|---|---|---|---|---|---|---|
| % Arrivals | 52 | 22 | 12 | 10 | 2 | 1 | 0.4 | 0.02 | 3139900 |

**Table 3.** Imported viral and bacterial diseases diagnosed in Tasmania

| | |
|---|---|
| AIDS | Typhoid[a] |
| Hepatitis B | Shigellosis |
| Rocky Mountain Spotted Fever[a] | Brucellosis[a] |
| LGV[a] | Tuberculosis |
| Chancroid | Leprosy[a] |
| Cholera[a] | Gonorrhoea (incl. PPNG) |

[a] Non-endemic diseases

associated with increasing overseas travel (Table 1) and especially with increased air travel (Goldsmid 1979, 1984, 1988).

An illustration of the significance of imported disease in Australia can be seen by looking at statistics for Tasmania – the small island state at the southernmost tip of the continent. This isolated state has a population of just over 450000. Only about 2% of overseas visitors to Australia visit the state and only 0.4% of international arrivals make this state their first point of contact (Table 2). Despite this, the range of imported infections and the geographical diversity of their origins is impressive (Tables 3, 4).

Although some of these imported diseases to Australia have become established to varying degrees (e.g. dengue, cholera and AIDS), in most cases such

**Table 4.** Imported parasitic infections diagnosed in Tasmania

| Species | Source |
|---|---|
| *Giardia lamblia* | India; Nepal; Vietnam |
| *Chilomastix mesnili*[a] | India; Vietnam |
| *Leishmania tropica*[a] | Middle East; Mediterranean |
| *Dientamoeba fragilis*[a] | Nepal |
| *Entamoeba histolytica*[a] | India; Nepal; Vietnam; Papua New Guinea |
| *Entamoeba coli* | Vietnam; Nepal; India; South Africa |
| *Entamoeba hartmanni*[a] | Nepal |
| *Iodamoeba bütschlii*[a] | Vietnam |
| *Endolimax nana* | India; Bangladesh; Vietnam; South Africa |
| *Blastocystis hominis* | Vietnam; Nepal Papua New Guinea |
| *Plasmodium falciparum*[a] | Kenya/Tanzania; Papua New Guinea |
| *P. vivax*[a] | Kenya/Tanzania; Ghana; Papua New Guinea; Indonesia; Solomon Islands; India; Bangladesh; Vietnam |
| *Fasciolopsis buski*[a] | Vietnam/Thailand |
| *Schistosoma mansoni*[a] | Kenya; Zimbabwe |
| *S. haematobium*[a] | Zimbabwe |
| *Hymenolepis nana*[a] | Bangladesh; Iran; Vietnam |
| *Taenia saginata*[a] | Lebanon |
| Hydatid | New Zealand |
| Hookworm[a] | Vietnam: Philippines; Egypt |
| Cutaneous larva migrans[a] | Pacific Islands; Malaysia |
| *Strongyloides stercoralis*[a] | Timor; Papua New Guinea; Vietnam; Kampuchea; India; Sri Lanka |
| *Trichuris trichiura* | India; Bangladesh; Maldives; Philippines |
| *Enterobius vermicularis* | India; Vietnam |
| *Ascaris lumbricoides* | India; Bangladesh; Maldives; Zimbabwe; Fiji; Philippines; Papua New Guinea |
| *Loa loa*[a] | Nigeria; West Africa |
| Tropical eosinophilia[a] | Maldives |
| *Wuchereria bancrofti*[a] | India; Tuvalu |
| *Cordylobia anthropophaga*[a] | Malawi |
| *Dermatobia hominis*[a] | South America |
| *Sarcoptes scabiei* | Vietnam |
| *Pediculus capitis* | Vietnam |

[a] Non-endemic species

diseases comprise primarily a diagnostic and therapeutic problem – a problem which we have to face and solve even in relatively isolated parts of the country.

A patient may present at any time, even in the smallest village, with some exotic disease acquired while travelling abroad. In these cases, specialist staff and facilities may not be readily available and the patient may die due to diagnostic ineptitude or simple lack of awareness by the clinician or laboratory.

How can this dilemma be overcome?

We cannot expect every little town or village to have expert facilities and staff trained in the so-called tropical diseases.

Australia is not alone in this concern – similar views have been expressed in the United States (IOM/NAS 1987) and the United Kingdom (Duggan 1982) regarding the decline in the specialty of tropical medicine and its practitioners. In Australia we have even seen the closure of the School of Tropical Medicine in Sydney by a short-sighted Federal Government.

Wright (1971) was aware of the increasing need for the general practitioner to be aware of imported disease, as was Maegraith (1971) when he advocated for inclusion in history taking from every patient, the two questions: Where have you been?

When were you there?

Browne (1978) expressed the dilemma as follows: "If we regard tropical medicine as a separate entity, then we shall fail to insinuate it in an already overcrowded curriculum; if we refrain from pushing its claims, then newly qualified doctors ... may be ill-prepared to face increasing calls on their diagnostic ability ... and many of our fellow citizens may suffer unnecessarily or even die from undiagnosed or misdiagnosed conditions that had their origin in tropical countries".

In conclusion I should like to advocate strongly, in the face of increasing disease importation and decreasing skills to deal with tropical diseases found in the developed countries today, the latter due largely to political ignorance and governmental parsimoniousness, that we must ensure that all medical undergraduates are taught, as routine, the elements of tropical medicine and are, at the very least, made aware of the importance of imported disease and the possibility of an exotic disease occurring in any patient consulting them and who has travelled overseas.

## References

Black R (1956) The epidemiology of malaria in the southwest Pacific: changes associated with increasing European contact. Oceania 27:136–142

Blainey G (1975) Triumph of the Nomads. MacMillan, Melbourne

Browne SG (1978) Tropical medicine – facing today's dilemma. Trans R Soc Trop Med Hyg 72:1–5

Cilento RW (1942) Tropical medicine in Australasia. Smith and Paterson, Brisbane

Cockburn A (1977) Where did our infectious diseases come from? The evolution of infectious disease. In: Hugh-Jones P (chairman) Health and disease in tribal societies. CIBA Symp No 49. Elsevier, Amsterdam, pp 103–113

Curson PH (1985) Times of crisis. Sydney University Press, Sydney
Duggan AJ (1982) Tropical medicine: a submerging art? Trans R Soc Trop Med Hyg 76:569–574
Feery B (1981) Impact of immunization on disease patterns in Australia. Med J Aust 2:172–174
Gandevia B (1978) Tears often shed. Charter Books. Gordan
Goldsmid JM (1979) The travel bug. University of Tasmania Occasional Paper No 17. University of Tasmania, Hobart
Goldsmid JM (1988) The deadly legacy. University of NSW Press, Sydney
Hollows FC (1986) Some aspects of Aboriginal health. Aust Fam Physician 15:884–887
IOM/NAS (1987) Institutes of Medicine/National Academy of Sciences Report. Trop Med Hyg News 36:39–40
Iveson JB (1977) *Salmonella* infections in wildlife in Western Australia: a natural barometer of environmental health. W.A. Nat Surveyor's Conference, Oct, pp 53–72
Maegraith B (1971) Imported disease in Europe. CIBA-Geigy, Basle
Moodie PM (1977) Medical aspects of Aboriginal health. Aust Fam Physician 6:1309–1313
O'Dea K (1986) Aboriginal health and changes in life style. Aust Fam Physician 15:875–881
Sandison T (1980) Treponemal infections in pre-European contact exhumed Aboriginal skeletons. 3rd European meeting, Paleopath Association Caen, France
Wright FJ (1971) Tropical disease and general medicine. Scot Med J 16:209–214

# A Review of Travel-Associated Illness

Jonathan H. Cossar

## Introduction

In 1973 an outbreak of pneumonia with three fatalities affecting a group of package holidaymakers returning from Benidorm to Glasgow was subsequently shown to be caused by Legionnaires' disease [1]. This example of the return of travellers within the incubation period of a then exotic disease which presented diagnostic difficulties and delay in the home country motivated the development of a collaborative study of illnesses associated with travel, conducted by the Communicable Diseases (Scotland) Unit (CDSU), the University of Glasgow Department of Infectious Diseases, the Department of Laboratory Medicine and the Regional Virus Laboratory (both at Ruchill Hospital) [2–22]. Over the past decade it has proved possible to establish a system which facilitates regular monitoring of the health experience of returning Scottish travellers and also the mounting of a specific enquiry into groups of travellers identified as being "at risk" following an alert about a possible health problem. Analysis was carried out on the information provided by travellers using a standard questionnaire [4] and serum samples were collected [4], enabling various antibody titres to be measured [11] (the methodologies are as detailed in the references quoted).

## Questionnaire Findings

Out of a total of 14 227 respondents 37% gave a history of illness with response rates amongst the different study groups ranging from 21% to 77%. The attack rates varied from a low of 19% amongst summer visitors to Scotland in 1980 [8] and 20% amongst winter package holidaymakers [9], to 75% amongst summer package holidaymakers to Romania in 1981 [12] and 78% amongst 375 tourists who selected themselves for study by writing or telephoning to the CDSU [4]. This followed media publicity on legionellosis and travel in 1977.

Comparing attack rates with the areas visited there is a general trend that the further south and to some extent the further east the travel the higher the rate. This remains generally true both in summer and in winter. Examples in support of this trend are the 77% attack rate reported by tourists staying in southern coastal areas of the Mediterranean in the summer and the 57% rate for those travelling to the east of Europe and also the 32% attack rate reported by winter tourists to north Africa. In addition attack rates in general are substantially lower in the winter than in the summer, the mean recorded attack

**Table 1.** Age distribution of travellers and reports of illness

| Age group (years) | Unwell | Totals | Overall |
|---|---|---|---|
| 0– 9 | 33% | 550 | (4%) |
| 10–19 | 41% | 1974 | (14%) |
| 20–29 | 48% | 3033 | (21%) |
| 30–39 | 38% | 2028 | (14%) |
| 40–49 | 32% | 2297 | (16%) |
| 50–59 | 28% | 2381 | (17%) |
| 60+ | 20% | 1239 | (9%) |
| Not known | 32% | 725 | (5%) |
| Totals | 37% | 14227 | (100%) |
| Range | (20%–48%) | | (4%–21%) |

rate for winter travellers being 20% compared with 37% for summer travellers.

Table 1 shows the distribution of travellers by age group and illness with the highest attack rates being recorded in the under-40 age groups; thereafter attack rates show a progressive diminution with increasing age.

Eighteen percent of the travellers reported alimentary symptoms, predominantly diarrhoea and vomiting. Taking all the symptom complexes which include alimentary symptoms, this figure rises to 28% of the total number of travellers and to 76% of all those who reported illness. The 20- to 29-year age group recorded the highest attack rate for alimentary problems.

Looking at attack rates in smokers compared with non-smokers overall 37% of 2784 smokers were unwell compared with 32% of 7294 non-smokers – this difference is statistically significant ($P<0.0001$).

## Serological Findings

Serological studies for poliomyelitis antibody were carried out on 470 of the travellers, which showed that only 2 (<1%) were without detectable antibody, 5% had antibody to one type and 14% had antibody to two types, i.e. 20% were incompletely immune.

Overall 75% of the 312 travellers tested had no evidence of successful immunization against *Salmonella typhi* (flagellar antibody titres $\geqq 1/40$) despite the fact that at the time of this study (1982) 63% of the visits carried out by United Kingdom residents were to countries where immunization was recommended.

Of the 761 samples tested for antibodies to *Legionella pneumophila*, less than 2% had a positive titre at a level of $\geqq 1/256$. All of these seropositive travellers had responded to nationwide publicity in the news media highlighting legionellosis in holidaymakers in Benidorm. They were therefore a highly self-selected group with histories of respiratory illness whilst on vacation in Spain [4].

Further studies in these travellers from the west of Scotland suggest that the population seropositivity to hepatitis A ranges from three out of ten for those aged under 20 years to almost nine out of ten for those aged over 60 years [17, 20]. These findings support the cost effectiveness of selective screening before giving immunoglobulin to older travellers at risk from hepatitis A [16].

## Comparative Studies

There are limitations in this type of survey due to non-respondents; therefore before drawing conclusions it is helpful to consider other comparable studies. Analysis of recent inpatient data (1985) from the Infectious Diseases (ID) wards at Ruchill Hospital, Glasgow, which is the major infectious diseases facility for the area, shows that 6% out of a total of 1265 ID admissions were travel associated, and Asian males accounted for greater than one in three of the total. Travel to the Indian subcontinent was associated with 60% of the admissions correlating with the higher attack rate seen in holidaymakers travelling further south and east. The 14% associated with travel to Spain probably reflects the sheer volume of United Kingdom holidaymakers to that country (5.6 million in 1985 [23]).

As with the questionnaire survey the 20- to 29-year age group had the highest proportion of admissions; however it gives cause for concern that 23% of the total admissions were aged <10 years.

Illnesses with alimentary symptomatology accounted for 38% of the admissions, the biggest single group with common symptomatology as occurred in the travel survey figures. It is of note that the largest single diagnosis was malaria, accounting for 37%.

Analysis of laboratory reports on isolates of pathogens from travellers collated at the CDSU show a fivefold increase in the annual total of reports between 1975 and 1986 and the proportion of isolates from travellers who were holidaymakers rose from 62% to 90% [24, 25]. During this same period cumulative review of the pathogens isolated reveals that infections associated with inadequate food handling and poor water supply or sanitation accounted for 87% of the reports.

Published studies on this subject from other researchers show attack rates from alimentary illnesses ranging from 18% to 41% [26–28]; those specifying the most affected age group are in agreement (20–29 years) [26, 28], and similarly where the area is specified travel to north Africa [26, 27] or to the east of Europe [28] is associated with the highest attack rates.

**Table 2.** Travellers "at risk" profile

| | |
|---|---|
| Package holidaymakers | >other travellers |
| Inexperienced travellers | >other travellers |
| Travellers further south, particularly north Africa | >other travellers |
| Summer travellers | >winter travellers |
| Younger age groups (specifically 20–29 years) | >older age groups |
| Smokers | >non-smokers |

This broad correlation in findings lends credibility in attempting definition of attack patterns in the studies detailed above and the largely identical methodology used encourages comparative rather than absolute analysis. From studies of the highest attack rates an "at risk" profile can be defined, summarized in Table 2, the features on the left side being associated with higher attack rates.

## Economic Considerations

From information supplied by 3049 travellers who became unwell whilst abroad, 1% required hospital admission in the United Kingdom and 14% consulted a doctor. The cost per travel-associated admission to Ruchill Hospital is given as approximately 500 pounds sterling.

Looking at the implications of these findings in terms of health economics, if the survey figures are revised assuming all non-responders to be "well", and the resulting "corrected attack rate" (12%) applied to the total number of United Kingdom holiday travellers in 1986 (17.9 million [29]), the following statistics are produced by extrapolation of the study findings – 2.2 million affected by illness, 0.5 million confined to bed, 0.3 million attended by a doctor and 21 500 admitted to hospital. This projection gives a figure of over 10 million pounds sterling for United Kingdom hospitalization costs alone in 1986 from travel-related illnesses.

## Conclusion

In conclusion this review shows that international travellers are vulnerable to minor illnesses, predominantly alimentary, with an attack rate approaching 40%. It helps define the medical and epidemiological perspective of travel-associated illnesses as well as the economic benefits which can accrue from effective pre-travel health education.

*Acknowledgments.* The help of Dr. D. Reid, Dr. R.J. Fallon, Miss M.H. Riding, Dr. E.J. Bell, Mr. R.D. Dewar, Professor N.R. Grist, Dr. J.C.M. Sharp, Dr. E.A.C. Follett, Mr. W.H. Abraham, Mr. J. Shearer, Dr. I. Pinkerton, Dr. C. Love, Dr. D. Kennedy, Dr. B. Datta, Dr. E. Walker, CDSU secretarial staff, Mr. H.N. Battersby and staff of the British Airport Authority, Mr. B.J. Forteath, Mr. J. MacPherson and colleagues of Renfrew District environmental health department, Mr. C. Sibbald and staff of Edinburgh City environmental health department, the family doctors of the travellers studied, and the travellers who gave their time to complete the questionnaire and agreed to give a blood sample, is greatly appreciated. This work was supported in part by the Chief Scientist Organization, Edinburgh.

## References

1. Lawson JH, Grist NR, Reid D, Wilson TS (1977) Legionnaires' disease. Lancet II:108
2. Reid D, Dewar RD, Fallon RJ, Cossar JH, Grist NR (1980) Infection and travel: the experience of package tourists and other travellers. J Infect 2:365–370

3. Bell EJ, Grist NR, Cossar JH, Dewar RD, Reid D (1981) Poliomyelitis worldwide. Br Med J 282:310
4. Cossar JH, Dewar RD, Fallon RJ, Grist NR, Reid D (1982) *Legionella pneumophila* in tourists. Practitioner 226:1543–1548
5. Grist NR, Cossar JH, Reid D (1982) Emporiatrics – travellers' health. Br Med J 285:894
6. Grist NR, Cossar JH, Reid D (1982) Travellers' infections. Update 25. 6:799–810
7. Reid D (1982) Tourism and illness. Proc R Soc Edinb 82B:23–25
8. Dewar RD, Cossar JH, Reid D, Grist NR (1983) Illness amongst travellers to Scotland: a pilot study. Health Bull (Edinb) 41/3:155–162
9. Cossar JH, Dewar RD, Reid D, Grist NR (1983) Travel and health: illness associated with winter package holidays. JR Coll Gen Pract 33:642–645
10. Cossar JH, Fallon RJ, Grist NR, Reid D (1983) Legionellosis. Update 27. 10:1433–1441
11. Cossar JH, Dewar RD, Fallon RJ, Reid D, Bell EJ, Riding MH, Grist NR (1984) Rapid response health surveillance of Scottish tourists. Travel Traffic Med Int 2:1,23–27
12. Grist NR, Cossar JH, Reid D, Dewar RD, Fallon RJ, Riding MH, Bell EJ (1985) Illness associated with a package holiday in Rumania. Scott Med J 30:156–160
13. Cossar JH, Reid D, Grist NR, Dewar RD, Fallon RJ, Riding MR, Bell EJ (1985) Illness associated with international travel: a ten year review. Travel Med Int 3:1,13–18
14. Reid D, Cossar JH, Ako TI, Dewar RD (1986) Do travel brochures give adequate advice on avoiding illness? Br Med J 293:1472
15. Walker E, Cossar JH, Dewar RD, Reid D (1987) Computerised advice on malaria prevention and immunisations. JR Coll Gen Pract 37:223
16. Cossar JH, Reid D (1987) Not all travellers need immunoglobulin for hepatitis A. Br Med J 294:1503
17. Cossar JH, Follett EAC, Riding MH, Reid D (1988) The use of immunoglobulin for travellers. CDS Weekly Rep 87/53:5–7
18. Cossar JH, Walker E, Reid D, Dewar RD (1988) Computerised advice on malaria prevention and immunisation. Br Med J 296:358
19. Cossar JH (1987) Studies on illnesses associated with travel. Thesis, University of Glasgow, Glasgow
20. Cossar JH, Follett EAC, Riding MH, Reid D (1989) How necessary is immunoglobulin for travellers going abroad? Community Med 11/1:9–12
21. Cossar JH (1988) Travel associated illnesses. JR Soc med 81:250–251
22. The Scottish Health Education Group (1986) Holiday information and checklist. (A guide to good health on holiday for travellers) Edinburgh
23. Central Statistical Office (1988) Social trends 18. Table 10.15. HMSO, London, p 165
24. Sharp JCM (1976) Imported infections into Scotland, 1975. CDS Weekly Report 76/26:v–vi
25. Campbell DM (1987) Imported infections in Scotland, 1986. CDS Weekly Rep 87/47:7–8
26. Steffen R, van der Linde F, Syr K, Schar M (1983) Epidemiology of diarrhoea in travellers. JAMA 249:1176–1180
27. Peltola H, Kyronseppa H, Holsa P (1983) Trips to the south – a health hazard. Scand J Infect Dis 15:375–381
28. McEwan A, Jackson MH (1987) Illness among Scots holidaymakers who had travelled abroad, summer 1983. CDS Weekly Rep 87/16:7–9
29. Business Statistics Office (1986) Business monitor annual statistics. Overseas travel and tourism, (MQ 6) table 8A. HMSO, London, p 13

# Fatalities of American Travelers – 1975, 1984

S. W. Hargarten, T. Baker, and K. Guptill

## Introduction

Over 27 million Americans travel abroad every year. By 1990, tourism is projected to be the United States' largest industry employing 7 million people and grossing a trillion dollars in revenue [1]. The morbidity experience of American travelers as well as European travelers is documented in the medical literature [2–6]. Health advice to travelers has been receiving increased attention in recent years [7–14]. American physicians should know the *mortality* risks as well as the *morbidity* risks to their patients who plan to travel overseas.

However, we could find no descriptions of the mortality experience of American travelers abroad. The deaths of United States Peace Corps volunteers working overseas has been recently studied by Hargarten and Baker [15]. Recently, the mortality statistics of commercial airline travel has been described in the literature [23]. A comparison article describing deaths to Americans both residing and traveling overseas has been submitted for publication [16]. We present this previously unpublished mortality data on Americans traveling outside the United States which should be of value to: physicians advising their patients who plan to travel overseas; international travelers' clinics; the insurance industry; the travel industry; the State Department; epidemiologists and vital statisticians.

## Sources of Data/Methodology

These deaths are *not* recorded or analyzed by the national Center of Health Statistics [17]. The deaths are reported to the United States Passport Office by the Consulor Representatives of the United States or their designated representatives in the various countries of the world. The Consuls send the death certificates to the United States Passport Office where the death registers have been maintained for approximately 12 years. The counsuls are notified by the local authorities in the event of the death of an individual who carries a United States passport.

We examined 2 years of death data in the passport section of the Department of State of Americans overseas. We selected the oldest year that was readily available, 1975, and the most current year that was complete, 1984. We analyzed all deaths under age 60 and randomly sampled 20% of the deaths in ages over 60.

Data on the American tourist population has been taken from the World Tourism Organization [18]. Conversion to an *annual exposure* was accomplished by calculating the "nights in hotels and other lodgings" for countries reporting to the WTO, extrapolating this number to all countries and dividing for "estimated nights stayed" per traveler by 365 days. This was then multiplied by the number of travelers to determine person years of exposure.

The death certificates data listing on the cause of death, country of death, age at death, sex, whether medically certified or not, whether death in hospital or home, whether resident or traveler, and occupation was transcribed and then tabulated with names and original residences in the United States eliminated to preserve confidentiality.

The ninth edition of the *International Causes of Disease (ICD Reference)* was our basis for coding of deaths. To obtain adequate number for analysis, we combined the codes to: cardiovascular, neoplastic, injuries (by type), all other and ill defined causes [19]. The quality of reporting varied considerably; however, the majority of reports were sufficiently accurate to permit coding.

Data from the World Bank was used for comparison of developed and developing countries [20]. Per capita GNP of less than US $2000 and male life expectancy in 1983 of less than 65 years were used to divide developed and undeveloped countries. Male life expectancy was used, as there were more males than females in the sample of deaths studied.

## Results

There were a total of 2463 deaths of American travelers during the study years. The distribution of those deaths according to causes was similar between the two comparative years and the average percentage is presented.

Cardiovascular diseases were the number one cause of death (49%), followed by intentional and unintentional injuries (25.0%). Infectious diseases (other than pneumonia) was the cause of death in only 25 cases (1.0%).

The age distribution of these deaths is presented in Table 1. The 65- to 74-year age group accounted for the greatest percentage (23.8%) of deaths. Travelers died in hospitals 41% of the time (1010 deaths). The deaths were

**Table 1.** Percent age death distribution of American travelers by age 1975/1984

| Age group | Frequency | Percent |
|---|---|---|
| Less than 15 | 56 | 2.3 |
| 15–24 | 108 | 4.4 |
| 25–34 | 193 | 7.8 |
| 35–44 | 176 | 7.1 |
| 45–54 | 327 | 13.3 |
| 55–64 | 558 | 22.6 |
| 65–74 | 585 | 23.8 |
| *75 and over* | *460* | *18.7* |
| Totals | 2463 | 100.0 |

medically certified 77% of the time (1893 deaths); certified by civil authorities 18% of the time (445 deaths); and not certified 5% of the time (125 deaths). Males accounted for 70.4% of the deaths. Tables 2 and 3 show the distribution of travel deaths by region and by selected countries for the study period. (Note: These distributions are not rates and reflect more the numbers of American travelers than the risk of death in these regions and countries. However, it is interesting to note that ten countries account for 58.5% of the deaths!)

There were 601 deaths due to injuries in the study period. Motor vehicle crashes (27%) were the most common cause of injury deaths, followed by drownings (16%) (Table 4). Homicides accounted for 52 deaths and suicides for 20 deaths. The category of poisoning includes acute alcoholic intoxication and drug overdoses.

Selected cause- and age-specific death rates for male travelers are shown in Table 5. Injury death rates for male travelers are consistently higher when compared with United States' rates. Cardiovascular death rates are lower then expected for ages over 44. (Note: Study years and developed and undeveloped country data were combined due to small numbers in certain age categories as

**Table 2.** Distribution of deaths (by regions – study years' average)

| Region | Percentage | Number |
|---|---|---|
| Western Europe | 48.0 | 1184 |
| Central America (includes Mexico) | 18.8 | 463 |
| Caribbean | 10.8 | 270 |
| Asia | 7.8 | 194 |
| Middle East | 6.4 | 157 |
| Eastern Europe | 2.5 | 63 |
| Australia (includes New Zealand and South Pacific) | 1.8 | 36 |
| *Africa* | *0.8* | *19* |
| Totals | 100 | 2463 |

**Table 3.** Distribution of traveler deaths (by country – study years' average)

| Country | Percentage | Number |
|---|---|---|
| Mexico | 16.0 | 396 |
| Federal Republic of Germany | 9.4 | 232 |
| Great Britain | 7.1 | 176 |
| Spain | 6.0 | 148 |
| Italy | 5.9 | 146 |
| Bahamas | 4.7 | 116 |
| France | 3.5 | 86 |
| Switzerland | 2.4 | 59 |
| Greece | 2.0 | 50 |
| *Bermuda* | *1.5* | *37* |
| Totals | 58.5 | 1446 |

**Table 4.** Injury deaths of American travelers – 1975, 1984

| Cause of death | No. of deaths 1975, 1984 | % of total |
|---|---|---|
| Motor vehicle crash | 163 | 27.1 |
| Drowning | 96 | 16.0 |
| Plane crash | 43 | 7.2 |
| Homicide | 52 | 8.7 |
| Poisoning | 39 | 6.5 |
| Suicide | 20 | 3.3 |
| Burns | 21 | 3.5 |
| Electrocution | 3 | 0.5 |
| *Others* | *164* | *27.2* |
| Totals | 601 | 100.0 |

**Table 5.** Injury control strategies for American tourists

1. Avoidance of motorcycles and small, less protective vehicles or at least use of helmets when using these vehicles
2. Use of seat belts, where available, including taxicabs
3. Use of larger in preference to smaller vehicles and not riding in the back of open trucks
4. Avoidance of small, nonscheduled aircraft
5. Careful selection of swimming areas, avoidance of alcohol while swimming
6. Avoidance of travel at night
7. Encouragement of travel in groups or pairs

**Table 6.** Mortality rates (male, by age) per 100000 (injury and cardiovascular)

| Cause | Age group | United States rate (1982) | Traveler rate |
|---|---|---|---|
| Injuries | 15–24 | 123.4 | 337.9 |
| Cardiovascular | | 4.3 | 48.9 |
| Injuries | 25–34 | 122.3 | 186.3 |
| Cardiovascular | | 14.9 | 43.4 |
| Injuries | 35–44 | 98.0 | 298.4 |
| Cardiovascular | | 73.2 | 93.9 |
| Injuries | 45–54 | 96.0 | 184.6 |
| Cardiovascular | | 300.7 | 295.4 |
| Injuries | 55–64 | 95.4 | 117.9 |
| Cardiovascular | | 808.9 | 793.2 |
| Injuries | 65–74 | 112.8 | 223.9 |
| Cardiovascular | | 1983.5 | 1692.3 |
| Injuries | 75 and over | 237.4 | 122.2 |
| Cardiovascular | | 5870.6 | 4141.3 |

well as denominator fluctuation.) Death rates due to injuries were consistently higher in less-developed countries when compared with developed countries (Table 6). Infectious disease accounted for 1% of the deaths ($n=25$) to American travelers. Malaria, typhoid and hepatitis B each accounted for one death in the study years.

Deaths of American travelers from "other" causes included animal mauling (shark, alligator and elephant) and falls from heights (mountains and buildings).

The most common "occupation" listed for travelers was "retired."

## Discussion

This is the first study describing the death pattern of Americans traveling outside the United States (excluding Canada). The distribution of deaths is quite different when compared with that of United States' residents who die "at home". Death due to injuries is ranked fourth in the United States, yet is the second most common cause of death of American travelers. Also, the mortality pattern is different from the morbidity pattern of travel. A recent study by Steffen et al. of Swiss travelers and their morbidity experience showed significant morbidity due to illness (15%), with injuries accounting for 0.5% of cases.

Deaths due to cardiovascular disease continue to be the number one killer in the United States and are reflected in the traveling population.

Higher death rates due to injuries particularly in less-developed countries suggest increased hazards on roadways and unfamiliarity with the environment as is the case of drowning. Use of motorcycles, mopeds and bicycles without protective gear poses grave dangers to travelers particularly to those inexperienced in their use [21].

The higher death rates due to injury in the study are particularly disturbing in that deaths due to injury in the United States are highest in lower socioeconomic groups [22]. American travelers are more affluent and less likely to die from injury in the United States.

Injury prevention strategies need to be emphasized. Examples of such advice appear in Table 5. Other strategies for injury prevention might include *requiring* rental agencies of cars and motorbikes to provide seat belts, car seats for infants, and helmets with requirement of their usage as part of the rental agreement.

Greater emphasis on prevention should be encouraged by travel agents and physicians through pre-travel evaluations particularly if over age 50 and if there are cardiovascular risk factors present. Appropriate immunizations and medication for travel with appropriate risk assessment for illnesses continue to be necessary as indicated by the three deaths from preventable infectious diseases.

Availability of physicians to travelers and emergency medical services in countries can affect the outcome once a traveler becomes ill or injured as suggested by the majority of deaths occurring outside hospitals. Providing names of physicians who assist travelers will be helpful to insure prompt diagnosis and treatment of illnesses and injuries.

## References

1. Lange RW (1987) Travel medicine resources for the primary care physician. Postgrad Med 81:293–300
2. Kendrick MA (1972) Study of illness among Americans returning from international travel. J Infect Dis 126:684–687
3. Cossar JH (1985) Illness associated with travel. Trav Med Int 3:13–18
4. Peltola H, Kyrönseppä H, Hölsä P (1983) Trips to the south – a health hazard. Scand J Infect Dis 15:375–381
5. Sharp JCM (1984) Infections acquired abroad. Practitioner 228:749–753
6. Steffen R, Rickenbach M, Wilhelm U, Helminger A, Schär M (1987) Health problems after travel to developing countries. J Infect Dis 156:84–91
7. Jong EC (1987) The travel and tropical medicine manual. WB Saunders, New York
8. Gangarosa EJ, Kendrick MA, Loewenstein MS, Merson MH, Mosley JW (1980) Travel and travelers health. Aviat Space Environ Med 51:265–270
9. Jong EC (1983) Recommendations for patients traveling. West J Med 138:746–751
10. Mann J (1983) Emporiatric policy and practice. JAMA 249:3323–3325
11. Peate WF, Push RE (1985) Health precautions for travelers in Mexico. South Med J 178:335–339
12. Sears SD, Sack RB (1987) Medical advice for international travelers
13. Weber SJ, Lefoch JL (1985) Health advice for international travelers. Am Fam Physician 32:165–169
14. Wolfe MS: Protection of travelers. Hunter's Tropical Medicine, 6th edn. Saunders, New York, pp 1698–1705
15. Hargarten SW, Baker SP (1985) Fatalities in peace corps. JAMA 254:1326–1329
16. Baker TD, Hargarten SW, Guptill KD (1989) The uncounted dead. Americans dying overseas. Submitted for publication
17. Personal communication brief of mortality statistics (1987) National Center for Mortality Statistics
18. World Tourism and Statistics (1985) Madrid. 37:1983
19. International Classification of Diseases (1980) US Department of Health
20. World Development Report of International Bank Reconstruction and Development (1985) Oxford University Press, Oxford
21. Baker SP, O'Neill R, Korpf RS (1984) Injury Fact Book. Lexington Books, Lexington, Mass0 22. New York Times, November 15, 1987
23. Cummins RO, Chapman PJC, Chamberlain DA, Schubach JA, Litwin PE (1988) In-flight deaths during commercial air travel. How big is the problem? JAMA 259:1983–1988

# Injury Deaths and American Travelers

S. W. Hargarten, T. Baker, and K. Guptill

## Summary

Injuries are the second most common cause of death of American travelers, accounting for 25% ($n=601$) of the deaths in the study years 1975 and 1984. Motor vehicle crashes were most common (27%) and were followed by drowning (16%) and homicides (9%). Less-developed countries accounted for 59% of unintentional travelers' injuries and deaths. Injury death rate for males was consistently higher in less-developed countries when compared with developed countries. Age and country distribution of motor vehicle crashes and drowning are presented. Preventive strategies are outlined.

## Results

There were 601 deaths of American travelers due to injuries, intentional and unintentional, in the study years 1975 and 1984. Motor vehicle crashes accounted for 27%, followed by drownings, 16%, and homicide, 9% (Fig. 1). Fifty-nine percent of the injury deaths occurred in less-developed countries.

Travelers who died of unintentional injuries expired outside the hospital setting 80.7% of the time. Motor vehicle crash deaths occurred 73% outside the hospital; 91% of the drownings were outside the hospital setting. Excluding Mexico, there were 351 deaths due to unintentional injury during our study years. Sixty percent were males; 35- to 44-year-old males were most frequently

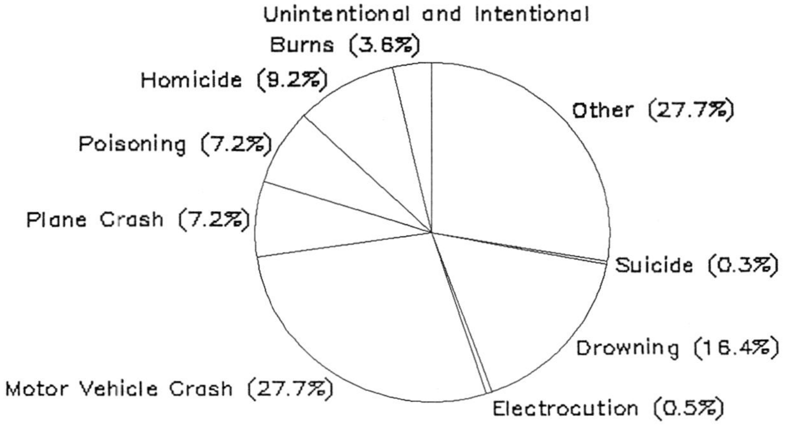


**Fig. 1.** Injury death of American travelers, unintentional and intentional

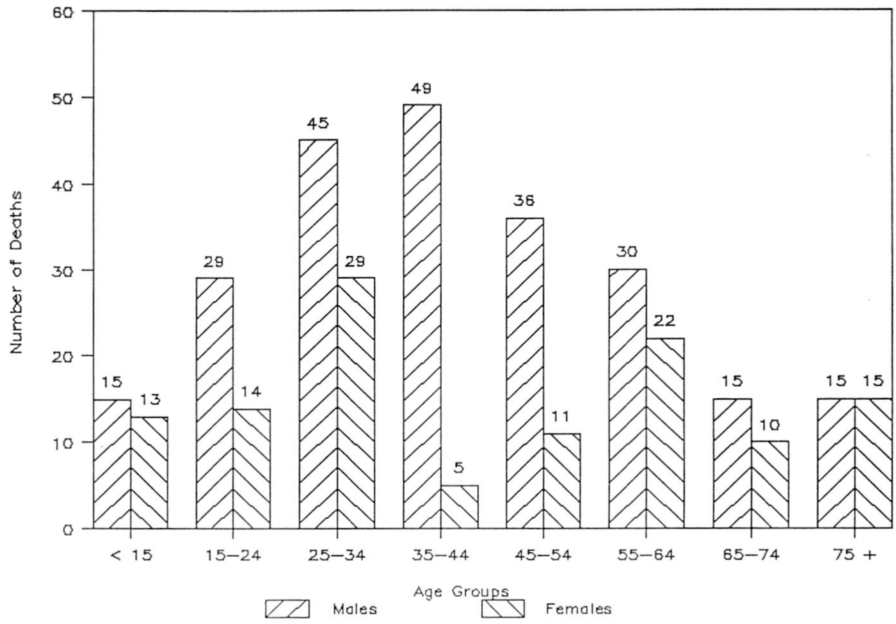


**Fig. 2.** Unintentional injury deaths by age and sex

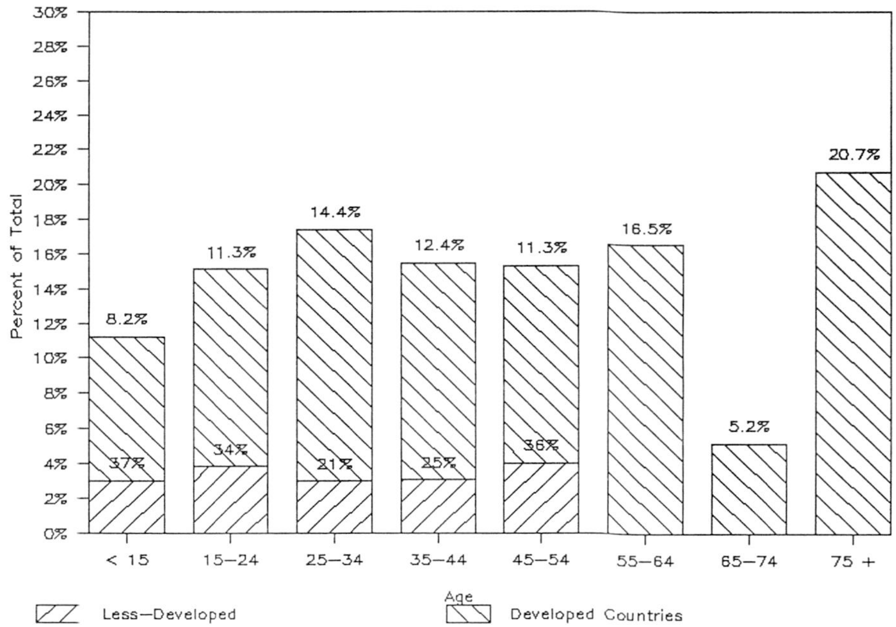


**Fig. 3.** Motor vehicle deaths by United States travelers by age and country ($n = 97$)

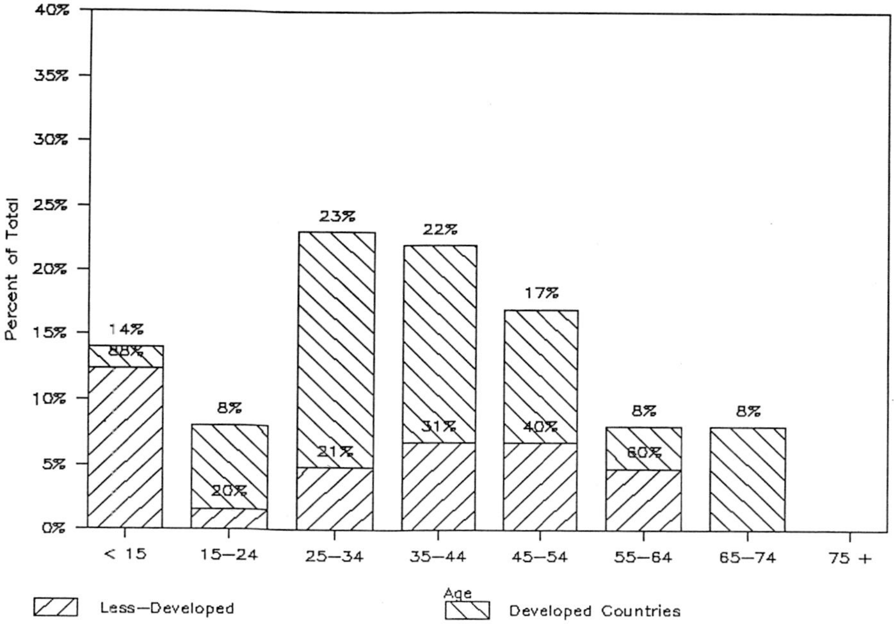


**Fig. 4.** Drowning deaths by United States travelers by age and country ($n=60$)

**Table 1.** Mexico injury deaths 1975, 1984

| Type of injury | No. of deaths | Percentage |
|---|---|---|
| Motor vehicle crash | 66 | 32.0 |
| Drowning | 36 | 17.6 |
| Homicides | 22 | 11.0 |
| Air crashes | 17 | 8.3 |
| Burns | 7 | 3.4 |
| Intoxication | 7 | 3.4 |
| Suicide | 4 | 1.8 |
| Electrocution | 3 | 1.5 |
| Others | 43 | 20.9 |
| Totals | 205 | 100.0 |

involved (Fig. 2). There were 30 homicides and 15 suicides during the study period. Males accounted for 83% of homicides and 73% of the suicides. In 1984, 7 of 15 homicides were in countries of Central and South America and the Caribbean.

Travelers to developed countries, ages 55 years and over, accounted for 42.4% of all motor vehicle crash deaths (Fig. 3). Travelers to less-developed countries who were under age 15 accounted for 88% of the drownings in that age group (Fig. 4). Mexico alone accounted for a total of 205 injury deaths.

**Table 2.** Injury control strategies for American tourists

1. Avoidance of motorcycles and small, less protective vehicles or at least use of helmets when using these vehicles
2. Use of seat belts, where available, including taxicabs
3. Use of larger in preference to smaller vehicles and not riding in the back of open trucks
4. Avoidance of small, nonscheduled aircraft
5. Careful selection of swimming areas, avoidance of alcohol while swimming
6. Avoidance of travel at night
7. Encouragement of travel in groups or pairs
8. Require rental agencies of cars, motorcycles and bicycles to provide seat belts for cars, car seats for infants and helmets for cyclists and motorcyclists
9. Require usage of protective equipment as a condition of rental

Motor vehicle crashes accounted for 32% of the deaths. This was followed by: drownings, 17.6%; and homicides, 11% (Table 1). Mexico accounted for 32% of all injury deaths to Americans traveling, 42% of the homicides and 38% of the drownings. We were not able to analyze age-specific death rates due to lack of denominator.

## Discussion

Injury prevention strategies should combine education to travelers about the risks of injury and travel, as well as efforts by emporiatric medical personnel to influence rental agencies of cars, motor bikes and bicycles to provide safety equipment such as seat belts, car seats for infants and helmets (Table 2).

Recent trends indicate greater use of car rentals by leisure travelers as airlines cooperate with rental agencies for transportation packages. Improved volume of travelers due to deregulation of airlines has resulted in more leisure travelers renting cars, and most discretionary renters keep their cars longer than business travelers. Deals made with airlines enable United States tourists to enjoy the use of rental cars for a week in Europe at low prices with unlimited mileage.

Regional variations in motor vehicle crash deaths are important when looking at trends and developing strategies as evidenced by European and Mexican travel of United States' citizens.

Homicides to United States' citizens traveling in the Americas may be an emerging problem. In 1984, there were 31 homicides to United States citizens, 74% occurring in the Americas and the Caribbean! In 1975, this region accounted for 43% of American traveler homicides.

# Mortality Amongst Overseas Travelers from Scotland

M. T. Paixao, J. H. Cossar and D. Reid

The rising numbers of travelers from the United Kingdom who report "illness" during their holidays or travel have been the focus of several surveys [1–3]. However, studies on death and the causes leading to it are few. This survey is an attempt to study the causes of mortality in overseas travellers, by looking at cause and place of death in persons whose death was registered in Scotland between July 1980 and December 1985.

## Survey Findings

Information was obtained on 395 persons (282 males and 113 females) whose ages ranged from 7 weeks to 89 years. A "death abroad" refers to any person dying while away from the United Kingdom and whose body was brought back to Scotland for cremation. The recorded mortality for the combined sexes in age groups 50–59 and 60–69 years was 202 (51.4% of the total). Combining age groups 0–9 and 10–19 years accounts for only 12 (3.0%) of the reported deaths, and the highest age group, over 80 years, had 11 (2.8%).

## Cause of Death

Cardiovascular disease or disease associated with the circulatory system was the commonest cause of death reported in both sexes. In males this was most notable in the 50–59 year age group (26.6%) followed by the 60–69 and 70–79 years age group (25.2%; 12.4%); amongst females, the peak from cardiovascular disease occurred in the 60–69 year age group.

Accidents, injuries, or their late effects, caused 21.3% of all deaths in males; motor vehicle, traffic accidents and unspecified "falls" were the leading causes in younger age groups and occurred particularly amongst those aged 20–29 years (10.3%).

## Countries Visited

Sixty-nine different countries were identified and grouped into major geographic areas. Most deaths (65.1%) occurred in Europe, 18.2% occurred in Spain and 13% in Majorca. The proportions attributable to other countries include France 7.2%, Federal Republic of Germany 5.2%, and the Canary Islands 4.1%. The most frequent country in the eastern European region where mortality occurred was Greece and its islands 7.8%, and in the Middle East region Saudi Arabia was the country with the highest number of cases 2.6%, followed by Abu Dhabi 1.3%.

The large "North America" region accounted for 5.8%; other deaths include 4 "at sea", 14 in Africa (3.5%), and 11 (2.8%) in the Channel Islands and the Isle of Man.

## Summary

The distribution of cases by region mostly relates to countries in southern Europe, predominantly Spain, its islands and other Mediterranean countries. The geographic and age distribution of deaths reflects various age-related health problems as well as those countries visited most often [4], which is likely to account for the large number of deaths reported from Spain. However, the significant association found between the grouped causes of death, namely cardiovascular diseases and accidents with age, suggests that there is scope for some preventative measures, and perhaps also a need for more guidance to those at special risk, e.g. elderly persons with cardiovascular disease.

*Acknowledgements.* We would like to thank the Scottish Home and Health Department, the Department of Community Medicine, University of Glasgow, and the Communicable Diseases (Scotland) Unit secretarial staff for their cooperation and assistance during this project.

## References

1. Reid D, Dewar RD, Fallon RJ, Cossar JH, Grist NR (1980) Infection and travel: the experience of package tourist and other travellers. J Infect 2:365–370
2. Grist NR, Cossar JH, Reid D, Dewar RD, Fallon RJ, Riding MH, Bell EJ (1985) Illness associated with a package holiday in Romania. Scott Med J 30:156–160
3. McEwan A, Jackson MH (1987) Illness among Scots holidaymakers who had travelled abroad, summer 1983. CDS Weekly Rep 87/16:7–9
4. Central Statistical Office (1986) Social trends. 16. Government Statistical Services, HMSO, London

# Health Risks of International Travel Among United States College Students

R. P. Smith, D. Smith, K. Bern, N. Mercer, and B. Conant-Sloane

International travel is a rite of passage for many United States college students, but the health risks of travelers from this population have not been studied. Surveys of short-term travelers to developing countries document high rates of minor illness [1–6]. College students, whose journeys are often spontaneous and adventurous, represent a potentially high risk group for travel-associated illness. This retrospective questionnaire study describes health risk behaviors and the frequency of illness and injury among United States college students traveling abroad.

## Methods

Four hundred and fifty-three students presenting to the student health service for pre-trip immunizations at the University of Pennsylvania and Dartmouth College in 1986–1987 were enrolled in the study. Dartmouth College students had attended a mandatory lecture on health advice for travelers; the University of Pennsylvania students received nonstandardized individual health advice. A 50-item questionnaire encompassing health risk behaviors and travel-associated illness and injury was mailed to participating students at the end of their trip. Nonresponders from the University of Pennsylvania group were sent a second mailing of the standard questionnaire.

Responses were compared between students traveling to western European countries (E) and to developing countries or the tropics (T).

Data were entered into the computer and analyzed using the SPSSX package.

## Results

Seventy-three percent of the western European travelers and 57% of tropical travelers had returned completed questionnaires after the first and second mailings. Mean duration of travel reported was 81 days (range 60–120 days) for E, and 74 days (range 7–474 days) for T. One-half of the tropical travelers visited Asia, with equal numbers of the remainder going to Africa, Central and South America, and to Mexico and eastern Europe. Pre-trip immunization rates were reported for typhoid (72% T, 20% E), immune serum globulins (77% T, 16% E) and cholera (40% T, 14% E). Students ate raw meat (2% T, 16% E), raw fish or shellfish (22% T, 17% E), raw vegetables (69% T, 63% E),

**Table 1.** Frequency of reported illness

| | Tropics (%) | Western Europe (%) |
|---|---|---|
| Diarrhea (>3 loose BMs/day)[b] | 62 | 18 |
| Upper respiratory infection | 39 | 42 |
| Febrile illness >1 day | 20 | 13 |
| Skin rash[a] | 10 | 3 |
| Severe sunburn | 8 | 16 |
| Heat illness | 8 | 3 |
| Altitude illness[a] | 9 | 1 |
| Motion sickness[a] | 7 | 18 |
| Dental problem | 3 | 11 |

[a] $\chi^2$ analysis, $p<0.05$
[b] $\chi^2$ analysis, $p<0.0001$

**Table 2.** Frequency of reported injuries

| | Tropics (%) | Western Europe (%) |
|---|---|---|
| Laceration | 10 | 5 |
| Animal bite | 3 | 4 |
| Sprain | 3 | 1 |
| Miscellaneous | 8 | 5 |

No significant differences by $\chi^2$ analysis

and unpeeled fruits (54% T, 75% E). A majority of students (57% T, 68% E) ate food purchased from street vendors.

Of the tropical travelers, 19% drank only untreated water, and 37% made no attempt to avoid ice. Thirty-six percent of T swam in freshwater lakes or ponds.

Of travelers to malarious countries, 39% were heavily bitten by mosquitos, but 67% reported rarely or never using mosquito netting, and 39% rarely or never used insect repellants. Thirty-three percent noted missed doses of chloroquine while traveling.

Fourteen percent of T used OTC medications obtained overseas, and 18% tried herbal or traditional remedies to treat illness. Two percent received needle injections.

Other potential health risk behaviors included frequent alcohol intoxication (16% T, 13% E), recreational drug use (11% T, 23% E) and moped or motorcycle travel (22% T, 9% E). Five percent of T and 8% of E were involved in motor vehicle accidents but no serious injuries resulted. Sexual activity with a new partner during the trip was reported (29% T, 19% E), often without the regular use of condoms (44% T, 73% E).

Minor illnesses were frequently reported (Table 1) as were minor injuries (Table 2). Of tropical travelers with diarrhea, 52% had two or more separate episodes, and 15% had episodes lasting more than 1 week. Five percent had blood diarrhea. No correlation could be demonstrated between risky dietary histories and diarrhea.

Serious morbidity occurred in 1,9% of all student travelers, and included one case each of appendicitis, severe allergic reaction, high-altitude cerebral edema, and presumed malaria. One student, known to be HIV-positive, died of encephalitis while traveling in India.

## Discussion

College students frequently reported behaviors during their trips that were a risk to their health. The seriousness of the risk associated with these behaviors cannot be assessed in this study, but failure to use standard protection from biting insects, the frequent use of recreational drugs and alcohol, and the frequent use of mopeds or motorcycles for travel are of particular concern to us. Motor vehicle crashes are the commonest cause of death among Peace Corps volunteers, and one-third of these deaths occur while riding motorcycles [7]. Involvement in a motor vehicle accident was reported by 5% (T) and 8% (E) of students in our study, though no serious injuries resulted. We did not evaluate the possible role of drug or alcohol use in these accidents in this study.

Minor illnesses, in particular diarrhea and upper respiratory infection, were the commonest problems reported, which is consistent with other studies of short-term travelers [1–6]. The frequency of heat and altitude illness in this student group probably reflects their athletic travel style and adventurous itineraries. Reported rates of injuries were higher than in other groups of travelers [3, 6], but our mean duration of travel was longer than in those other studies, and incidence data were not evaluable for our group. Comparison of rates of illness and injury between travelers to developing countries and to western Europe were not significantly different except for diarrhea, altitude sickness, skin rashes, and motion sickness (Table 1).

Possible biases in this study include a nonresponse bias, particularly for the tropical travelers, and recall bias, which may account for the lack of correlation between dietary risks and diarrhea [8]. Our study group was too small accurately to assess the frequency of serious morbidity in United States college students traveling abroad, but the results support the need for more epidemiologic data on this group of high-risk travelers. With such data in hand, illness and injury prevention strategies can be more effectively designed and tested.

## References

1. Kendrick MA (1972) Study of illness among Americans returning from international travel. J Infect Dis 126:684–685
2. Gangarosa EJ, Kendrick MA, Lownestein MS et al. (1980) Global travel and the traveler's health. Aviat Space Environ Med 51:265–270
3. Steffen R, Van der Linde F, Meyer HE (1978) Erkrankungsrisiken bei 10500 Tropen- und 1300 Nordamerika-Touristen. Schweiz Med Wochenschr 108:1485–1495

4. Peltola H, Kyronseppa H, Holsa P (1983) Trips to the South – a health hazard. Scand J Infect Dis 15:375–381
5. Reid D, Dewar RD, Fallon RJ et al. (1980) Infection and travel: the experience of package tourists and other travellers. J Infect 2:365–370
6. Steffen R, Rickenbach M, Wilhelm J et al. (1987) Health problems after travel to developing countries. J Infect Dis 156:84–91
7. Hargarten S, Baker S (1985) Fatalities in the Peace Corps. JAMA 254:1326–1329
8. Kozicki M, Steffen R, Schar M (1985) "Boil it, cook it, peel it or forget it": does this rule prevent traveler's diarrhea? Int J Epidemiol 14:169–172

# Survey of International Travel Medicine Work at Beijing Capital Airport and Beijing City

Xu Hua

## Introduction

Beijing is the capital of the People's Republic of China (PRC). The airport, located 25 km northeast of Beijing, is the largest international airport in China, serving 110 scheduled flights per week. The Beijing Health and Quarantine Service is responsible for international travel medicine in Beijing, enforcing the International Health Regulations and the Frontier Health and Quarantine Law of the PRC, including vector and rodent surveillance and control at the airport and on aircraft. In addition, the Quarantine Service conducts disease surveillance, and provides health advice and immunizations for international travelers.

## Vector and Rodent Surveillance and Control on Aircraft

To prevent transportation of potentially harmful insects and rodents, such vectors need to be identified quickly. The temperature and humidity during the summer months are conducive for growth and multiplication of vectors and rodents. The vector and rodent surveillance and control is conducted by seven doctors and several sanitary inspectors at the airport. Each arriving plane is required to have a disinsecting certificate and all aircraft are inspected. During the past 10 years no vector or rodent has been found on planes of Swissair, Quantas, and Pan American. These flights have their Health Declarations available together with the empty dispensers of aerosol. Unfortunately, conditions on some aircraft are not always satisfactory. For instance, in 1977 a stewardess on a plane from Bombay had been bitten by a rat during the flight. The plane was deratted after arrival with poison bait. The cabins were examined after 6 h and 5% of the baits had been eaten by rats.

In recent years insect vectors found on arriving flights have included flies, mosquitoes, cockroaches, and rats (Table 1). In those cases fines are levied and the planes are disinsected or deratted. Rats are most commonly found in bar boxes, and in the luggage and carge space.

Departing planes are inspected. If any vectors are found, the disinsecting certificate is not issued until disinsection has been completed. Insecticides used were aerosols containing pyrethrum or phtalthrin.

**Table 1.** Vectors found on arriving planes at Beijing Capital Airport January 1982–June 1985

| From | Airline | Number of flights |
|---|---|---|
| I. Flies (*Musca domestica*) | | |
| Baghdad | IQ | 1 |
| Bangkok | TG | 1 |
| Bombay | ET | 1 |
| Bombay | Extra | 1 |
| Hongkong | CA | 3 |
| Karachi | CA | 3 |
| Karachi | PK | 1 |
| Karachi | AF | 1 |
| Moscow | SU | 1 |
| Pyongyang | JS | 1 |
| Pyongyang | Extra | 1 |
| Sharjah | CA | 5 |
| Teheran | IR | 3 |
| Tokyo | JL | 1 |
| II. Mosquitoes (*Culex*) | | |
| Baghdad | IQ | 1 |
| Bombay | ET | 2 |
| Bombay | ET | 2 |
| Hongkong | BA | 1 |
| Karachi | CA | 2 |
| Karachi | RQ | 1 |
| Karachi | AF | 1 |
| III. Rodents | | |
| Bangkok | CA | 1 |
| Hongkong | CA | 1 |
| Karachi | CA | 1 |
| Sharjah | CA | 1 |
| IV. Cockroach | | |
| Tokyo | JL | 1 |

## Vector and Rodent Surveillance and Control at the Airport

Surveys for the presence and density of insect vectors and rodents are conducted periodically at and around the airport. The environmental sanitation activities are coordinated by the Committee of Public Health Campaign which consists of all units at the airport. The leader of the airport is appointed as head of the committee. The Quarantine Station is in charge of the technical guidance. The committee conducts the routine sanitary inspection of the airport area and the health education activities. The environmental sanitation is improved by modifying public open-air lavatories, removing pigsties and eliminating breeding places, routine insecticidal spraying of the terminal building, and deratting and anti-cockroach measures three to four times per year.

These control efforts have been very successful: the rat density in the field was reduced from 10.04% to 0.51%; the indoor reduction was from 6.7% to 0.05%. The international airport was the first airport in China to be declared to be without rat infestation.

## Sanitary Supervision of Food and Water

Bacteriological examinations are carried out regularly on random samples of potable water and food in restaurants, bars, and catering services for the airport and the planes. All phases of the food preparations are inspected. All deficiences need to be corrected within a specified time limit or service is suspended. All personnel engaged in food or water supplies receive a physical examination every year and a health certificate is issued. A health certificate is a condition for work.

## Disease Surveillance at the Airport and in Beijing

Disease surveillance is conducted by surveillance of arriving passengers and the establishment of an epidemic reporting system. This system consists of the quarantine service, large hospitals, hotels, international travel agency and units in charge of foreign affairs. Each suspected or diagnosed case of an infectious disease is reported to the quarantine service. An epidemiologic investigation is then conducted and preventive or control measures are instituted. Table 2 indicates the number of imported cases of infectious diseases in Beijing detected through the epidemic reporting system. In addition, the quarantine service provides the reporting system units with information on infectious diseases abroad.

**Table 2.** Imported cases of infectious diseases in beijing (January 1984 to June 1985)

| Diseases | Detected at airport | Detected after entering |
|---|---|---|
| Malaria | 4 | |
| Dysentery | | 8 |
| Hepatitis | 19 | 14 |
| Typhoid fever | 1 | |
| Tuberculosis | 5 | |
| AIDS | | 1 |
| Total | 29 | 23 |

## Health Advice and Immunizations

From the quarantine service international travelers can obtain information on the occurrence of infectious diseases abroad, the possible health risks in the areas of destination, and advice on preventive measures. Lectures are given by the staff on travel and health, and information is provided to the news media.

Since 1983, 300 000 leaflets and booklets pertaining to health and international travel have been published and distributed to international travellers. This includes information about prevention of AIDS.

About 30 000 travellers are immunized every year. The immunizations include those for yellow fever, cholera, tetanus, diphtheria, typhoid, poliomyelitis, Japanese encephalitis, gammaglobulin, and hepatitis B. Chemoprophylaxis against malaria and insect repellents are given annually to 15 000 travellers going to malarious areas. Physical examinations are provided for international business travellers and persons who are going to study or live abroad.

# Reported Illness and Compliance in United States Travelers Attending an Immunization Facility

E. Hilton, B. Edwards, and C. Singer

In a retrospective study conducted at Long Island Jewish Medical Center in New York City, 214 travelers were interviewed by telephone. Data collected included the following: age, duration of trip, month of departure, countries visited, purpose of trip, vaccinations prior to traveling, illnesses and symptoms during their trip, visits to foreign physicians or hospitals, need for antidiarrheal antibiotics, duration of diarrhea, number of mosquito bites suffered, use of insect repellent, and assessment of chloroquine compliance. In addition, women of menstrual age were questioned regarding menstrual irregularities during or after their trip.

Of the 214 travelers surveyed, 79 were males and 135 females. The median age was 49 years (range 4–78 years). The mean length of stay was 21.3 days (range 8–330 days). The areas visited included: East Africa 89, West Africa 15, China 10, other Southeast Asia 28, India and Nepal 31, South America 36, Egypt 3, and multiple destinations 2. The incidence of diarrhea was as follows: East Africa 44% (mean duration 3.1 days); West Africa 13% (mean duration 1.5 days); China no incidence of diarrhea; other Southeast Asia 42% (mean duration 3 days); India and Nepal 22% (mean duration of 2.8 days); South America 36% (mean duration of 6.6 days); and Egypt 33% (mean duration 2 days).

Other illnesses reported were: East Africa one rash, one upper respiratory tract infection, one upper GI infection; West Africa one upper respiratory tract infection; China four upper respiratory tract infections; and other Southeast Asia one rash. There was one episode of pharyngitis in a traveler to India and Nepal and one episode of altitude illness in a traveler to South America.

Most patients reported very few mosquito bites. The following reflect greater than five mosquito bites per traveler: East Africa none of 89; West Africa 1 of 15; Mainland China none of 10; other Southeast Asia 3 of 28; India and Nepal none of 31; and South America 3 of 36. Repellent was used infrequently; one patient travelling in West Africa and one patient to South America used Cutters.

Antimalarial compliance was assessed. In patients under the age of 40 there were 72 patients on chloroquine. The number completing the full recommended course was 43 or 59%. The number with premature cessation of chloroquine was 29 or 41%. Over the age of 40 there were 128 patients. The number completing a full course was 104 or 81% and the number with premature cessation was 24 or 19%. Of women of menstruating age, 35 women were on chloroquine and 4 women were not. Eight of the 35 on chloroquine (22.8%) had menstrual irregularities including delayed menses (one), premature menses (one), heavy menses (three), and skipped menses (three). In addition, two patients attending our travel clinic during the period of the last 2 years developed malaria. One had traveled to Egypt with a Nile cruise and was noncompliant with malaria prophylaxis. The other developed *Plasmodium falciparum* malaria while traveling in Ghana. He had been taking chloroquine prophylactically.

In summary, we conducted a retrospective study evaluating illness during and after travel, compliance with antimalarial medications, and possible chloroquine adverse reactions. Further study is needed to investigate the possible association of menstrual irregularities with chloroquine. We continue to stress the importance of compliance with antimalarial medication.

# Prevention and Control of Infections in Tourists in the Mediterranean Area

W. Pasini

The Società Italiana di Medicina del Turismo (SIMT), the World Health Organization (WHO), and the World Tourism Organization (WTO) jointly convened an interregional meeting in Rimini, Italy, from 8 to 11 February 1988, to discuss the prevention and control of infections in tourists in the Mediterranean area.

With the recent tremendous development of tourism and the new health risks involved, the promotion and protection of tourists' health deserves special attention.

Although the more serious infectious diseases (typhoid fever, malaria, schistosomiasis, louse-borne typhus, anthrax) have been eliminated or brought under control, a low endemicity of these diseases still exists in some parts of the Mediterranean area. Currently, the most frequent infections to which tourists are exposed include: diarrhoeas, other gastrointestinal infections, intoxications, acute respiratory infections, sexually transmitted diseases, zoonoses and some parasitic diseases.

The tourist should be made aware of the health risks specific to the area to be visited and of simple methods of avoiding them. Informational material should be based on the latest epidemiological situation which should be made known to physicians and others who give advice to tourists.

Unfortunately, there have been many instances of reluctance to disseminate surveillance information freely for fear of scaring away tourists when important hazards were identified.

The exchange of disease surveillance information between the Mediterranean countries and those from which the tourists come is often slow or absent.

There is a need to re-examine the problem of disease surveillance from the point of view of contemporary tourism and increasing international travel.

The meeting stressed that the protection and promotion of the health of tourists requires the combined efforts of several disciplines and professions such as medicine, environmental health and other health sciences, civil engineering, transport, hotel, catering and tourist industires as well as governmental and non-governmental agencies.

It was proposed that "tourist health" be recognized as a specialized branch of public health and that the three organizing agencies of this meeting (SIMT, WHO, WTO) should consider holding an expert consultation in order to define this discipline and to plan education and training in various participating fields/sectors and advise on organization of services and coordination of multisectorial contributions at different levels and on other related matters.

These agencies should also prepare guidelines, monographs, textbooks and self-care advice material including audiovisual devices. Where appropriate, existing guides and codes of practice should be updated.

The SIMT office in Rimini was designated as the focal point to implement the recommendations of the meeting and to facilitate cooperation between national bodies dealing with protection of health of the tourist and touristic medicine in the Mediterranean basin and possibly other areas.

## Reference

World Health Organization (1988) Report of the International Meeting on Prevention and Control of Infections in Tourists in the Mediterranean area. Rimini, Italy, 8–11 February 1988. Weekly Epidemiol Rec 63:10

# Malaria

# Malaria and Use of Prevention Measures Among United States Travelers

H. O. Lobel

## Summary

Each year between 7 and 8 million United States citizens travel to countries with malaria. The spread of drug-resistant *Plasmodium falciparum* malaria and the limited array of safe and effective drugs for prophylaxis have resulted in an increased risk of infection for United States travelers to many of these countries. This risk is high (1 per 50 to 1 per 1 000 000 travelers) for travelers to Africa and Oceania, and during the past decade it has increased more than fivefold for travelers to Kenya. The risk is intermediate (1 per 5 000 000 to 1 per 12 000 000) for travelers to Haiti and the Indian subcontinent, and low (less than 1 per 50 000 000) for travelers to Asia and Central and South America.

Risk factors for malaria include the itinerary, length of travel, and the use and efficacy of preventive measures. Traveler surveys indicate that chemoprophylaxis is used by more than 80% of United States travelers to Africa, but by only one-third of travelers to Haiti, and less than 10% of travelers to rural areas of Southeast Asia. Prophylaxis-specific attack rates in travelers in 1986 suggest that chloroquine prophylaxis was of limited efficacy in suppressing *P. falciparum* infections in travelers to East Africa, but was highly effective for travelers to Nigeria. Travelers to East and Central Africa are advised to carry a presumptive treatment dose of Fansidar, but only one-third of travelers comply with this recommendation. In recent years use of antimosquito measures has been emphasized; 55% of travelers to Africa use these. Malaria risk can be reduced by modifying the behavior of travelers. Detailed information is essential for targeting and evaluating prevention efforts.

## Introduction

Malaria is a serious, life-threatening infection of increasing importance. Malaria transmission is prevalent throughout the tropics, and an increase of imported malaria has occurred in most nonmalarious countries. Prophylaxis with chloroquine effectively suppressed malaria infections until the late 1950s, when chloroquine-resistant *Plasmodium falciparum* was identified in Colombia and Thailand. However, drug-resistant *P. falciparum* malaria was not a major problem for most United States travelers until 1978 when it emerged in East Africa and subsequently spread throughout most of Africa. Chloroquine-resistance is now present in all areas where *P. falciparum* occurs except Haiti, the Dominican Republic, Central America, and the Middle East. The other human malaria species have thus far remained sensitive to chloroquine [16].

Several alternative drugs, such as pyrimethamine combinations with sulfadoxine and other sulfonamides, amodiaquine, proguanil, and doxycycline, have since been employed for malaria prophylaxis. However, none are both totally effective and without adverse reactions [5].

The increase of *P. falciparum* infections in travelers, the spread of drug-resistant falciparum malaria, and the absence of safe and effective drugs for prophylaxis have required the development and continuous evaluation of malaria prevention strategies that balance the risk of malaria infection against the risks and benefits of prevention measures. To reduce the incidence of malaria and minimize the risk of adverse reactions, malaria prevention strategies must be targeted at travelers who are at risk of infection, especially with chloroquine-resistant *P. falciparum*.

The number of United States travelers visiting malarious countries, their risk of infection, and the risk factors for malaria must be determined. In addition, mechanisms are needed to assess the efficacy of malaria prevention measures and detect adverse reactions associated with drugs used for prophylaxis. To influence the behavior of travelers, we must assess what travelers know about malaria, their use of antimalaria measures, their sources of information, and how malaria prevention recommendations influence their behavior [17].

## Malaria in United States Travelers

In the last few years, 45% of all imported malaria infections in United States travelers were caused by *P. falciparum*. Seventy percent of all *P. falciparum* infections are acquired in Africa, although fewer than 10% of all United States travelers visit this continent. Imported *P. falciparum* infections acquired in Africa have increased 21-fold between 1975 and 1983 [7]. This rise may, in part, be due to an increase of travel, but the risk of infection has also increased as demonstrated by the increase of the attack rates of imported *P. falciparum* infections in United States travelers returning from travel to Kenya from 21 cases per 100000 travelers in 1977 to 120 cases in 1987.

*P. falciparum* infections in nonimmune persons are often fatal unless diagnosed and treated promptly. Of 1723 American travelers with imported *P. falciparum* infections reported in 1966 to 1987, 64 died (case-fatality rate of 4%). Because cases are underreported and deaths are not, 2% is a more realistic estimate of the case-fatality rate. The age of the patient was a risk factor: the age-specific case-fatality rate increased from 0% in persons under 20 years of age to 8% in those 50 years of age and older. Lack of prompt and adequate medical care contributed to many deaths. Only 54% of the patients who died sought medical attention within 6 days after onset of illness. An average of 3 days elapsed between obtaining medical care and the time of diagnosis. Physicians had included malaria in the differential diagnosis of only 37% of the patients. Not using any chemoprophylaxis also contributed to the deaths: only 9% of the patients who died had used chemoprophylaxis while abroad, as compared with 47% of patients who did not die. Whereas suboptimal chemoprophylaxis may not prevent parasitemia or illness, it may reduce the risk of dying from a *P. falciparum* infection [6].

## United States Travelers

To target intervention strategies at travelers at risk of infection, we must know the number of travelers to malarious countries, the length and reasons of travel, and the risk of acquiring malaria. It is estimated that approximately 7 million North Americans travel to countries with malaria each year, but a more realistic estimate is probably 1 million or less because itineraries often include several countries and not all areas within a country present a malaria risk. Certainly, only few of the 220 000 travelers to China, the 470 000 travelers to Southeast Asia, and the 400 000 travelers to South America are at risk since they visit predominantly urban areas or rural areas with a low level of transmission. Surveys indicate that travelers to East Africa and Haiti are predominantly tourists traveling for less than 3 weeks, whereas travelers to West Africa go predominantly for business or to visit friends and relatives.

## Risk of Malaria Infection

For travelers the risk of acquiring malaria depends on the intensity of malaria transmission in the country visited, the season, altitude, habits of the traveler, length of visit, and the use and efficacy of protective measures. We estimated this risk for United States travelers to various countries based on the country in which these travelers acquired malaria and the number of United States travelers to that country. Malaria risk for United States travelers after their return to the United States was highest for travelers to Africa and Papua New Guinea, ranging from 1 : 190 for travelers to Papuas New Guinea, to 1 : 210 for travelers to Nigeria, to 1 : 926 for travelers to Kenya. The risk of acquiring malaria was much less for United States travelers to India (1 : 1450), Pakistan (1 : 5263), and Haiti (1 : 4762). United States travelers to other countries of Asia had a negligible risk of developing malaria (less than 1 : 50 000). The risk of malaria after return to the United States underestimates the real risk, especially for those who travel for more than a few weeks.

An excellent source of information about the risk of developing malaria overseas is provided by the disease surveillance system of the US Peace Corps. In Peace Corps Volunteers (PCVs) in Africa in 1987 the attack rates of *P. falciparum*/100 PCVs/month were high, with an average monthly attack rate of 1%/month. In contrast, the risk of malaria was very low or absent in Latin America, the Near East, North Africa, Asia, and the Pacific Region. Only in Oceania was the risk comparable to that in Africa.

## Efficacy of Prophylaxis

The prophylactic efficacy of a drug is usually inferred from its therapeutic effect because controlled prophylactic drug trials are expensive, time-consuming and labor-intensive [5]. Prophylaxis trials are therefore done infrequently, and often include relatively small, semi-immune populations. However, malaria surveillance data, in conjunction with traveler statistics and surveys of travelers, can provide an estimate of the efficacy of drugs in different countries [9]. The attack rates of *P. falciparum* in United States travelers who used no prophylaxis were compared with those in travelers who used drugs to prevent malaria. In 1984, the number of cases per 100 000 travelers who did not take prophylaxis was 1619 in those who went to Nigeria and 282 in travelers to Kenya. The attack rate in travelers to Haiti who did not use chemoprophylaxis was 20 cases per 100 000 travelers. The attack rate in travelers to Thailand was negligible (less than 1/100 000), whether they used prophylaxis or not. Using chloroquine for prophylaxis reduced the attack rate tenfold for travelers to Nigeria, from 1619 to 168, and it eliminated the risk for travelers to Haiti, but in Kenya the incidence in chloroquine users was only half of that in travelers who did not use any chemoprophylaxis (158 and 282, respectively). Prophylaxis with Fansidar (Pyrimethamine/sulfadoxine; Roche) and chloroquine reduced the risk tenfold for travelers to Kenya.

## Adverse Reactions

When it became necessary to use alternative drugs to chloroquine to prevent *P. falciparum* infections, serious adverse reactions were noted. Two recent examples concern Fansidar and amodiaquine. Three years after Fansidar became available to United States travelers, several cases of serious cutaneous adverse reactions were reported. Subsequent investigations demonstrated that the risk of such reactions ranges from 1 in 5000 to 1 in 9000 users. The risk of a fatal reaction was between 1 in 11 000 and 1 in 25 000 users [10]. Similar rates have been observed in Scandinavia, the United Kingdom, and Australia. In Switzerland, however, this risk appeared to be much lower than in other countries [14]. These serious cutaneous adverse reactions were due to the long-acting sulfa component of Fansidar, sulfadoxine. When Fansidar could no longer be used for prophylaxis, several countries began to recommend amodiaquine because it seemed somewhat more effective than chloroquine in East Africa [13]. However, the occurrence of agranulocytosis and hepatic toxicity reported from Switzerland and the United Kingdom in association with amodiaquine [3, 11] demonstrated again that drugs given to hundreds of thousands of healthy travelers, who may be exposed to a readily treatable disease, need to be extremely safe.

Many travelers reported experiencing side effects to drugs. Surveys of United States travelers indicated that the frequency of sideeffects ranged from 10% to 20% but hospitalization was seldom required. These reactions not only detract from the pleasure of foreign travel, but, more importantly, they significantly reduce compliance with prophylaxis.

Adverse reactions are seldom identified during the premarketing drug trials because such trials do not involve large numbers of people. Postmarketing surveillance is therefore absolutely essential. Reporting of adverse drug reactions to the manufacturers and to regulating agencies is grossly deficient. Such reactions are often reported to those who develop the recommendations for chemoprophylaxis, such as national public health agencies, because they may, in part, be held responsible for the adverse reactions. Such organizations can and should play an important role in the surveillance of adverse reactions.

## Use of Prevention Measures

To guide the behavior of travelers effectively, we must determine their knowledge about malaria, their use of antimalaria measures, their sources of information, and how our actions influence their behavior. What do travelers know about malaria risk and what do they do about it? Surveys indicate that 89% of travelers to Africa were aware of the malaria risk and that 71%–84% used chemoprophylaxis regularly [8]. In contrast, only 55% of travelers to Haiti and 25% of travelers to Southeast Asia were aware of the malaria risk. Chemoprophylaxis was used regularly by only 17% of travelers to Haiti and by less than 10% of travelers to rural areas of Southeast Asia.

Because of the limited efficacy of chemoprophylaxis, antimosquito measures for reducing the risk of exposure are now emphasized [2], but 44% of United States travelers to Africa used no antimosquito measures (Table 1).

**Table 1.** Use of protective measures by 1796 persons. (CDC Traveller Surveys 1986) ($n=1796$)

| Measures to reduce exposure | [%] | |
|---|---|---|
| Applied insect repellent | 36.3 | 56,5 |
| Sprayed insecticide | 32.2 | |
| Used mosquito net | 25.1 | |
| Wore long clothes in evening | 25.4 | |
| Avoided evening walks | 12.5 | |
| Other | 2.4 | |

**Table 2.** Sources of malaria risk information; 97.4% of travelers had been informed of malaria risk ($n=1796$)

| Source of Information | [%] | |
|---|---|---|
| Family MD | 18.7 | 52.9% |
| MD at workplace | 12.3 | |
| Travel clinic | 10.5 | |
| Health Dept./CDC | 24.4 | |
| Travel Agent | 23.9 | 28.3% |
| Tourism Brochures | 12.2 | |
| Friend | 20.7 | 61.8% |
| Knew beforehand | 41.4 | |
| Other | 12.3 | |

## Sources of Information

Travelers use a wide range of medical and nonmedical sources of health information (Table 2). Almost half of the United States travelers to Africa sought no medical advice before their travel, thus limiting the contribution that the medical profession can make in protecting the health of travelers. However, even if more travelers sought medical attention, there is no guarantee that their information would be accurate. Investigations in Canada, Switzerland, and the United Kingdom indicate that physicians are remarkably ill informed about health risks abroad and the use of appropriate protection measures [4, 12, 15].

## Impact of Recommendations

In April 1985 the US Centers for Disease Control (CDC) recommended that Fansidar no longer be used for routine prophylaxis for all travelers to areas with chloroquine-resistant *P. falciparum* [1]. Such travelers were advised to use chloroquine and to carry a treatment dose of Fansidar to be used in the event of a febrile illness if medical care is not readily available. Also, because totally safe and effective drugs for chemoprophylaxis were no longer available, increasing emphasis was placed on use of antimosquito measures, although their efficacy has not adequately been determined. The effect of these changes in the recommendations on the behavior of United States travelers to East Africa is shown in Fig. 1 and 2. Use of chemoprophylaxis remained at a very high level from 1984 to 1987, whereas carrying of a drug for presumptive treatment and use of antimosquito measures increased from 1986 to 1987 (Fig. 1). Major

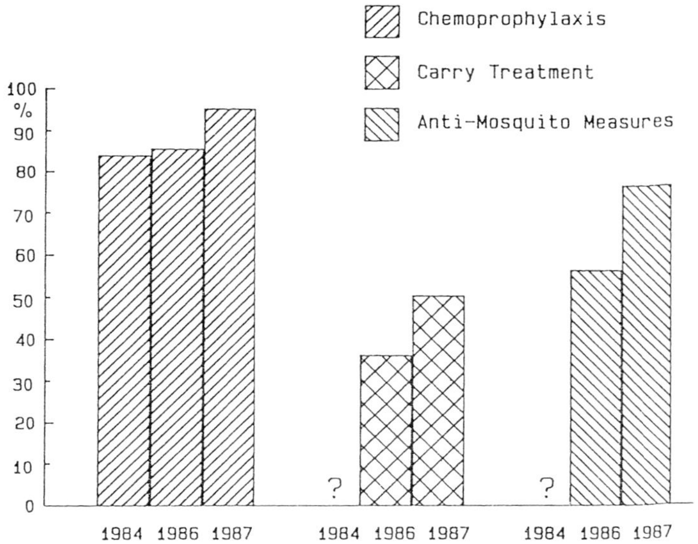


**Fig. 1.** Antimalaria measures used by United States travelers to East Africa 1984–1987

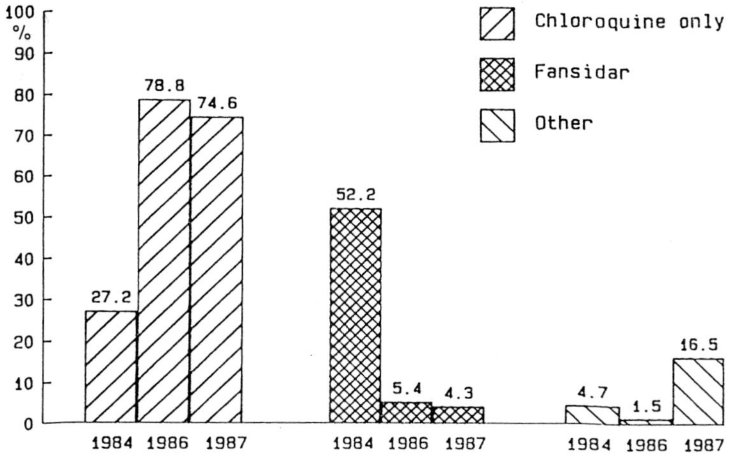


**Fig. 2.** Drugs used for prophylaxis by United States travelers to East Africa 1984–1987

changes were observed in the use of drugs for prophylaxis; use of chloroquine alone increased markedly from 1984 to 1986 and 1987, whereas use of Fansidar for prophylaxis declined dramatically from 1984 to 1986 and 1987 (Fig. 2).

## Conclusions

Two major issues are involved in limiting malaria risk in travelers: providing recommendations for prevention of malaria, and communicating accurate advice to the traveler. At present there is contained chaos around the world on how to prevent malaria in travelers. There are about as many recommended regimens as there are institutions making the recommendations. During a recent survey in Kenya of 8000 travelers from 72 countries, we found that more than 80 different drugs or drug combinations were used. The urgency is not so much to develop new prophylactic drugs, but to use a systematic approach to the formulation and evaluation of strategies for minimizing malaria risk in travelers. The risk of malaria must be balanced quantitatively against the risks and benefits of chemoprophylaxis to ensure that the risks of prevention do not outweigh the risks of infection. To achieve this, the industrialized countries must compare data on the risk of infection for travelers, the incidence rate of adverse reactions to drugs, and the efficacy of chemoprophylactic regimens. No such comparisons are now possible because few countries use comparable surveillance systems.

The other major issue concerns the health advice travelers receive. Many travelers depart without accurate health information despite considerable efforts by local and state health departments, the CDC, and many private physicians.

The four groups involved with health information are the medical profession, the travel industry, the press, and the travelers themselves. The medical profession must be accurately informed about risks of infection and the optimal protection measures for travelers at risk. The travel industry, including travel agents, tour companies, and airlines, has a special responsibility. The industry's interest in selling travel could profitably be combined with demonstrations of interest in their customers' safety by advising their clients to seek medical consultation for preventive health measures. Unfortunately, only few airlines and travel companies are now demonstrating this interest. Hotels and the tourist boards of countries with a high malaria risk should inform travelers of the need for protective measures. The press can, and often is, playing an important role providing health advice by noting the potential of malaria infection in tropical countries. A very large proportion of travelers get their information from the written press. Finally, the travelers themselves are responsible for following the advice and most appear to do so. Travelers who are aware of potential malaria risk are much more likely to use malaria prevention measures than those who are not aware of this risk.

## References


1. Centers for Disease Control (1985) Revised recommendations for preventing malaria in travelers to areas with chloroquine-resistant *Plasmodium falciparum*. MMWR 34:185–195
2. Centers for Disease Control (1987) Health information for international travel 1987. HHS Publication No (CDC) 85–8280
3. Hatton CSR, Bunch C, Peto TEA et al. (1986) Frequency of severe neutropenia associated with amodiaquine prophylaxis against malaria. Lancet I:411–414
4. Keystone JS, Lawee D, McIntyre L et al. (1984) Counseling travelers about malaria. Can Med Assoc J 131:715–716
5. Lobel HO, Campbell CC (1986) Malaria prophylaxis and distribution of drug resistance. In: Strickland GT (ed) Clinics in tropical medicine and communicable diseases, vol 1/1. Saunders, London, pp 225–242
6. Lobel HO, Campbell CC, Roberts JM (1985) Fatal malaria in U.S. civilians. Lancet I:873
7. Lobel HO, Campbell CC, Schwartz IK, Roberts JM (1985) Recent trends in the importation of malaria caused by *Plasmodium falciparum* into the United States from Africa. J Infect Dis 152:613–617
8. Lobel HO, Campbell CC, Pappaioanou M, Huong AY (1987) Use of prophylaxis for malaria by American travelers to Africa and Haiti. JAMA 257:2626–2627
9. Lobel HO, Roberts JM, Somaini B, Steffen R (1987) Efficacy of malaria prophylaxis in American and Swiss travelers to Kenya. J Infect Dis 155:1205–1209
10. Miller KD, Lobel HO, Satriale RF et al. (1986) Severe cutaneous reactions among American travelers using pyrimethamine-sulfadoxine (Fansidar) for malaria prophylaxis. Am J Trop Med Hyg 35:451–458
11. Neftel KA, Woodtly W, Schmid M et al. (1986) Amodiaquine induced agranulocytosis and liver damage. Br Med J 292:721–723
12. Raeber PA, Scheidegger C, Vodoz A et al. (1982) Enquete sur les recommendations prodguees aux voyageurs en zone tropicale. Med Soc Prev 27:266–267
13. Spencer H (1985) Drug-resistant malaria-changing patterns mean difficult decisions. Trans R Soc Trop Med Hyg 32:922–925
14. Steffen R, Somaini B (1986) Severe cutaneous reactions to sulfadoxine-pyrimethamine in Switzerland. Lancet I:610

15. Williams A, Lewis DJM (1987) Malaria prophylaxis: postal questionnaire survey of general practitioners in south east Wales. Br Med J 295:1449–1452
16. World Health Organization (1987) The epidemiology of drug resistance of malaria parasites: memorandum from a WHO Meeting. Bull WHO 65:797–816
17. World Health Organization (1988) Development of recommendations for the protection of short-stay travellers to malaria endemicareas: memorandum from two WHO meetings. Bull WHO 66:177–196

# Epidemiology of Malaria in European Travelers

P. A. Phillips-Howard and D. J. Bradley

## Malaria Risk in Travelers

Malaria imposes an increasing risk to travelers, due primarily to the expansion of travel to highly endemic areas. Concomitantly, the spread of resistance to safe chemoprophylaxis and the diminished use of more efficacious drug combinations, because of toxicity, necessitates comprehensive and systematic appraisal of malaria risk [1]. In order to develop optimal recommendations to protect European travelers, we need to classify who is at risk and why. A series of questions need to be addressed as a basis for action:

1. *Clarification of the problem:* What is the distribution of malaria in different groups of European travelers in terms of both incidence and incidence rates?
2. *Postulated reasons:* What risk factors are strongly associated with malaria in the different groups?
3. *Modifying influences:* How efficient are the protective measures in modifying risk and under what conditions?
4. *Motivating factors:* What methods enhance maximum uptake and compliance with potentially efficacious measures?
5. *Implementation:* How can results be applied to achieve maximum effect?

## Characteristics of Risk

Postulated characteristics of risk to be measured may be classified as risk markers, determinants and modifiers. Risk markers are characteristics that are associated with increased risk but do not, themselves, cause disease. These include age, sex, ethnicity, reason for travel, and occupational class. Markers classify groups for targetting specific recommendations. Determinants characterise travelers' potential exposure to infection. These are the country and place of visit, duration of visit and its temporal association with seasonal endemicity. Modifiers directly influence acquistion of infection and outcome. Principal modifiers are (1) malaria chemoprophylactic drugs, measured with respect to the type and dose, regimen and regularity of use, (2) behavioural and environmental components which inhibit or enhance exposure, including the use of antimosquito measures, (3) immune status which can be discounted as protective for the majority of European travelers, and (4) behaviour and health care intervention if symptoms are manifest.

## Survey Designs Used To Collect Data on Travelers

Many different study designs may be used to survey travelers. The main types of studies are (1) Ongoing surveillance either of malaria or of travelers. These can be conducted locally, nationally or internationally. (2) Cross sectional studies monitor travelers to describe their knowledge, attitudes and practices and can provide an estimate of malaria infection. (3) Longitudinal studies use cohorts or repeated cross sectional surveys to detect the impact of preventive advice, the changing pattern of health of travelers, their compliance and determinants that influence compliance. (4) Case control studies measure associations of risk but have limited use when investigating malaria in travelers. (5) Case base linkage studies combine together the denominators and numerators collated from other studies. Limitations of the survey designs and the restrictions imposed by finances and manpower resources, especially in European countries, reduce the methods for investigation of malaria in travelers principally to ongoing surveillance and cross sectional surveys. Measurement of rates is essential to interpret risk of infection in different groups; therefore incidence data need to be applied to denominators. Case base linkage provides the only feasible method of doing this on a large scale. Ongoing surveillance of imported malaria is, therefore, crucial for the determination of risk in travelers. The information collected on each case and the coverage of the surveillance system need to be of the highest calibre attainable to prevent spurious conclusions.

# Pattern of Imported Malaria in Europe

## Imported Malaria Statistics

Data used to illustrate the malaria situation in Europe originate from the information collected by 27 countries. These have been collated from two sources: (1) a survey of national surveillance systems during 1986–1987 and (2) data collected by the World Health Organisation (WHO).

1. The survey was conducted between 1986 and 1987, by primarily tracing the person responsible for malaria surveillance in each European country. This was achieved by contacting three informants; the Minister of Health, the Chief Epidemiologist of the Department of Health and the Chief of Infectious and Tropical Diseases. A follow-up questionnaire was then sent to the key person responsible requesting a summary of malaria surveillance data compiled for all of the preceding 5 years. A copy of current prevention advice and a description of statistics collected routinely by the national surveillance system was also requested. Twenty-four (88%) of the 27 countries provided information on malaria cases; 60% of them were unable to supply data for the five preceding years. Twenty-three (85%) countries completed the question sheets on prevention advice and routinely collected surveillance data.

2. Secondly a request was made to the Epidemiological Methodology and Evaluation Unit, Malaria Action Programme, WHO, in Geneva, for malaria

surveillance data routinely sent to WHO by the European countries. Two datasets were collated: incidence data over the last 10 years to illustrate the changing pattern of malaria and country-specific surveillance data for 1986, to supplement the survey. After collation, data were sent to each country for verification. Individual countries supplied data that were missing from tabulations, and requested changes to the existing datasets.

## Incidence of Malaria in Europe

Table 1 shows the 44945 cases of imported malaria that have been recorded throughout Europe over the preceding 10 years. Annual reports to WHO are not, however, complete. Of the 27 countries, 7 omitted reports to WHO for 1 year and a further 4 for 2 or more years. Intracountry annual variation also

**Table 1.** Malaria cases imported into Europe[a], 1977–1986. (WHO, Epidemiological Methodology and Evaluation, Malaria Action Programme data supplemented and modified during surveillance survey, 1987)

| | 1977 | 1978 | 1979 | 1980 | 1981 | 1982 | 1983 | 1984 | 1985 | 1986 | Total |
|---|---|---|---|---|---|---|---|---|---|---|---|
| Albania | 3 | 0 | | 0 | 0 | 1 | 0 | | | | 4 |
| Austria | 33 | 94 | 35 | 44 | 54 | 60 | 86 | 58 | 77 | 89 | 630 |
| Belgium | 40 | 35 | 56 | 59 | 30 | 24 | 108[b] | 146[b] | 44 | 154 | 696 |
| Bulgaria | 90 | 101 | 101 | 128 | 417 | 368 | 242 | 269 | | 95 | 1811 |
| Czechoslovakia | 4 | | 6 | 15 | 2 | 37 | 29 | 25 | 9 | 11 | 138 |
| Denmark | 49 | 54 | 110 | 70 | 104 | 102 | 87 | 122 | 128 | 178 | 1004 |
| Finland | 3 | 10 | 13 | 13 | 14 | 33 | 34 | 31 | 30 | 28 | 209 |
| France | 232 | 535 | 99 | 111 | 77 | 108 | 75 | 51 | 1640 | | 2928 |
| GDR | 17 | 18 | 24 | 16 | 36 | 82 | 44 | 61 | 61 | 38 | 397 |
| GFR | 337 | 534 | 486 | 570 | 390 | 514 | 447 | 481 | 530 | 1099 | 5388 |
| Greece | 39 | 64 | 35 | 41 | 52 | 65 | 39 | 51 | 34 | 39 | 459 |
| Hungary | 4 | 8 | 13 | 6 | 34 | 25 | 15 | 25 | 17 | 18 | 165 |
| Ireland | 32 | 26 | 32 | 22 | 25 | 21 | 17 | 12 | 22 | 21 | 230 |
| Italy | 205 | 243 | 162 | 176 | 143 | 155 | 155 | 181 | 178 | 191 | 1789 |
| Luxembourg | | 0 | | | 7 | 4 | 4 | 1 | 9 | 7 | 32 |
| Malta | 0 | 0 | 0 | 0 | 1 | | 7 | 4 | 4 | 4 | 20 |
| Netherlands | 107 | 109 | 113 | 101 | 128 | 119 | 143 | 123 | 137 | 167 | 1247 |
| Norway | 16 | 20 | 32 | 25 | 35 | 35 | 69 | 69 | 53 | 68 | 422 |
| Poland | 27 | 35 | 23 | 16 | 29 | 16 | 12 | 15 | 15 | 14 | 202 |
| Portugal | 133 | 52 | 45 | 25 | 27 | 18 | 36 | 49 | 62 | 95 | 542 |
| Romania | 17 | 17 | 13 | 12 | 18 | 20 | 15 | 14 | 10 | 8 | 144 |
| Spain | 57 | 32 | 52 | 90 | 68 | 81 | 101 | 124 | 112 | 179 | 896 |
| Sweden | 78 | 79 | 104 | 97 | 123 | 121 | 108 | 129 | 140 | 147 | 1126 |
| Switzerland | 48 | 112 | 93 | 95 | 138 | 130 | 162 | 153 | 200 | 196 | 1327 |
| UK | 1528 | 1909 | 2053 | 1668 | 1575 | 1470 | 1707 | 1927 | 2208 | 2306 | 18351 |
| USSR | 350 | 408 | 399 | 386 | 304 | 441 | 450 | 447 | 462 | 537 | 4184 |
| Yugoslavia | 60 | 50 | 53 | 82 | 56 | 51 | 69 | 51 | 57 | 75 | 604 |
| Total | 3509 | 4545 | 4152 | 3868 | 3887 | 4101 | 4261 | 4619 | 6239 | 5764 | 44945 |

0, cases reported as zero; blank space: cases not reported

[a] Excludes indigenous, induced, cryptic and congenital cases

[b] Cases from laboratory based reporting system

suggests flaws in case ascertainment in some countries, reducing confidence in reports and interpretation of malaria incidence in Europe [2]. Under the present pattern of reporting 41% of cases occurred in the United Kingdom, 12% in the Federal Republic of Germany and 7% in France.

## Pattern of Malaria Distribution

Case reports to WHO have increased by 61% over the past 10 years. The pattern of change is not uniform between countries. Five countries reported a reduction in cases, two reported an incidence similar to their 1977 figures, a small relative increase (under threefold) was reported in eight countries, and ten reported a substantial rise (over threefold).

## Malaria Incidence in Individual Countries

Incidence ranges a thousandfold between countries. These extremes are illustrated with the 1986 dataset, when 4 cases were reported by Malta, and 2306 cases by the United Kingdom (Table 2). An average annual figure of 100 cases or less are reported by 17 (63%) of countries, 100–200 cases in six (22%) countries, a range between 200 and 1000 in 3 (11%) countries and the United Kingdom alone regularly reports over 1000 cases.

## *Plasmodium falciparum* Infections

The proportion of *P. falciparum* cases to other species is 1:1 in Europe. The ratio differs considerably by country (Table 2). In 1986, *P. falciparum* was the predominant species in 11 (41%) countries. The proportion of *P. falciparum* cases equated with other species in 7 (26%) countries, and in the remaining countries, other species, principally *P. vivax*, predominated. Mortality associated with malaria is relatively uncommon in Europe. Two hundred and seventy-two deaths have been attributed to malaria in the last 10 years (Table 3) giving a non-specific case fatality rate (CFR) of 0.6%. Rates are not always proportional to the relative levels of *P. falciparum*. The *P. falciparum*-specific CFR in 1986 was 1.1%. A tenfold difference in CFR existed between the seven countries reporting deaths, ranging from 0.4% in the USSR to 3.9% in Spain. Nevertheless, there has been a dramatic decline of the *P. falciparum* CFR since 1970, when a rate of 8.1% was recorded [3].

## Regions of Acquisition of Malaria

Over half (55%) of all cases of imported malaria in Europe are in travelers who have visited Africa (Table 4). Of the 17 countries who provided data on country of infection, 8 reported infection from Africa in 75% of their cases, and a further seven countries indicated that over 50% of their cases are acquired in Africa. Only two countries reported Asia as the principal source of malaria. The main Africa countries visited by travelers who acquire malaria are Kenya, Nigeria, Zaire and Ghana. Malaria imported from Asia originates from India and Pakistan. Countries of acquisition vary with the European country of or-

**Table 2.** Species of malaria cases imported into Europe and mortality from imported malaria, 1986. (Data collected during surveillance survey, 1987, supplemented by WHO, Epidemiological Methodology and Evaluation, Malaria Action Programme

| Country | Total All spp. | *P.f* | % *P.f* (known sp.) | *P.v.* | *P.m.* | *P.o* | Mx | Uncl. | Deaths | CFR # %*P.f* | Ratio *P.f*: Other spp. |
|---|---|---|---|---|---|---|---|---|---|---|---|
| Austria | 89 | 44 | 52 | 35 | 1 | 2 | 2 | 5 | 0 | – | 1:1 |
| Belgium [a] | 303 | 218 | 75 | 40 | 6 | 24 | 3 | 12 | 1 | 0.5 | 3:1 |
| Bulgaria | 95 | 44 | 46 | 43 | 0 | 2 | 6 | 0 | 0 | – | 1:1 |
| Czechoslovakia | 11 | 2 | 20 | 6 | 1 | 1 | 0 | 1 | 0 | – | 1:4 |
| Denmark | 178 | 57 | 32 | 98 | 0 | 23 | 0 | 0 | 0 | – | 1:2 |
| Finland | 28 | 13 | 48 | 111 | 0 | 2 | 1 | 1 | 0 | – | 1:1 |
| GDR | 38 | 18 | 47 | 16 | 1 | 3 | 0 | 0 | 0 | – | 1:1 |
| GFR | 1099 | 578 | 57 | 345 | 21 | 40 | 25 | 90 | 15 | 2.6 | 3:2 |
| Greece | 39 | 22 | 58 | 16 | 0 | 0 | 0 | 1 | 0 | – | 3:2 |
| Hungary | 18 | 13 | 72 | 2 | 0 | 1 | 2 | 0 | 0 | – | 9:2 |
| Ireland | 21 | 9 | 56 | 3 | 0 | 4 | 0 | 5 | 0 | – | 1:1 |
| Italy | 191 | 135 | 71 | 48 | 6 | 2 | 0 | 0 | 1 | 0.7 | 5:2 |
| Luxembourg | 7 | 6 | 86 | 1 | 0 | 0 | 0 | 0 | 0 | – | 6:1 |
| Malta | 4 | 0 | – | 3 | 0 | 0 | 0 | 1 | 1 | ? | – |
| Netherlands | 167 | 71 | 43 | 81 | 1 | 13 | 1 | 0 | 0 | – | 2:3 |
| Norway | 68 | 14 | 22 | 44 | 0 | 2 | 3 | 5 | 0 | – | 1:3 |
| Poland | 14 | 3 | 38 | 3 | 0 | 1 | 1 | 6 | 0 | – | 1:1 |
| Portugal | 95 | 86 | 93 | 2 | 1 | 2 | 1 | 3 | 2 | 2.3 | 17:1 |
| Romania | 8 | 1 | 13 | 1 | 2 | 2 | 2 | 0 | 0 | – | 1:5 |
| Spain | 179 | 101 | 77 | 23 | 3 | 2 | 2 | 48 | 4 | 3.9 | 9:2 |
| Sweden | 147 | 66 | 45 | 58 | 3 | 16 | 4 | 0 | 0 | – | 1:1 |
| Switzerland | 196 | 115 | 64 | 49 | 1 | 11 | 3 | 17 | 0 | – | 2:1 |
| UK | 2306 | 717 | 32 | 1403 | 30 | 64 | 22 | 70 | 4 | 0.6 | 1:2 |
| USSR | 537 | 236 | 44 | 226 | 4 | 63 | 8 | 0 | 1 | 0.4 | 1:1 |
| Yugoslavia | 75 | 41 | 57 | 19 | 3 | 2 | 7 | 3 | 0 | – | 3:2 |
| Total | 5913 | 2610 | 46 | 2576 | 84 | 282 | 93 | 268 | 29 | 1.1 | 1:1 |

CFR #, case fatality rate in *P. falciparum* infections; *P.f., Plasmodium falciparum; P.v., P. vivax; P.m., P. malariae; P.o., P. ovale*

[a] Cases from laboratory-based reporting system

Table 3. Mortality associated with malaria in Europe, 1977–1986. (WHO, Epidemiological Methodology and Evaluation, Malaria Action Programme data supplimented and modified during surveillance survey, 1987)

| | 1977 | 1978 | 1979 | 1980 | 1981 | 1982 | 1983 | 1984 | 1985 | 1986 | Total | CFR # | Management indicator |
|---|---|---|---|---|---|---|---|---|---|---|---|---|---|
| Albania | 0 | | | | | 0 | 0 | | | | 0 | | |
| Austria | | 9 | | 1 | 1 | | | | 1 | | 12 | 1.9% | 3.6 |
| Belgium | | | 1 | | 1 | | 1 | 0 | | 1 | 4 | 0.6% | 0.8 |
| Bulgaria | 1 | | | | 1 | 1 | 1 | | | | 4 | 0.2% | 0.4 |
| Czechoslovakia | | | | | | 0 | 0 | 0 | 0 | 0 | 0 | | |
| Denmark | | | | | 1 | | 0 | | 1 | 0 | 2 | 0.2% | 0.6 |
| Finland | | | | | 1 | | 0 | 0 | 0 | 0 | 1 | 0.5% | 1.0 |
| France | | | | | | 0 | 1 | | 10 | | 11 | 0.4% | |
| GDR | 0 | 0 | 0 | 0 | 1 | 1 | 1 | 0 | 1 | 0 | 4 | 1.0% | 2.1 |
| GFR | 10 | 11 | 5 | 7 | 5 | 10 | 8 | 8 | 17 | 15 | 96 | 1.8% | 3.1 |
| Greece | | | | | 1 | | | | | | 1 | 0.2% | 0.3 |
| Hungary | | | | 1 | | | | 0 | | | 1 | 0.6% | 0.8 |
| Ireland | 0 | | | | | 0 | 0 | 0 | 0 | 0 | 0 | | |
| Italy | 2 | 3 | | 1 | 5 | 4 | 1 | 2 | 2 | 1 | 21 | 1.2% | 1.7 |
| Luxembourg | | | | | 1 | 0 | 0 | 0 | 0 | 0 | 1 | 3.1% | 3.6 |
| Malta | | | | | | | 0 | 0 | | + | + | 5.0% | |
| Netherlands | | 0 | 3 | 0 | 0 | 0 | 1 | 0 | 0 | ? | 4 | 0.3% | 0.7 |
| Norway | | | | | | | 0 | 0 | 0 | 0 | 0 | | |
| Poland | 0 | 0 | 0 | 0 | 0 | 0 | 0 | 1 | 0 | 0 | 1 | 0.5% | 1.3 |
| Portugal | | | | 1 | | | | | 1 | 2 | 4 | 0.7% | 0.8 |
| Romania | | | | 0 | 0 | 0 | 0 | 0 | 0 | 0 | 0 | | |
| Spain | 2 | 1 | | | | 3 | 3 | 3 | 2 | 4 | 18 | 2.0% | 2.6 |
| Sweden | 1 | | 1 | | | | | | | | 2 | 0.2% | 0.4 |
| Switzerland | 3 | 5 | 0 | 1 | 2 | 0 | 1 | 0 | 2 | 1 | 15 | 1.1% | 1.7 |
| UK | 7 | 10 | 6 | 9 | 2 | 12 | 6 | 6 | 5 | 4 | 67 | 0.4% | 1.3 |
| USSR | | 1 | | | | 0 | 0 | | 0 | 1 | 2 | 0.05% | 0.1 |
| Yugoslavia | | | | 1 | | | | 0 | 0 | | 1 | 0.2% | 0.4 |
| Total | 26 | 40 | 16 | 22 | 22 | 31 | 24 | 20 | 42 | 29 | 272 | 0.6% | 2.0 |

0, death as zero; blank space; no deaths reported; +, one death reported during survey; CFR #, case fatality rate in all species
Management indicator: CFR/% *Plasmodium falciparum* to correct for species

**Table 4.** Imported malaria by region of acquisition, 1986. (Data collected during surveillance survey, 1987)

| | Total | Africa (% known) | Asia | Other | Unknown |
|---|---|---|---|---|---|
| Austria | 89 | 59 (67) | 21 | 8 | 1 |
| Belgium | 303 | 241 (90) | 23 | 3 | 36 |
| Bulgaria | 95 | 72 (75) | 2 | 21 | 0 |
| Denmark | 178 | 89 (50) | 87 | 2 | 0 |
| Finland | 28 | 14 (56) | 7 | 4 | 3 |
| GDR | 38 | 34 (89) | 4 | 0 | 0 |
| GFR | 1099 | 701 (66) | 311 | 50 | 37 |
| Greece | 39 | 23 (59) | 16 | 0 | 0 |
| Ireland | 21 | 20 (95) | 1 | 0 | 0 |
| Luxembourg | 7 | 6 (86) | 1 | 0 | 0 |
| Malta | 4 | 2 | 0 | 0 | 2 |
| Netherlands | 167 | 94 (60) | 50 | 13 | 10 |
| Norway | 68 | 21 (32) | 43 | 1 | 3 |
| Portugal | 95 | 95 (100) | 0 | 0 | 0 |
| Spain | 179 | 156 (87) | 7 | 14 | 2 |
| Switzerland | 196 | 141 (72) | 42 | 13 | 0 |
| UK | 2306 | 813 (37) | 1308 | 99 | 86 |
| Yugoslavia | 75 | 69 (92) | 4 | 2 | 0 |
| Total | 4987 | 2650 (55) | 1927 | 230 | 180 |

igin. For example, a high proportion of travelers from the Federal German Republic, Austria and Switzerland acquire malaria from Kenya, the Belgians from Zaire, the Spanish from Equatorial Guinea, the Portuguese from Angola and the United Kingdom from India, Pakistan and Nigeria.

### Population Groups

The main reasons for travel are broadly described as tourist, business, immigrants, crew and other travelers. Proportionately the highest incidence occurs in tourists, 37%, and settled immigrant groups, 29% (Table 5). High incidence in specific categories varies by country; for example, sea- and aircrew import malaria into Greece, Poland, Spain and the USSR, tourists into the Federal German Republic, the Netherlands and Switzerland, overseas residents on home leave into Portugal and work-related visits into the GDR, the USSR and Italy. Settled immigrant populations constitute a substantial proportion of cases imported into Bulgaria, Denmark, France, Norway, Sweden and the United Kingdom.

## Limitations Imposed on Determining Risk

The data currently available to WHO provide a general picture of the epidemiology of malaria in European travelers. Absolute identification of which travelers are at highest risk and why calls for more definitive data. A survey

**Table 5.** Population groups importing malaria, 1986. (Data collected during surveillance survey, 1987, supplemented by WHO, Epidemiological Methodology and Evaluation, Malaria Action Programme)

| | Total | Imm | Work | Crew | Mil | Visit | Other | Unknown |
|---|---|---|---|---|---|---|---|---|
| Bulgaria | 95 | – | 19 | 8 | – | – | 68 | – |
| Czechoslovakia | 11 | – | 6 | – | – | – | 5 | – |
| Denmark | 178 | 94 | ← | | | 84[a] | | → |
| GDR | 38 | – | 35 | 1 | – | 2 | – | – |
| GFR | 1099 | 297 | 170 | 16 | – | 578 | 14 | 24 |
| Greece | 49 | – | 26 | 7 | – | 3 | 13 | – |
| Hungary | 18 | – | 1 | – | – | 4 | 13 | – |
| Ireland | 21 | – | 20 | – | – | – | 1 | – |
| Italy | 191 | – | 100 | 9 | – | 71 | 11 | – |
| Luxembourg | 7 | 1 | 3 | – | – | 3 | – | – |
| Malta | 4 | – | 1 | – | – | 1 | – | 2 |
| Netherlands | 167 | 3 | 58 | 13 | – | 74 | 18 | 1 |
| Norway | 68 | 68 | – | – | – | – | – | – |
| Poland | 14 | – | 3 | – | – | 2 | 9 | – |
| Portugal | 95 | 6 | 23 | 1 | – | 61 | 4 | – |
| Romania | 8 | – | 8 | – | – | – | – | – |
| Sweden | 147 | 66 | 18 | – | 2 | 46 | 15 | – |
| Switzerland | 194 | 17 | 29 | – | – | 105 | 7 | 36 |
| UK | 2306 | 962 | 172 | 1 | 9 | 741 | 14 | 407 |
| USSR | 537 | – | 120 | 44 | – | 52 | 321 | – |
| Yugoslavia | 75 | – | 40 | 4 | – | 3 | 28 | – |
| Total | 5322 | 1514 | 852 | 104 | 11 | 1830 | 541 | 470 |
| Total known | 4852 | 31% | 18% | 2% | | 38% | 11% | – |

Imm, immigrant; Mil, military; Visit, short visits
Each category includes both residents and visitors
[a] Pooled data

was conducted to establish whether other determinants were collected by ongoing surveillance systems for extending analysis.

## Data Collected by National Surveillance Systems

The survey revealed heterogeneity in types of data routinely collected (Fig. 1). For analysis, data were classified as; always collected (100% of countries), usually collected (at least 75% of countries), not always collected (above 50% of countries) and less frequently collected (less than 50% of countries).

*Always Collected.* Age.

*Usually Collected.* Sex, name, address, nationality, use of unnamed chemoprophylaxis (CP), country of infection, date of onset, species, place, date and method of diagnosis, recovery and record of deaths.

*Not Always Collected.* Reason for travel, occupation, resident status, days between onset and treatment, name of CP and regimen, date of return and verification of deaths.

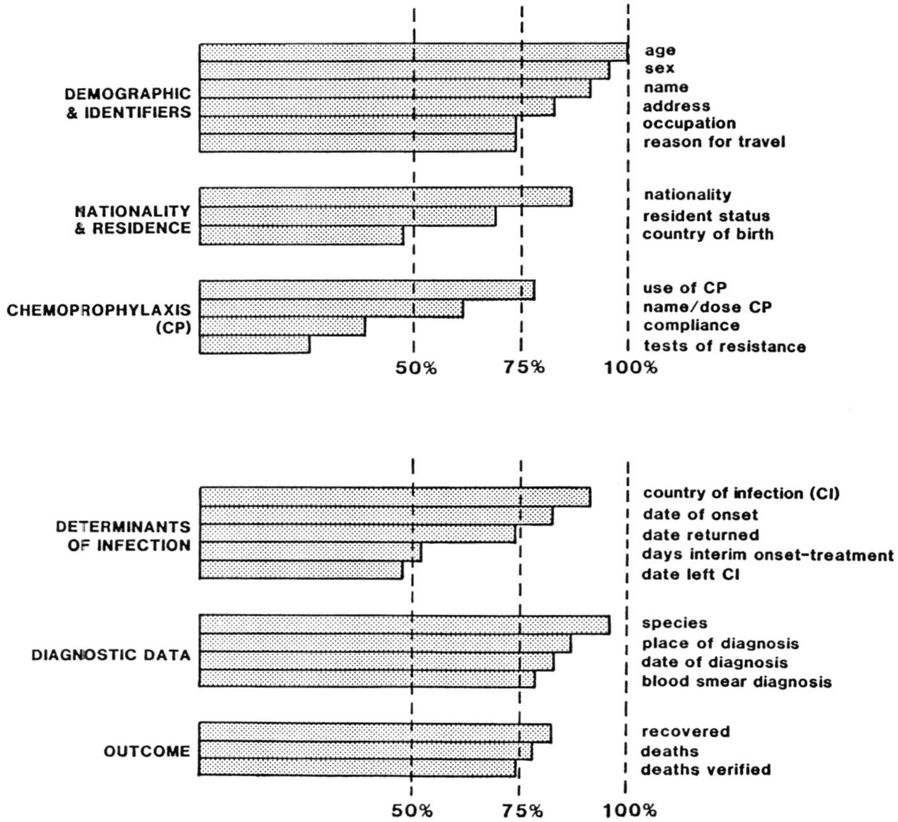


**Fig. 1.** Surveillance data routinely collected by countries in Europe 1986–1987

*Infrequently Collected.* Country of birth, date left malarious country, compliance with CP and biological assays of resistance.

If we assume that a variable collected by 75% or more of countries adequately represents a characteristic of risk, the present surveillance systems provide adequate data on most of the specified risk markers, but only adequately records the country of infection as a determinant. Few modifiers are described.

## Incompatibility of Definitions

Where date are common to ongoing surveillance systems, analysis remains limited because definitions and measures are incompatible. The categories that differ markedly are nationality, resident status, reasons for travel, the grouping of malarious regions and levels of compliance. Measurement scales are also diverse, particularly for age, period of residence, duration of travel overseas and epidemiological dates.

## Reporting Artefacts

Development of a standard European form would minimise this diversity. However, other limiting factors must also be addressed. Foremost of these are artefacts in surveillance of both numerators and denominators.

*1. Numerators.* To be effective, surveillance systems need to describe the characteristics of the groups they purport to monitor. High coverage is reported in Eastern Block countries, like Hungary, Yugoslavia and Bulgaria, where surveillance is mandatory [4]. However, surveillance systems in many European countries have not been investigated. Whilst incomplete case ascertainment is acceptable for measuring risk of malaria if cases reported are representative, studies in the United Kingdom suggest that case reporting is biased. Disparity exists in regional notifications and reports are biased towards *P. falciparum*, severe and hospitalised cases (Phillips-Howard, unpublished data). Not all countries have developed national reporting networks; some, like France, are in the process of development. Others, such as Belgium and the United Kingdom, have two or three independent surveillance systems, providing disparate datasets.

*2. Denominators.* The monitoring of travelers receives less attention than the surveillance of malaria cases. However, poor enumeration remains a major obstacle to risk analysis.

Where European government services collate travel statistics, calculations of attack rates by country and reason for visit are facilitated [5]. Data are available in the United Kingdom, and calculations of rates illustrate a 20-fold variation between travel categories. More generally European countries must rely on data from host countries, compiled by international agents like the World Tourism Organisation (WTO) [6] or embassies. Travel statistics are not comprehensive. About one-third of malarious countries submit data; datasets from Africa focus on tourists and exclude settled immigrants; European countries may be pooled into regions, for example Eastern Block or "Scandinavian" countries; definitions of national status are inconsistent; and, lastly, few definitive data are available on characteristics of risk.

## Attack Rates in European Travellers to Kenya

One country that can be studied is Kenya because travelers there are unusually homogeneous, visiting for holiday or business. Travel statistics collated by WTO from government statistics are therefore representative. Malaria attack rates were compared for European countries between 1984 and 1986 (Table 6). These resemble the rate of 160/100000 calculated for Swiss and American travelers [7]. Travellers from the Federal Republic of Germany appear to be at increased risk. Further interpretation of risk may be achieved through case base linkage using data generated from cross sectional studies.

**Table 6.** Malaria attack rates (per 100000) in Europeans visiting Kenya, 1984–1986. (Source: denominators: Kenyan Embassy; numerators: survey 1986–1987)

| | 1984 | | | 1985 | | | 1986 | | |
|---|---|---|---|---|---|---|---|---|---|
| | Travellers | Cases | Rate | Travellers | Cases | Rate | Travellers | Cases | Rate |
| GFR | 76400 | 99 | 130 | 100300 | 132 | 132 | 111700 | 340 | 304 |
| UK | 53800 | 100 | 186 | 65000 | 128 | 197 | 73100 | 84 | 115 |
| Switzerland | 32300 | 43 | 133 | 31700 | 39 | 123 | 49500 | 59 | 119 |
| Italy | 25700 | | | 34200 | 34 | 99 | 38100 | | |
| France | 19300 | | | 26600 | 14[b] | – | 27100 | | |
| Scandinavia | 12800 | 18 | 141 | 13400 | 10[a] | 75 | 15100 | 26[a] | 172 |
| Other Europe | 30300 | 34 | 112 | 35800 | 47 | 131 | 39800 | 65 | 163 |
| Total | 250600 | | | 318500 | 404 | 129 | 354500 | | |
| Without Italy and France | 205600 | 294 | 143 | 257700 | 356 | 138 | 289300 | 574 | 198 |

[a] Data from Sweden missing
[b] French data for 1985 for half year, French nationals only
NB: Countries grouped according to the denominators available

## Conclusions

Malaria will continue to threaten the health of international travelers. Data collected by national malaria surveillance systems in Europe are essential to determine which European travelers are at highest risk of infection. The quality and content of these data are, however, questionable. The coverage of reporting is unknown, not all countries report annually to WHO, records are incomplete and important variables are missed. Furthermore, data that are collected cannot be collated because definitions are often incompatbile. Finally, enumeration of travelers to malarious areas is inadequate.

The WHO are sponsoring a meeting of those responsible for surveillance in Europe in order to address these problems. Primarily, representatives will focus attention on a standard European report form to ensure that surveillance of malaria cases in Europe is comprehensive and data are compatible. The WHO annual report form requires modification to include the key variables collected by European countries.

Other issues which require collective attention concern reporting artefacts. The sensitivity of surveillance systems is generally unknown, but study methods and data generated from countries who have facilities to investigate reporting can provide useful guidelines for other countries. Where countries have duplicate reporting systems, reports need to be collated nationally before data are sent to WHO. The participation of countries that fail to report annually to WHO can be enhanced by active follow-up and also if the data are shown to be applied constructively.

Surveillance of travelers has received scant attention in the past, but is essential for analysis of rates. Systems that collate international travel statistics need to be developed. These rely on support from the governments of both host and resident countries. Airline data that enumerate returning Europeans could be made more accessible.

Surveys of travelers through cross sectional and cohort studies provide considerable help in understanding why some travelers are at great risk of malaria. Regular surveys are recommended at local and national level and, where possible, linked internationally with other European countries. Pooled understanding and commitment will best enable the countries of Europe to cope successfully with the problem of malaria in travelers.

*Acknowledgments.* We would like to thank the epidemiological, clinical and research staff of each European country for their large contribution towards the collection of data for this review. The project was financially supported by the World Health Organisation. Mr Hempel, of the Epidemiological Methodology and Evaluation Unit, Division of the Malaria Action Programme, WHO, is gratefully acknowledged for his competent assistance. Julia Mitchell skillfully typed the manuscript.

## References

1. WHO (1987) Bases for development of recommendations on protection for short term travelers against malaria. WHO/MAL/87.1040, Geneva
2. WHO (1987) Malaria risk for travelers. Report of a WHO working group. EUR/ICP/MAL 012, Geneva
3. WHO (1977) Imported malaria in Europe. Weekly Epid Rec 52:89–90
4. Varnai F, Banhegyi D (1986) Experiences with malaria chemoprophylaxis. Ann Trop Med Parasitol 80:279–283
5. Phillips-Howard PA, Breeze E, Lakin C, Bradley DJ (1988) Short term travel to malarious areas: risk to UK residents. Travel Med Int: 6, 2, 51–60
6. WTO (1986) Yearbook of tourism statistics, vol I and II, 39th issue. World Tourism Organisation, Madrid
7. Lobel HO, Roberts JM, Somaini B, Steffen R (1987) Efficacy of malaria prophylaxis in American and Swiss travelers to Kenya. J Infect Dis 155:1205–1209

# Advantages and Disadvantages of Antimalarials for Chemoprophylaxis

J. S. Keystone

## Introduction

With the increased spread of chloroquine-resistant *P. falciparum* malaria and mounting evidence for lack of efficacy and toxicity of alternate drugs, it has become extremely difficult to propose simple, widely applicable and uniformly acceptable recommendations for malaria chemoprophylaxis [1]. In addition, contradictory information in the lieterature has created considerable confusion as to the most efficacious prophylactic measures.

A recent unpublished WHO report listed five criteria required for the development of guidelines for malaria prevention [2]. These criteria included: (1) risk of infection, (2) risk of fatal outcome, (3) efficacy of prophylaxis (4) drug toxicity, and (5) efficacy of personal protection measures against mosquito bites. This review will concentrate on efficacy of prophylaxis and drug toxicity. However, there are a number of problems with our present knowledge base with respect to these two areas. Many studies on drug efficacy are out of date, based on therapeutic rather than prophylaxis trials, and deal with semi-immune populations and hence may not be applicable to non-immune travellers. Similarly, drug toxicity information has often been derived from therapeutic or short-term prophylaxis studies involving few subjects. There are very little data in the literature on long-term safety of chemoprophylaxis regimens.

## Chloroquine

Chloroquine, a 4-aminoquinoline, has been the mainstay of malaria chemotherapy until the late 1950s when clinical treatment failures were noted in Thailand and soon after in South America [3–4]. Its rapid action against the asexual blood-stages of all sensitive human malaria parasites made it a very appealing drug for chemoprophylaxis. Chloroquine has no effect on the exo-erythrocytic stages in the liver. Chloroquine alone has very little role to play in the prevention of *P. falciparum* malaria because of widespread chloroquine resistance. The only areas of the world which remain sensitive are Central America, Haiti, North Africa and the Middle East. However, a recent survey on cases imported into the Netherland suggested that chloroquine may reduce the severity of chloroquine resistant *P. falciparum* (CRPF) malaria although complete prevention does not occur [5]. Of the 10 patients who took no chemoprophylaxis, 50% were seriously ill compared with only 11% of the 41 patients who took chloroquine.

Chloroquine is well tolerated and safe for use by pregnant women and children when taken at the recommended dosage [6]. It does, however, have a narrow margin of safety and overdose is dangerous, particularly in children. Minor side effects such as gastrointestinal disturbance and difficulty with visual accomodation occur frequently. Pruritis in dark-skinned individuals is common. Rarely, photosensitization, aplastic anemia, agranulocytosis, myopathy, neuropsychiatric disturbances and irreversible retinopathy occur [7].

## Amodiaquine

Amodiaquine, another 4-aminoquinoline, has been used as an antimalarial and antirheumatic medication for more than 30 years. It came into greater use in Europe in 1985 following several studies which showed that amodiaquine had greater therapeutic efficacy than chloroquine in the treatment of CRPF malaria [8–10]. Up until 1985, there were only 13 published cases of agranulocytosis of which three were associated with amodiaquine use in the recommended dose for malaria chemoprophylaxis in the absence of other drugs which had the potential for marrow suppression. In 1986, a review by the Centres for Disease Control in Atlanta reported 7 fatalities out of 25 cases which developed in British, American and Swiss travellers [11–13]. Marrow suppression developed within 3–24 weeks of drug use. Rhodes et al. demonstrated that amodiaquine alone was able to produce colony growth inhibtion of bone marrow cultures. The estimated risk of agranulocytosis was 1:2000 users [14]. The lid on the amodiaquine coffin was nailed shut by a report of seven cases of hepatitis by Larrey et al. from France in 1986 [15].

## Proguanil

Proguanil, a dihydrofolate-reductase inhibitor developed in 1945, was favoured as a prophylactic agent by British physicians in spite of well-documented resistance by *P. vivax* and *P. falciparum* [16]. Proguanil is known to develop cross resistance with pyrimethamine. Increased interest in the use of proguanil developed because proguanil was found to retain its prophylactic effect against *P. falciparum* despite erythrocytic schizont resistance in the same strains [17]. Proguanil is known to act on the primary erythrocytic cycles of all species except for *P. malariae*. The drug is considered to be one of the safest antimalarials, although mouth ulcers have been reported recently.

Data on proguanil efficacy have been difficult to come by. McLarty et al. in Tanzania stimulated increased interest in proguanil for use in CRPF malaria when they described a 91% protective efficacy of 200 mg daily proguanil in a retrospective study of chemoprophylaxis use in expatriates [18]. Flaws in study design were highlighted by the fact that 100 mg proguanil daily produced 0% protective efficacy.

Watkins and his colleagues in Kenya recently completed a trial of chlorproguanil in 118 schoolchildren in Kenya [19]. the protective efficacy of an adult equivalent dose of 40 mg/week was only 36%. Further studies on chlorproguanil pharmacokinetics showed that the elimination profile for the active metabolite of chlorproguanil, chlorcycloguanil, indicated partition of drug into more than one compartment [20]. Abnormally low chlorcycloguanil plasma levels in several volunteers probably explains the low protective efficacy in this study.

Nevill and his colleagues from Nairobi carried out a prophylaxis study of proguanil in 190 schoolchildren in rural Kenya. The low protective efficacy of 77% might be explained by poor compliance by some subjects [21]. In the same study, mosquito nets were found to have a 97% protective efficacy. Fogh and his colleagues from Copenhagen carried out an uncontrolled study comparing chloroquine and proguanil with chloroquine and Fansidar in 767 expatriate travellers, the majority of whom stayed less than 4 weeks in Kenya and Tanzania [22]. One percent of each of the study groups developed documented *P. falciparum* malaria. The results of the above studies suggest that proguanil provides moderately good protective efficacy in East Africa but additional confirmatory data are needed.

Studies on proguanil efficacy in Southeast Asia are more definitive. Early studies in South Vietnam between 1967 and 1968 showed a relatively high degree of efficacy of proguanil used as prophylaxis by the Australian Army [23]. In the period 1969–1971 the addition of dapsone to a proguanil regimen resulted in a dramatic fall in malaria incidence. In a more recent study in Papua New Guinea, Henderson et al. documented failure of malaria chemoprophylaxis with a proguanil-chloroquine combination [24]. Fifteen out of 120 British Army soldiers on a 7-week jungle exercise in Papua New Guinea developed either falciparum malaria alone or a mixed infection with *P. vivax* after the chloroquine had been stopped. A more recent unpublished study in 186 semi-immune children living in a malaria endemic area along the Thai-Burmese border showed a significant failure rate with the equivalent of 200 mg proguanil used daily for prophylaxis [25]. Over a 3-month period, 18% of the proguanil group broke through with *P. falciparum* and 12% with *P. vivax* malaria. In contrast, 28% of the chloroquine prophylaxis group developed falciparum while 1% developed vivax malaria. Available data suggest therefore that proguanil alone is not likely to be efficacious in Southeast Asia and Oceania.

## Pyrimethamine

Pyrimethamine, another dihydrofolate-reductase inhibitor developed in the mid-1940s, is no longer indicated as sole prophylactic agent for malaria because of widespread resistance to *P. falciparum* and *P. vivax*. This resistance developed rapidly within the first 2 years of its introduction as a chemoprophylactic and therapeutic agent.

## Pyrimethamine/Sulfadoxine

Pyrimethamine/sulfadoxine (Fansidar) is a combination of dihydrofolate reductase and dihydroopterate inhibitors which act synergistically in the folic acid cycle. Fansidar chemoprophylaxis trials began in the 1960s and within 10 years resistance was documented along the Thai-Cambodian border [26]. Widespread resistance is now well established in Southeast Asia, Bangladesh, Oceania, the Amazon area of Brazil and parts of East Africa [27–31]. A study by Lobel et al. of travellers to Kenya in 1983 and 1984 showed that the combination of Chloroquine and Fansidar had a 90% prophylactic efficacy compared with 42% for chloroquine alone [32]. A follow-up study in East Africa by Steffen et al. in 1985–1986 showed that the prophylactic efficacy of chloroquine and Fansidar dropped slightly to 82% [33].

Post-marketing reports of severe cutaneous adverse reaction (SCAR) to Fansidar caused the CDC in Atlanta to revise its recommendations concerning weekly Fansidar use in travellers [34]. Between 1982 and 1985, 24 travellers developed toxic epidermal necrolysis, Stevens-Johnson syndrome or erythema multiforme within 2–7 weeks of starting the drug. The incidence of SCAR was 1 : 5000–8000 users and the mortality rate was 1 : 11 000–25 000 [35]. These data have since been confirmed in the United Kingdom, Australia and Sweden [36]. Although the data in Swiss travellers showed a much lower incidence, 1 : 150 000 users [37], Steffen and his colleagues have since revised these figures down to approximately 1 : 50 000 users. No deaths were reported in Swiss travellers who developed SCAR.

Sulfadoxine appears to be the drug component responsible for SCAR. When 2 g sulfadoxine was used alone for cholera prophylaxis in Mozambique in 1981, the incidence of SCAR was 1 : 7000 with a fatality rate of 1 : 50 000 users [38]. Similarly, when multiple doses of sulfadoxine were given for meningococcus prophylaxis in Morocco in 1968, the fatality rate was 1 : 7250 users [39].

On the basis of the above data, pyrimethamine/sulphadoxine should not be used as a first-line drug for malaria chemoprophylaxis but may have a role as a presumptive treatment agent.

## Pyrimethamine/Dapsone

The combination of pyrimethamine and dapsone (Maloprim) was introduced in 1968 for malaria chemoprophylaxis. The combination was notable for the discrepancy in half-lives of the two components. The half-life of pyrimethamine is 100 h compared with a 22-h half-life for dapsone. On theoretical grounds, by the end of 1 week, most of the dapsone would have been excreted, leaving pyrimethamine as the only antimalarial drug in the circulation.

Most of the efficacy data on maloprim were obtained by studies conducted in the early and mid 1970s [40–42]. A well-controlled trial of maloprim suppression in semi-immune Thais in 1973 showed a protective efficacy of 70% for *P. falciparum* and 83% for *P. vivax* when compared with the previous years' controls [43]. Cook recently reported ten cases of *P. vivax* in army personnel who had been taking regular prophylaxis with pyrimethamine and dapsone in Papua New Guinea [44]. He recommended that chloroquine be added to maloprim in areas where *P. vivax* and chloroquine-resistant *P. falciparum* malaria were prevalent.

Little toxicity was noted with maloprim use during the first 11 years of product marketing. Between 1979 and 1982 in Europe and particularly in the United Kingdom, maloprim was recommended as a twice weekly dosage because of the discrepancy in half-lives of its component drugs. Between 1979 and 1982, 17 cases of agranulocytosis were reported with maloprim use and all but two of these were associated with the twice weekly dose. In a review of cases by Hutchinson et al. in 1986 it was noted that 12 of 18 cases occurred with the twice weekly dose and 50% of these patients died [45]. In contrast, only 6 of the 18 developed agranulocytosis when taking a weekly dose of maloprim and one of these patients died. The estimated incidence of agranulocytosis with maloprim is 1:2000–5000 users when the twice weekly dose is used. No data are available on the risk of agranulocytosis when the weekly dose is used. Hutchinson felt that agranulocytosis was an idiosyncratic reaction to dapsone which was exacerbated by pyrimethamine.

Long-term safety of maloprim was evaluated by Cook and Kish in a study of 373 Papua New Guinean soldiers who took maloprim weekly for 5 years [46]. Compared with controls the soldiers showed a significant decrease in hematological parameters none of which were clinically significant. On the other hand, when maloprim use was evaluated in 159 white persons who had taken the drug for 15–34 months (average, 18 months) there was a significant drop in hemoglobin, white count and polymorphonuclear leucocytes. Seven individuals developed anemia and two had leucopenia.

The above review points out the paucity of current information on maloprim efficacy in CRPF areas and the need for the drug to be used in combination with chloroquine. Also, hematological parameters should be monitored (perhaps every 6 months) during long-term use of the drug.

## Doxycycline

Coatney and Greenberg in 1952 first reported efficacy of chlortetracycline against malaria parasites [47]. The drug was not considered to be valuable because of its slow therapeutic effect. In the 1970s, the tetracyclines were reconsidered as antimalarial drugs because of the progressive worldwide spread of chloroquine resistance.

Tetracyclines were found to exhibit a strong causal prophylactic effect against the pre-erythrocytic stages of chloroquine-resistant *P. falciparum* in human volunteers inoculated by infected mosquitos (Table 1) [48, 49]. The data on tetracyclines as a casual prophylactic agent against *P. vivax* were much less clear [50, 51].

Pang and his colleagues reported recently that doxycycline showed an 87% protective efficacy as a suppressive agent of *P. falciparum* in semi-immune children in eastern Thailand [52]. When the same dose, equivalent to 100 mg in adults was given to another group of children, the protecture efficacy for *P. falciparum* and vivax was 88% and 95% respectively [53]. The protective efficacy for *P. vivax* was reduced to 76% while that for *P. falciparum* remained 88% when the dose of doxycycline was reduced to the adult equivalent of

**Table 1.** Effect of tetracycline against pre-erythrocytic stages of *P. falciparum* and *P. vivax*

| Parasites | Drugs | Drug schedule (day) | No. of persons | |
|---|---|---|---|---|
| | | | Treated | Protected |
| *P. falciparum* | Tetracycline | 0– 3 | 6 | 6 |
| | Minocycline | −1– 5 | 9 | 9 |
| | | 0– 4 | 3 | 3 |
| | | 0– 3 | 3 | 3 |
| *P. vivax* | Tetracycline | 0–31 | 2 | 1 |
| | Doxycycline | 0–13 | 2 | 1 |
| | Minocycline | −1– 4 | 2 | 0 |

Modified from references [48–51]

50 mg/day. The causal prophylactic effect of doxycycline on *P. falciparum* and its efficacy in suppressing *P. vivax* malaria suggest that doxycycline can be discontinued when travellers depart from malarious endemic areas. Although chloroquine need not be combined with doxycycline to prevent *P. vivax* malaria during exposure, it should be continued for 4 weeks after exposure since the causal effect of doxycycline on *P. vivax* has not been established. From a practical point of view, it is probably better to add chloroquine to doxycycline during exposure than to start it after exposure when the latter is discontinued.

The most common adverse reactions of doxycycline are gastrointestinal upset, occurring in 3%–7% of users, and phototoxicity, which requires excessive (several hours) sun exposure [54, 55]. Peptobismol and antacids decrease doxycycline bioavailability [56].

## Mefloquine

Mefloquine is a 4-quinolinemethanol compound which underwent clinical trials in 1972. The first suppressive prophylaxis field trial in the late 1970s by Pearlman et al. showed almost 100% efficacy in semi-immunes in Thailand [57]. The drug has a very long half-life (6–33 days) and is a rapidly acting schizonticide. It is highly efficacious against both *P. vivax* and *P. falciparum* malaria [58]. Recently, in vitro resistance has been reported in areas where the drug has not yet been used [59] and in vivo resistance has been documented in a few cases [60, 61]. The main problem with mefloquine is its lack of availability. A combination of mefloquine with Fansidar (Fansimef) has been shown to be highly efficacious as a prophylactic agent. However, this combination is not very practical considering the severe adverse reactions associated with Fansidar use.

The most common side effects associated with mefloquine are nausea, vomiting, diarrhea and dizziness [58]. In a recent unpublished study of Swiss travellers to East Africa, Steffen showed that 20% of mefloquine users developed mild side effects while 2% needed to consult a doctor [33]. These side effects in short-term travellers compared favourably with those associated with chloroquine and chloroquine/Fansidar use.

## Conclusions

As can be seen from the above review, there is no present-day antimalarial which is uniformly safe, effective and widely available (Table 2). In spite of the shortcomings of antimalarials used as prophylactic agents, supplying travellers with a course of curative therapy remains a controversial issue. Most travellers who develop malaria on return home are first seen by health care professionals who have little experience with this infection. My personal preference would be to encourage prophylaxis for areas where the risk of malaria is high. Standby treatment or none at all might be considered for travellers at low risk for malaria or as a backup medication where the prophylactic agent of choice has less well documented protective efficacy (Table 3).

In Table 4, I have outlined my preferred and alternative regimens according to geographic area. Although mefloquine is listed as the drug of choice in

**Table 2.** Summary of drug review

| Drug | Advantage | Disadvantages |
|---|---|---|
| Amodiaquine | More effective than chloroquine in Rx CRPF | Agranulocytosis hepatitis |
| Chloroquine | *P.v.*, *P.o.*, *P.m.* sensitivity; safety | *P.f.* resistance; GI, eye toxicity |
| Doxycycline | Efficacy CRPF ± *P.v.* | Photosensitivity contra-I children |
| Mefloquine | Efficacy CRPF + *P.v.* | Limited long-term safety data, limited availability |
| Proguanil | Safety; efficacy CRPF (Africa) | Limited efficacy data, ↓ efficacy in Southeast Asia and Oceania |
| Pyrimethamine | Safety | Widespread resistance |
| Pyr/dapsone | ? Efficacy CRPF | Limited efficacy data, agranulocytosis, ↓ efficacy *P.v.* |
| Pyr/sulfadoxine | Presumptive treatment | Widespread *P.f.* resistance, ↓ efficacy *P.v.*, SCAR |

**Table 3.** Drugs or bugs?

| | | | Drug resistance | |
|---|---|---|---|---|
| | | | Low | High |
| Risk of Malaria | Low | Long | Chloroquine + standby treatment | Standby treatment |
| | | Short | None | None |
| | High | | Prophylaxis | Prophylaxis |

**Table 4.** What makes sense?

| Regimen | Drug of choice | Alternative |
|---|---|---|
| 1. Chloroquine sensitive<br>Central America<br>Carribbean<br>Middle East, etc. | Chloroquine | Proguanil (200 mg) |
| 2. Chloroquine resistant | | |
| a) South America | Chloroquine + Fansidar treatment | Chloroquine + maloprim |
| Amazon (Brazil) | Mefloquine | Chloroquine + doxycycline |
| b) Asia | Chloroquine + fansidar treatment | Chloroquine + maloprim |
| c) Africa (sub Saharan) | Chloroquine + proguanil + fansidar treatment | Chloroquine + maloprim<br>Mefloquine |
| d) Southeast Asia and Oceania | Mefloquine | Chloroquine + doxycycline<br>Chloroquine + maloprim |

areas where chloroquine and Fansidar resistance coexist, its lack of availability makes doxycycline the practical alternative. When using this table, the reader should note that, with few exceptions, malaria risk is absent in urban areas of South America and Southeast Asia. Travellers to these regions require antimalarials only if they plan to stay overnight in rural areas.

Regardless of the method used to prevent malaria, travellers must be informed that no present-day drug guarantees protection against malaria. In addition to emphasizing the need for personal protection measures (insect repellents, knock-down insecticides, bed nets and long-sleeved clothing) travel counsellors must point out that fever in a returning traveller should be considered a medical emergency requiring attention from a health care professional as soon as possible. As pointed out by Snoopy while sitting on his dog house, the only way to avoid malaria is to stay away from airports ... and to stay home (provided that home is not in a malaria endemic area!)

## References


1. Spencer HC (1985) Drug resistant malaria – changing patterns means difficult decisions. Trans R Soc Trop Med Hyg 79:748–758
2. Anon (1987) Bases for development of recommendations on protection for short-term travellers against malaria. WHO/MAL/87.1040, WHO Geneva
3. Harinasuta T, Migasena S, Boonag D (1962) Chloroquine-resistance in *Plasmodium falciparum* in Thailand. First regional symposium on scientific knowledge of tropical parasites, Singapore, 5–9 November 1962. University of Singapore, pp 148–153
4. Young MD, More DV (1961) Chloroquine resistance in *Plasmodium falciparum*. Am J Trop Med Hyg 10:317–320
5. Weststeyn JCFM, DeGeus A (1985) Bull WHO 63:107–108
6. Wolfe M, Cordus JF (1985) Safety of chloroquine in chemosuppression of malaria in pregnancy. Br Med J 290:1466–1467
7. Wittes R (1987) Adverse reactions to chloroquine and amodiaquine as used for malaria prophylaxis: a review of the literature. Can Fam Physician 33:2644–2649

8. Watkins WM, Sixsmith DG, Spencer HC et al. (1984) Effectiveness of amodiaquine as treatment for chloroquine-resistant *Plasmodium falciparum* infections in Kenya. Lancet I:357–359
9. Deloron P, Le Bras J, Ramanamirija JA (1984) Amodiaquine and chloroquine efficacy against *Plasmodium falciparum* in Madagascar. Lancet I:1303–1304
10. Looareesuwan S, Phillips RE, White NJ et al. (1985) Intravenous amodiaquine and oral amodiaquine/erythromycin in the treatment of chloroquine resistant falciparum malaria. Lancet II:805–808
11. Anon (1986) Agranulocytosis associated with the use of amodiaquine for malaria prophylaxis. MMWR 35:165–166
12. Hatton CSR, Peto TEA, Bunch C et al. (1986) Frequency of severe neutropenia associated with amodiauquine prophylaxis against malaria. Lancet I:411–414
13. Neftel KA, Woodthy W, Schmid M et al. (1986) Amodiaquine induced agranulocytosis and liver damage. Br Med J 292:721–723
14. Rhodes EGH, Ball J, Franklin IM (1986) Amodiaquine induced agranulocytosis: inhibition of colony growth in bone marrow by antimalarial agents. Br Med J 292:717–718
15. Larrey D, Castot A, Pessayre D et al. (1986) Amodiaquine-induced hepatitis. Ann Intern Med 104:801–803
16. Avery-Jones S (1958) Mass treatment with pyrimethamine. A study of resistance and cross resulting from a field trial in the hyperendemic malarious area of Makueni, Kenya, September 1952–September 1953. Trans R Soc Trop Med Hyg 52:547–561
17. Davey DG, Robertson GI (1957) Experiments with antimalarial drugs in man IV. An experiment to investigate the prophylactic value of proguanil against a strain of *Plasmodium falciparum* known to be resistant to therapeutic treatment. Trans R Soc Trop Med Hyg 51:463–466
18. McLarty DG, Webber RH, Jaatinen M et al. (1984) Chemoprophylaxis of malaria in non-immune residents in Dar es Salaam, Tanzania. Lancet II:656–659
19. Watkins WM, Brandling-Bennett AD, Oloo AJ et al. (1987) Inadequancy of chlorproguanil 20 mg per week as chemoprophylaxis for falciparum malaria in Kenya. Lancet II:125–127
20. Watkins WM, Chulay JD, Sixsmith DG et al. (1987) A preliminary pharmacokinetic study of the antimalarial drugs, proguanil and chlorproguanil. J Pharm Pharmacol 39:261–265
21. Nevill CG, Watkins WM, Carter JY et al (1988) Comparison of mosquito nets, proguanil hydrochloride and placeboto prevent malaria. Br Med J 297:401–403
22. Fogh S, Schapira A, Bygbjerg IC et al. (1988) Malaria chemoprophylaxis in travellers to East Africa: a comparative prospective study of chloroquine plus proguanil and chloroquine plus sulphadoxine/pyrimethamine. Br Med J 296:820–822
23. Black RH (1973) Malaria in the Australian army in South Vietnam: successful use of proguanil-dapsone combination for chemoprophylaxis of chloroquine-resistant falciparum malaria. Med J Aust 1:1265–1270
24. Henderson A, Simon JW, Melia W (1986) Failure of malaria chemoprophylaxis with proguanil-chloroquine combination in Papua New Guinea. Trans R Soc Trop Med Hyg 80:838–840
25. Limsomwong N, Pang LW, Singharaj P (1988) Malaria prophylaxis with proguanil in children living in a malaria endemic area. (Unpublished study)
26. Hurwitz ES, Johnson D, Campbell CC (1981) Resistance of *Plasmodium falciparum* malaria to sulfadoxine/pyrimethamine (Fansidar) in a refugee camp in Thailand. Lancet I:168–170
27. Doberstyn EB (1984) Resistance of *Plasmodium falciparum*. Experientia 40:1211–1217
28. Timmermanns PM, Hess U, Jones ME (1982) Pyrimethamine-sulfadoxine resistant falciparum malaria in East Africa. Lancet I:1118

29. Weniger BC, Blumberg RS, Campbell CC et al. (1982) High level chloroquine resistance of *Plasmodium falciparum* acquired in Kenya. N Engl J Med 307:1560–1562
30. Pinichpongse S, Doberstyn EB, Cullen JR et al. (1982) An evaluation of five regimens for the outpatient therapy of falciparum malaria in Thailand 1980–1981. Bull WHO 60:907–912
31. Farraroni JJ, Alencar FH, Shrimpton R (1983) Multiple drug resistance from Brazil. Trans R Soc Trop Med Hyg 77:138–139
32. Lobel HO, Roberts JM, Somaini B, Steffen R (1987) Efficacy of malaria prophylaxis in American and Swiss travellers to Kenya. J Infect Dis 155:1205–1209
33. Steffen R, Heusser R, Hofmann AM et al. (1988) Use, safety and efficacy of malaria chemoprophylaxis in travellers to Africa. (Unpublished study)
34. Anon (1985) Revised recommendations for preventing malaria in travelers to area with chloroquine-resistant *Plasmodium falciparum*. MMWR 34:185–190
35. Miller K, Lobel HD, Satriale RF et al. (1986) Severe cutaneous reactions among American travelers using pyrimethamine-sulfadoxine (Fansidar) for malaria prophylaxis. Am J Trop Med 35:451–458
36. Hellgren U, Rombo L, Berg B (1987) Adverse reactions to sulphadoxine pyrimethamine in Swedish travellers: implications for prophylaxis. Br Med J 295:365–366
37. Steffen R, Somaini B (1986) Severe cutaneous adverse reactions to sulfadoxine-pyrimethamine in Switzerland. lancet I:610
38. Hernborg A (1985) Stevens-Johnson syndrome after mass prophylaxis with sulfadoxine for cholera in Mozambique. Lancet II:1072–1073
39. Bergoend H, Loffer A, Maleville J (1968) Reactions cutaneés sur venues au cours de la prophylaxie de masse de la meningite cerebro-spinale par un sulfamide long-retard. Ann Dermatol 95:481–490
40. Harwin RM (1972) A field trial of pyrimethamine combined with dapsone in the chemoprophylaxis of malaria. Cent Afr J Med 18:201–204
41. Lucas A, Hendrickse R, Okubadejo O et al. (1969) The suppression of malaria parasitemia by pyrimethamine in combination with dapsone or sulformethoxine. Trans R Soc Trop Med Hyg 63:216–229
42. O'Holohan D, Hugoe-Matthews J (1971) Malaria suppression and prophylaxis on a Malayan rubber estate. Southeast Asian J Trop Med Public Health 2:164–168
43. Segal HE, Pearlman EJ, Thiemanun W (1973) The suppression of *Plasmodium falciparum* and PLASMODIUM VIVAX parasitemias by a dapsone-pyrimethamine combination. J Trop Med Hyg 76:285–290
44. Cook IF (1985) Inadequate prophylaxis of malaria with dapsone-pyrimethamine. Med J Aust 142:340–342
45. Hutchinson DBA, Whiteman PD, Farquhar JA (1986) Agranulocytosis associated with maloprim: review of cases. Hum Toxicol 5:221–227
46. Cook IF, Kish MY (1985) Haematological safety of long-term malarial prophylaxis with dapsone-pyrimethamine. Med J Aust 143:129–141
47. Coatney GR, Greenberg J (1952) The use of antibiotics in the treatment of malaria. Ann NY Acad Sci 55:1075–1081
48. Williamson D, Rieckmann KH, Carson PE (1972) Effects of minocycline against chloroquine-resistant falciparum malaria. Am J Trop Med Hyg 21:857–862
49. Rieckmann KH, Willerson WD, Carson PE et al. (1972) Effects of tetracycline against drug-resistant *P. falciparum* malaria. Proc Helminthol Soc Wash 39:339–347
50. Cycle DF, Miller RM, DuPont HL (1971) Antimalarial effect of tetracycline in man. J Trop Med Hyg 74:238–242
51. Rieckmann KH (1984) Antibiotics. In: Peters W, Richards WHG (ed) Antimalarial drugs. Springer, Berlin Heidelberg New York, pp 443–470 (Handbook of experimental pharmacology, vol 68/II)
52. Pang LW, Limsomwong N, Boudreau EF Doxycycline prophylaxis for falciparum malaria. Lancet I:1161–1164

53. Pang LW, Limsomwong N, Sinharaj P Vivax and falciparum malaria prophylaxis with low dose doxycycline. (Unpublished study)
54. Akers WA, Mailbach HI (1976) Relative safety of long-term administration of tetracycline in acne vulgaris. Cutis 17:531
55. Frost P, Wienstein GD, Gomez EC (1972) Phototoxic potential of minocycline and doxycycline. Arch Dermatol 105:681–683
56. Anon (1981) The Medical Letter 23:26–27
57. Pearlman EJ, Doberstyn EB, Somphong S (1980) Chemosuppressive field trials in Thailand IV. The suppression of *Plasmodium falciparum* and *Plasmodium vivax* parasitemias by Mefloquine. Am J Trop Med Hyg 29:1121–1137
58. World Health Organization (1984) Advances in malaria chemotherapy. WHO Tech Rep Ser 711:101–125
59. Oduola AMJ, Milhous WK, Salako LA et al. (1987) Reduced in-vitro susceptibility to Mefloquine in West Africa isolates of *Plasmodium falciparum.* Lancet II:1304–1305
60. Boudreau EF (1982) Type II Melfoquine-resistance in Thailand. Lancet II:1335
61. Bygberg IC, Schapira A, Flachs H, Gomme G (1983) Mefloquine-resistance of falciparum malaria from Tanzania enhanced by treatment. Lancet I:774–775

# Measures Against Mosquito Bites

P. F. Beales and R. L. Kouznetsov

## Introduction

In the past before the advent of synthetic antimalarial drugs individual protective measures against mosquitos were important means of personal protection against malaria. But as such drugs became more widely available these measures tended to be neglected in favour of chemoprophylaxis, even though it is not fully protective against *Plasmodium vivax*. However, over the past decade the rapid spread of chloroquine-resistant *P. falciparum* and the mounting evidence of toxicity to some alternative drugs has compromised the primary role of chemoprophylaxis and again underlines the unremitting importance of personal protective measures against mosquito bites. Such measures are also essential for protection against mosquito-borne diseases other than malaria, which in some circumstances may be even more important, for instance, dengue hemorrhagic fever, Japanese encephalitis and other mosquito-borne infections.

Past experience indicates that with the exception of small well-organized groups personal protection measures are not always properly and fully utilized. This may be due to inadequate knowledge of the protective value of various measures, limited availability, unacceptability and the relatively high cost to the individual.

Today, persons travelling to malaria endemic countries need to be well informed about the risks and consequences of contracting this disease, the limitations of chemoprophylaxis, and the importance of personal protective measures that can and should be taken. This will depend upon a knowledge of the area being visited. The promotion of travelers' awareness of the risk of malaria and of using protective measures is the joint responsibility of the national health authorities and medical practitioners in both the travelers' home country and the host country, as well as the organizations, industries, airlines and tourist agencies responsible for their travel. Information needs to be provided on the choice of protective measures according to the local conditions, where supplies may be obtained, and on what to do if the person develops fever during his or her stay in, or return from, malarious areas.

## Avoidance of Risk

The risk of contracting malaria might well be avoided in some instances. Careful consideration should be given by individuals travelling from non-endemic areas to malarious areas as to the necessity for such travel versus the risk of contracting potentially fatal *P. falciparum* malaria. This will necessitate the availability of well-informed medical persons who can be consulted before travel. Such consultations should result in advice to the traveller regarding their individual state of health and particular conditions which could predispose to serious consequences of a malaria infection or reaction to chemoprophylaxis. Especially at risk are persons who are taking immunosuppressant drugs, who have had a splenectomy, who are suffering from immunodeficiency conditions, and who have a history of drug allergies. Those individuals in perfect health need also to reconsider the necessity of exposing themselves and their young children to the risks of mosquito bites and of contracting mosquito-borne diseases. This is especially important during pregnancy which is time-limited, in which case it might often be possible to postpone the visit particularly when proposing to visit areas of multidrug-resistant *P. falciparum*.

## Reduction of Risk

Malaria is often a focal and seasonal disease and therefore travelers need to be sufficiently well informed to be able to select the best time to travel and the most appropriate location for their stay to reduce the risk of contracting infection.

Travelers also need to be provided with basic facts about malaria in order to be able intelligently to select their living accomodation, assess its safety with regard to mosquito penetration and to introduce, whenever necessary, additional protective measures. Living in a tropical environment, even for a short time, may necessitate a change in life-style and endurance of some inconvenience if diseases are to be avoided.

### Selection of Accommodation

Travelers need to pay more attention to the selection of living accommodation in malarious areas with respect to its proximity to mosquito breeding sites and the extent to which accommodation can be and is protected against mosquito intrusion.

Tourist holiday packages that are trying to be increasingly more economical have the danger of accommodating clients in badly located and protected accommodation as far as malaria vectors are concerned. In addition adventurous travelers are becoming more interested in visiting places “off the beaten track”, which puts them in greater danger of contracting malaria. Groups engaging in camping and trekking holidays should be guided on where to site their camps.

When selecting accommodation, preference should be given, if possible, to accommodation located in the more well developed parts of the town or at least 1 km away from any obvious major sources of mosquito breeding. Comparatively well constructed and well maintained buildings and mosquito-proofed rooms with or without air-conditioning are preferable. However, in air-conditioned accommodation great care needs to be taken to keep the rooms free from mosquitos as there is a tendency for mosquitos to breed in or enter through the air-conditioning system and to be trapped inside so that very localized transmission is possible. Another source of entry for mosquitos is from unscreened bathrooms, air vents, and gaps under doors, as well as holes in badly maintained screens.

## Bednets

Mosquito bednets are a time-honoured, simple and effective means of preventing mosquito bites (Port and Boreham 1982) and reducing malaria morbidity (Bradley et al. 1986). The bednet has the advantage that it can be set up in a few minutes over any bed, a mat placed on the floor, a hammock and even outside, and can be an effective protection for travelers. To be effective a mosquito net should:

1. Be made of a thread (natural or synthetic) of adequate thickness, woven or knitted into a net with a mesh of 23–26 holes/cm$^2$ (150–235 holes/in$^2$) or more and there should be no tears (Bruce-Chwatt 1985)
2. Preferably be of a rectangular pattern, especially at the base although other patterns such as pyramidal and conical may be found, and provided they have a rectangular base are useful if only one or two fixation points are possible

Impregnation of bednets with fast-acting insecticides, for example, synthetic pyrethroids such as permethrin or deltamethrin could further increase their effectiveness (Hervy and Sales 1980; Curtis and Lines 1985; Lines et al. 1985) in two ways:

1. By diminishing the number of mosquitos that can bite parts of the human body that come into close contact with the mosquito net during sleep or that try to enter the bednet at night through existing tears
2. By killing mosquitos that have entered the sleeping room during the day time through unscreened openings

Recent studies have indicated that bednets impregnated with a 20% solution of permethrin at the rate of 0.08 g/m$^2$ have proved highly effective in reducing man-vector contact even in the most mosquito-infested areas (Darriet et al. 1984). However, 0.2 g/m$^2$ or even 0.5 g/m$^2$ have been proposed for longer-lasting effectiveness (Schreck and Self 1985). The use of bednets impregnated with insecticide eliminates the need for pre-dusk spraying with insecticidal aerosols and utilization of various other devices aimed at repelling and/or killing mosquitos which have managed to penetrate the room before the person retires to bed. However, at the present time, bednets impregnated with repellents or synthetic pyrethroids are not commercially available, although the treatment of bednets with synthetic pyrethroids is not difficult or expensive and its effects have been known to last from at least 6 months to a year. Suggestions were made that travelers may themselves spray the bednets with commercially available aerosols containing synthetic pyrethroids. However, in the absence of any studies on the effectiveness and the residual effect of such a method of treatment, the diversity of commercial preparations on the market and determination of the most efficient technique to use, further investigations on this topic are needed.

Some other aspects for research include:

1. Development of bednets from light, inexpensive fabrics impregnated with synthetic pyrethroids which could be easily disposed of by the short-term traveller at the end of the journey
2. Assessment of the effectiveness of using easily installed insecticide impregnated "curtains" at the doors and windows. This method has proved to be as effective as bednets in reducing man-vector contact under the rural conditions of tropical Africa (Majori et al. 1987), but needs to be evaluated under various conditions and in areas with different vectors

## Indoor Disinsection

This measure is required when living quarters are unscreened or their protection against mosquito penetration is not assured as a result of faulty design, bad maintenance of screening devices or negligence in their utilization.

When living quarters, and especially bedrooms, are well protected but the risk of entry by mosquitos prior to their utilization cannot be ruled out, disinsection could be achieved by space spraying with a knockdown insecticide before the dusk hours. Various commercial products are available such as aerosols containing synthetic pyrethroids or other fast-acting insecticides. If economy is essential and commercial preparations are not available or if for environmental reasons aerosols are to be avoided, then a simple inexpensive "flit gun" could be employed using a 0.25% solution of pyrethrum prepared by diluting a commercial standardized 25% pyrethrum concentrate in an appropriate amount of kerosene.

When there is a risk that mosquitos could enter the sleeping quarters during the evening and night hours interior residual fumigation can be employed using dichlorvos (DDVP) dispensers containing 200 g/kg (20%) active ingredients in various plastic resins. One dispenser will cover 2.8–8.5 $m^3$. This has a fumigant action and will kill mosquitos entering the room. It can be suspended from the ceiling and be effective for up to 6 weeks (WHO 1984).

More recently impregnated pads have become available which can be heated by a spirit lamp or electricity and which have a similar fumigant/repellent effect (Chadwick and Lord 1977). The mats are coloured and may be perfumed. As the insecticide is released mosquitos already in the room are killed and others are prevented from entering. When the mat is spent it changes colour, indicating that a replacement is necessary.

Felt tip pens are also available which contain a liquid insecticide with a fumigant action. This is useful for short-term travelers and can be used in temporary accommodation in out of the way places.

Pyrethrum mosquito coils and sticks are used throughout Asia and other parts of the world. They burn slowly over a period of 2 or more hours and have been shown to be effective in generally reducing the number of anopheline mosquitos coming to bite (Chadwick 1975; Charlwood and Jolley 1984; Birley et al. 1987). Innovative ways of using these can be devised to reduce the chances of being bitten by mosquitos whilst outdoors.

## Appropriate Clothing

The use of appropriate clothing during the biting period of the malaria vectors can provide some protection. By "appropriate" is meant those garments which would leave a minimum area of skin exposed to the bites of the mosquito, which are of an appropriate thickness and texture through which the mosquito is less likely to bite and which are of a colour that is less likely to attract the vectors of disease (generally lighter rather than the dark colours).

In one country protective clothing for the upper part of the body is available consisting of two components: (a) an undervest with long sleeves made from a wide-mesh material, which is as thick as the length of a mosquito proboscis and (b) a long-sleeved shirt made of a finer net which still allows a good aeration of the body. The principle is that blood-sucking insects will be unable to reach the skin or penetrate it sufficiently with their mouth parts.

Clothing can also be impregnated and in particular impregnated socks, stockings and anklet bands can be effective (WHO 1984; Lines et al. 1985; Curtis et al. 1986). However, travelers should keep impregnated mosquito nets and clothing in sealed plastic bags when not in use to preserve the insecticide. More research could usefully be done on developing a set of knitted bands such as those used by tennis players for the exposed and most vulnerable parts of the body – the head, wrists and ankles. These bands could be made in such a way that only the outside is impregnated with a pyrethroid insecticide or repellant while the inside in contact with the skin is not impregnated. If effective in reducing or eliminating *Anopheles* mosquito bites they could be made commercially available in attractive colours to be worn in the evenings. Other methods of repelling mosquitos have been proposed for individual personal protection. Two of these are the use of vitamin $B_1$ and the use of battery-operated electronic devices.

Vitamin $B_1$ taken orally has been said to render oneself repellent to mosquitos (Shannon 1943) based on studies carried out in adults and children. Shannon used a loading dose of thiamine chloride (120 mg in adults) followed by a small daily dose (10–20 mg in adults). He found it either gave complete protection or it reduced the mosquito biting rate (no mention of the species) and reduced the irritation reaction to bites. Since that study there have been several published reports, some of studies using various doses of thiamine chloride and some of opinions and observations on the effect of vitamin $B_1$ as a repellent for mosquitos (*Aedes, Culex* and *Anophelines*) and fleas (Wilson et al. 1944; Eder 1945; von Rahm 1958; Müting 1958; Kunze 1960; Ritschel and Ritschel-Beurlin 1963; Bruun 1964; Khan et al. 1969; Sauerbrey 1970; Maldonado and Tamay 1973; Maasch 1973). In reviewing this literature it is apparent that few if any of the studies reported are comparable. Some claim a significant effect, most cannot show any statistical significant differences when $B_1$ is used and not used, and only one paper categorically states that *Anopheles* mosquitos (*A. gambiae*) were tested. There are several confounding factors for such studies, among them the known individual variation in natural attraction to mosquitos, the effect of diet on attractability to mosquitos, the variation in absorption and metabolism of vitamin $B_1$ and skin surface excretion, individual variation in perspiration, the state of "starvation" of the mosquitos and so on. It is clear that a well-designed and carefully conducted study is required to decide whether or not the oral intake of vitamin $B_1$ can be considered a reliable personal protection measure against the bite of the vectors of malaria (*Anopheles* spp.). It would seem therefore that with the scientific information available today vitamin $B_1$ taken orally cannot be relied upon to protect against the bite of the malaria-carrying species of mosquitos.

A more definite situation prevails with respect to electronic devices that have been, and still are, marketed in some countries as mosquito repellents. These devices emit sound waves of ultrasonic frequencies varying from low to high peak (Belton 1981; Schreck et al. 1984 b) and in one study sound pressure levels were from 65 to 96 db at 0.5 m (Schreck et al. 1984 b), which did not meet the US Occupational Safety and Health Act guidelines for human tolerance of sound radiation. Various manufacturers suggest that the sound waves generated ward off most female mosquitos for distances of 1–2.5 m, based upon the claim that certain sound waves attract male mosquitos but the fertilized female mosquito seeking a blood meal is repelled (Kunze 1974; Singleton 1977). There have been several carefully controlled studies on the effects of different makes of these devices, some conducted under laboratory conditions others in the field, directed against a variety of mosquitos (and cockroaches) including *Anopheles* species (Rasnitsyn et al. 1974; Kunze 1974; Schreck et al. 1977; Singleton 1977; Snow 1977; Schreck et al. 1984 b; Foster and Lutes 1985).

None of these studies or those reviewed by Foster and Lutes (1985) demonstrated any significant mosquito repellency effect of any of the devices that were tested. Two brands of buzzer sold as mosquito repellents have been taken off the market in the United Kingdom after prosecutions under the Trades Description Act (Curtis 1986).

## Mosquito Repellents

Since the 1930s the classical anti-mosquito repellent for application to the skin, oil of citronella, has been replaced in some areas by synthetic repellents, such as benzyl-benzoate, butyl ethyl propanediol, *NB*-diethyl-3-tolnamide (deet), dibutyl phthalate, dimethyl carbate, dimethyl phthalate, ethyl hexanediol, beetopy zonoxyl and 2-chlorodiethylbenzamide (WHO 1984). In recent years a number of alicyclic carbomoximides of heterocyclic amines which are very effective as clothing and skin repellents have been developed. Permethrin applied to clothing is also effective (Schreck et al. 1978, 1979, 1984 a). Repellents are available in the form of liquids, lotions, solid waxes (stick-type formulations), creams, foams, impregnated wipe-on towelettes and in pressurized containers. Unfortunately they have the disadvantage of irritating mucous membranes and they affect plastic materials including watch glasses, pens, spectacle frames, plastic lenses, some synthetic fabrics and possibly contact lenses, and repellent sprays from a pressurized can may cause damage to the eyes if used improperly. The most effective repellents against *Anopheles* species are dimethyl phthalate and deet. The latter is usually available as a 50% alcohol solution, and remains active for 6–13 h depending upon the mosquito species, rate of perspiration and other factors. These repellents can be used for impregnating clothing and bednets but are relatively expensive and comparatively short lasting and therefore the use of synthetic pyrethroids is now being explored with the expectation that they will be more economical and will last longer.

### Personal Hygiene

Not all individuals are equally attractive to *Anopheles* mosquitos and all the precise reasons are not known. However, it is known that $CO_2$ and body odours especially those produced by amines are good attractants. This fact has been put to use for mosquito collections in the field whereby bait is more attractive to mosquitos after eating bananas or meat for example. By adding a $CO_2$ device to a light trap more specimens of some mosquito species can be caught than with the trap alone. Thus bathing before dusk, especially after a hot and sticky day, may significantly reduce the attraction of the individual to mosquitos. Bars resembling soap are available containing 20% deet plus permethrin either 0.5% or 1.0%, for personal protection (Yap 1986). They are not soap but are one method of applying a repellent formulation. Reasonably good protection against *Anopheles* and other genera has been demonstrated. However, further careful studies are indicated, especially on efficacy, formulation, toxicity and acceptability.

## Costs and Choice of Method

The individual may or may not have control over the choice among the many methods of self and family protection mentioned in the aforegoing. In principle, a combination of all methods would provide the best protection. However, undoubtedly cost and availability are major influencing factors.

Costs vary considerably from one part of the world to another. The price of mosquito nets for instance can range from US $2–3 each in some countries of Asia, up to US $35 in Africa and US $50 in Europe and the United States, depending on the size and quality. An average single size net is about 10 $m^2$. The cost of impregnating it with permethrin to give 0.5 $gm/m^2$ is approximately US $0.30 (MacCormack et al. 1989), and this could last from 6 months to a year even if washed. The cost of repellents for application also varies according to the chemical used. On average 100 ml costs from US $1.5 to US

\$ 5 to the skin, and if perfumed and if dispensed as an aerosol then the cost will be considerably higher. Aerosols used as knockdown sprays cost from US \$ 1.5 to US \$ 5, whilst pyrethrum coils cost from US \$ 0.10 to US \$ 1/coil depending on the country of manufacture and sale, which pyrethroid is used, and whether they are perfumed. The cost of impregnated curtains would depend on the local material used and the size. There is clearly a need to bring the costs of some of these products down to a more affordable level and for them to be packaged in a convenient form for travelers to purchase at airports, railway stations, sea ports and through travel agencies.

## Health Information

There are numerous potential outlets for health information, many of which are not at present fully utilized as far as malaria is concerned. The WHO Malaria Action Programme provides information in the *Weekly Epidemiological Record* and also directly to the International Travel Agency Association. It is desirable that pamphlets and leaflets on malaria risk and personal protection measures are made available to the public through travel agents, airlines and transport companies in general. More health authorities in malaria endemic countries could provide incoming travelers at the point of entry with information on local malaria risk, location of health facilities for diagnosis and treatment, and guidance on how to prevent infection. In addition to health information, industry could provide employees with the necessary protective measures at very low cost or free of charge as part of their responsibility for the health care of their workers.

There are other important means of providing information on malaria prevention. One is on the vaccination certificate card which is used by travelers to record their immunizations. Another means is through the monthly airline magazines that most people read in all sections on the aeroplane. A health page or section could be suggested to the airlines as a regular feature. It would have to take into account all destinations since often the same monthly magazine covers all routes. However, in the same way that information is provided on duty-free sales and allowances, and on plane safety, so information on the risk of malaria and means of prevention could be provided in an equally "eye-catching" manner.

There is much that can, and should be, done to reduce the traveller's risk of catching malaria and other mosquito-borne infections which may be fatal. First and foremost it is an individual responsibility, but not entirely, and all those involved in one way or another in the travel industry could contribute significantly in reducing the health risks to their clients.

## References

Belton P (1981) An acoustic evaluation of electronic mosquito repellers. Mosq News 51(4):751–755
Birley MH, Mutero CM, Turner IF, Chadwick PR (1987) The effectiveness of mosquito coils containing esbiothrin under laboratory and field conditions. Ann Trop Med Parasitol 81(2):163–171
Bradley AK, Greenwood BM, Greenwood AM, Marsh K, Byass P, Tulloch S, Hayes R (1986) Bednets (mosquito nets) and morbidity from malaria. Lancet II:204–207
Bruce-Chwatt LJ (1985) Essential malariology, 2nd edn. Heinemann, London
Bruun J (1964) Thiamine as a remedy against mosquitos. Nord Med 71:650–651
Chadwick PR (1975) The activity of some pyrethroids, DDT and lindane in smoke from coils for biting inhibition, knockdown and kill of mosquitoes (Diptera, Culicidae). Bull Entomol Res 65(1):97–107
Chadwick PR, Lord LJ (1977) Tests of pyrethroid vaporizing mats against *Aedes aegypti* (L) (Diptera: Culicidae). Bull Entomol Res 67(4):667–674
Charlwood JD, Jolley D (1984) The coil works (against mosquitoes in Papua New Guinea). Trans R Soc Trop Med Hyg 78(5):678
Curtis CF (1986) Fact and fiction in mosquito attraction and repulsion. Parasitology Today 2 (11):316–318
Curtis CF, Lines JD (1985) Impregnated fabrics against malaria mosquitoes. Parasitology Today 1:147
Curtis CF, Ijumba J, Lines JD, Hill N, Callaghan A (1986) Mosquitos repellent anklets and a theory of relativity. Trans R Soc Trop Hyg 80:841–842
Darriet F, Robert V, Tho Vien N, Carnevale P (1984) Evaluation of the efficacy of permethrin-impregnated intact and perforated mosquito nets against vectors of malaria. (Unpublished document WHO/VBC/84.899 WHO/MAL/84.1008)
Eder HL (1945) Prevention and treatment with thiamine chloride in children against flea bites. Arch Paediatr 62:300–301
Foster WA, Lutes KI (1985) Tests of ultrasonic emissions on mosquito attraction to hosts in a flight chamber. J Am Mosq Control Assoc 1:199–202
Hervy JP, Sales S (1980) Evaluation de la rémanence de deux pyrethrinoides de synthèse OMS-1821 et OMS-1998, après imprégnation du différents tissus entrant dans le confection de moustiquaires. Doc. multigr Centre Muraz Bobo-Dioulasso No 7353/80/Doc Tech OCCGE No 04/ENT/80 du 8.2.1980
Khan AA, Maibach HI, Strauss WG, Fenley WR (1969) Vitamin $B_1$ is not a systemic mosquito repellent in man. Trans St. John's Hosp Dermatol Soc 55(1):99–102
Kunze W (1960) Letter to the editor. Med Klin 55:1339–1340
Kunze FW (1974) Evaluations of an electronic mosquito repelling device. Mosq News 34(4):369–375
Lines JD, Curtis CF, Myamba J, Njau R (1985) Tests of repellents or insecticide impregnated curtains, bednets and anklets against malaria vectors in Tanzania. (Unpublished document WHO/VBC/85.920)
Lunsford C (1949) Flea problem in California. Arch Dermatology Syphilol 60:1184
MacCormack CP, Snow RW, Greenwood BM (1989) Use of insecticide-impregnated bed nets in Gambian primary health case: economic aspects. Bulletin World Health Organization 67(2):209–214
Maasch HJ (1973) Investigations on the repellent effect of vitamin $B_1$. Z Tropenmed Parasitol 4:119–122
Majori G, Sabatinelli G, Coluzzi M (1987) Efficacy of permethrin-impregnated curtains for malaria vector control. (Unpublished document WHO/MAL/87.1037 WHO/VBC/87.944)
Maldonado RR, Tamayo L (1973) Treatment of 100 children with papular urticaria with thiamine chloride. Int J Dermatol 12:258–260
Müting D (1958) Über die Verhütung von Mückenstichen durch Einnahme von Vitamin $B_1$. Med Klin 53(23):1023

Port GR, Boreham PFL (1982) The effect of bed nets on feeding by *Anopheles gambiae* Giles (Dipteria: Culicidae). Bull Entomol Res 72:483–488
Rasnitsyn SP, Alekseev AN, Gornostreva RM, Kupriyanna ES, Potapov AA, Razumova OV (1974) Negative results of a test of examples of sound generators intended to repel mosquitos. Med Parazitol Parazit Bolezni 43:706–708
Ritschel WA, Ritschel-Beurlin G (1963) Sunderbans-Expedition. Dtsch Apoth Zeitung 103:1098–1103
Sauerbrey W (1970) Letter. Z Allgemeinmed 46:1000
Schreck CE, Self LS (1985) Treating mosquito nets for better protection from bites and mosquito-borne disease. (Unpublished document WHO/VBC/85.914)
Schreck CE, Weidhaas DE, Smith N (1977) Evaluation of electronic sound-producing devices against *Aedes taeniorhynchus* and *Ae. sollicitans*. Mosq News 37(3):529–531
Schreck CE, Posey D, Smith D (1978) Durability of permethrin as a potential clothing treatment to protect against blood-feeding arthropods. J Econ Entomol 71(3):397–400
Schreck CE, Kune DL, Smith N (1979) Protection afforded by the insect repellent jacket against four species of biting midge (Diptera: Culicidae). Mosq News 39(4):739–742
Schreck CE, Haile DG, Kline DL (1984a) The effectiveness of permethrin and deet, alone or in combination, for protection against *Aedes taeniorhynchus*. Am J Trop Med Hyg 33(4):725–730
Schreck CE, Webb JC, Burden GS (1984b) Ultrasonic devices: evaluation of repellency to cockroaches and mosquitoes and measurement of sound output. J Environ Sci Health A19(5):521–531
Shannon W (1943) Thiamine chloride as an aid in the solution of the mosquito problem. Minn Med 26:799–802
Singleton RE (1977) Evaluation of two mosquito-repelling devices. Mosq News 37(2):195–199
Snow WF (1977) Trials with an electronic mosquito-repelling device in West Africa. Trans R Soc Trop Med Hyg 71:449–450
Von Rahm U (1958) Besitzt Vitamin $B_1$ insektenabhaltende Eigenschaften? Schweiz Med Wochenschr 88 (26):634–635
WHO (1984) Chemical methods for the control of arthropod vectors and pests of public health importance. WHO, Geneva
Wilson CS, Mathieson DR, Jachowski LA (1944) Ingested thiamine chloride as a mosquito repellent. Science 100:147
Yap HH (1986) Effectiveness of soap formulations containing deet and permethrin as personal protection against outdoor mosquitoes in Malaysia. J Am Mosq Control Assoc 2(1):63–67

# Induced and Imported Malaria: Then and Now!

L. J. Bruce-Chwatt †

## Summary

Summaries of the world malaria situation published periodically by the World Health Organisation indicate that this disease continues to remain a major public health problem in developing countries. The latest reports indicate that there were roughly 2.5 million cases in Southeast Asia, 1.1 million in the South Pacific, 0.9 million in the Americas, 0.3 million in the eastern Mediterranean and 0.03 million in the European region comprising mainly Asian Turkey. There is no reliable information from the WHO African region, which has a total population of about 420 million and forms the core of the global reservoir of malaria. It is estimated that the annual number of clinical cases of malaria is between 80 and 120 million, but the period prevalence of the infection is close to 90% of the population. Transfusion malaria is a form of indirectly imported disease and any shortage of blood donors increases the difficulty of proper screening of donors. A number of technical, administrative and other aspects of screening of voluntary blood donors have arisen recently and their importance must not be underestimated. Any modifications of the present regulation must take into account the epidemiological conditions of the countries concerned. The presence of chloroquine resistance in *Plasmodium falciparum* requires special considerations.

## Introduction

The term induced malaria has been defined as follows: *Malaria infection transmitted not by a mosquito bite in nature but by a deliberate inoculation (as in malariatherapy or scientific experiment)* or *accidentally as in blood transfusion or other form of parenteral transfer of the specific pathogen.*

The history of induced malaria could be divided into two periods: that from 1884 to 1950 and that from 1950 to the present time.

The first period covers the early experimental studies following Laveran's discovery of malaria parasites and Wagner-Jauregg's method of malariatherapy of syphilis of the CNS. The second period refers almost exclusively to malaria due to accidental blood transfusion. In this respect it may be considered as a form of tropical disease seen mostly in non-endemic countries.

## Therapeutic Malaria

Malaria was recognized by Hippocrates as a fever that may result in a cure of other diseases. In the *57th Aphorism*, 4th section, the Greek physician stated some 2400 years ago: *Fever in a patient suffering from epilepsy or tetanus may be cured by it.* Boisseau (1832) [1] in his *Treatise on Fevers* advised a visit to the famous Pontine marshes where the fever indigenous in that part of Italy may cure epilepsy, gout, mania and paralysis.

However, Boisseau was preceded by James MacCulloch [2], who in his book of 1827 under the title *Malaria – an essay about the production and propagation of this poison* stated that the fever can cure a number of chronic afflictions. In 1876, four years before the discovery of malaria parasites by Laveran, a Russian neurologist Rosenblum from Odessa attempted to treat patients with mental diseases by injection of blood from malarious patients [3, 4]. Ross (1911) points out that Dochman, another Russian physician, inoculated in 1880 two persons with a serum of a herpetic blister from a malaria patient and thus transmitted the infection [5]. However, both Ross and Laveran rejected this observation as unreliable. It appears that Laveran was urged in 1880 to carry out such a demonstration of his discovery of the malaria parasite, but refused to do it for ethical reasons [6].

Other workers repeated this experiment with similar results; among these one must mention Saharov in Russia, who drew the malarial blood by leeches, kept them on ice for 4 days and infected himself with *Plasmodium falciparum* after an incubation period of 16 days [4].

In 1902 Favr (then in Tbilisi) transmitted to himself *P. falciparum* by the bite of *Anopheles claviger* infected experimentally from a patient; after a 12-day incubation period Favr had a severe attack of malaria [7].

Outside Russia the first deliberate blood transmission of falciparum malaria from a human case to a healthy person took place in 1882 and was carried out in Germany by Gerhardt, who injected 1 ml blood of a patient with quotidian fever into two healthy subjects and transmitted malaria with 6–10 days incubation period [8].

Although Wagner-Jauregg, a Viennese physician, reported in 1887 on the good effects of fever in some mental diseases, it was only in 1917 that he started using deliberate inoculations of benign tertian malaria for such patients [9]. His success was such that in 1927 he was given the Nobel Prize for the practice of malariatherapy for the general paralysis of syphilitic origin [10–11]. Since then several thousand patients have been treated by this method alone or combined with chemotherapy using arsenicals and bismuth preparations [12].

The practice of malariatherapy was soon extended to other centres such as Paris (Mollaret), Sokola – Bucarest (Ciuca), Columbia SC (Young), Talahassee (Boyd), Liverpool (Yorke), and especially Horton Hospital, Epsom, where James's, Covell's, Garnham's, Nicol's and P. G. Shute's contribution to the technique of induced malaria was enormous.

Since 1925 the Mott Clinic was established by S. P. James at Horton Hospital, Epsom; there during the next 25 years over 8500 patients were treated and much new knowledge on the clinical course of induced malaria and some important parasitological aspects of it was gained [13].

It was in 1922 that Warrington Yorke in Liverpool was the first to start inducing malaria by mosquito transmission and in 1923 malariatherapy by this method was put on a routine basis. The English indigenous *A. atroparvus* was found to be an efficient vector of the Madagascar strain of *P. vivax* [14].

The main advantage of mosquito transmission of induced malaria is the avoidance of some viral diseases like hepatitis B, which is possible when blood inoculations are used from cryptic carriers of this or other infections. Today the long-term preservation in the blood of any of the developmental forms of plasmodia is possible by freezing them in liquid nitrogen. Induced malaria appeared to be a valuable method for treatment of paresis, syphilitic optic atrophy, and meningovascular syphilis. Myocardial, hepatic and renal lesions are a contraindication [12–15, 17–19].

The benefits derived from malariatherapy depend on the degree of pyrexia and the number of paroxyms; usually 10–12 of the latter were required for treatment. Still better results were obtained when specific antisyphilitic therapy by penicillin or organic arsenicals was combined. The rationale of malariatherapy for cerebral syphilis is uncertain; the fact that malaria, like syphilis, can produce positive Kahn's or Wasserman reaction points to some immunological defence mechanism [16].

In 1943 the United States Government set up the *Imported Malaria Studies Programme*, the purpose of which was concerned with the possibility of malaria imported by the returning troops to introduce the infection through the agency of American anophelines [17].

A few points related to the medical and scientific achievements of the method of treatment of neurosyphilis ought to be mentioned here for historical and epidemiological reasons, related to the present problems of transfusion malaria.

The benefits of therapeutic malaria, however relative, were nevertheless undeniable. Generally speaking (and subject to various factors such as the age or condition of the patient, phase of the specific pathological process, previous exposure, etc.) during the period 1920–1950, when several thousand syphilitics were treated by this method, some 15% fully recovered, 20% greatly improved and about 50% did not respond, died or were lost from the records [12–18].

Today malariatherapy has been largely abandoned because of the success of penicillin treatment. However, the amount of new knowledge that this method provided was immense. The solution of the former mystery of exo-erythrocytic stages [18, 19], the longevity of specific malaria infection in nature, the dynamics of recrudescenses or relapses and the screening of candidate antiplasmodial compounds depended on the use of this technique in patients and in human volunteers. Hamilton Fairley's masterly and heroic studies on paludrine in Australian Army volunteers in 1943–1945 are a milestone in the annals of chemotherapy of malaria [20].

The same appreciation applies to the remarkable research programme of 1941–1952 or other similar studies carried out in the United States and United Kingdom in which human volunteers have been involved. Russell deservedly described them in glowing terms [21]. There is no doubt of the scientific merit of this splendid work.

Experimental monkey malaria formed another, perhaps less heroic but scientifically not less important, chapter of experimental chemotherapy [22–25].

The discovery of rodent malaria in 1948 by Vincke was of value, but it did not fully replace the advantage of studies of other primate mammalian hosts.

## Malaria Therapy and Its Contribution to Parasitology

Studies on induced human malaria for treatment of neurosyphilis carried out by the Horton Hospital covered 3 decades; their longitudinal character was most valuable.

From the early days of vector-transmitted malariatherapy there was some controversy whether blood-induced or sporozoite-induced malaria are preferable. With blood-induced infection the usual dosage of *P. vivax* is between 0.5 and one million parasites, although 200–1000 plasmodia were often sufficient to produce an infection, when given intravenously, depending on the species of the parasite, its degree of virulence and the host's immune status. *Plasmodium vivax* (Madagascar strain) was used more than any other species because of its relatively benign infection easily transmissible by *A. atroparvus*. The isolate of this strain was obtained in 1925 from an Indian "lascar" whose ship left Madagascar and during the voyage the man developed clinical symptoms of *P. vivax* malaria. This strain, first used for malariatherapy at Horton in 1925, was still maintained after 26 years and was transmitted through 25 000 *A. atroparvus*. The minimum number of male and female gametocytes to produce a mosquito infection was 6–12/μl blood. To produce a good infection 100–200 ripe male gametocytes are necessary and at 23–25 °C about 400–1000 oocysts may be formed in a single female *Anopheles*. If each oocyst develops 1000 sporozoites then the infected mosquito may have well over one million sporozoites. At the optimum temperature of 23–25 °C sporozoites will be formed in 9–10 days. Such heavily infected *Anopheles* may transmit the infection for at least 1 month. In one case a single *Anopheles* transmitted the infection to 15 patients when fed on alternate days.

An interesting observation was that all species of malaria parasites, if regularly transmitted by blood, may lose after some time the ability to form gametocytes and cannot infect mosquitos.

When a small number of sporozoites of *P. vivax* were injected, a period of latency of 28 weeks was common and this suggested that in some strains tissue forms must be present in the liver [18, 19]. Incidentally, it was evident that black patients have a degree of natural immunity that prevents the infection or mitigates it. We know today that this is due to the absence of Duffy blood group antigen.

Until 1930 only *P. vivax* was used for malariatherapy at Horton but some patients did not fully benefit from a full course of *P. vivax* infection and could not get re-infected with the same strain. However, when *A. stephensi* of Indian origin was colonized it was found that *P. falciparum* of Romanian or Italian origin can be easily transmitted to man by this species of *Anopheles*. Such refractoriness of European *Anopheles* was later confirmed in *A. labranchiae*, which failed to become infected by a West African *P. falciparum*.

Infection with *P. falciparum* is often dangerous and has to be carefully monitored so that the parasitaemia should not exceed 100 000/µl; *P. ovale* was used at Horton in the 1930s; the infections are relatively mild and may terminate spontaneously. The simian *P. knowlesi* was quite often used by Ciuca in Bucarest [26]. It is benign with few relapses and some individuals resist the infection altogether.

In an untreated primary attack of vivax malaria the initial stage lasting 2–5 days presents as an irregular remittent fever without rigors. In the next stage the fever is high, the rigors common but often quotidian and the disease becomes truly tertian only after 2–3 weeks. Then there is the latent period and about 50%–60% of patients have relapses between 190 and 270 days after the primary attack. This was the first pointer to the existence of hypnozoites [27, 28].

It was at Horton that the range of immunospecificity of strains of vivax and falciparum malaria was demonstrated. Thus the infection with the Madagascar *P. vivax* gave little or no protection against a later infection of *P. vivax* from British Guyana. Also a patient who had a primary attack of an Indian *P. falciparum* (following a mild attack on reinfection with the same parasite, and then a complete protection on reinoculation of this parasite) developed severe malaria when given a Sardinian strain of *P. falciparum* [18, 19, 28].

Finally, there is no need to remind us that in 1948 a human volunteer at Horton, who had had malariatherapy, was subjected to massive sporozoite homologous infection 2 years later by the madagascar strain of *P. vivax* through the bites of 2000 *Anopheles* and the intravenous injection of 200 infected salivary glands. Altogether in this case of induced malaria about 20 million sporozoites were inoculated [18, 19].

Some isolates of *P. falciparum* studied at Horton were biologically distinct by their virulence of immunological characteristics. Their incubation period varied between 7 and 14 days but there was no long latency as in benign tertian malaria. Already in 1898 the Italians observed that the infection in the south of Italy was more severe than in northern Italy. Koch noted 50 years ago, and James [13] confirmed it later, that African and Indian falciparum infections respond better to treatment than those from Italy. The amount of quinine needed to control primary attack caused by a Roman or Sardinian strain was eight times higher than in malaria due to other geographical strains. Studies on response to various antimalarials were carried out in 1940–1960 in the United States on human volunteers or in neurosyphilitic patients. This opened the way to experimental methodology of drug resistance fully developed by Schmidt [25].

A list of various "strains" is long (Coker, Panama, Santee-Cooper, McLendon, Costa, etc.) and their study opened the way to the present knowledge of resistance of various isolates to chloroquine and other modern antimalarials [29–32].

*Quartan malaria* is characterized by the difficulty of mosquito transmission and a long pre-patent period (29–40 days). At Horton success was achieved only in 1949 using *A. stephensi* from India. The clinical picture was as described by ancient authors and no nephrosis was evident in the few patients. A strain (VS) isolated in Romania in 1962 produced an infection easily curable by chloroquine alone. There are also different responses of various geographical strains to primaquine (Papua New Guinea, Korea, etc.).

*Plasmodium ovale*, originally described in 1922 from East Africa by Stephens, caused some controversy as many doubts were expressed as to its being truly a new species. In 1931 Yorke supplied the Horton centre with blood of a patient from the Belgian Congo. *A. atroparvus* was infected and several passages confirmed its distinct features such as a pre-patent period of 11–16 days and the morphology of blood stages [14].

These studies and others that used the method of induced malaria in man and on simian primates revealed the fact that some species of anopheline vectors are resistant and others particularly susceptible to the infection by certain species and strains of malaria parasites. Moreover, they showed that the immunity to malaria is species specific and partly strain specific. It is also stage specific, mainly against blood stages, whether the latter are induced by blood inoculation or by sporozoites.[1] The importance of these findings for the understanding of clinical, biological and epidemiological aspects of malaria in a human community was and still is enormous [33, 34].

## Imported Malaria and Blood Transfusion

*The resurgence of malaria* in the tropical world continues to threaten the health of developing countries but the growing reservoir of malaria infection presents also serious problems for the western world. There has been a steady increase of the number of passengers flying between countries and continents during the past 20 years [36]. For the first time in the history of aviation the total number of passengers on scheduled airline flights exceeded 800 million in 1980.[2] In terms of passenger/kilometres the relevant figure for 1982 was 1057000 million (including USSR). Taking into account that unscheduled (viz. charter) flights carry at least 10%–15% of scheduled services, the total number of airline passengers in 1980 was over 900 million [36, 37].

Of this overall number about one-quarter were tourists; their estimated number was 259 million in 1978 and close to 300 million in 1980. The recent

[1] Although the treatment of neurosyphilis by induced malaria was given up already in the 1960s, its use for other affections continued for some time by a few enthusiasts such as Corelli. Believing that any febrile attack acts as a non-specific stimulus, which liberates certain factors of hypothalamic, anti-inflammatory or neurohormonal origin, these clinicians employed induced malaria for treatment of progressive scleroderma, lipid nephrosis, peptic ulcer, herpetiform dermatitis and especially Burger's disease (thromboangeiitis obliterans) with results ranging from indifferent to satisfactory. Today, reserpine and sympathectomy are the main, relatively successful methods for treatment of these conditions [35).

[2] According to most recent estimates (*The Economist*, 27 February 1988) the world passenger jet-fleet has been increasing during the past decade by 4.5%/annum. During that period the figure of world-passenger/kilometres went up from 1000 billion in 1980 to nearly 2000 billion in 1987 and it is likely that it will reach 3000 billion in the year 2000.

trends show significant increases in air travel to Asia and the Far East (from 12% to 22% over the decade), and to Africa, Middle East and Latin America.

The forecast for the next decade shows about 5% annual growth of the world air traffic and it is estimated that during the 1980s the airlines will invest some US $ 700 billion in developing their means of air transport and ground facilities [37].

It has been estimated that during the period 1950–1980 the total number of recorded cases of accidental transfusion malaria was of the order of 3000; this represents probably less than one-half of the true number of such cases [36–40]. According to data available to the WHO, 536 cases of transfusion malaria occurred in some 35 countries during the period 1978–1982. There is good evidence that many instances of malaria (and also some other blood-transmitted diseases) have not been reported, even if the origin of the infection was known.[3]

Problems related to blood transfusion are at present of growing complexity and importance. An expression of the opinion of a few members of an international forum convened by Dr. A. Hässig of Berne in 1987 indicated the difficulties that the medical profession has to deal with at the present time [41].

Notification of malaria is not often complied with, even in advanced countries, let alone in endemic malarious areas. The true incidence of transfusion malaria is a matter of guesswork. The wide range of between 0.2 and 50 cases/million of blood transfusion units, estimated 10 years ago, is a good indicator of the difference between the situation in various countries.

The situation in the United States was described by Guerrero et al. [42], whose report indicates that during the decade 1972–1981 at least 26 cases of transfusion malaria were recorded, giving an estimated risk of 0.25 cases/million donor units. This compares favourably with the previous incidence of 32 cases during the 5-year period 1967–1971. A global survey of transfusion malaria covering the period 1950–1972 [38–40, 42] showed that *P. malariae* (48%) was the most prevalent species of the parasite involved at that time. This ratio was followed by *P. vivax* (19%), *P. falciparum* (5%) and rare cases of *P. ovale*; in nearly 30% of cases the species of the parasite was not determined. A more

---

[3] Two aspects of accidental and imported malaria have not been given in detail in the present survey, though they have been discussed by other authors. One concerns some unusual hospital or laboratory accidental infections known as "needle malaria" or "stick injury" seen in nursing staff and caused by a prick of an infected needle contaminated by a minute amount of blood of a patient with malaria. This occurrence is common among drug addicts and cases have been reported in Germany, Italy, Poland, the United Kingdom and U.S.S.R. The present frequency of congenital malaria in newborn, whose mothers (often recent immigrants from endemic parts of the world) were exposed to infection on their visits to the country of origin, also causes much concern.

The second, relatively new, problem is that of airport malaria, in which the air-carrier becomes a true and not metaphorical vector of the infection, classified as imported or introduced. Some 20 occurrences of cases in persons living near or working at large international airports have been recorded during the past decade in France, Belgium, Holland and Switzerland. Two such cases were observed in the United Kingdom and two other ones (somewhat cryptic) might have been brought from Ethiopia.

recent survey of the period 1973–1980 [40] indicated that *P. vivax* has become more common (42%) than *P. malariae* (38%), but *P. falciparum* frequency has quadrupled to 20%. These data are very relative, because over half of all cases of transfusion malaria have not been identified as to the species involved. The shift to *P. vivax* and *P. falciparum* is certainly due to closer contacts of many present and prospective blood donors with highly malarious parts of the world.

In the United States, 17% of blood donors during the period 1972–1981 were of foreign origin, and of the 17 cases in which the infected donor was traced, 8 came from Africa, 3 from Vietnam, 2 from Mexico, 2 from Europe and 1 from India; 6 of them denied having ever had malaria [43].

The present situation of imported malaria in the United Kingdom was outlined and commented upon by Phillips-Howard et al. [44] but it appears that the problems of blood transfusion had not greatly changed.

Two recent cases of transfusion malaria were reported in the United Kingdom. However, over the period of the past 50 years, when an estimated total of 36 million transfused blood units (equivalent to about 14 million litres or 3.7 million US gallons) of blood were used, the total number of known cases of accidentally induced malaria was eight, of which two reported in 1977 and 1978 are uncertain as the patients might have been naturally infected in the past.

Deaths caused by transfusion malaria are rare but fatal cases have occurred in the United States and elsewhere. The problem of responsibility for death or for additional suffering caused by accidental infection of the patient who received the contaminated blood have rarely been subjected to legal procedure and may be difficult to judge. However, in the new social climate of antimedical litigation to extract from the doctor the highest possible financial compensation for any true or alleged professional fault, the situation may be expected to change [40].

In highly endemic malarious areas of the world the problem is of great complexity. The majority of the prospective blood donors are infected and most of them are asymptomatic carriers of malaria parasites. Studies in Nigeria, Zambia and Papua New Guinea showed that in some parts of these countries up to 10% of donors have malaria parasites detectable by simple microscopy. As most adult inhabitants show a high degree of immunity to one or more species of prevalent plasmodia, the person to person transfer of malaria parasites has limited if any clinical consequences in immune recipients. However, in countries like India, Sri Lanka, Thailand and other parts of the world where some areas have little or no malaria while others are highly endemic, and accidental infection of non-immunes by blood from asymptomatic carriers may be serious.[4]

---

[4] Categories of travellers for individual protection from malaria were estimated by the World Health Organization in 1987. This report indicated that some 9 million residents of France, one million each of British and United States citizens, about half a million Swiss and the same number of other European travellers will be visiting endemic malarious countries each year.

Major national and cultural differences in the appreciation of the risk involved and in the knowledge of preventive measures and their application were evident [55].

*Prevention of transfusion malaria* depends largely on the awareness of asymptomatic carrier-state of plasmodia in persons previously exposed to the disease. The consensus of expert opinion supports the view that a single infection with *P. falciparum* does not persist in the body of its human host for more than 2 years; *P. vivax* and *P. ovale* usually die out within 3 years, but *P. malariae* of quartan periodicity may show recrudescences with or without symptoms for very long periods of up to 40–50 years. The limits of survival of *P. falciparum* and *P. vivax* may be exceeded in subjects who lived in endemic areas most of their lives, and these infections may also be quite discrete in their delayed reappearance in such immune carriers. The smallest number of plasmodia that can result in a human infection is not known, but vivax malaria has been successfully transmitted with only 10 parasites/μl. The blood donor may have a discrete infection of 1–2 parasites/μl; a patient given 1 unit of this blood would receive about half a million parasites [45].

It is well known that direct microscopic examination of blood for the possible presence of malaria infection in donors is of no value whatsoever, for reasons mentioned before, namely that scanty parasitaemia, of the order of less than 100 parasites/μl blood, is not readily detectable on routine microscopy.

The value and practice of serological methods of malaria diagnosis such as the indirect fluorescent antibody test (IFA) or the enzyme-linked immunosorbent assay (ELISA) was discussed by many authors [37–41, 45–49] and this is now the most dependable screening test, although it requires experience, suitable instrumentation and trained laboratory staff [41–49]. some newer immunological and molecular methods may detect the presence of as few as 10 parasites/million red blood cells, but they are not ready for general use.

One of these methods is the radioimmunoassay; the other is the DNA probe. The first exploits the ability of soluble red cell antigen to bind to malaria antibodies and thus to inhibit the antibody reaction with malaria antigens coated on a plastic surface; monoclonal antibodies provide high specificity but require radioactive isotopes (such as iodine-151) for labelling.

The DNA probe is based on the binding (hybridization) of nucleic acid single strands with another single strand containing a complementary nucleotide base sequence. These methods are of great potential value for epidemiological studies rather than for single tests [48].

*Screening of potentially infected donors* of whole blood or of erythrocyte, leucocyte and platelet concentrates is of paramount importance. The interview of the donor is the simplest but also the most fallible method, especially in countries where there is a financial gain for giving blood.

A few cases of malaria transmitted from donors or organ transplants who were born and raised in countries where malaria is endemic drew attention to this rare but possible source of infection [50–52].

The current standards in the United States are that persons who travelled in endemic malarious areas may be accepted as whole blood donors 6 months after their return to non-endemic areas, providing that they have been free of febrile symptoms and have not taken during that time any preventive antimalarial drugs. Those who had a confirmed malaria infection on their return or immigration into the United States should be excluded from whole blood donation for 3 years after becoming asymptomatic or after stopping the administration of antimalarial drugs. Immigrants or visitors from endemic areas may be accepted as blood donors 3 years after their departure from these areas, if they have shown no symptoms of malaria during that time. In view of the fact that some infections, especially with quartan malaria, may be present in an asymptomatic form for 40–50 years, the above time limit of 3 years is a compromise. In order not to eliminate most of the prospective but suspected donors, the risk of some cases of transfusion malaria had to be accepted in the hope that the 3-year limit will minimize the occurrence of *P. falciparum* and *P. vivax* infections.

Regulations concerning the acceptance or rejection of blood donors possibly infected with malaria vary from country to country and some of them are extremely vague. In the United Kingdom new regulations have been introduced; the decision whether or not to accept blood donations from persons who have lived in endemic malarious areas or have visited them depends largely on the availability of serological tests for the presence of antibodies in the blood of potential donors. Thus, if the facilities for such tests are not available, blood donors who have had malaria should be deferred for at least 6 months and then accepted for plasma fractions only. Donors born in endemic malarious areas, or former residents or visitors to such areas, should be deferred for 6 months after their arrival or return to the United Kingdom, but their blood can be taken for plasma fractions after that time; if they have not visited endemic malarious areas for 5 years their donation of whole blood is acceptable. However, if the serological test is negative after 6 months since their return, donation of whole blood is acceptable.

The introduction of the indirect fluorescent antibody (IFA) test has been a great advance. The value of this test for detection of immune response to previous infection in individual donors is beyond any doubt. However, several investigators indicated the need for caution, since the proper technique of the IFA test is of paramount importance. The main requirement is the availability of three homologous antigens (*P. falciparum, P. vivax* and *P. malariae*). The last two are difficult to obtain but *P. falciparum* can now be maintained in culture and an excellent test kit has been developed (Falciparum Spot IF) commercially by the Institute Mérieux in Lyon. It consists of a glass slide on which there are ten round spots of human blood infected with *P. falciparum* in culture. A recent comparative study carried out in France [47] confirmed the value of this method, which appears to be rapid and reliable although relatively expensive.

Recent studies [48–50] extended their survey of transfusion malaria in France, by covering the whole period 1980–1985, during which the authors analysed the collection of 158 788 units of blood from potential donors [48–50]. Subjects who have travelled to endemic malarious areas were screened using the IFA test with the culture in vitro of *P. falciparum* as antigen (Spot IF Bio-Merieux); the threshold positive dilution of serum was 1/20. Of the 1747 subjects who were a possible risk (as judged from verbal inquiry), 107 were positive, representing 6.1% of tested sera; thus only 0.67% of all blood units collected were rejected from total blood donation. A repeated testing of positives showed long persistence of positive results or the so-called *cicatrice serologique palustre* ("serological malaria scar"). The use of one antigen limits the specificity of this test, when it comes to infections with *P. vivax, P. ovale* and *P. malariae*; however, these plasmodia usually show some cross-reactivity with *P. falciparum* and, if the threshold of positivity is arbitrarily determined as 1:20, then the test may be of indicative value. It should be remembered, however, that a positive IFA test with a titre of over 1:64 reflects an immune response to the infection, but does not necessarily confirm the presence of circulating parasites in the blood of the donor. It is the negative IFA test with a proper primate antigen that indicates with a high degree of probability the freedom from malaria. The advantage of the IFA test lies not only in that it may pick up the possibly infected donor; its equal if not greater advantage is that, when negative, it allows the use as blood donors those subjects who might have been rejected on a selection interview. The methodology of serological as well as enzyme-linked immunosorbent assay (ELISA) techniques have been adapted for screening of large numbers of sera [46].*Prevention of transfusion malaria by chemoprophylaxis* is one of the methods of dealing with this problem commonly used in the past. Chloroquine was the most reliable drug of the 4-aminoquinoline series and the administration of the single or repeated dosage of chloroquine base up to 1500 mg in 3 days, to the recipient of blood, possibly containing malaria parasites, was the standard method of prevention. This was important in some tropical countries where most of the prospective donors were carriers of plasmodia. Today this procedure is less reliable because of the development of *P. falciparum* resistance to chloroquine and other drugs of the groups of 4-aminoquinolines as well as to some other compounds.

The geographical extension of *Plasmodium falciparum* strains resistant to chloroquine has been quite rapid since 1960 when it was first observed in Thailand and in Colombia. During the past 10 years resistant strains of this parasite species have appeared in large areas of Southeast Asia and also in several countries of Central and South America. By 1980 the situation in Asia was quite complex and constantly changing. The WHO is responsible for monitoring the progress of chloroquine resistance and the relevant reports are useful for prophylactic or therapeutic guidance [53–54].

Thus, in cases of donors suspected of being asymptomatic carriers of malaria that originated in Southeast Asia or northern parts of South America or Central America or East Africa the protection of recipients of whole blood would have to depend on the use of sulphadoxine-pyrimethamine or mefloquine. Even then it may be useful to use the standard dosage of chloroquine, since *P. vivax* and *P. ovale* are less susceptible to sulphadoxine-pyrimethamine than to chloroquine. On the other hand there is no need to give to the recipient of suspected blood any 8-aminoquinolines such as primaquine because blood-induced malaria does not involve any extra-erythrocytic liver stages, which are responsible for relapses of *P. vivax* or *P. malariae*.

Premedication of donors suspected of asymptomatic malaria in highly malarious areas (where screening for non-infected donors would have been of little practical value) has been used in some countries in Southeast Asia. However, as chloroquine appears to be the only suitable long-term chemoprophylactic in these situations and since chloroquine resistance is on the increase this advice calls for more caution.

## Envoi

Only 2 decades ago the method of induced malaria in man was virtually the only means to assess the subtle biological relationship of that infection between the human host, the plasmodium and the invertebrate vector. Our present knowledge of these aspects is very much greater and more complex. Parasite determinants of transmission, biology of the various stages of the life cycle, antigenic characteristics of each stage, the role of cellular membranes, genetic profile of the vertebrate host and of the pathogen, metabolism of nutrients, problems of drug resistance, new methods of diagnosis, in vitro cultivation, advances of molecular biology, DNA probe developments and other more or less abstruse subjects – all this takes us deeper and deeper into fundamental science where we often lose sight of the wood for admiring so many splendid trees. The technical progress expanded the boundaries of global travel beyond imagination but this opened the way for a flood of human infections that were formerly confined to populations of tropical areas. In the meantime, the burden of malaria in the Third World is on the increase and our means of fighting it are diminishing. There must be a moral and social lesson in this, somewhere!!

## References


1. Boisseau FG (1832) A treatise on fevers. Carey and Lee, Philadelphia
2. MacCulloch J (1827) Malaria – an essay on the production and propagation of this poison. Longman, London
3. Boyd M (1969) Malariology, 2 vols. Saunders, Philadelphia
4. Zasuhin DN (1951) Outstanding achievements of national scientists in the field of malaria (in Russian). Government Publishing House, Moscow
5. Ross R (1911) The prevention of malaria. Murray, London
6. Laveran A (1907) Traite du paludisme. Masson, Paris
7. Favr VV (1903) Studies on malaria in Russia. Kharhov
8. Gerhardt C (1884) Über Intermittents Impfungen. Z Klin Med 7:372–378
9. Wagner-Jauregg J (1887) Über die Einwirkung fieberhafter Erkrankungen auf Psychosea. Jahrb Psychiatr Neurol 7:94–102
10. Wagner-Jauregg J (1922) The treatment of general paralysis by inoculation of malaria. J Nerv Ment Dis 55:369–375
11. Wagner-Jauregg J (1939) Derzeitige Behandlung der progressiven Paralyse. Wien Wochenschr 52:1075–1080
12. Becker FT (1949) Induced malaria as a therapeutic agent. In: Boyd M (ed) Malariology, vol 2, pp 1145–1157
13. James SP (1931) Some general results of induced malaria in England. Trans R Soc Trop Med Hyg 2:341

14. York W, McFie JW (1925) Observations on malaria during the treatment of general paresis. Trans R Soc Trop Med Hyg 18:13–21; 19:108–115
15. Covell G, Nicol WD (1951) Studies on induced malaria. Br Med Bull 8:51–55
16. Russell PF et al. (1963) Practical malariology. Oxford University Press, London
17. Young M et al. (1945) Studies on imported malarias. J Nat Malar Soc 4:127–134
18. Shortt HE, Garnham PCC, Covell G, Shute PG (1948) The pre-erythrocytic stages of human malaria: *P. vivax*. Br Med J 1:547
19. Shute PG (1951) Mosquito infection in artifically induced malaria. Br Med Bull 8:56–63
20. Fairley NH (1947) Sidelights on malaria in man obtained by sub-inoculation experiments. Trans Soc Trop Med Hyg 40:621–676
21. Russell PF (1955) Man's mastery of malaria. Oxford University Press, London
22. Bray RS (1963) The malaria parasites of anthropoid apes. J Parasitol 49:888–891
23. Bray RS (1969) Malaria in chimpanzees. Chimpanzee 1:413–424
24. Coatney GR et al. (1971) The primate malarias. U.S. Government Printing Office, Washington D.C.
25. Schmidt LH et al. (1973) Infection with *P. falciparum* and *P. vivax* in the owl monkey. Trans R Soc Trop Med Hyg 67:446–474
26. Ciuca M (1966) Eradication du paludisme en Roumanie. Editions Medicales, Bucarest
27. Bray RS, Garnham PCC (1982) Life cycle of primate malaria parasites. Br Med Bull 38:117–122
28. Krotoski WA, Garnham PCC, Bray RS (1982) Observations on early and late post-sporozoite tissue stages in primate malaria. Am J Trop Med Hyg 31:24–35
29. Peters W (1970) Chemotherapy and drug resistance in malaria. Academic Press, London
30. Peters W (1982) Antimalarial drug resistance: an increasing problem. Br Med Bull 38:187–192
31. Peters W, Richards WHR (1986) Chemotherapy and drug resistance in malaria. Academic Press, London
32. Bruce-Chwatt LJ et al. (1982) Chemotherapy of malaria, 2nd edn. World Health Organization, Geneva
33. World Health Organization (1984) Advances in malaria chemotherapy. Techn Rep Ser No 711. WHO, Geneva
34. World Health Organization (1987) The biology of malaria parasites. Techn Rep Ser No 743. WHO, Geneva
35. Corelli F (1974) Symposium on malaria research: present day applications of malariatherapy. World Health Organization, Rabat. WHO.MDP/SMR/74/3
36. International Civil Aviation Organisation (1980) Air traffic 1979. ICAO Bull 35–37
37. Bruce-Chwatt LJ (1972) Blood transfusion and tropical disease. Trop Dis Bull 69:825–862
38. Bruce-Chwatt LJ (1974) Transfusion malaria. Bull WHO 50:340–347
39. Bruce-Chwatt LJ (1982) Transfusion malaria revisited. Trop Dis Bull 79:827–840
40. Bruce-Chwatt LJ (1981) Imported malaria; an ininvited guest. Br Med Bull 38:179–186
41. Hässig A (1987) Which are the appropriate modifications of existing regulations? Vox Sanguinis 52:138–148
42. Guerrero IC, Weniger BG, Schultz MG (1983) Transfusion malaria in the United States 1972–1981. Ann Intern Med 99:221–226
43. Lobel HO, Campbell CC (1986) Malaria prophylaxis and distribution of drug resistance. In: Strickland GT (ed) Clinics in tropical medicine. Saunders, Philadelphia
44. Phillips-Howard PH, Bradley DJ, Blaze M, Hurn M (1988) Malaria in Britain 1977–1986. Br Med J 296:245–248
45. Bruce-Chwatt LJ (1985) Essential malariology, 2nd edn. Heinemann, London

46. Voller A, Draper CC (1982) Immunodiagnosis and seroepidemiology of malaria. Br Med Bull 38:173–178
47. Deroff P, Regner M, Simitsis AM (1982) Screening of blood doors likely to transmit malaria. Rev Fr Transfus 25:3–10
48. Bruce-Chwatt LJ (1988) From Laveran's discovery to DNA probes: new trends in diagnosis of malaria. Lancet II:1509–1511
49. Saleun JP, Deroff P, imitsis AM et al. (1987) Paludisme post-transfusionnel. Ann Parasitol Hum Comp 62:9–16
50. Jeannel D, Bard D, Gentilini M (1987) Le paludisme d'importation en France. Ann Soc Belge Med Trop 57:177–127
51. Lefavour GS, Pierce JC, Frame JD (1980) Renal transplant-associated malaria. Am Med Assoc 244:1820–1821
52. Johnston IDA (1981) Possible transmission of malaria by renal transplantation. Br Med J 282:780
53. Peto TE, Gilks CF (1986) Strategies for prevention of malaria in travellers. Lancet I:680–681
54. World Health Organisation (1988) Vaccination certificate for international travel and health advice to travellers. WHO, Geneva
55. World Health Organisation (1987) Bases for development of recommendations on protection for short-term travellers against malaria. WHO/Mal./87.10405

# Chloroquine-Resistant Malaria in West Africa

J. S. Moran and K. W. Bernard

Chloroquine-resistant *Plasmodium falciparum* (CRPF) malaria is a potential threat to the health of approximately 1000 Amcerican Peace Corps Volunteers (PCVs) in West Africa. Minimizing that threat requires accurate and up-to-date information on the geographical extent of CRPF so that prophylaxis recommendations and treatment protocols can be based on the risk of CRPF in specific areas. Experience with spreading CRPF in East [1] and Central [2] Africa, as well as in Asia [3], has shown that chloroquine prophylaxis failure in nonimmunes often becomes widespread before chloroquine resistance is detected by standardized in vivo or in vitro sensitivity testing. To best define the extent of the risk of CRPF to PCVs in West Africa, we surveyed for evidence of chloroquine prophylaxis failure in nine West African countries between September 1985 and February 1988.

## Methods

Peace Corps Volunteers work in West Africa in education, agriculture, rural development and a variety of other occupations. Most live in villages or small towns. Nearly all have bed nets and/or screened sleeping quarters but few have electric fans and almost none have air conditioning. Thus their exposure to mosquitoes is much higher than that of many expatriate residents of West Africa. All are required to take chloroquine phosphate, 500 mg weekly, as antimalarial prophylaxis. The average number of PCVs serving in surveyed countries in 1986–1987 was: Benin, 55; Gambia, 52; Ghana, 75; Liberia, 130; Mali, 104; Niger, 140; Senegal, 105; Sierra Leone, 195; Togo, 123. Most PCVs serve for 2 years, although some leave service early and some extend their service beyond the usual 2-year term.

When sick, PCVs treat themselves, seek local medical care, or report to the Peace Corps Medical Officer (PCMO) for their country, depending on the nature of their illness and their proximity to the PCMO or other source of medical care. PCVs are instructed to report all illnesses to their PCMO and, in the case of suspected malaria, to make thick and thin blood slides (using Peace Corps-provided materials) to be sent to the PCMO for examination.

Each month, each PCMO sends to Peace Corps's office of medical services in Washington DC a standard report of the incidence of certain illnesses (including malaria) and injuries among PCVs in the country. Included are: the total number of PCVs in country on the 15th of the month, the number of

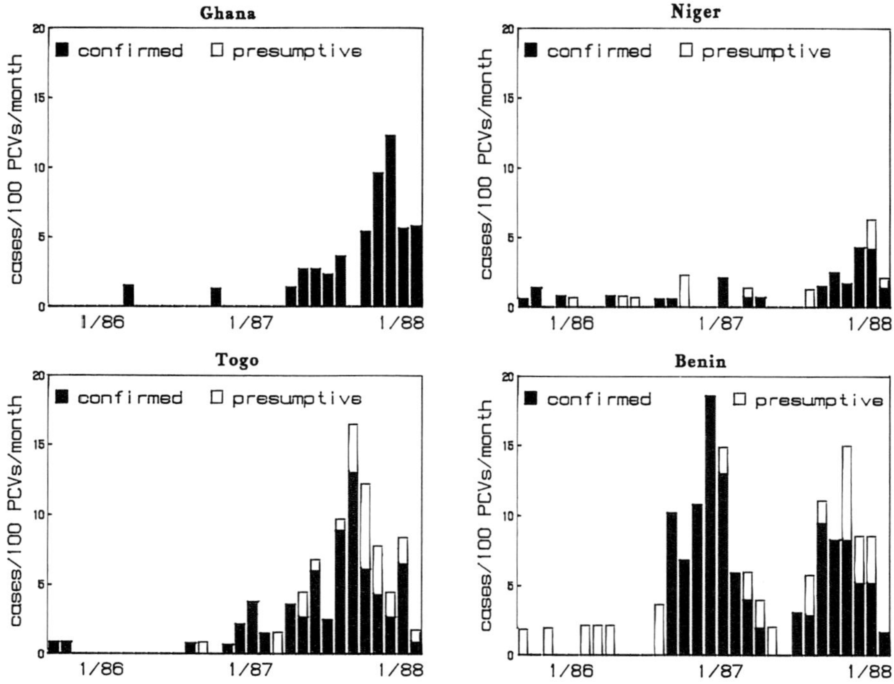


**Fig. 1.** Incidence of confirmed falciparum malaria and presumptive malaria in Peace Corps Volunteers in Benin, Togo, Ghana and Niger, September 1985–February 1988

slide-confirmed cases of falciparum malaria, and the number of cases of presumptive malaria cases of suspected malaria, not confirmed by a reliable laboratory, for which antimalarial treatment was given). Confirmed cases of non-falciparum malaria are also reported but are very rare.

## Results

In the first 3 months of the study period, September–November 1985, there were 7 confirmed cases of falciparum malaria among 1002 PCVs or an incidence of 0.2/100 PCVs per month. In the last 3 months, December 1987–February 1988, there were 53 cases among 998 PCVs or an incidence of 1.8/100 PCVs per month, a ninefold increase. The increase was not uniform in the nine countries surveyed, but occurred earliest in the most easterly country, Benin, a few months later in Togo (which borders Benin on the west) and a few months later in Ghana (which borders Togo on the west) (Fig. 1). A small increase was observed in Niger (which borders Benin on the north) in late 1987. There was no clear-cut pattern of increasing incidence in the five surveyed countries to the west of Ghana (Fig. 2).

The reported incidence of presumptive malaria showed a similar increase in several countries but the pattern of increase was much less distinct (Figs. 1, 2).

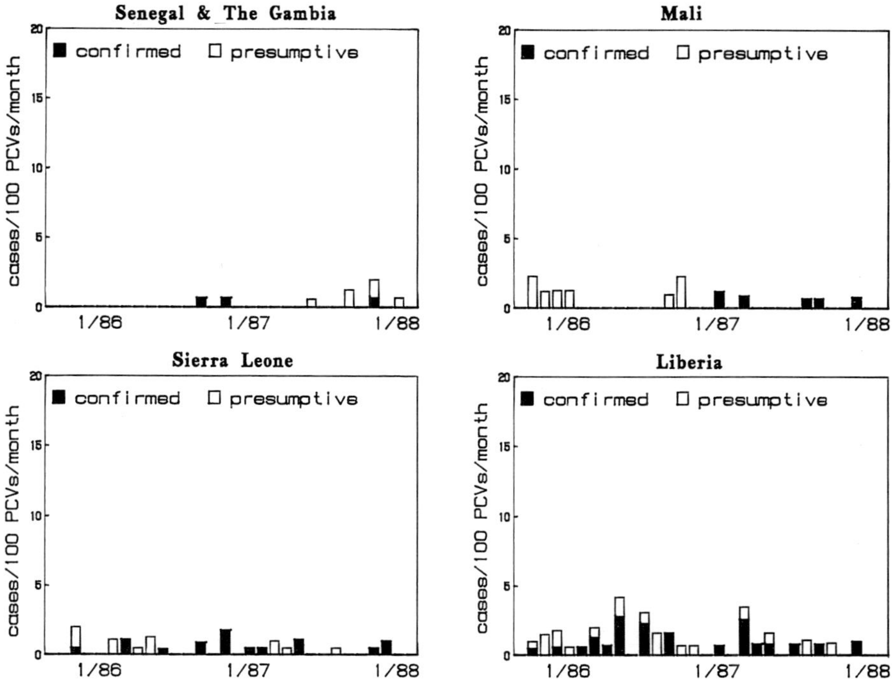


**Fig. 2.** Incidence of confirmed falciparum malaria and presumptive malaria in Peace Corps Volunteers in Liberia, Sierra Leone, Mali, Senegal and The Gambia, September 1985–February 1988

## Discussion

During the 1st year of the study period, cases of confirmed malaria were sporadic and occurred with a similar, low frequency (less than 3 cases/100 PCVs per month) in all countries. These cases included PCVs who missed doses of their chloroquine prophylaxis as well as a few cases associated with travel to known areas of CRPF. These cases can be considered to represent a "background level" of falciparum malaria in PCVs residing in areas without CRPF. The sudden increase in cases in Benin in September 1986, occurring in the absence of any similar sudden increase in any other country, can be best explained as being due to the appearance of CRPF resulting in widespread chloroquine prophylaxis failure. Alternative explanations, such as a sudden decrease in compliance with chloroquine prophylaxis recommendations, limited to Benin PCVs, or a sudden increase in unreported travel by Benin PCVs to CRPF areas, are much less likely. Supporting the hypothesis that the September increase represented the appearance of CRPF in Benin is the isolation by Le Bras et al. of *P. falciparum* parasites resistant in vitro to chloroquine, from patients exposed to malaria in Benin in the same month [4].

The sudden increase in cases in Togo, west of Benin, occurring in December 1986, can likewise be explained as being due to the appearance of CRPF in Togo [5]. The increase in Ghana, west of Togo, in April 1987 follows the pattern in Benin and Togo.

The smaller increase in incidence reported from Niger in September 1987 is also probably due to CRPF. [Three of the cases in Niger were confirmed to be chloroquine prophylaxis failures (JS Moran, unpublished).]

All countries that experienced an abrupt rise in *P. falciparum* infection incidence also later experienced a more gradual decrease in incidence temporally coinciding with the expanded use of additional prophylactic measures including better protection from mosquitoes and increased use of Fansidar and proguanil for prophylaxis.

The persistent low incidence and sporadic occurrence of confirmed cases of *P. falciparum* among PCVs in Liberia, Mali, Sierra Leone, Senegal and The Gambia suggests that CRPF, if it exists in those countries, is not widespread and is not, as a February 1988, a major threat to travellers to those countries.

The malaria surveillance system described here continues to function and should detect the spread of CRPF to far west Africa when it occurs. The same system has also been adapted to collect country-specific data on failure rates of chloroquine + Fansidar and chloroquine + proguanil prophylaxis regimens.

## References

1. Spencer HC, Masaba SC, Kiaraho D (1982) Sensitivity of *Plasmodium falciparum* isolates to chloroquine in Kisumu and Malindi, Kenya. Am J Trop Med Hyg 31:902–906
2. Moran JS (1983) Failure of chloroquine prophylaxis in *Plasmodium falciparum* in Zaire. Lancet II:171–172
3. Lewis AN, Dondero TJ Jr, Ponnanpalam JT (1973) Falciparum malaria resistant to chloroquine suppression but sensitive to chloroquine treatment in West Malaysia. Trans R Soc Trop Med Hyg 67:310–312
4. Le Bras J, Hatin I, Bouree P et al. (1986) Chloroquine-resistant falciparum malaria in Benin. Lancet II:1043–1044
5. Moran JS, Bernard KW, Greenberg AE, Patchen L, Waterman S, Bennett HS (1987) Failure of chloroquine treatment to prevent malaria in Americans in West Africa. JAMA 258:2378–2379

# Malaria Chemoprophylaxis in 28712 European Travelers to Africa: A Follow-up Study

R. Steffen, R. Heusser, R. Mächler, U. Naef, and B. Somaini

Those in charge of formulating recommendations for malaria prophylaxis in short-term travelers must know the:
- Incidence rate of (falciparum) malaria in travelers to various destinations
- Case fatality rate of *Plasmodium falciparum* infection
- Toxicity of the drugs used
- Chemoprophylactic efficacy

Many of these data are not yet available.

## Method

Since May 1985 passengers of two charter (Balair, LTU) and of one scheduled airline (Swissair) were invited to complete a questionnaire (Q1) during their return flight from East Africa (Kenya) or West Africa (eight countries). These questionnaires were distributed and collected by cabin crews. A second questionnaire (Q2) was mailed 12 weeks later to all respondents because malaria and adverse reactions may occur after return. All reported episodes of malaria diagnosed by blood examination and of hospitalizations for adverse reactions were verified by contacting the treating physicians.

## Results

### Population

So far 36367 airline passengers (31890 from East and 4477 from West Africa) completed Q1; 28712 (24795 and 3917 respectively) completed Q2. The response rate for Q1 was 80% of all passengers aboard, and that for Q2 was 78% of the respondents to Q1. The vast majority of the travelers (93%) were vacationers. The male: female ratio was 49% : 51%; 52% were below 40 years of age, 9% were older than 60 years.

### Knowledge, Attitudes and Practices

More than 99% of the travelers were informed about the risk of malaria; 10% (usually business persons) never consulted a medical source but relied on information by friends or on the experience of previous journeys. Only 50% of travelers had been informed by travel agencies about the risk of infection.

Only half of the travelers applied one or more measures against mosquito bites, but less than 1% used a mosquito net *and* repellents *and* insecticides *and* long clothing in the evening.

Overall 90% of the travelers had taken their prophylactic drugs regularly; only few refused to take any medication or stopped taking it while abroad. Side effects were the reason for discontinuing chemoprophylaxis in just about half of these latter cases. There are significant differences in compliance depending on the drug regimen: weekly medication was taken regularly significantly more often than any other regimen.

Many travelers discontinued chemoprophylaxis after return earlier than advised.

## Side Effects

All prophylactic agents were associated with side effects. Single drugs, mainly proguanil and Fansidar, caused fewer side effects than combinations of *two* drugs (Fig. 1). A treatment dose of three tablets of Fansidar or of three to six tablets of mefloquine was used by 4% of those who had carried these standby drugs. Fansidar was well tolerated, but mefloquine caused vertigo and nausea in more than 30% of the patients. Fifteen patients were hospitalized for adverse reactions. Five such cases (two gastrointestinal, one thrombocytopenia, one skin reaction, one encephalopathy) were attributed to chloroquine ($n=$

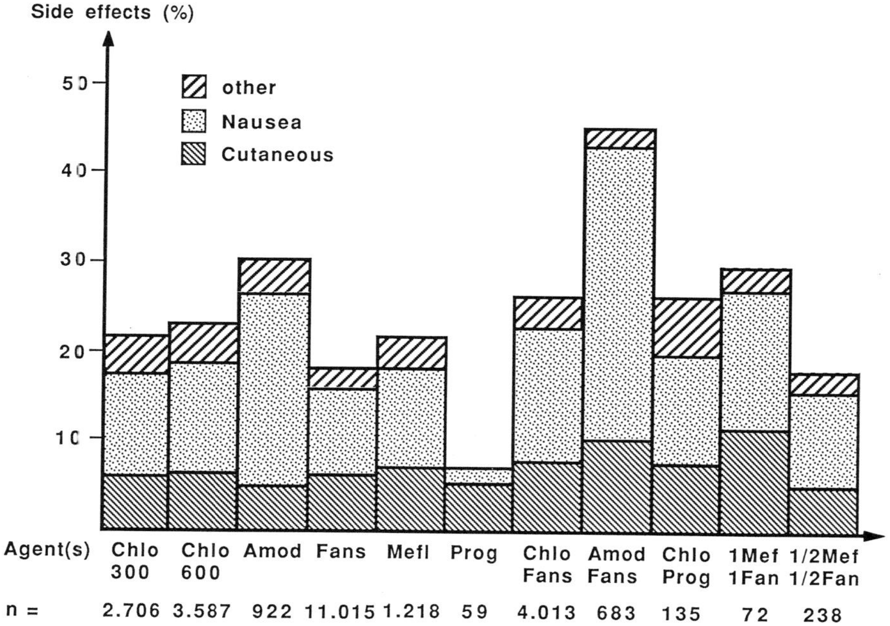


**Fig. 1.** Side effects attributed to malaria chemoprophylaxis. "MALPRO", March 1988, $n=27{,}906$ (3258 excluded, Q1+Q2)

11 458 travelers having used this drug); all recovered. Amodiaquine ($n=1013$) was associated with four cases of agranulocytosis (two fatal) and one case of toxic hepatitis. Fansidar ($n=11\,770$) was associated with one case each of toxic hepatitis, nausea and skin rash. Additionally one patient died of Lyell's syndrome after having used chloroquine plus Fansidar ($n=4013$) plus three double-strength sulfamethoxazole/trimethoprim tablets daily.

## Malaria Incidence in Africa

In 167 cases of malaria diagnosed by a blood smear, 73 were excluded (Africans, duration of stay longer than a year, etc.). Thus, only 94 were evaluated, of which 86% were due to *P. falciparum*. Many cases were diagnosed and treated abroad. Two patients *died* despite regularly using chloroquine for prophylaxis. The monthly incidence rate among travelers who did not take any chemoprophylaxis is estimated to be in West Africa: 18.9/1000, in East Africa: 12.3/1000. These rates are similar to those in US Peace Corps Volunteers (unpublished data). They do *not* include cases of "clinical malaria" diagnosed without a blood film.

## Efficacy of Chemoprophylaxis

The efficacy of chemoprophylaxis in those with good compliance is shown in Table 1.

**Table 1.** Monthly incidence rate of malaria per 1000 non-African travelers with good chemoprophylaxis compliance

| Chemoprophylaxis | Malaria cases | Person-month exposure | Incidence per month | Prophylactic efficacy (%) |
|---|---|---|---|---|
| *East Africa* | | | | |
| None | 6 | 486 | 12.3 | 0 |
| Chloroquine 300–450 mg base/week | 9 | 583 | 15.4 | − 25.2 |
| Chloroquine 600–700 mg base/week | 2 | 758 | 2.6 | 78.6 |
| Amodiaquine | 4 | 316 | 12.7 | − 2.8 |
| Fansidar | 10 | 3866 | 2.6 | 78.9 |
| Mefloquine | 0 | 415 | 0 | 100.0 |
| Chloroquine + Fansidar | 3 | 1397 | 2.1 | 82.6 |
| Amodiaquine + Fansidar | 1 | 276 | 3.6 | 70.6 |
| *West Africa* | | | | |
| None | 4 | 211 | 18.9 | 0 |
| Chloroquine 300–450 mg base/week | 10 | 413 | 24.2 | − 28.0 |
| Chloroquine 600–700 mg base/week | 2 | 264 | 7.6 | 60.0 |

## Conclusions

1. Systematic application of measures against mosquito bites must be instructed and enforced.
2. Continuation of chemoprophylaxis in the 4 weeks after leaving the malaria endemic area must be enforced.
3. All prophylactic agents cause side effects in 7%–45% of users.
4. Mefloquine taken for presumptive therapy (750–1500 mg/24 h) often causes considerable vertigo and nausea.
5. The malaria surveillance systems in industrialized nations underestimate the true incidence of malaria in travelers, because many cases are diagnosed and treated abroad.
6. None of the currently recommended chemoprophylactic regimens (possibly except mefloquine) grants efficacy near 100% in East or in West Africa.
7. Chloroquine 300 mg base/week may give a lower protection than 600 mg base/week, but this must be assessed by a controlled study.

# Malaria Protection for Swissair Crews

R. Wyss

Malaria is a problem in most tropical and subtropical areas of the world. The major problems in providing adequate protection against malaria for aircrews include the widespread resistance of *Plasmodium falciparum* to some antimalarial drugs and the occurrence of adverse reactions in association with prophylactic use of drugs such as amodiaquine and sulfadoxine-pyrimethamine (Fansidar). Recommendations for malaria chemoprophylaxis also have to take into account the reluctance of crews with frequent assignments to tropical routes to use chemoprophylaxis.

## Recommendations for Malaria Protection

Guidelines issued in 1985 recommended chemoprophylaxis only for crews flying to high-risk areas (sub-Saharan Africa) with a greater likelihood of exposure (e.g., several night-stops, lack of air-conditioned rooms). Use of antimosquito measures was considered to provide adequate protection for crews in other parts of the world, including parts of sub-Saharan Africa with reduced exposure to mosquito bites. All crews were advised to carry with them a treatment dose of sulfadoxine-pyrimethamine-mefloquine (Fansimef) to be taken in the event of a febrile illness when professional medical care is not readily available. Those with a history of sulfonamide intolerance were given a treatment dose of mefloquine (Lariam).

## Malaria in Swissair Crews

Data on the incidence of malaria in crews were derived from the Swissair medical certificate of absence from work, which includes a diagnosis, the insurance companies which compensate for occupational diseases, and the distribution of Fansimef to crew.

Malaria was diagnosed in 10 crew members in 1983, 8 in 1984, 11 in 1985, and 14 in 1986. *P. falciparum* parasites were found in 10 of the cases in 1986.

## Use of Prophylaxis and Presumptive Treatment

Between 1982 and 1984, 107000 tablets/year were issued to crew members for chemoprophylaxis. A survey among crew members in 1984 revealed that only 25% regularly used chemoprophylaxis. Between 1985 and 1987, 62000 tablets were issued each year, a reduction of 45000 tablets/year. A treatment dose of Fansimef had been taken by 43 of the 2500 crew members who flew to the tropics in 1986.

## Conclusions

No significant increase of malaria among Swissair crew members has been noted since the introduction of our policy of giving preference to chemotherapy over chemoprophylaxis. This may be due to the relatively low risk for most crew members because they stay mostly in low-risk areas, and in very good hotels in urban areas.

# Long-Term Tolerance of the Triple-Combination Fansimef™ (Mefloquine + Sulfadoxine + Pyrimethamine): Results of a Double-blind Field Trial in Nigeria

H. Kollaritsch, H. Stemberger, H. Mailer, R. Kollaritsch, R. Leimer, and G. Wiedermann

When in 1972 the Walter Reed Army Institute of Research introduced the quinolinemethanol mefloquine, many specialists thought that our problems concerning resistance of *Plasmodium falciparum* would be solved for the next few years.

However, preclinical studies showed that resistance against mefloquine in the *P. berghei*-mouse model could be induced within a short period [1]. In particular, long-term suppressive medication with mefloquine alone bears a relatively high risk of resistance development in vitro as well as in vivo [2]. To overcome this risk of resistance induction, a fixed combination of Mefloquine + Fansidar, Fansimef, was developed. This combination of 250 mg mefloquine plus 500 mg sulfadoxine plus 25 mg pyrimethamine exhibited a gross delay of possible resistance induction. Prophylactic use of Fansidar has been associated with severe side effects in the United States, the United Kingdom, Scandinavia and Australia, but the incidence seems to be low in Switzerland [3, 4].

Fansimef proved to be an effective tool in the treatment of severe and multidrug-resistant *P. falciparum* infections and in the chemosuppression of multidrug-resistant falciparum malaria in semi-immune volunteers in the southeastern part of Burma bordering Thailand [5].

No data on long-term tolerance of Fansimef in Europeans are available; therefore we investigated in a randomized double-blind field trial the side effects of this triple combination during controlled long-term chemoprophylaxis versus chloroquine. The study was conducted in Warri/Benin State, Nigeria, with German and Austrian industrial workers employed at Delta Steel Plant Nigeria.

The volunteers received at random either one tablet Fansimef or one tablet chloroquine, corresponding to 300 mg chloroquine base/week. Of 211 volunteers included in the study, data of 171 participants could be used for statistical analysis as volunteers with only baseline values due to short duration of prophylaxis were excluded.

Volunteers were checked 3-monthly for red and white cell count, platelet and differential count, GOT and GPT, gamma-GT and alkaline phosphatase. To provide information on side effects according to self-observation, detailed questionnaires had to be completed by the volunteers. Mean duration of prophylaxis exceeded 41 weeks in both groups. In total, 37 volunteers taking Fansimef and 42 taking chloroquine were observed for more than 1 year. The main reason for premature termination of chemoprophylaxis was departure from

Nigeria. No acute cases of malaria occurred in either group during suppressive medication. In all cases of intercurrent episodes of fever malaria was excluded parasitologically.

Hematological and biochemical parameters showed only minor deviations assumed not to be of clinical relevance. Significant deviations of liver enzymes could be found, however, within both groups at different times after the start of the trial. Differences between the two groups could not be detected, except at month 3 when GOT and gamma-GT levels increased significantly more in the Fansimef group than in the chloroquine-control group. This observation is also thought not to be of clinical relevance since after 6 months no differences could be found between the two groups and relative to pre-study values. In one patient of the chloroquine group a steady decrease of white cell count occurred during the chemoprophylaxis but complete hematological examination, including sternal puncture, did not show any toxic depression of bone marrow.

Regarding individual tolerance as recorded by the participants various complaints were reported (Table 1). Nine out of 81 volunteers of the Fansimef group complained of side effects; 7 discontinued their prophylaxis because of the adverse reactions. Main complaints were headache, often concomitantly with eye-burning, insomnia, palpitations, and nausea. In all cases of moderate

**Table 1.** Adverse reactions

| Adverse reaction | Intensity | Onset (week of study) | Cessation of prophylaxis (week of study) | Relation to test medication |
|---|---|---|---|---|
| Fansimef group ($n=81$) | | | | |
| Headache | Moderate | 3 | Yes 3 | Remote |
| Headache, eye-burning | Moderate | 1st dose | Yes 3 | Possible |
| Eye-burning | Moderate | 2 | Yes 2 | Possible |
| Palpitations, insomnia | Severe | 3 | Yes 4 | Possible |
| Insomnia nausea | Moderate | 2 | Yes 2 | Possible |
| Palpitations, dizziness | Moderate | 26 | Yes 25 | Improbable |
| Nausea, dizziness | Mild | 22 | Yes 25 | Improbable |
| Nausea | Mild | 35–40 | No – | Improbable |
| Heartburn | Mild | 1st dose | No – | Possible |
| Chloroquine group ($n=90$) | | | | |
| Headache, loss of hair | Mild – moderate | ? | Yes 3 | Possible |
| Nausea, dizziness, vomiting | Moderate | 26–40 | Yes 40 | Possible |
| Headache | Mild | 1st dose | No – | Possible |
| Gastralgia | Mild | ? | No – | Possible |
| Fatigue | Mild | Weeks 1–4 | No – | Improbable |

or severe side effects, no clinical abnormalities could be documented, although ECG and complete clinical examination of these volunteers was performed. Mild complaints reported concerned two cases of nausea and one case of transient gastralgia.

In comparison with the individual results obtained from the volunteers of the chloroquine group (Table 1), Fansimef seems to be less tolerated. Although the differences are statistically not significant, it should be noted that only two participants taking chloroquine discontinued prophylaxis because of side effects, and that insomnia and palpitations exclusively occurred in the Fansimef group. In general, the frequency of adverse reactions seemed to be lower in the chloroquine group. Interestingly, most of the adverse reactions in the Fansimef group leading to cessation of prophylaxis were noted after a short period of intake (median after 2.3 weeks). Considering the pharmacological properties of mefloquine (cumulation factor and steady state are reached after 8–12 weeks [6], a decrease of tolerance should be expected only after maximal cumulation of mefloquine.

We tried to elucidate which component of our triple combination used may cause the specific adverse reactions. Therefore we compared our data with a previous study of long-term tolerance of Fansidar versus chloroquine (Table 2). This study was performed in 1982–1984 in the same region [7]. The study design was completely identical and some 30% of participants included in the first study participated also in this recent field trial. According to these results, the mefloquine component in our Fansimef preparation may be considered to be the cause for most of the moderate or severe side effects, in particular for severe headache, insomnia and palpitations. In several studies

**Table 2.** Comparison of subjective tolerability of Fansimef and Fansidar

| Adverse reaction | Fansimef ($n=81$) | Fansidar (Stemberger et al. 1984) ($n=86$) |
|---|---|---|
| Headache | 2 | – |
| Eye-burning | 2 | – |
| Palpitations | 2 | – |
| Insomnia | 2 | – |
| Nausea | 2 | 1 |
| Dizziness | 2 | – |
| Heartburn | 1 | – |
| Gastralgia | – | 2 |
| Skin rash, erythema | – | 2 |
| Visual disturbance | – | 1 |
| Total of adverse events | 13[a] | 6 |
| No. of volunteers with adverse reactions | 9 | 6 |
| Cessation of prophylaxis because of adverse reactions | 7 | 1 |

[a] In 5 volunteers of the Fansimef group two adverse events occurred concomitantly

evaluating tolerance of mefloquine monotherapy during treatment of *P. falciparum* infections, these complaints were also reported as major problems [8].

In summary, we could not find clinically relevant deviations of laboratory parameters and no evidence for drug-related liver damage, although the subjective tolerance of Fansimef seems to be less than that of chloroquine. Nevertheless the value of this combination should not be ignored. Taking into account adverse side effects, the use of this combination may be restricted to nonimmune persons traveling for a period for more than 3 months to regions with high endemicity of multidrug-resistant *P. falciparum* strains, as for example industrial workers under insufficient medical supervision. In these cases tolerance should be assessed individually, implying that use should start at least 4 weeks prior to departure to evaluate possible side effects under optimal supervision. Furthermore, a different dosage strategy should be considered since the fixed combination used in our trial leads to an extensive and unnecessary cumulation of mefloquine not required for effective suppression of *P. falciparum* parasitemia. It should be emphasized that, because of the relatively small number of participants in our study, we were not able to assess the occurrence of severe cutaneous reactions as reported for Fansidar prophylaxis. Fansimef will clearly be as toxic as Fansidar alone because mefloquine does not suppress adverse reactions caused by sulfonamides.

## References

1. Merkli B, Richle R (1980) Studies on the resistance to single and combined antimalarials in the *Plasmodium berghei* mouse model. Acta Trop (Basel) 37:228–231
2. Merkli B, Richle R (1983) Experimentally derived stable mefloquine resistance in *Plasmodium yoelii nigeriensis*. Trans R Soc Trop Med Hyg 77(1):141–142
3. Miller KD, Lobel HO, Satriale RF et al. (1986) Severe cutaneous reactions among American travelers using pyrimethamine-sulfadoxine (Fansidar) for malaria prophylaxis. Am J Trop Med Hyg 35:451–458
4. Steffen R, Somaini B (1986) Severe cutaneous reactions to sulfadoxine-pyrimethamine in Switzerland. Lancet I:610
5. Win Kyaw Lwin TT, Thwe Y, Win Khin (1985) Combination of mefloquine with sulfadoxine-pyrimethamine compared with two sulfadoxine-pyrimethamine combinations in malaria chemoprophylaxis. Lancet II:694–695
6. Mimica I, Fry W, Eckert G, Schwartz DE (1983) Multiple-dose kinetic study of mefloquine in healthy male volunteers. Chemotherapy 29:184–187
7. Stemberger H, Leimer R, Wiedermann G (1984) Tolerability of long-term prophylaxis with Fansidar: a randomized double-blind study in Nigeria. Acta Trop (Basel) 41:391–399
8. Fernex M, Leimer R (1984) Fortschritte in der Chemoprophylaxe und -therapie der Malaria. Schwerpunktmedizin 7:44–52

# Imported Malaria at Barcelona University Hospital, 1983–1987

G. Añaños, J. Mas, M. E. Valls, M. Corachan, and M. L. Roldan

The Tropical Medicine Unit was established in January 1983 at the University Hospital, Barcelona. Malaria was soon one of the main problems presented by patients attending the unit. The parasitic and epidemiological data for 98 cases seen at the hospital over a 5-year period are presented in Tables 1 and 2. Five cases came from South America, 75 from Africa, and 18 from India and Pakistan.

All 62 cases from West Africa were residents of Equatorial Guinea. Most cases were in tourists from East Africa and India. Tourism to East Africa is a recent development in Spain. The African origin of the cases explains the high proportion of *P. falciparum* (62%). Most of the *P. vivax* cases came from the Indian subcontinent. However, finding seven cases of this species from

**Table 1.** Species distribution

| *Plasmodium falciparum* | | *P. vivax* | | *P. ovale* | | *P. malariae* | |
|---|---|---|---|---|---|---|---|
| West Africa | 48 | West Africa | 7 | West Africa | 5 | West Africa | 7 |
| East Africa | 5 | North Africa | 1 | Central Africa | 2 | | |
| Central Africa | 6 | Pakistan | 6 | India | 1 | | |
| India | 2 | India | 9 | | | | |
| | | Latin America | 5 | | | | |
| | 61 | | 28 | | 8 | | 7 |

Undetermined species two cases
Mixed infections, eight cases

**Table 2.** Prophylaxis of the 63 European cases

| | No. cases |
|---|---|
| No prophylaxis | 12 |
| Correct prophylaxis (but infected by *Plasmodium vivax* | 9 |
| Incorrect prophylaxis | |
| Patients' lack of discipline | 26 |
| Ill advised | |
| Insufficient chloroquine dose (less than 5 mg/kg/week) | 8 |
| Using only chloroquine (in a *P. falciparum* resistant area) | 8 |
| Total of ill-advised patients 25% | |

Equatorial Guinea was unexpected. Therefore a survey concerning Duffy erythrocytic antigenic characteristics has been undertaken in that country. In two cases the *Plasmodium* species could not be determined.

*Prophylactic Measures.* Incomplete compliance was recorded in 26 cases: 16 discontinued prophylaxis before 4 weeks while in Europe and 10 patients took it irregularly. Eight falciparum cases were found in patients who were advised to take less than 5 mg/kg per week.

Many patients from Equatorial Guinea presented to our clinic with bizarre treatment schedules combining quinine and chloroquine at unorthodox dosages (e.g., 400 mg quinine sulfate/day plus 300 mg chloroquine base/day for 5 days).

The results of our experience show that Spain needs to update its health structures dealing with imported diseases. Education is needed on subjects related to with travel and tropical medicine at several levels: travel agencies, general practitioners and medical students. The personnel in charge of vaccination centres and of traveler's clinics should be trained in advising individuals.

# Seasonal Pattern of *Plasmodium vivax* Malaria in Scotland

E. Walker, C. M. Crawford, and G. Urwin

This is an update of an earlier publication [1]. The 193 cases of *Plasmodium vivax* malaria imported into Glasgow from India and Pakistan over 10 years showed a dramatic seasonal pattern, with 85% of cases occurring between May and October of each year regardless of the time of return to Britain. Analysis of the cases shows that the "hypnozoite" stage of the infection varies in length according to the season of the year when exposure occurs. If the infection is contracted during the first 6 months of each year illness is likely to occur during the same year. If infection is contracted during the last 6 months of the year infection is likely to be delayed until the summer of the following year. This is probably the major factor explaining why the time between exposure and illness can extend up to 12 months but not often longer after exposure has taken place. It seems likely that some adaptation of the parasite has taken place which encourages parasites to be present in the blood during the monsoon season in the Punjab of India at the time when mosquito prevalence is at its height. This seasonal pattern of *P. vivax* in cases from India and Pakistan does not appear to be present with *P. vivax* infections from other parts of the world with a less-pronounced monsoon season.

## Reference

1. Walker E (1983) The seasonal pattern of *Plasmodium vivax* malaria in Scotland. J Infect 7:227–230

# Malaria Chemoprophylaxis Among Temporary Residents in Tanzania

C. Hatz and E. Burnier

## Introduction

Until 1984, chloroquine was the universally prescribed drug for chemoprophylaxis and treatment of malaria for expatriates coming to Ifakara (Burnier, unpublished information). However, because *Plasmodium falciparum* strains may be resistant to chloroquine [1], chloroquine is no longer prescribed as the sole prophylaxis and alternative protective measures are needed. Malaria is endemic in Tanzania, which is of great concern to temporary residents [2]. Due to the wide choice of chemoprophylactic drugs currently available and the efficacy of individual protective measures, there is much discussion at any social gathering as to the individual merits of the various protection measures. This also reflects the lack of a consensus among malaria experts.

This report presents the results of a retrospective survey in mid-1987 among temporary residents in Ifakara, southeastern Tanzania, on use of malaria chemoprophylaxis. Malaria is hyper- to holoendemic in this area.

## Methods

A questionnaire was given to all expatriates who had lived for less than 6 years in the Ifakara area. On occasion, blood slides were taken to confirm clinical attacks.

## Results

### Duration of Stay and Age Distribution

The 44 respondents lived in Ifakara between 1 and 55 months (average 23 months). The average age was 25 years. Fifteen respondents were children below 10 years of age and 29 were adults between 26 and 50 years of age. The male to female ratio was 21 : 23. Ten subjects who had lived in Ifakara for more than 7–40 years were excluded from the study because no reliable data could be obtained. The age distribution is typical for expatriate communities in the tropics, the majority being families with young children.

## Advice

Few people followed the advice concerning chemoprophylaxis received from physicians or institutes in their home country. Most temporary residents took a prophylactic regimen that was recommended by a physician in Tanzania or, more often, followed advice of friends in Tanzania. It is very common to change the prophylactic regimen several times during a stay abroad depending on personal experience (Stifl, unpublished data 1987; Nordic Clinic, Dar es Salaam, personal communication).

## Prophylactic Regimens

All but one of the respondents used regular chemoprophylaxis at some stage of their stay in Ifakara. Twenty-two persons had changed their prophylaxis at least once since arrival. Ten different regimens were used. Five persons reported side effects of their regimen: visual disturbance in one person, bad dreams in two persons taking chloroquine and bad dreams and mild skin lesions in one each taking proguanil + amodiaquine.

At the time of the survey, ten persons were not taking any chemoprophylaxis (Table 1). Chloroquine weekly alone or a combination of daily proguanil and weekly chloroquine prophylaxis accounted for the majority of regimes used. Two persons took chlorproguanil twice weekly, one took proguanil daily, and one person took daily chloroquine

These observations differ from those of a survey carried out in 1984 in Ifakara when 49 persons were asked about their chemoprophylaxis: 41 persons (84%) used chloroquine (35 once or twice weekly, 6 daily or on alternate days). Four persons used amodiaquine and only two used proguanil.

**Table 1.** Chemoprophylaxis used by expatriates ($n = 44$)

| Drug used | Number | Percent |
|---|---|---|
| None | 10 | 22.7 |
| Chloroquine | 15 | 34.1 |
| Proguanil + chloroquine | 15 | 34.1 |
| Other drugs | 4 | 9.1 |

## Malaria Infection Rates

A total of 46 malaria attacks were recorded in 25 persons. Of these, 25 attacks were confirmed by blood slide examination. Twenty-two of 34 persons who took a prophylactic drug had 36 malaria attacks (63 person-years). Three of 10 persons without chemoprophylaxis had 10 malaria attacks (19 person-years). Individual rates of malaria attacks are shown in Figs. 1 and 2. The infection rates in people using no chemoprophylaxis, chloroquine alone and in combination with proguanil are listed in Table 2. The number of person-years

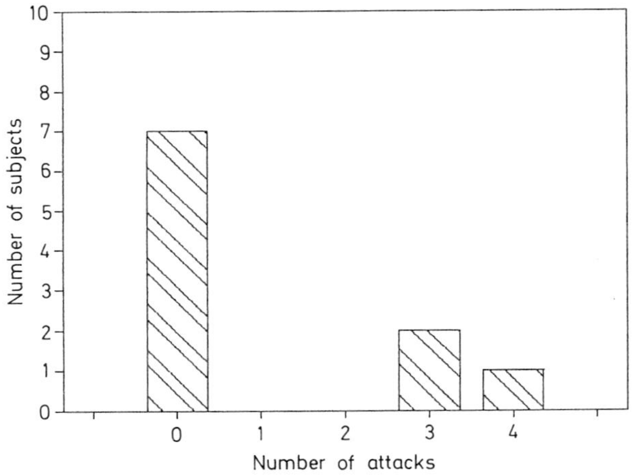


**Fig. 1.** Malaria attacks in individuals without chemoprophylaxis ($n=10$)

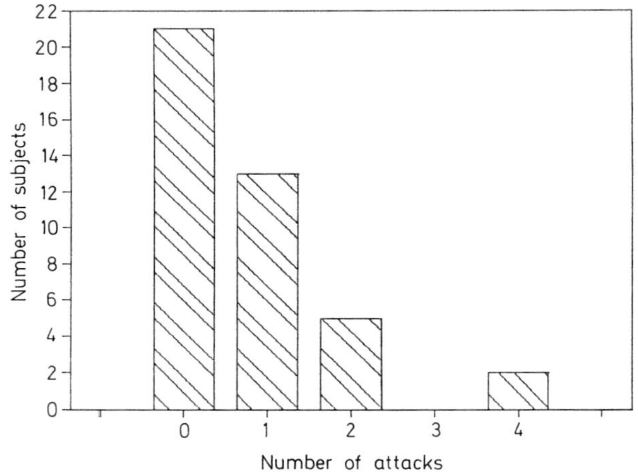


**Fig. 2.** Malaria attacks in individuals under chemoprophylaxis ($n=34$)

for each regimen was calculated by adding the length of time each regimen was used. The malaria infection rate was calculated from the number of malaria attacks per number of person-years times 100.

Statistical analysis showed a significantly lower relative risk of being attacked by malaria in persons using proguanil plus chloroquine than in those using chloroquine alone in an area where chloroquine resistance is present but not abundant. The relative risk of a malaria attack is lower for persons taking proguanil plus chloroquine than for those without chemoprophylaxis. Persons using chloroquine alone appear to have more attacks than people taking no chemoprophylaxis. The influence of personal protective measures could not be

**Table 2.** Malaria infection rates with different chemosuppressive regimens used by 44 persons living in Ifakara for more than 6 years

| | Number of malaria attacks | | | Infection rate by person-years (person-years) |
|---|---|---|---|---|
| | Total | Confirmed | Not confirmed | |
| No prophylaxis | 10 | 6 | 4 | 51.8% (19.3) |
| Chloroquine (weekly/twice weekly) | 24 | 13 | 11 | 75.5% (31.6) |
| Proguanil daily/ chloroquine weekly | 5 | 1 | 4 | 27.3% (18.3) |

Relative risk no prophylaxis vs. proguanil+chloroquine: 1874 (90% CI 0.6–7.4)
Relative risk chloroquine vs. proguanil+chloroquine: 5113 (90% CI 1.9–17.3)

assessed. All persons used bednets at night, most houses had adequate mosquito screens, and repellents were regularly used. Entomological parameters were not assessed.

## Conclusions

The combination of proguanil and chloroquine proved the most effective method of preventing malaria attacks. The advantage of taking chloroquine in addition to proguanil is unclear and requires further study. Malaria attacks in individuals taking no chemoprophylaxis were dispersed, suggesting that some individuals are more exposed to infection. This may be due to behavioral or immunological factors.

There is considerable confusion as to which protective measure should be used in a high-risk malaria area. The present study demonstrates that chloroquine alone provides insufficient protection, a situation that has apparently changed since 1984 when it was almost exclusively recommended and used.

## References

1. Burnier E, Tanner M (1984) Preliminary investigations on the resistance of malaria to chloroquine at St Francis hospital, Ifakara. Proceedings of the Meeting of the Italian Medical Team, Tanzania, 8–10 February, Tosamaganga
2. McLarty D, Webber R, Jaatinen M, Murru M (1984) Chemoprophylaxis of malaria in non-immune residents in Dar es Salaam, Tanzania. Lancet II:656–658

# Time Limits in the Initiation of Treatment of Falciparum Malaria

I. Ebisawa

Serious or fatal cases of malaria are usually due to *Plasmodium falciparum*. We feel it important to emphasize that there is a time limit within which falciparum malaria patients can be safely treated.

## The Patients

A total of 116 cases of infection with *P. falciparum* came to our attention during the period 1966–1987. Included were 7 females, and the patients' ages ranged from 20 to 65 years, with a median of 32 years. A total of 68 patients were infected in Africa, 32 in Southeast Asia, 9 in the Indian subcontinent, and 7 in Oceania. In all, 91 cases recovered uneventfully (age range, 20–65 years with a median of 32 years); however, 25 patients developed serious complications, including disseminated intravascular coagulation, renal failure, and hemoglobinuria, singly or in association with more than one complication. The age range of these patients was 23–53 years, with a median of 35 years.

## Results

*Group 1: Moribound, Seriously Ill, or Fatal Cases.* Of the 25 patients in this group, 8 patients survived, 10 patients died within a mean of 3 days without any improvement of their general condition and 7 patients were diagnosed as having falciparum malaria postmortem. In all these cases serious complica-

**Table 1.** Day of disease on which treatment was started vs. prognosis

| Day of disease treatment was started or died undiagnosed | Moribund or fatal | | | Uneventful recovery | Total |
|---|---|---|---|---|---|
| | Moribund but survived | Treated but died | Died untreated | | |
| 1– 5 | 1 (5th) | | | 45 | 46 |
| 6–10 | 6 | 7 | 3 | 25 | 41 |
| 11–25 | | 3 | 3 | 11 | 17 |
| 16–20 | 1 | | | 4 | 5 |
| 21–67 | | | 1 (23rd) | 6 | 7 |
| Total | 8 | 10 | 7 | 91 | 116 |

tions developed or the patient died on the 5th day or later of illness; the treatment was either then started, or the patient died undiagnosed. Of the cases with serious complications, these developed on day 5 in 1 case (survived); between 6 and 10 in 16 cases (6 survived, 7 were treated but died, and 3 died untreated); between days 11 and 15 in 6 cases (3 treated but died, and 3 died untreated); and between days 16 and 23 in 2 cases (1 survived and 1 died untreated ) (Table 1).

Treatment was started in ten patients after they had developed serious complications and all died. The average day on which the treatment was started in these patients was $8.9 \pm 2.1$ days after the onset of illness, and the average survival time was 3 days after treatment was started.

*Group 2: Uneventful Cases.* Ninety eight percent of the patients recovered uneventfully when treatment was started within 5 days after the onset of illness and 73% when treatment was started 6 days or more after the onset of illness.

## Conclusion

The treatment of falciparum malaria must be started by the 4th day after the onset of illness. This is occasionally difficult because of the insidious nature of falciparum malaria. The importance of educating travelers to malaria endemic areas as well as general physicians about the early symptoms of falciparum malaria is stressed.

# Splenic Infarction: A Complication of *Plasmodium Falciparum* Malaria

J. M. Estavoyer, J. Leroy, D. Amsallem, R. T. Chambers, P. Balvay, and A. le Mouel

The limited efficacy of *Plasmodium falciparum* prophylaxis has resulted in an increase in the number of malaria attacks following travel in tropical areas. In patients who do not take the correct preventive measures, the severity of this particular form is primarily related to the risk of developing cerebral malaria. Other life-threatening complications occur less frequently.

A 29-year-old male, without any significant medical history, spent 15 days in Zaire in 1987. Three days after returning to France, despite chloroquine prophylaxis, he presented with fever (40 °C) and splenomegaly without altered consciousness.

Laboratory tests revealed moderate anemia, 3 100 000 RBC/mm$^3$, hemoglobin 10.6 g/dl; hemolysis, total bilirubin 21 µmol/liter ($N \leqq 18$ µmol/liter), haptoglobin 0.3 g/liter ($N$, 0.5–2.7 g/liter); leukopenia, 2800/mm$^3$; thrombocytopenia, 33 000/mm$^3$ without associated hemostasis abnormality. Thick and thin smears showed *P. falciparum*. Blood cultures, coprocultures and other parasitic studies were normal.

Apyrexia was achieved after 48 h of treatment with iv. quinine. Recovery was satisfactory until the 7th day, at which time the patient presented with se-

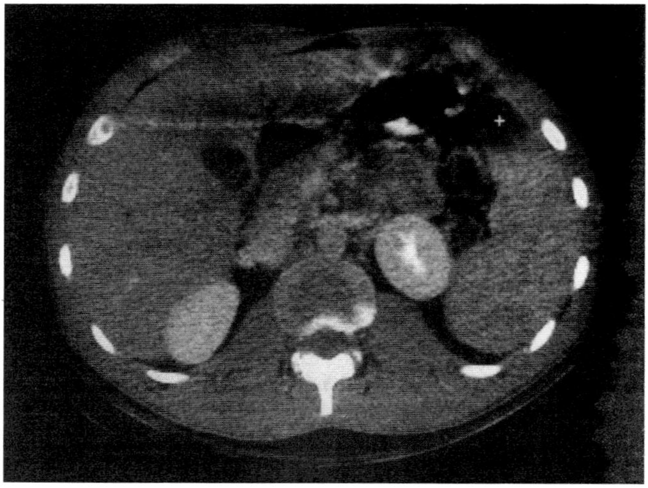

**Fig. 1.** Computed tomography scan: hypodensity without contrast enhancement in the anterioinferior region of the spleen

vere left upper quadrant pain without shock. An abdominal ultrasound study demonstrated a hypoecogenic area, 2.5 cm in diameter, in the anteroinferior region of the spleen. A CT scan of the same region (Fig. 1) showed a hypodense area without contrast enhancement. These images were consistent with splenic infarction.

Splenic infarction is a rare complication of malaria [1, 2]. It may go unrecognized and occasionally precedes splenic rupture. The physiopathology, which is not yet fully understood, appears to involve two mechanisms: microcirculation abnormalities due to agglutination (sludge effect) and lysis of red blood cells, and a cytotoxic anoxia phenomenon due to Maegraïth toxin.

The diagnosis of splenic infarction due to malaria should be considered in patients who have traveled in endemic zones presenting with fever and left upper quadrant pain, after ruling out sickle cell disease and salmonella infection.

## References

1. Christoforov B, Chiche B, Duflo B, Laffitte M, Fresneau M, Pequignot H (1976) Infarctus splénique au cours d'une primo-invasion à *Plasmodium falciparum*. Ann Med Interne (Paris ) 127:47–49
2. Manson-Bahr PEC, Apted FIC (1982) Malaria and babesiosis. In: Manson's tropical disease. Bailliere-Tindall, London, p 51

# Cellular and Molecular Aspects of Phagocytosis in Mice Treated with Pyran and Infected with *Plasmodium Yoelii*

V. Radha Krishna, M. M. Fouant, and S. G. Bradley

The polyanion, pyran copolymer, is formed by the polymerization of divinyl ether and maleic anhydride. This agent has numerous immunomodulatory effects (Shopp and Munson 1984) including induction of interferon, complement, enhanced antiviral activity, antineoplastic activity and priming of macrophages. Effects on the reticuloendothelial system (RES) are often biphasic with a suppression of RES activity followed by an enhancement of the RES (Munson et al. 1981).

Treatment of female B6C3F1 mice with pyran copolymer i.v. on days −4 and −3 elicited a modest reticulocytosis (9.4% ± 0.6% vs. 4.8% ± 0.3% for untreated mice) and provoked a modest anemia ($4.3 \pm 0.8 \times 10^6/\text{mm}^3$ vs. $9.5 \pm 0.5 \times 10^6/\text{mm}^3$) 6 days after drug administration. Mice treated with pyran i.v. on days −4 and −3 before challenge with *P. yoelii* developed a more severe parasitemia on day 14 and the parasitemia persisted on day 17 as compared with vehicle-treated infected control mice. Similarly, anemia was more severe and persisted longer in pyran-treated infected mice than in vehicle-treated infected mice. Moreover, mice treated with 25 mg/kg pyran i.v. on days −3 and −2 and challenged with *P. yoelii* on day 0 developed a more severe parasitemia than vehicle-treated mice, and the parasitemia persisted longer.

Mice treated with pyran i.p. on days −4 and −3 before challenge displayed slightly higher levels of parasitemia than vehicle-treated *P. yoelii*-infected mice. Similarly, the anemia in pyran-treated mice was more severe than that in vehicle-treated *P. yoelii*-infected mice. All mice recovered from *P. yoelii* infections. Mice treated with pyran i.v. on days −3 and −2 before challenge with *P. berghei* developed a more severe parasitemia than vehicle-treated infected mice. Severe anemia developed earlier in pyran-treated infected mice than in vehicle-treated infected mice. All mice infected with *P. berghei* died.

Mice treated i.v. with pyran on days −3 and −2 before challenge with *L. monocytogenes* showed the same susceptibility as vehicle-treated infected mice. Conversely mice treated i.p. with pyran on days −3 and −2 before challenge were protected from a lethal challenge. Peritoneal exudate cells (PECs) from mice treated with pyran i.p. showed enhanced zymosan-induced chemiluminiscence but mice treated with pyran i.v. did not. Similarly phagocytosis of Covaspheres by PECs was enhanced more by pyran i.p. than by pyran i.v. Adherent splenocytes from mice treated with pyran i.p. or i.v. showed enhanced zymosan-induced chemiluminiscence as compared with those from untreated mice.

Membranes of resident PECs possessed proteolytic activity as measured by digestion of azocasein at pH 8.5. The azocaseinase activity was completely inhibited by phenylmethylsulfonyl fluoride (2 m*M*) and soya bean trypsin inhibitor (2 m*M*) and partially inhibited by ethylenediaminetetraacetate (10 m*M*) and phenanthroline (10 m*M*). Comparable membrane preparations of PECs from pyran-treated mice have markedly reduced levels of azocaseinase activity.

The membrane-bound azocaseinase activity appears to be a serine protease. Serine proteases localized within the cytoplasmic granules have been related to target killing by cytotoxic T-lymphocytes (Redmond et al. 1987). The macrophage membrane serine protease activity is lost upon priming the peritoneal exudate cell population with pyran. This protease has no role in host resistance to *Listeria* but might afford some protection in murine malaria.

Macrophage priming appears to play a paradoxical role in susceptibility to murine malaria as compared with susceptibility to *L. monocytogenes*. Host resistance to murine malaria is impaired by giving pyran i.p. or i.v. Brown and Kreier (1986) have observed that macrophages activated by *Corynebacterium parvum in vivo* have decreased capability to bind to free *Plasmodium* in vitro in the presence of normal serum as compared with resident macrophages. These results are consistent with our unpublished observations that phagocytosis by PECs from i.v. treated and infected mice is lower than that by the untreated and uninfected mice of by untreated and infected mice or by i.v. treated and uninfected mice.

## References

Brown KM, Kreier JP (1986) Effect of macrophage activation on phagocyte-*Plasmodium* interaction. Infect Immun 51:744–749

Munson AE, White KL Jr, Klykken PC (1981) Pharmacology of MVE polymers. In: Hersh EM, Chirigos MA, Mastrangelo MJ (eds) Augmenting agents in cancer therapy. Raven, New York, pp 329–343

Redmond MJ, Letellier M, Parker JMR, Lobe C, Havele C, Paetkau, Bleackley RC (1987) A serine protease (ccpi) is sequestered in the cytoplasmic granules of cytotoxic T lymphocytes. J Immunol 139:3184–3188

Shopp GM, Munson AE (1984) Modification of the pharmacokinetics of MVE-2 to enhance its effects on host resistance. In: Kende M, Gainer J, Chirigos M (eds) Chemical regulation of immunity in veterinary medicine. Lix, New York, pp 501–509

# Round Table Discussion

## Recommendations for Malaria Prevention in European Countries

D. J. Bradley (Chairman and Rapporteur)
and P. Phillips-Howard (Rapporteur)

In the course of studies on the reporting of malaria imported into European countries, we made inquiries of the regimes of malaria prophylaxis recommended for use by each country, or the practice generally followed for travel-

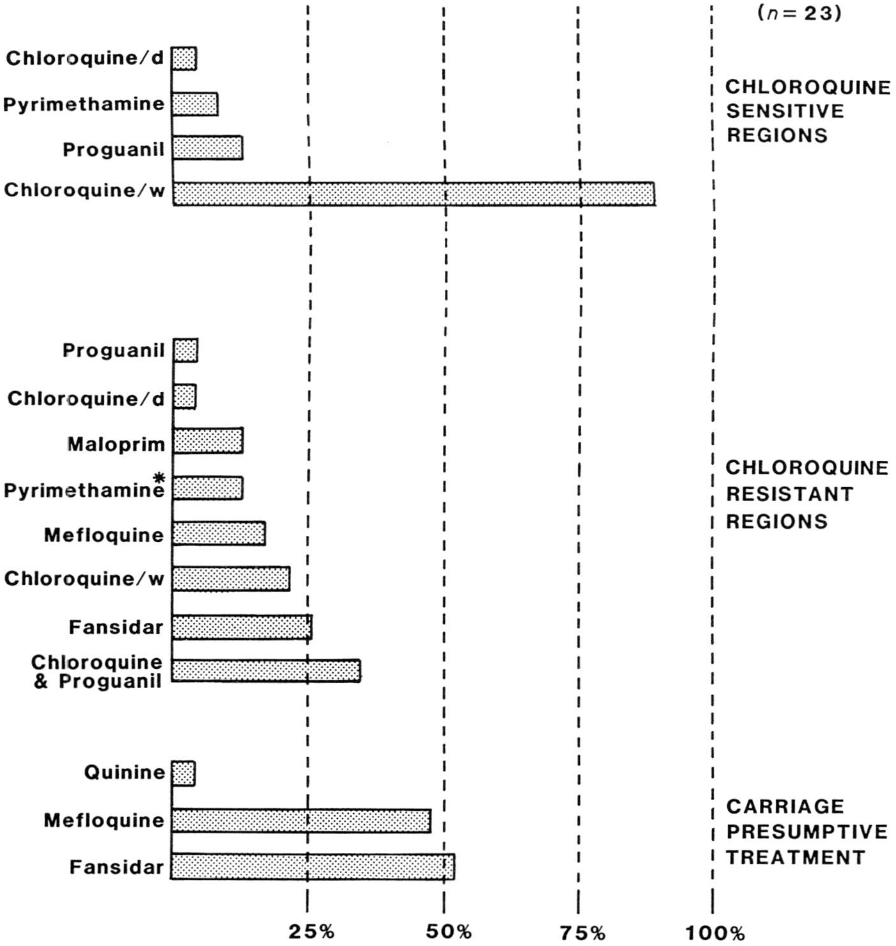


**Fig. 1.** Recommended malaria chemoprophylaxis for European travellers

… [Data collected during surveillance survey (Phillips-Howard and Bradley 1988)]

| Regimens | Ireland | Spain | Italy | Greece | Hungary | Portugal | Netherlands | UK | Finland | Denmark | Sweden | Malta | Belgium | GDR | Luxembourg | Norway | Poland | Switzerland | Bulgaria | Austria | France | GFR | Yugoslavia |
|---|---|---|---|---|---|---|---|---|---|---|---|---|---|---|---|---|---|---|---|---|---|---|---|
| 1. *CQSPF* | | | | | | | | | | | | | | | | | | | | | | | |
| Py 25/w–50/w | × | × | | | | | | | | | | | | | | | | | | | | | |
| P 100/d | × | | | | | | × | | | | | | | | | | | | | | | | |
| Py 50/w + P 100/d | × | | | | | | | | | | | | | | | | | | | | | | |
| P 200/d | | | | | | | | × | | | | | | | | | | | | | | | |
| CQ 300/w | | × | × | × | × | × | ×* | × | × | × | × | × | × | × | × | × | × | × | × | × | | × | × |
| CQ 100/d # | | | | | | | | | | | | | | | | | | | | | × | | |
| 2. *CQRPF* | | | | | | | | | | | | | | | | | | | | | | | |
| P 200/d | | | | | | | | | | | | | | | | | | | | | | | |
| CQ 300/w | × | | × | | | × | | | | | | | | × | × | | | | | | | | |
| CQ 100/d | | | | | | | | | | | | | | | | | | | | | × | | |
| CQ 300/w × 2 | | × | | | | | | | | | | | | | | | | | | | | | |
| CQ 300/w + P 100/d | | | | | | | ×* | | | | | | × | | | | | | | | | | |
| CQ 300/w + P 200/d | | | | | | | | × | × | × | × | × | | | × | | | | | | | | |
| M 1/w | × | | | | | × | | | | | | | | | | | | | | | | | |
| M 1/w + P 200/d | × | | | | | | | | | | | | | | | | | | | | | | |
| M 1/w + CQ 300/w | | | | | | | | × | | | | | | | | | | | | | | | |
| Py 100 × 2/w | | × | | | | | | | | | | | | | | | | | | | | | |
| CQ 300/w + Py > 50/w | | | | × | × | | | | | | | | | | | | | | | | | | |
| F 1/w | | | | | | | | | | | | | | | | | × | × | × | × | | | × |
| F 2/2w | | | | | | | | | | | | | | | | | | | × | | | | |
| F 1/w + CQ 300/w | | | | | | | | | | | | | | | | × | | | | | | | |
| Mf 1/w | | | | | | | | | | | | | | | × | | | | | × | × | × | |
| 3. *Carriage* | | | | | | | | | | | | | | | | | | | | | | | |
| F 3/od | | | | | × | | × | | | × | × | × | × | × | | × | | × | | × | × | × | |
| Mf 3/od | | | | | | | | | | × | × | × | × | | × | × | | × | | × | × | × | |
| Q | | | | | | | | | | | | | | | | | | | | | × | | |

P, proguanil; CQ, chloroquine; Py, pyrimethamine; M, Maloprim; F, Fansidar; Mf, mefloquine; Q, quinine; d, day; w, week; *, bolus CQ 600 mg; #, 6 days a week; 100, 100 mg; 200, 200 mg; 300, 300 mg; 1, 1 tablet; /2w, a fortnight; w × 2, twice weekly; /od, once only; 2, 2 tablets; CQSPF, areas with chloroquine-sensitive *P. falciparum;* CQRPF, areas with chloroquine-resistant *P. falciparum* lers from that country to malarious areas. For simplicity of presentation we have considered three categories of advice: chemoprophylaxis for areas where malaria is prevalent but *Plasmodium falciparum* is sensitive to chloroquine; chemoprophylaxis for areas with chloroquine-resistant *P. falciparum*; and for countries which recommend the carriage of an antimalarial for self-treatment in difficult circumstances and where chloroquine resistance occurs, the drug recommended to be carried.

The detailed results of our inquiries are summarized in Table 1. It is seen that there is substantial consistency of advice for visiting places without chloroquine resistance and on the drugs to be carried (if any). Over chemoprophylaxis for preventing chloroquine-resistant falciparum malaria there is far from any uniformity or consistency.

This is illustrated in Fig. 1, which shows clearly the preponderance of chloroquine as the drug of choice in susceptible areas and the confusion over recommendations in chloroquine-resistant areas. The diagram underestimates the consistency over carriage of presumptive treatment in that about half the countries recommend this and the majority of that half recommend both Fansidar and mefloquine (but the traveller to take one of them with him or her).

The data are not adequate for a clear rational decision for one regime for chloroquine-resistant malarious areas, but, even if they were, consistency between countries would be limited because several of the drugs are registered only in some of the countries of Europe.

This material provided a factual basis for the subsequent discussion.

# Vaccine Preventable Diseases, Vaccines, Immune Globulins

# General Use Immunizations for Travelers

S. R. Preblud, E. W. Brink, and W. A. Orenstein

## Summary

Immunizations for travelers can be divided into two categories: those required solely by various country regulations (cholera and yellow fever vaccines), and those recommended specifically for the health and well-being of the traveler. Some immunizations in the second category are recommended only under special circumstances (e.g., typhoid, meningococcal, Japanese encephalitis, and yellow fever vaccines). Others are recommended on a more routine basis since they are included in the routine immunization schedule of a particular country. The latter are "general-use" immunizations and include diphtheria and tetanus toxoids and pertussis vaccine (DTP); pediatric and adult diphtheria and tetanus toxoids (DT and Td, respectively); and measles and polio vaccines. Rubella, BCG, and mumps vaccines may also be included in this classification. In contrast with many other travel-related immunizations, recommendations for these "general-use" immunizations are relatively straightforward. They are usually indicated for any traveler who does not have documented immunity, provided there are no contraindications to their administration. The issues most frequently raised regarding administration of the "general-use" immunizations include (1) the criteria for immunity, (2) the simultaneous administration of these and other immunizations, (3) the minimum interval required between doses when departure necessitates an accelerated immunization schedule, and (4) the minimum age at which they can be administered to infants. As the number of international travelers increases, and as countries strive both to safeguard the health of travelers and to limit the importation and spread of vaccine-preventable diseases, attention to these "general-use" immunizations becomes increasingly important.

## Introduction

Every year, millions of persons travel outside their country of origin. Many venture to exotic and exciting lands which may place them at risk for maladies not usually encountered at home [1–3]. Some of the illnesses that the traveler may encounter can be prevented by immunizations. These immunizations can be divided into two general categories: those required solely by various country regulations (cholera and yellow fever vaccines) and those recommended specifically for the health and well-being of the traveler. Some immunizations in the second category are recommended only under special circumstances [e.g., typhoid, meningococcal, Japanese encephalitis, and yellow fever vaccines and immune globulin (IG)]. Others are recommended on a more routine basis since they are included in the routine immunization schedule of a particular country. The latter are "general-use" immunizations and include diphtheria and tetanus toxoids and pertussis vaccine (DTP); pediatric and adult diphtheria and tetanus toxoids (DT and Td, respectively); and polio and measles vaccines. Depending on the country, rubella, mumps, *Haemophilus influenzae* type b (Hib), and BCG vaccines may also be included in this classification.

In contrast with many other travel-related immunizations, recommendations to administer these "general-use" immunizations are relatively straightforward. They are usually indicated for any traveler who does not have documented immunity, provided there are no contraindications to their administration.

## General Considerations

To facilitate this discussion, a few generic comments on contraindications and simultaneous administration that apply to these immunizations are necessary. Minor illnesses, such as mild upper-respiratory infections with or without low-grade fever, should not be a reason to defer vaccination. However, infants and children who have an illness accompanied by a high temperature usually should have their immunization postponed until they have recovered. In general, vaccines are contraindicated in persons with a history of an anaphylactic reaction to vaccine components. Finally, live attenuated vaccines usually should not be administered to pregnant women or immunocompromised persons [4, 5].

Regarding simultaneous administration, based on currently available data, these antigens can be administered simultaneously with no impaired antibody responses or increased rates of adverse reactions [6–8]. It also appears that simultaneous administration of any of these vaccines with other combinations of live and inactivated vaccines can be recommended. Finally, since IG may interfere with replication of live attenuated viruses, parenterally administered live vaccines should not be given within 6 weeks, and preferably 3 months, after IG use. If IG is given after a live vaccine preparation, it should be given no sooner than 2 weeks later. Since there is little interaction between IG preparations and inactivated preparations, the latter can be given simultaneously or at any time interval before or after IG is used.

## Diphtheria, Tetanus Toxiods and Pertussis Vaccine

### Indications and Use

Diphtheria is a serious disease that is endemic in many developing countries. Tetanus is ubiquitous worldwide. Pertussis is common in developing countries and in some developed countries where routine immunization is not practiced as widely as in other countries, for example the United States and Canada. Because of the risk of contracting these diseases while traveling abroad, travelers should be as well immunized as possible before departure. In the United States, equal emphasis is placed on preventing all three of these infections [9, 10].

Immunization is indicated for any person without documentation of age-appropriate vaccination if there are no contraindications. Because the incidence and severity of pertussis decreases with age and because the vaccine causes side effects and adverse reactions, routine pertussis immunization is not routinely recommended for persons 7 years of age or older. If the recommended immunization schedule has been interrupted, there is no need to restart a series regardless of the time elapsed between doses since there is no reduction in immunity. Pertussis vaccination is not necessary following culture-proven pertussis. In contrast, previous infection with tetanus, and probably diphtheria (to provide a margin of safety), does not obviate the need for vaccination.

Unimmunized infants and children traveling to areas where diphtheria or pertussis are endemic or epidemic preferably should receive three doses of DTP, the first no sooner than 6 weeks of age and the next two doses at intervals of no less than 4 weeks [11]. While two doses of DTP received at intervals of at least 4 weeks probably provide protection against diphtheria and tetanus, three doses may be advisable for infants; three doses are needed for good protection against pertussis [12, 13]. Infants and other children less than 7 years of age who at the time of travel have received less than three doses of DTP and who will remain for extended periods in areas of increased risk of exposure to pertussis or diphtheria should complete their remaining doses at 4-week intervals (instead of the more customary 8-week intervals). A fourth dose to help maintain immunity against diphtheria, tetanus, and pertussis should be administered for infants and children traveling internationally or remaining in areas of high risk. While the interval between the third and fourth dose is customarily 6–12 months, reducing the interval to 6 months may be considered.

For children under 7 years old with a contraindication to pertussis vaccine, and for persons 7 years of age and older, DT or Td, respectively, should be used instead of DTP if there are no other contraindications. Three doses of diphtheria and tetanus toxoids provide protection (although four doses may be optimal for unimmunized infants receiving their first DT dose). The first two doses of diphtheria and tetanus toxoid containing preparations are commonly administered 4–8 weeks apart with the third dose administered 6–12 months later. As with DTP, the shorter intervals may be used if the risk of exposure is great. While there are varying opinions, United States travelers are advised to receive a Td booster every 10 years.

## Side Effects and Adverse Reactions

Local reactions, generally erythema and induration with or without tenderness, are common after receipt of DTP, DT, and Td (in up to 50% or more of vaccinees). Mild systemic reactions such as fever, drowsiness, fretfullness, and anorexia occur in up to one-half of DTP vaccinees. More severe systemic events such as fever $\geqq 40.5$ °C, persistent or unusual high-pitched crying, and collapse (hypotonic hyporesponsive episode) or convulsions occur relatively infrequently (approximately 1/330, 1/100, 1/900, and 1/1750 DTP doses, respectively). Rarely, severe neurologic events such as prolonged seizures or encephalopathy have occurred after receipt of DTP. The estimated risk of acute serious neurologic illness occurring within 7 days of DTP is approximately 1/140000 doses; for permanent neurologic damage, approximately 1/330000 doses [14].

Rarely, an anaphylactic reaction has been reported after receiving one of these preparations. Arthus-type hypersensitivity reactions, characterized by severe local reactions, may follow administration of tetanus toxoid, particularly in adults who have received frequent boosters of tetanus toxoid. Current data indicate that DTP is not causally related to sudden infant death syndrome or infantile spasms.

## Precautions and Contraindications

There is not total agreement on the adverse events following DTP vaccination that should be considered absolute contraindications to further vaccination with pertussis antigen. However, many authorities agree on the following: (1) allergic hypersensitivity, (2) fever of $\geqq 40.5$ °C within 48 h, (3) collapse or shock-like state (hypotonic-hyporesponsive episode) within 48 h, (4) persisting, inconsolable crying lasting 3 h or more or an unusual, high-pitched cry occurring within 48 h, (5) convulsions with or without fever occurring within 3 days, or (6) encephalopathy within 7 days. In the United States, a personal history of a seizure occurring more than 3 days after receipt of DTP, a personal history of an unrelated seizure disorder, or a first-degree family (i.e., siblings or parents) history of convulsions are not considered absolute contraindications to further DTP vaccination. In addition, vaccine is indicated for children with stable, resolved, or corrected neurologic disorders.

The only contraindication to tetanus and diphtheria toxoids is a history of a neurologic or a severe hypersensitivity reaction following a previous dose. Persons with a history of anaphylaxis to diphtheria or tetanus toxoids, or to vaccine components such as thimerosol, may benefit from intradermal skin testing. If a contraindication to tetanus toxoid exists, tetanus immune globulin (TIG), preferably, or tetanus antitoxin (TAT) should be used in wound management.

These preparations are not contraindicated in immunocompromised individuals. Although there is no evidence that tetanus and diptheria toxoids are teratogenic, postponing administration of Td until the second trimester may be considered to minimize any theoretical concern if time permits. Td is particularly important for unimmunized pregnant women who may deliver in a developing country because of the possible increased risk of neonatal tetanus.

# Polio Vaccine

## Indications and Use

In developed countries such as Japan, Australia, New Zealand, the United States, Canada, Japan, and the eastern or western European countries, the risk of acquiring poliomyelitis is quite low. In contrast, all developing countries should, in general, be considered endemic for poliomyelitis. Therefore, travelers to such countries are, in general, at increased risk of exposure to polioviruses and should be immune.

Polio immunization [with oral polio vaccine (OPV), conventional or enhanced-potency inactivated polio vaccine (IPV), or combinations thereof] is indicated for any person without documentation of age-appropriate vaccination if there are no contraindications [15, 16]. As with the diphtheria-, tetanus-, and pertussis-containing antigens, there is no need to restart a series regardless of the time elapsed between doses if the recommended immunization schedule has been interrupted.

Because of the variety of polio vaccines in use and the great variation in immunization schedules (both in terms of the types of vaccines and numbers of doses used in the primary series) among developed countries, it is beyond the scope of this presentation to discuss polio immunization schedules in detail. However, some generic points will be made. In general, virtually all vaccinees seroconvert to the three serotypes of polio virus following three doses of either OPV or enhanced-potency IPV or four doses of conventional IPV [11, 12, 17]. However, for travel to an endemic area, an additional dose of vaccine is advisable. The need for further additional doses has not been established.

While OPV is the recommended vaccine for primary immunization in many countries, including the United States, the usual vaccine of choice for adults (e.g., those $\geqq 18$ years of age) who may need immunization against polio is an IPV preparation. The availability of the enhanced-potency IPV may lead to changes in the few existing recommendations to administer OPV to adults. An example is the previous recommendation in the United States to give one dose of OPV to unimmunized adults if time does not permit receipt of at least two doses of conventional IPV; enhanced-potency IPV may now be given instead of OPV.

Although polio immunization is frequently started at 6–12 weeks of age, a dose of OPV can be administered in the newborn period, e.g., at birth or before 6 weeks of age as recommended by the Expanded Programme on Immunization (EPI) of the World Health Organization [11, 18]. However, this dose does not count in the primary immunization series. Based on the EPI recommendations, the three-dose OPV primary series can be administered at 4-week intervals instead of the longer intervals customarily recommended. In the United States, enhanced-potency IPV is recommended at 8 weeks of age with the second and third doses given 8 weeks and 12 months later, respectively. However, the immunization can be begun as early as 6 weeks of age with 4-week intervals between subsequent doses. These recommendations are useful for infants traveling to endemic areas and who will remain at risk.

### Side Effects and Adverse Reactions

In rare instances, administration of OPV has been associated with paralysis in healthy recipients (1/7.8 million doses) and their contacts (1/5.5 million) [19]. No serious side effects of the IPV preparations have been documented.

### Precautions and Contraindications

Neither immunoglobulin nor breast milk have been shown to interfere with OPV. OPV is contraindicated in persons who are themselves immunocompromised or who are in close contact with immunocompromised persons. In these situations, IPV is the vaccine of choice. Since IPV preparations may contain trace amounts of antibiotics such as streptomycin and neomycin, persons with a history of an anaphylactic reaction following administration of these antibiotics should not be vaccinated.

There is no convincing evidence that either OPV or conventional IPV are teratogenic; there are no data for enhanced-potency IPV. On theoretical grounds, it is best to avoid vaccinating pregnant women. However, if vaccination is indicated, OPV is the vaccine of choice in the United States.

## Measles Vaccine

### Indications and Use

Measles is endemic in many developing countries and in some developed countries where measles immunization is not routinely practiced. Although vaccination against measles is not a requirement for entry into any country, persons traveling abroad should be immune since measles is often severe, particularly in young children and adults [20]. Adults who may have received killed measles vaccine and have not been revaccinated with live vaccine have the additional risk of developing atypical measles. In the United States, persons are considered susceptible to measles if they lack documentation of appropriate immunization with live measles vaccine on or after the first birthday, physician-diagnosed measles, or laboratory evidence of immunity [21].

Based on the trends in reported measles cases in the United States following licensure of measles vaccine in 1963, most persons born in that country before 1957 are likely to have been naturally infected and generally are not considered to be susceptible. However, since measles vaccine is not 100% effective and since the risk of exposure to measles abroad may be substantially greater than in the United States, the Center for Disease Control (CDC) has recommended that persons born after 1956 who travel abroad receive a one-time dose of vaccine regardless of their previous vaccination status.

Vaccine is indicated for all susceptible persons if there are no contraindications. Measles vaccine can be administered alone or in combination with rubella and mumps vaccine in vaccinees 12 months of age and older. In some countries, combined measles, mumps, and rubella (MMR) vaccine is administered routinely.

The age at vaccination should be lowered for those children traveling to areas where measles is endemic or epidemic. In the United States where MMR is administered routinely at 15 months of age, MMR may be administered at 12–14 months of age before departure [22]. Children 6–11 months of age should receive a dose of single measles antigen vaccine before departure and subsequently should be revaccinated (with MMR vaccine if that is the usual practice). While the optimal age at revaccination is considered to be 15 months in the United States, the age at revaccination may be as low as 12 months if the child remains in a high-risk area. Since virtually all infants less than 6 months of age will be protected by maternally derived antibodies, no additional means to provide protection against measles is generally necessary.

## Side Effects and Adverse Reactions

Primary vaccination may be associated with a transient rash in 5% and fever of ≧39.4 °C in 5%–15% of vaccinees. The rash usually starts 7–10 days after vaccination and lasts 2–4 days. The fever usually begins about the 5th–6th day following immunization and lasts approximately 2 days. Encephalitis and encephalopathy have been reported with a frequency of 0.3 cases/million doses of vaccine administered (1 case/3.6 million doses) (unpublished CDC data). This rate is lower than that noted for severe neurologic disorders of unknown etiology, suggesting that chance temporal association rather than cause-and-effect accounts for some if not all cases. Persons with a personal or first-degree family (i.e., siblings or parents) history of convulsions have an increased risk of a febrile seizure following measles vaccination. However, the risk is small and it does not preclude vaccination. There is no evidence that vaccination of persons who are already immune to measles, either from vaccination or natural disease, is associated with an increased risk of vaccine-associated adverse events. Thus, routine prevaccination antibody testing for susceptibility is not necessary.

## Precautions and Contraindications

Based on theoretical considerations, vaccine should not be administered to pregnant women. Furthermore, conception should be prevented for 3 months after vaccination. A history of an anaphylactic reaction to vaccine components such as neomycin is also a contraindication to vaccination. Since there is no evidence that measles vaccine exacerbates tuberculosis, tuberculin skin testing does not need to be performed before vaccination. Although immunosuppression is also a contraindication to measles vaccination, the CDC has recommended that measles vaccine (as well as mumps and rubella vaccines) should be administered to persons with asymptomatic human immunodeficiency virus (HIV) infection and considered for those with symptomatic infection [23–25]. These recommendations are consistent with those of the WHO [26].

Egg allergy is a relative contraindication. Persons with a history of anaphylactic reactions following egg ingestion may be vaccinated but only with extreme caution. A protocol for vaccinating such persons has been developed

[27]. Persons with nonanaphylactic reactions to eggs, or allergies to chickens or feathers, may be vaccinated as usual.

Immune globulin should be administered to persons with a contraindication to vaccination following a known exposure. The dose recommended in the United States is 0.25 ml/kg for immunocompetent persons and 0.5 ml/kg for immunocompromised individuals (the maximum dose is 15 ml in all cases). High doses of intravenous immunoglobulin administered at regular intervals may be protective, but there are no efficacy data and this regimen would be very expensive.

## Rubella Vaccine

### Indications and Use

Rubella infection may be associated with significant morbidity in adults and is associated with a high rate of fetal wastage or defects if contracted in the early months of gestation [28]. Since the risk of exposure may be high in many developing countries and in some developed countries where rubella immunization is either not routinely practiced or intended to interrupt transmission, persons traveling abroad, particularly women of childbearing age, should be immune, even though rubella vaccination is not a requirement for entry into any country. In the United States persons are considered susceptible to rubella if they lack documentation of appropriate immunization with rubella vaccine on or after the first birthday, or laboratory evidence of immunity. A clinical diagnosis of rubella is unreliable and should not be considered in assessing immune status [29].

A single dose of rubella vaccine is indicated for all susceptible persons if there are no contraindications. Vaccine can be administered alone or in combination with measles and mumps vaccines in vaccinees 12 months of age or older. The risk of serious disease with rubella infection in infants is so small that there is no need to administer rubella vaccine below 12 months of age.

### Side Effects and Adverse Reactions

Primary vaccination of children is sometimes associated with low-grade fever, rash, and lymphadenopathy. Up to 40% of vaccinees in large-scale field trials have experienced joint pain, but frank arthritis has generally been reported in fewer than 2%. Arthralgia and transient arthritis occur more frequently and are more likely to occur in susceptible women (e.g., 10%–20%) than children (e.g., 3%) [30]. Transient peripheral neuritic complaints, such as paresthesias and pain in the extremities, have also occurred rarely [31]. These vaccine-related effects generally begin 3–25 days after immunization and persist for 1–11 days. They rarely recur or persist [30, 32–34]. Because the vast majority of data indicate that only susceptible vaccinees have side effects and that persons who have previously either been vaccinated or had rubella are apparently not at any increased risk of local or systemic reactions, routine antibody testing for susceptibility is not necessary.

### Precautions and Contraindications

The same precautions and contraindications regarding hypersensitivity to vaccine components, immunosuppression, and pregnancy noted above for measles vaccine apply to rubella vaccine. Concerns about egg allergy are not relevant for the Cendehill and RA 27/3 vaccines since they are produced in rabbit and human tissue, respectively; they are applicable only to the duck embryo vaccine (HPV:77-DE:5).

A few specific comments on the risk of rubella vaccine to the developing fetus should be made. Although rubella vaccine viruses have been demonstrated to cross the placenta and infect the fetus, they have not yet been shown to be associated with any defects consistent with congenital rubella infection. None of approximately 400 infants born to susceptible mothers who had received rubella vaccine in the United States, the United Kingdom, or Germany, had anomalies consistent with congenital rubella [35]. However, the maximal theoretical risk could be approximately 1%. Thus, based on theoretical concerns, rubella vaccine still should not be administered to pregnant women and pregnancy should still be avoided for 3 months after vaccination. On the other hand, since it appears that the risk of vaccine-associated defects is so small as to be negligible, fetal exposure to the vaccine virus is not ordinarily considered to be a reason to interrupt pregnancy in the United States.

These data have also led to CDC recommendations that routine rubella serology and pregnancy testing not be done before vaccinating postpubertal females who do not have evidence of immunity (as defined above). Rather, they are asked if they are pregnant, and if they say they are not, they are vaccinated and counseled to avoid pregnancy for 3 months.

Breastfeeding is not a contraindication for vaccination. While the vaccine virus has been isolated from breast milk, there are no conclusive data to suggest that exposure is harmful to the neonate [32–34].

## Mumps Vaccine

### Indications and Use

While generally a mild, self-limited disease, mumps can be moderately debilitating. Since mumps is prevalent worldwide, mumps vaccination can be of particular value for children approaching puberty and for adolescents and adults – particularly males, 20% or so of whom may experience orchitis – who have not had mumps. In the United States, persons are considered susceptible to mumps if they lack documentation of appropriate immunization with rubella vaccine on or after the first birthday, physician-diagnosed mumps, or laboratory evidence of immunity. However, most adults can be considered to be immune [36].

A single dose of mumps vaccine is indicated for all susceptible persons if there are no contraindications. Vaccine can be administered alone or in combination with measles and mumps vaccines in vaccinees 12 months of age or older. The risk of serious disease with mumps infection in infants is so small that there is no need to administer mumps vaccine below 12 months of age.

## Side Effects and Adverse Reactions

Mumps is one of the safest vaccines currently available. Parotitis temporally associated to vaccination has been reported rarely. Very rarely, manifestations of CNS involvement, such as febrile seizures, unilateral nerve deafness, and encephalitis within 30 days of vaccination, are reported. However, there is no way to rule out temporal association. The frequency of reported CNS events following mumps vaccination is lower than the observed background incidence rate of CNS dysfunction in the normal population. As with measles and rubella vaccines, there is no evidence that vaccination of persons who are already immune to mumps, either from vaccination or natural disease, is associated with an increased risk of vaccine-associated adverse events. Thus, routine prevaccination antibody testing for susceptibility is not necessary.

## Precautions and Contraindications

The same precautions and contraindications regarding hypersensitivity to vaccine components, immunosuppression, and pregnancy noted above for measles vaccine apply to mumps vaccine.

# *Haemophilus influenzae* Type b Vaccine

## Indications and Use

*Haemophilus influenzae* type b infection causes meningitis and other serious invasive illness (sepsis, pneumonia, septic arthritis, and epiglottis), primarily in children less than 5 years of age. Disease can be especially severe in infants and young children. In the United States, administration of *Haemophilus influenzae* type b vaccine became routine in 1985 when the polysaccharide vaccine was licensed; it was routinely given to children 24 months of age although children 18–23 months of age who were at high risk could be vaccinated, with revaccination to follow [37]. The diphtheria conjugate vaccine was licensed at the end of 1987 and is now the preferred vaccine, and will probably eventually replace the polysaccharide vaccine [38]. It is intended for all children 18 months of age. All children 19–23 months should also be vaccinated. Based on the epidemiology of invasive *Haemophilus influenzae* type b infection in the United States, the vaccine is not routinely recommended beyond the 5th year of life. Children 18–23 months of age who have already received the polysaccharide vaccine should be revaccinated with the conjugate vaccine. Since the risk of Hib infection while traveling outside the United States is comparable to that within the United States, the CDC recommends that all children old enough to be vaccinated receive vaccine before departure. Similar recommendations may be issued by other countries when they introduce the vaccine. This process will be accelerated if the conjugate vaccine is licensed for use in infants [8].

### Side Effects and Adverse Reactions

The vaccines appear to be quite safe. Local reactions at the injection site and fever (temperature >39.0 °C) have been noted in approximately 10% and 1% of vaccinees, respectively. Although there has been some concern about an increased risk of *Haemophilus influenzae* type b infection shortly after receipt of the polysaccharide vaccine, this problem has not been observed with the conjugate vaccine.

### Precautions and Contraindications

The vaccine should not be administered if there is a history of anaphylaxis to diphtheria toxoid or other vaccine components like thimerosol. Since vaccine does not prevent carriage and since it is not 100% effective, vaccination does not preclude use of rifampin when indicated.

## Conclusion

The information presented indicate that the "general-use" vaccines are safe and effective. Furthermore, they are highly cost effective means of prevention. While the list of these vaccines is relatively small and varies by country, new vaccines will undoubtedly be added and more countries will eventually recommend their use.

As the number of international travelers increases, and as countries strive both to safeguard the health of travelers and to limit the importation and spread of vaccine-preventable diseases, attention to these "general-use" immunizations becomes increasingly important [39]. This is particularly true when considering the increased global interest in eradication of measles and polio [40, 41]. Perhaps in the future, a discussion of some, or even all, of the "general-use" immunizations will not be necessary since the risk of the diseases will have disappeared.

## References


1. Mann JM (1983) Emporiatric policy and practice: protecting the health of Americans abroad. JAMA 249:3323–3325
2. Rust RE, Peate WF, Cordes DH (1986) Comprehensive care of travelers. J Fam Pract 23:572–579
3. Steffan R, Rickenbach M, Wilhelm U, Helminger A, Schar M (1987) Health problems after travel to developing countries. J Infect Dis 156:84–91
4. CDC (1987) Health information for international travel 1988. CDC, Washington DHHS publ no (CDC) 88–8280
5. CDC (1989) Recommendations of the Immunization Practices Advisory Committee (ACIP). General recommendations on immunizations. MMWR 38:205–214, 219–227
6. CDC (1986) Recommendations of the Immunization Practices Advisory Committee (ACIP). New recommended schedule for active immunization of normal infants and children. MMWR 35:577–579

7. Deforest A, Long SS, Lischner HW et al. (1988) Simultaneous administration of measles-mumps-rubella vaccine with booster doses of diphtheria-tetanus-pertussis and poliovirus vaccines. Pediatrics 81:237–246
8. Eskola J, Peltola H, Takala AK et al. (1987) Efficacy of *Haemophilus influenzae* type b-polysaccharide diphtheria toxoid conjugate vaccine in infancy. N Engl J Med 317:717–722
9. CDC (1985) Recommendations of the Immunization Practices Advisory Committee (ACIP). Diphtheria, tetanus, and pertussis: guidelines for vaccine prophylaxis and other preventive measures. MMWR 34:405–414, 419–426
10. CDC (1987) Recommendations of the Immunization Practices Advisory Committee (ACIP). Pertussis immunization; family history of convulsions and use of antipyretics – Supplementary ACIP statement. MMWR 36:281–282
11. Halsey N, Galazka A (1985) The efficacy of DTP and oral poliomyelitis immunization schedules initiated from birth to 12 weeks of age. Bull WHO 63:1151–1169
12. Orenstein WA, Weisfeld JS, Halsey NA (1983) Diphtheria and tetanus toxoids and pertussis vaccine, combined. In: Halsey NA, de Quadros CA (eds) Recent advances in immunization: a bibliographic review. Pan American Health Organization, pp 30–51 (Scientific publ no 451)
13. Barkin RM, Samuleson JS, Gotlin LP (1984) DTP reactions and serologic response with a reduced dose schedule. J Pediatr 105:189–194
14. Ross E, Miller D (1986) Risk and pertussis vaccine (Letter). Arch Dis Child 61:98–99
15. CDC (1982) Recommendations of the Immunization Practices Advisory Committee (ACIP). Poliomyelitis prevention. MMWR 31:22–26, 31–34
16. CDC (1987) Recommendations of the Immunization Practices Advisory Committee (ACIP). Poliomyelitis prevention: enhanced-potency inactivated poliomyelitis vaccine – Supplementary statement. MMWR 36:795–798
17. Bernier RH (1986) Improved inactivated poliovirus vaccine: an update. Pediatr Infect Dis 5:289–292
18. Expanded Program on Immunization (1985) Global advisory group. Weekly Epidemiol Rec 60:13–16
19. Nkwane BM, Wassilak SGF, Orenstein WA, Bart KJ, Schoenberger LB, Hinman AR, Kew O (1987) Vaccine-associated paralytic poliomyelitis. United States: 1974 through 1984. JAMA 257:1335–1340
20. Miller DL (1964) Frequency of complications of measles, 1963. Report on a national inquiry by the Public Health Laboratory Service in collaboration with the Society of Medical Officers of Health. Br Med J 2:75–78
21. CDC (1987) Recommendations of the Immunization Practices Advisory Committee (ACIP). Measles prevention. MMWR 36:409–418, 423–425
22. Orenstein WA, Markowitz L, Preblud SR, Hinman AR, Tomasi A, Bart KJ (1986) Appropriate age for measles vaccination in the United States. Dev Biol Stand 65:13–21
23. CDC (1986) Recommendations of the Immunization Practices Advisory Committee (ACIP). Immunization of children infected with human T-lymphotrophic virus type III/lymphadenopathy associated virus. MMWR 35:595–598, 603–606
24. CDC (1988) Recommendations of the Immunization Practices Advisory Committee (ACIP). Immunization of children infected with human immunodeficiency virus – Supplementary ACIP statement. MMWR 37:181–183
25. CDC (1988) Measles in HIV-infected children, United States. MMWR 37:183–186
26. Von Reyn CF, Clements CJ, Mann JM (1987) Human immunodeficiency virus infection and routine childhood immunisation. Lancet II:669–672
27. Herman JJ, Radin R, Schneiderman R (1983) Allergic reactions to measles (rubeola) vaccine in patients hypersensitive to egg protein. J Pediatr 102:196–199
28. Miller E, Cradock-Watson JE, Pollock TM (1982) Consequences of confirmed maternal rubella at successive stages of pregnancy. Lancet II:781–784

29. CDC (1984) Recommendations of the Immunization Practices Advisory Committee (ACIP). Rubella prevention. MMWR 33:301–310, 315–318
30. Preblud SR (1985) Some current issues relating to rubella vaccine. JAMA 254:253–256
31. Preblud SR, Serdula MK, Frank JA Jr, Brandling-Bennett AD, Hinman AR (1980) Rubella vaccination in the United States: a ten-year review. Epidemiol Rev 2:171–194
32. Tingle AJ, Chantler JK, Pot KH, Paty DW, Ford DK (1985) Postpartum rubella immunization: association with development of prolonged arthritis, neurological sequelae, and chronic rubella viremia. J Infect Dis 254:253–256
33. Preblud SR, Orenstein WA, Lopez CL, Herrmann KL, Hinman AR (1986) Postpartum rubella immunization (Letter). J Infect Dis 154:367–368
34. Tingle AJ (1986) Postpartum rubella immunization (Letter). J Infect Dis 154:368–369
35. CDC (1989) Rubella vaccination during pregnancy – United States, 1971–1988. MMWR 38:289–293
36. CDC (1982) Recommendations of the Immunization Practices Advisory Committee (ACIP). Mumps vaccine. MMWR 31:617–620, 625
37. CDC (1985) Recommendations of the Immunization Practices Advisory Committee (ACIP). Polysaccharide vaccine for prevention of *Haemophilus influenzae* type b disease. MMWR 34:201–205
38. CDC (1988) Recommendations of the Immunization Practices Advisory Committee (ACIP). Update: prevention of *Haemophilus influenzae* type b disease. MMWR 37:13–16
39. Markowitz LE, Tomasi A, Hawkins CE, Preblud SR, Orenstein WA, Hinman AR (1987) International measles importations: United States, 1980–1985. Int J Epidemiol 17:101–105
40. Hinman AR (1985) Costs of not eradicating measles. Am J Public Health 75:713–714
41. Hinman AR, Foege WH, de Quadros CA, Patriarca PA, Orenstein WA, Brink EW (1987) The case for global eradication of poliomyelitis. Bull WHO 65:835–840

# Special-Use Immunobiologics for Travelers

M. G. Schultz

## Introduction

This paper describes the special-use immunobiologics for travelers. This group includes biologic products for the prevention of cholera, hepatitis A, hepatitis B, Japane encephalitis, meningococcal meningitis, plague, rabies, typhoid and yellow fever. Each of the diseases and immunobiologics discussed in this paper have at least seven important facets. They are: the products available; criteria for administering the product to travelers; use in pregnant travelers; use in children who travel; primary and booster immunization schedule; precautions and contraindications; and side effects and adverse reactions. There are other important factors that the health care provider must consider before administering any of these immunobiologics. He or she must decide: What is the risk of the disease to the traveler? What is the traveler's susceptibility to the disease? Is there time available for immunization? Will there be simultaneous or non-simultaneous administration? To help make these decisions there are some key questions that should be asked of each traveler. They are: Where are you going? How long will you be there? What will you be doing there? How soon are you leaving? What is your prior immunization history? Do you have any special risk factors? When answers to these questions are in hand (and a test for antibody performed in special circumstances), an appropriate course of special-use immunobiologics can be prescribed.

The content of this paper is derived mainly from the statements of the Advisory Committee for Immunization Practices that are published in the Morbidity and Mortality Weekly Reports (MMWRs) by the Centers for Diseases Control (CDC). Hence the paper represents a North American point of view about immunizations for travelers.

## Cholera Immunization for Travelers

Currently available cholera vaccines, whether prepared from Classic or El Tor strains, are of limited usefulness [1]. In field trials conducted in areas with endemic cholera, vaccines have been shown to provide only about 50% effectiveness in reducing the incidence of clinical illness for a period of 3–6 months. They do not prevent transmission of infection. Vaccine available in the United States is prepared from a combination of phenol-inactivated suspensions of classic Inaba and Ogawa strains of *Vibrio cholerae* grown on agar or in broth.

The risk of cholera to most international travelers is so low that it is questionable whether vaccination is of any benefit [2]. Persons following the usual tourist itinerary who use standard accommodations in countries affected by cholera are at virtually no risk of infection. The traveler's best protection against cholera, as well as against many enteric diseases, is to avoid food and water that might be contaminated.

Even though the Twenty-Sixth World Health Assembly in 1973 amended the International Health Regulations so that a cholera vaccination certificate should not be required of any traveler, and the World Health Organization no longer recommends cholera vaccination for travel to or from cholera-infected areas some countries, particularly countries affected or threatened by cholera require evidence of cholera vaccination for entry. For persons anticipating travel to such countries, a single dose of vaccine is sufficient to satisfy International Health Regulations. With the threat or occurrence of epidemic cholera, health authorities of some countries may require evidence of a complete primary series of two doses or a booster dose within 6 months before arrival. The complete primary series is otherwise suggested only for special high-risk groups that work and live in highly endemic areas under less than sanitary conditions. WHO does report those countries that require cholera vaccination in *Vaccination Certificate Requirements and Health Advice for International Travel* and the *Weekly Epidemiologic Record.* These requirements are reproduced in CDC's *Health Information for International Travel* and *Bi-Weekly Summary of Countries with Areas Infected with Quarantinable Diseases.*

Physicians administering vaccine to travelers should emphasize that an International Certificate of Vaccination against cholera must be validated for it to be acceptable to quarantine authorities. Failure to secure validation may cause travelers to be revaccinated or quarantined. A properly documented certificate is valid for 6 months beginning 6 days after vaccination or beginning on the date of revaccination, if this is within 6 months of a previous injection.

Specific information is not available on the safety of cholera vaccine during pregnancy. Therefore, it is prudent on theoretical grounds to avoid vaccinating pregnant women.

No data are available concerning the efficacy or side effects of cholera vaccine in children less than 6 months of age. Cholera vaccine is not recommended for children less than 6 months of age. Breast-feeding is protective against cholera; careful preparation of formula and food from safe water and foodstuffs should protect nonbreast-fed infants. If a child less than 6 months of age is to travel to areas requiring cholera immunization, a medical waiver should be obtained before travel. For older infants and children traveling to countries that require vaccination, a single dose of vaccine is sufficient to satisfy International Health Regulations.

Complete primary immunization consists of two doses of vaccine given 1 week to 1 month or more apart. Dose volume by age group and by route of administration is shown in Table 1. The intradermal route is satisfactory for persons 5 years of age and older. Booster doses may be given every 6 months

**Table 1.** Recommended doses, by volume (ml), for immunization against cholera

| Dose number | Route and age | | | |
|---|---|---|---|---|
| | Intradermal[a] 5 years and over | Subcutaneous or intramuscular | | |
| | | 6 months–4 years | 5–10 years | Over 10 years |
| 1 and 2 | 0.2 ml | 0.2 ml | 0.3 ml | 0.5 ml |
| Boosters | 0.2 ml | 0.2 ml | 0.3 ml | 0.5 ml |

[a] Higher levels of protection (antibody) may be achieved in children less than 5 years old by the subcutaneous or intramuscular routes

if necessary for travel or for residence in highly endemic, unsanitary areas. In areas where cholera occurs in a 2-to-3-month "season," protection is best if the booster dose is given at the beginning of the season. The primary series does not ever need to be repeated for booster doses to be effective. Simultaneous administration of yellow fever and cholera vaccines may result in lower-than-normal antibody responses to both vaccines (see paragraph on simultaneous vaccination).

Vaccination often results in 1–2 days of pain, erythema, and induration at the site of injection. The local reaction may be accompanied by fever, malaise, and headache. Serious reactions following cholera vaccination are extremely rare. If a person has experienced a serious reaction to the vaccine, revaccination is not advisable. Most governments will permit an unvaccinated traveler to proceed if he or she carries a physician's statement of medical contraindication.

## Hepatitis A Prophylaxis

Immune globulin (IG) (formerly called "immune serume globulin," ISG, or "gamma globulin") produced in the United States contains antibodies against the hepatitis A virus (anti-HAV) and the hepatitis B surface antigen (anti-HBs). Tests of IG lots prepared since 1977 indicate that both types of antibody have uniformly been present. Numerous field studies conducted in the past 4 decades confirm that IG given before exposure or during the incubation period of hepatitis A is protective against clinical illness [3]. Its prophylactic value is greatest (80%–90%) when given early in the incubation period and declines thereafter [4].

The risk of acquiring hepatitis A for persons traveling abroad varies with living conditions, length of stay, and the incidence of hepatitis A in the area visited. Travelers to developed countries in Europe, Japan, Australia and New Zealand are at no greater risk of acquiring hepatitis A than they are in North America. For travelers to developing countries, risk of infection can vary greatly. It is commonly believed that the highest attack rates occur in travelers who live in or visit rural areas, who trek in back country, or who frequently eat and drink in settings of poor sanitation. A recent, as yet unpublished, study by CDC has, however, shown that many cases of travel-related hepatitis A occur in travelers with so-called "standard" tourist itineraries, accommodations and food consumption behaviors.

Immune globulin is generally recommended for travelers to developing countries if they will be eating in settings of poor or uncertain sanitation or will be visiting extensively with local persons, especially young children. Persons who plan to reside in developing areas under such conditions for long periods should receive IG regularly.

For persons who might require repeated IG prophylaxis, screening for total anti-HAV antibodies before travel may be useful to define susceptibility and eliminate unnecessary doses of IG in those who are immune. A policy of selective screening of travelers to determine if they have antibody to hepatitis A (anti-HAV) has recently been suggested [5], and a formula has been devised that enables the cost-benefit to be calculated [6]. In general, the benefit of testing accrues with increasing age of the traveler, length of stay abroad, and frequency of visits abroad. The place of residence of the traveler is an important factor because even within developed countries the expected prevalence of anti-HAV positivity is highly variable [7].

Pregnancy is not a contraindication to using immune globulin.

Infants and children traveling to developing countries are at increased risk of acquiring hepatitis A, especially if their travel is outside usual tourist routes, if they will be eating food or drinking water in settings of questionable sanitation, or if they will be in contact with local young children in settings of poor sanitation. Although hepatitis is rarely severe in children under age 5 years, infected children efficiently transmit infection to older children and adults. Immune globulin (IG) should be given to infants and children in the same schedule as recommended for adults.

A single dose of IG of 0.02 ml/kg is recommended if the traveler will have exposure of 3 months or less. For prolonged travel, 0.06 ml/kg should be given every 5 months.

Immune globulins prepared in the United States have few side effects (primarily soreness at the injection site) and have never been shown to transmit infectious agents [hepatitis B, non-A non-B hepatitis, or human immunodeficiency virus (HIV)]. Recent specific laboratory studies have additionally shown that immune globulins prepared by the Cohn-Oncley procedure carry no risk of transmission of AIDS.

Live attenuated vaccine viruses might not successfully replicate and antibody response could be diminished when the vaccine is given with IG preparations. In general, parenterally administered live vaccines, e.g., measles-mumps-rubella vaccine (MMR), should not be given for at least 6 weeks, and preferably 3 months, after IG administration. However, IG does not interfere with immune response to either oral polio vaccine (OPV) or yellow fever vaccine, and this recommendation does not apply to these vaccines.

If IG administration becomes necessary after a live vaccine has been given, interference may occur. In general, vaccine virus replication and stimulation of immunity will occur within 7–10 days. Thus, if the interval between vaccine and IG is less than 14 days, vaccine should be repeated at least 3 months after IG was given, unless serologic testing indicates that antibodies have been produced; if the interval was longer, vaccine need not be readministered. If administration of IG becomes necessary because of the imminent exposure to disease, live virus vaccines may be administered simultaneously with IG, with the recognition that vaccine-induced immunity may be compromised. The vaccine should be administered in a site remote from that chosen for the IG inoculation. Vaccination should be repeated about 3 months later, unless serologic testing indicates antibodies have been produced.

In general, there is little interaction between IG preparations and inactivated vaccines. Therefore, inactivated vaccines can be given simultaneously or at any time interval after or before an IG product is used. However, vaccines should be administered at sites different than the IG product.

## Hepatitis B Immunization

Two different hepatitis B vaccines are currently in use. The vaccine produced from plasma of hepatitis B carriers has been available since 1982. The second is produced from common bakers' yeast into which the gene for hepatitis B surface antigen has been inserted through recombinant DNA technology. The two vaccines when given in recommended dosages have comparable immunogenicity and efficacy, and may be considered equivalent for primary vaccination [8, 9].

Hepatitis B immunization is currently recommended for all persons who work in health care fields (medical, dental, laboratory or other) which entail exposure to human blood.

Hepatitis B immunization should also be considered for persons who plan to reside (greater than 6 months) in areas with high levels of endemic hepatitis B, and who will have the types of contact with the local population that are likely to transmit hepatitis B infection. In particular, persons who anticipate sexual contact with the local population, who will live in rural areas and/or have intimate contact with local populations; and persons who are likely to seek medical, dental or other treatment in local facilities during their stay, should receive the vaccine. Circumstances in which disease transmission could occur also include receipt of blood transfusions not screened for HBsAg, exposure to unsterilized needles (or other medical/dental equipment) in local health facilities, or open skin lesions (impetigo, scabies, scratched insect bites). Immunization for hepatitis B should be considered for short-term travelers (less than 6 months) who will have direct contact with blood, or sexual contact with residents of areas with high levels of endemic hepatitis B infection.

The prevalence of HBV carriers is high (5%–20%) in all socioeconomic groups in certain areas of the world: all of sub-Saharan Africa, Southeast Asia including China, Korea, and Indonesia, South Pacific Islands, interior Amazon Basin, and Haiti and the Dominican Republic in the Caribbean. It is moderate (1%–5%) in North Africa, south central and southwest Asia, Japan, eastern and southern Europe and the USSR, and most of Central and South America. In northern and western Europe, North America, Australia and New Zealand, HBV carrier prevalence is low (less than 1%) in the general population.

Specific data are not available on the safety of the vaccine for the developing fetus, but, because it contains only noninfectious HBsAg particles, administration of vaccine to pregnant women is not considered to constitute a risk to the fetus. In contrast, HBV infection in a pregnant woman may result in serious disease for the mother and chronic infection for the newborn. Pregnancy is not a contraindication to the use of this vaccine for persons at risk.

Children who expect to live in an HBV endemic area for 6 or more months and who are expected to be at risk should receive the hepatitis B vaccine in three doses of 10 μg (0.5 ml) plasma-derived vaccine or 5 μg (0.5 ml) recombinant DNA vaccine, by the same schedule as recommended for adults.

Primary adult immunization consists of three intramuscular doses of vaccine; each adult dose is 20 μg plasma-derived vaccine or 10 μg recombinant DNA vaccine. The second dose should be given 1 month after the first dose, and the third dose 6 months after the first. Vaccine doses administered at longer intervals provide equally satisfactory protection, but optimal protection is not conferred until after the third dose. Immunization should ideally begin at least 6 months before travel in order to complete the full vaccine series prior to departure. However, since some protection is provided by one or two doses, the vaccine series should be initiated, if indicated, even if it cannot be completed prior to departure. The optimal site of injection in adults is the deltoid muscle; vaccination in the buttocks results in poorer antibody response. There is no evidence of interference between HB vaccine and other simultaneously administered vaccines or with immunoglobulin. Because the vaccines are so new, the duration of protection and the need for booster doses have not yet been determined [10].

The major side effects observed with hepatitis B vaccines during 5 years use have been soreness and redness at the site of injection. Serious adverse reactions, including neurological events, have been reported rarely. The production process for the plasma-derived vaccine has been shown to inactivate representatives of all classes of viruses found in blood, including the causative agent of AIDS (HIV) [11].

## Japanese Encephalitis Immunization

Formalin-inactivated vaccines for Japanese encephalitis (JE) have been manufactured and used in Japan and China for many years, and during the last decade in the Republic of Korea. The Japanese and Korean vaccines are made in adult mouse brain, the Chinese vaccine in primary hamster kidney tissue culture. The inactivated mouse-brain preparation as used in Japan was field tested in 400 000 Taiwanese children. The seroconversion rate was 90%–100% one month after the second of two inoculations a month apart, and its protective efficacy was 80%; a booster dose 1 year later maintained neutralizing antibody for at least 3 years [12]. In 71 000 Chinese children, four doses of the Chinese hamster kidney vaccine gave a protective efficacy of 95% [13]. Side effects with both vaccines were negligible; less than 1% had systemic reactions, including fever, and the frequency of allergic reactions was less than 0.02% [12, 13]. The World Health Organization is considering formulating requirements for JE vaccine and for establishing a reference standard preparation [14].

In the United States, the Centers for Disease Control have been sponsoring the evaluation of an inactivated highly purified mouse brain JE vaccine manufactured by Biken Laboratories, Osaka, Japan. The initial evaluation of the Biken JE vaccine in the United States demonstrated a low level of response to the two-dose primary vaccination schedule (recommended by the manufacturer and was considered unsatisfactory (72% of 68 participants seroconverted with a post-vaccination titer of less than 8). Evaluation of a three-dose primary vaccination schedule on 72 participants showed acceptable serological responses – 99% developed titers of 16 or greater, and 93% developed titers of 64 or greater.

The risk of Japanese encephalitis to short-term travelers and persons who confine their travel to urban centers is low. Persons at greatest risk are those living for prolonged periods in endemic or epidemic areas. In temperate areas where the disease may occur in epidemics in late summer and autumn, the risk of transmission during the winter months is negligible. This includes areas such as China and Japan, and the northern part of the tropical zones of Bangladesh, Burma, India, Kampuchea, Laos, Nepal, Thailand, Vietnam, and eastern areas of the USSR. In subtropical and tropical areas, such as south India, Indonesia, Malaysia, Philippines, Singapore, Sri Lanka, Taiwan, and south Thailand, the risk of transmission is present throughout the year, but it is accentuated during the rainy season and early dry season when mosquito populations are highest. Travel in rural areas where rice culture and pig farming are common increases the risk of contracting JE.

Vaccination for JE should be considered for persons who plan long-term residence in areas experiencing epidemic JE especially when the travelers' activity will include trips into rural farming areas or sleeping in unscreened quarters. Short-term travelers (less than 1 month), especially those restricting their visits to major urban areas and staying in mosquito-proof quarters, are at negligible risk of JE infection.

There are several problems associated with the use of Japanese encephalitis vaccine in developed countries. One problem is availability of the product [15]. No vaccine for Japanese encephalitis is licensed for use in the United States and the Japanese manufacturer has not applied to the Food and Drug Administration for licensure of their vaccine, mainly because of the small market and the risk of litigation. At the moment this issue is unresolved, but there is reasonable hope that it can be solved in the near future.

The use of this inactivated vaccine during pregnancy has not been studied and the vaccine should not be given to pregnant women. No lower age limit is specified by the manufacturer.

**Table 2.** Japanese encephalitis vaccine

| Doses | Subcutaneous route | | Comments |
|---|---|---|---|
| | Less than 3 years of age | More than 3 years of age | |
| Primary series 1, 2, and 3[a] | 0.5 ml | 1.0 ml | Give 1–2 weeks apart |
| Booster | | | One dose at 12–18 months, and at 4-year intervals thereafter if risk continues |

[a] Manufacturer's recommendations vary from two to three doses. Recent limited study in the United States suggests a three-dose primary series may be preferable

Table 2 provides dose information about JE vaccine. JE vaccine should not be administered to persons acutely ill with fever and/or active infections, those with cardiac, renal, or hepatic disorders, leukemia, lymphoma, or other generalized malignancies, those with a history of hypersensitivities, and pregnant females. However, except for known hypersensitivity, most of these hypothetical contraindications should not preclude vaccination under medical supervision if the risk of exposure to the virus is significant.

At the time of the latest evaluation of the CDC protocol for administering JE vaccine (1987), 1328 people had received 3552 doses of the vaccine, 8% experienced local reactions (tenderness or erythema), 2% experienced generalized symptoms, and 2% experienced severe reactions (most of this group were concurrently receiving other vaccines). This is considerably more morbidity than previously reported [13].

## Meningococcal Immunization

The recently licensed quadrivalent A,C,Y,W-135 vaccine is the meningococcal polysaccharide vaccine that is currently available in the United States. The vaccine consists of 50 μg each of the respective purified bacterial capsular polysaccharides. The serogroup A vaccine has been shown to have a clinical efficacy of 85%–95% and to be of use in controlling epidemics. A similar level of clinical efficacy has been demonstrated for the serogroup C vaccine, both in American military recruits and in an epidemic. The group Y and W-135 polysaccharides have been shown to be safe and immunogenic in adults [17] and in children over 2 years of age; clinical protection has not been demonstrated directly, but is assumed, based on the production of bactericidal antibody, which for group C has been correlated with clinical protection. The antibody responses to each of the four polysaccharides in the quadrivalent vaccine are serogroup specific and independent.

Antibodies against the group A and C polysaccharides decline markedly over the first 3 years following a single dose of vaccine [18, 19]. This antibody decline is more rapid in infants and young children than in adults. Similarly, while vaccine-induced clinical protection probably persists in schoolchildren and adults for at least 3 years, a study in Africa demonstrated a marked decline in the efficacy of the group A vaccine in young children over time.

Vaccination against meningococcal disease is not a requirement for entry into any country. Meningococcal disease is endemic throughout the world. Vaccine may be of benefit for some travelers to countries recognized as having epidemic meningococcal disease. Cases of meningococcal disease in short-term travelers are uncommon; however, prolonged contact with the local populace could enhance the risk of infection and make vaccination a reasonable precaution. Serogroup A is the most common cause of epidemics outside the United States, but serogroup C and, on rare occasions, serogroup B, can also cause epidemic disease.

One area of the world recognized as having recurrent epidemics of meningococcal disease is the so-called "meningitis belt" of sub-Saharan Africa, which extends from Mauritania in the west to Ethiopia in the east. Epidemics of meningococcal meningitis have occurred in many other parts of the world; epidemics have recently been reported in India, Nepal, the Sudan, and in Haj pilgrims returning to home from Saudi Arabia [20]. In the absence of an effective global surveillance network, travelers and their physicians are at a considerable disadvantage. The recognition and prompt reporting of these epidemics is weak. Equally problematic is knowing when the risk created by an epidemic has subsided.

On theoretical grounds, it is prudent not to immunize pregnant women unless there is a substantial risk of infection. However, evaluation of the vaccine in pregnant women during an epidemic in Brazil demonstrated no adverse effects. Further, antibody studies in these women showed good antibody levels in maternal and cord blood following vaccination during any trimester; antibody levels in the infants declined over the first few months and did not affect their subsequent response to immunization [21].

The serogroup A polysaccharide induces antibody in some children as young as 3 months of age, although a response comparable to that seen in adults is not achieved until 4 or 5 years of age; the serogroup C component does not induce an antibody response before age 18–24 months [22].

Primary immunization for both adults and children is a single 0.5-ml dose of vaccine administered subcutaneously. The vaccine can be given at the same time as other immunizations, if needed. Good antibody levels are achieved within 10–14 days after vaccination. Revaccination may be indicated for individuals at high risk of infection, particularly children who were first immunized under 4 years of age; such children should be considered for revaccination after 2 or 3 years if they remain at high risk. The need for revaccination in older children and adults remains unknown. The dose volume depends on the directions of the manufacturer.

Adverse reactions to meningococcal vaccine are mild and infrequent, consisting principally of localized erythema lasting 1–2 days. Up to 2% of young children develop fever transiently after vaccination.

## Plague Immunization

The plague vaccine licensed for use in the United States is prepared from *Yersinia pestis* organisms grown in artificial media, inactivated with formaldehyde, and preserved in 0.5% phenol. The vaccine contains trace amounts of beef-heart extract, yeast extract, agar, and peptones and peptides of soya and casein. The effectiveness of plague vaccine has never been measured precisely [23, 24]. Field experience indicates that vaccination with plague vaccine reduces the incidence and severity of disease resulting from the bite of infected fleas. The degree of protection afforded against primary pneumonic infection is not known.

Vaccination against plague is not required by any country as a condition for entry. There is no need to vaccinate persons other than those who are at particularly high risk of exposure because of research activities or certain field activities in epizootic areas. In most of the countries of Africa, Asia, and Americas where plague is reported, the risk of exposure exists primarily in rural mountainous or upland areas. Vaccination is not indicated for most travelers to countries reporting cases, particularly if their travel is limited to urban areas with modern hotel accommodations.

Selective vaccination might be considered for persons who will have direct contact with wild rodents or rabbits in plague-epizootic areas, persons who will reside in plague-enzootic rural areas where avoidance of rodents and fleas is difficult, or laboratory personnel who work regularly with *Yersinia pestis* organisms or plague-infected rodents.

The safety or efficacy of vaccination with plague vaccine during pregnancy has not been determined, and therefore it should not be used unless there is a substantial risk of infection.

Primary immunization for adults and children 11 years of age or older consists of three doses of vaccine. The first dose, 1.0 ml, is followed by the second dose, 0.2 ml, 4 weeks later. The third dose, 0.2 ml, is administered 6 months after the first dose. If an accelerated schedule is essential, three doses of 0.5 ml each, administered at least 1 week apart, may be given. The efficacy of this schedule has not been determined. Primary immunization for children 10 years of age or less is also three doses of vaccine, but the doses are smaller (Table 3). The intervals between injections are the same as for adults.

When needed because of continuing exposure, three booster doses should be given at approximately 6-month intervals. Thereafter, antibody levels decline slowly and booster doses at 1- to 2-year intervals, depending on the degree of continuing exposure, should provide good protection. The recommended booster dosages for children and adults are the same as the second and third doses in the primary series. However, if serious side effects to the vaccine occur, their severity may be reduced by using half the usual dose. The primary series need never be repeated for booster doses to be effective (Table 3).

Plague vaccine should not be administered to anyone with a known hypersensitivity to any of the constituents, such as beef protein, soya, casein, and phenol. Patients who have had severe local or systemic reactions to plague vaccine should not be revaccinated.

**Table 3.** Plague vaccine

| Dose | Dose volume[a] | | | | Comments |
|---|---|---|---|---|---|
| | <1 year of age | 1–4 years of age | 5–10 years of age | >10 years of age | |
| Primary series | | | | | Give doses 1 and 2, 4 weeks apart; give dose 3, 3–6 months after dose 2 |
| 1 | 0.2 ml | 0.4 ml | 0.6 ml | 1.0 ml | |
| 2+3 | 0.04 ml | 0.08 ml | 0.12 ml | 0.2 ml | |
| Booster | 0.02 ml | 0.04 ml | 0.06 ml | 0.1 ml | Give two booster doses 6 months apart: thereafter, one booster dose at 1- to 2-year intervals if risk of exposure persists |

[a] For intramuscular injection

Primary immunization may result in general malaise, headache, fever, mild lymphadenopathy, and erythema and induration at the injection site in about 10% of recipients. These reactions occur more commonly with repeated injections. Sterile abscesses occur rarely. Rare cases of sensitivity reactions manifested by urticarial and asthmatic phenomena have been reported.

## Rabies Immunization

Human diploid cell rabies vaccine (HDCV) is an inactivated virus vaccine prepared from fixed rabies virus grown either in WI-38 (American-made vaccine) or MRC-5 (European-made vaccine) human diploid cell culture. Both vaccines are supplied as 1.0-ml single-dose vials of lyophilized vaccine with accompanying diluent. Both HDCV vaccines are considered equally efficacious and safe when used as indicated on the labels. Only the European-made HDCV vaccine has been evaluated by the intradermal (ID) route for preexposure immunization. A new cell culture derived rabies vaccine, called Rabies Vaccine Adsorbed (RVA), has been developed for use in humans by the Michigan Department of Public Health. RVA may be licensed in the near future for both preexposure and postexposure prophylaxis. RVA is made with a different virus strain, cell line and concentration process than HDCV, and it is alum adsorbed and therefore liquid, rather than lyophilized.

Preexposure vaccination with HDCV is recommended for travelers who will be living or visiting countries (for more than 30 days) where rabies is a constant threat. The risk of rabies is highest in countries where dog rabies remains highly endemic, including many countries of Africa, Asia, and Central and South America, except as noted in Table 4. Table 4 lists countries which have reported no cases of rabies during the most recent 2-year period for which information is available (formerly referred to as "rabies-free countries").

**Table 4.** Countries reporting no cases of rabies[a]

The following countries and political units stated that rabies was not present:

Africa
Mauritius[b]

Americas
*North:* Bermuda; St. Pierre and Miquelon
*Caribbean:* Anguilla; Antigua and Barbuda; Bahamas; Barbados; Cayman Islands; Dominica; Guadeloupe; Jamaica; Martinique; Montserrat; Netherlands Antilles (Aruba, Bonaire, Curaçao, Saba, St. Maarten, and St. Eustatius); Redonda; St. Christopher (St. Kitts) and Nevis; St. Lucia; St. Martin; St. Vincent; Turks and Caicos Islands; Virgin Islands (UK and USA)
*South:* Uruguay[b]

Asia
Bahrain; Brunei Darussalam; Japan; Kuwait; Malaysia (Malaysia-Sabah[b]); Maldives[b]; Oman[b]; Singapore; Taiwan

Europe
Bulgaria[b]; Faroe Islands; Finland; Iceland; Ireland; Malta; Norway; Portugal[b]; Sweden; United Kingdom

Oceania
American Samoa; Australia; Belau (Palau); Cook Islands; Federated States of Micronesia (Kosrae, Ponape, Truk, and Yap); Fiji; French Polynesia; Guam; Kiribati; New Caledonia; New Zealand; Niue; Northern Mariana Islands; Papua New Guinea; Samoa; Solomon Islands; Tonga; Vanuatu
Most of Pacific Oceania is "rabies-free." For information on specific islands not listed above, contact Centers for Disease Control, Division of Quarantine

[a] Bat rabies should be considered separately
[b] Countries that have only recently reported cases of rabies; these classifications should be considered provisional

For international travelers, preexposure prophylaxis may provide protection when there is an inapparent or unrecognized exposure to rabies and when postexposure therapy is delayed. This is of particular importance for persons at high risk of being exposed in countries where the available rabies immunizing products carry a high risk of adverse reactions. *Preexposure vaccination does not eliminate the need for additional therapy after a rabies exposure* but simplifies postexposure treatment by eliminating the need for rabies immune globulin (RIG) and by decreasing the number of doses of vaccine required.

If there is a substantial risk of exposure to rabies, preexposure prophylaxis may be indicated during pregnancy. Because of the potential consequences of inadequately treated rabies exposure and limited data that indicate that fetal abnormalities have not been associated with rabies vaccination, pregnancy is not considered a contraindication to postexposure prophylaxis.

In infants and children, the dose of HDCV for preexposure or postexposure prophylaxis is the same as that recommended for adults.

Preexposure immunization consists of three doses of HDCV, 1.0 ml i.m. (i.e., deltoid area), one each on days 0, 7, and 28. HDCV may be administered to travelers by the intradermal (i.d.) dose/route (0.1 ml i.d. on days 0, 7, and

21 or 28) if the three-dose series is completed 30 days or more before departure. If this is not possible, the i.m. dose/route should be used. Preexposure immunization of immunosuppressed persons is not recommended.

For travelers who have continuing risk of exposure to rabies, a booster immunization or serologic test should be performed every 2 years. Preexposure booster immunization consists of one 1.0-ml dose of HDCV, i.m. (deltoid area).

Routine serologic testing is not necessary for persons who receive the recommended preexposure or postexposure regimen with HDCV. For those travelers who received preexposure immunization and have continuing exposure, an acceptible antibody level is 1:5 titer (complete inhibition in RFFIT at 1:5 dilution). A booster should be given if the titer falls below 1:5. Persons previously vaccinated with vaccines other than HDCV should receive the complete postexposure regimen with HDCV unless they developed a laboratory-confirmed antibody response to the primary vaccination. Serologic testing is still recommended for persons whose immune response might be diminished by drug therapy or by diseases. Rabies preexposure prophylaxis is rarely indicated for travelers to the countries listed in Table 4, and postexposure treatment is rarely necessary after exposures to terrestrial animals in these countries.

Postexposure immunization should be preceded by the immediate, thorough cleansing of all wounds with soap and water. For persons who have been previously immunized, two doses of HDCV, 1.0 ml, i.m. (i.e., deltoid area), one each on days 0 and 3, should be given; RIG should not be administered. For persons not previously immunized, RIG, 20 IG/kg body weight, should be given with one half infiltrated at the bite site (if possible), and the remainder given i.m.; and five doses of HDCV, 1.0 ml i.m. (i.e., deltoid area), one each on days 0, 3, 7, 14, and 28 should be given. *The i.d. route should not be used for postexposure prophylaxis* [25].

Chloroquine phosphate (administered for malaria prophylaxis) and other unknown factors encountered by persons traveling to developing countries may interfere with the antibody response to HDCV [26, 27]. The i.m. dose/route of preexposure prophylaxis, however, provides a sufficient margin of safety in this setting. HDCV should not be administered by the i.d. dose/route when chloroquine or other drugs which may interfere with the immune response are being used.

Persons who have received HDCV may experience local reactions such as pain, erythema, and swelling or itching at the injection site, or mild systemic reactions, such as headache, nausea, abdominal pain, muscle aches, and dizziness. Approximately 6% of persons receiving booster vaccinations experience an immune complex-like reaction characterized by urticaria, pruritis, and malaise [28, 29]. This problem of serum sickness-like allergic reactions may be reduced when Rabies Vaccine Adsorbed (RVA) is more widely used since less than 1% of recipients of RVA experienced systemic allergic reactions. Once initiated, rabies postexposure prophylaxis should not be interrupted or discontinued because of local or mild systemic reactions to rabies vaccine.

## Typhoid Immunization

Two different kinds of typhoid vaccines are currently manufactured: the new oral typhoid vaccine, live attenuated Ty 21a (Swiss Serum and Vaccine Institute) and a parenteral heat-phenol-inactivated vaccine (Wyeth) which has been in use for many years. The oral vaccine is not yet licensed in the United States, but it is anticipated that it will be in the near future. Several different preparations of parenteral killed vaccine have been shown to protect 70%–90% of recipients, depending in part on the degree of their subsequent exposure [30, 31]. Parathyphoid A and B vaccines are not effective and are not licensed in many industrialized countries.

Three doses of the oral live vaccine have been shown to provide about 67% protection for at least 3 years against clinical infection in controlled field trials conducted in endemic areas (95% confidence interval 47%–79%) [32]. The incidence of clinical typhoid was significantly lower in the persons receiving four doses of vaccine compared with two or three doses; no placebo group was included in that trial, so vaccine efficacy could not be calculated. A primary series of two doses of heat-phenol-inactivated typhoid vaccine, very similar but not identical to the currently available parenteral vaccine, has demonstrated 50%–77% efficacy in several field trials [33].

Parenteral killed vaccine and live attenuated Ty 21a oral vaccine have never been directly compared in a field trial, but in separate studies, the live attenuated Ty 21a oral vaccine shows similar efficacy and fewer adverse reactions than the parenteral killed vaccine. There is limited experience with the use of live attenuated oral vaccine in persons from nonendemic areas and in children under 5 years of age and there is no experience with its use in persons previously vaccinated with parenteral vaccine.

Immunization should be considered for travelers to areas where there is a recognized risk of exposure to typhoid [34]. The risk of typhoid fever is greatest to travelers who have prolonged exposure to potentially contaminated food and water [35]. Typhoid vaccination, however, is not a substitute for the careful selection of food and drink.

Neither the safety of parenteral killed whole cell vaccine nor live attenuated Ty 21a oral vaccine has been demonstrated in pregnancy. Their use in pregnant women who are traveling should reflect the actual risks of disease and probable benefits of the vaccine.

No data are available concerning the efficacy or side effects of typhoid vaccines in infants, although vaccine is probably immunogenic in this age group. Breast-feeding is likely to be protective against typhoid; careful preparation of formula and food from safe water and foodstuffs should protect nonbreast-fed infants. Typhoid vaccine is recommended for older children traveling to areas where there is a recognized risk of exposure to *Salmonella typhi*.

Primary immunization of adults and children 10 years and older with inactivated parenteral vaccine consists of 0.5 ml subcutaneously, given on two occasions, separated by 4 or more weeks. Primary immunization of children less than 10 years old with inactivated parenteral vaccine consists of 0.25 ml sub-

**Table 5.** Typhoid vaccine

| Doses | Subcutaneous route | | Intradermal route | |
|---|---|---|---|---|
| | Less than 10 years of age | 10 years of age or older | All ages | Comments |
| Primary series 1 and 2 | 0.25 ml | 0.50 ml | | Give 4 or more weeks apart |
| Booster | 0.25 ml | 0.50 ml | 0.1 ml[a] | One dose at least every 3 years under conditions of continued or repeated exposure |

[a] Generally less reaction follows vaccination by the intradermal route, except when acetone-killed and dried vaccine is used. (Acetone-killed and dried vaccine should not be given intradermally)

cutaneously, given on two occasions, separated by 4 or more weeks. If the physician has chosen to use parenteral vaccine and there is not sufficient time for two doses at the specified interval, it has been common practice to give three doses in the volumes cited above at weekly intervals, although it is recognized that this schedule may be less effective. Table 5 provides dose information about inactivated parenteral typhoid vaccine.

Primary immunization of adults and children 10 years and older with live attenuated Ty 21a oral vaccine presently consists of one enteric coated capsule taken on three occasions with cool liquid no warmer than 37 °C on alternate days. The capsules must be kept refrigerated and all three doses must be taken to achieve maximum efficacy. Primary immunization of children less than 10 years with live attenuated Ty 21a oral vaccine also consists of one enteric coated capsule taken on three occasions with cool liquid no warmer than 37 °C on alternate days. The capsules must be kept refrigerated and all three doses must be taken to achieve maximum efficacy.

Under conditions of continued or repeated exposure to typhoid, a booster dose of parenteral inactivated vaccine should be given every 3 years. The optimal booster schedule for live attenuated Ty 21a oral vaccine has not been determined, although efficacy was shown to persist at 4 years with the four-dose regimen, and there is no experience with using live attenuated oral vaccine as a booster in persons who were previously immunized with parenteral vaccine. Alternate routes and dosages of parenteral vaccine for booster immunization are shown in Table 5 and can be expected to produce comparable antibody responses. Even when more than 3 years has elapsed since the prior immunization, a single booster dose of parenteral vaccine is sufficient.

The only contraindication to parenteral typhoid vaccination is a history of severe local or systemic reactions following a previous dose. Live bacterial vaccines such as live attenuated Ty 21a should probably not be used in immunocompromised persons.

During volunteer trials and field studies of oral vaccination with Ty 21a in enteric coated tablets, side effects were very rare and consisted of abdominal discomfort, diarrhea, headache, or rash. Vaccination with parenteral killed whole cell vaccine frequently results in 1–2 days of discomfort at the injection site, often accompanied by fever, malaise and headache. More severe reactions have been reported, including hypotension, chest pain and shock.

## Yellow Fever Immunization

Yellow fever vaccine is a live, attenuated virus preparation made from the 17D yellow fever virus strain [36]. The 17D vaccine has proven to be extremely safe and effective [37]. It is grown in chick embryos inoculated with a seed virus of a fixed-passage level. The vaccine is freeze-dried supernate of centrifuged embryo homogenate, packaged in one-dose and five-dose vials for domestic use. Vaccine should be stored at temperatures between 5 °C and −30 °C – preferably frozen, below 0 °C – until it is reconstituted by the addition of diluent, sterile physiologic saline supplied by the manufacturer. Multiple dose vials of reconstituted vaccine should be held at 5°–10 °C; unused vaccine should be discarded with 1 h after reconstitution.

Yellow fever vaccine is administered to travelers for two indications: (1) for personal health protection and (2) to meet the requirements of the International Health Regulations.

*For personal health protection*: Persons 9 months of age or older traveling in rural areas of South America and Africa where yellow fever infection is officially reported should be vaccinated. Information on known or probable infected areas is available from the WHO, the Pan American Health Organization (PAHO), and the Division of Vector-Borne Diseases, Center for Infectious Diseases, Centers for Disease Control (CDC), Fort Collins Colorado, Tel. 303-221-6400; and in the *Bi-Weekly Summary of Countries with Areas Infected with Quarantinable Diseases*, published by the Division of Quarantine, Center for Prevention Services, Centers for Disease Control (CDC), Atlanta, Georgia. Vaccination is also recommended for travel outside the urban areas of countries which do not officially report the disease, but which lie in the yellow fever endemic zone (see WHO and CDC maps). It should be emphasized that the actual areas of yellow fever virus activity far exceed the infected zones officially reported and that, in recent years, fatal cases of yellow fever have occurred in unvaccinated tourists [38].

*To meet the requirements of the International health Regulations*: Yellow fever vaccination for international travel may be required for travelers visiting certain countries. These countries are reported in WHO's *Vaccination Certificate Requirements and Health Advice for International Travel*, and are reproduced in CDCs *Health Information for International Travel*. Travel agencies, international airlines, and/or shipping lines should also have up-to-date information, as published in the *Travel Information Manual (TIM)*.

Although specific information is not available concerning side effects of yellow fever vaccine on the developing fetus, it is prudent on theoretical grounds to avoid vaccinating pregnant women and to postpone travel to areas where yellow fever is present until after delivery. If international travel requirements constitute the only reason to vaccinate a pregnant woman, rather than an increased risk of infection, the traveler's physician should provide a waiver letter. Pregnant women who must travel to areas where the risk of yellow fever is high should be vaccinated. It is believed that under these circumstances the small theoretical risk for mother and fetus from vaccination is far outweighed by the risk of yellow fever infection. Children who are 9 months of age or older may be immunized; however, children who are visiting or residing in urban areas (of yellow fever endemic countries) who do not go to rural areas may be immunized at 12 months of age. Infants under 9 months of age should be considered for vaccination if they are traveling to areas undergoing ongoing epidemic yellow fever when travel cannot be postponed and a high level of prevention against mosquito exposure is not feasible. Infants under 4 months of age are more susceptible to serious adverse reactions (encephalitis) than older children. The risk of this complication appears to be age related; whenever possible, immunization should be delayed until 9 months. In no instance should infants under 4 months of age receive yellow fever vaccine.

Primary immunization for yellow fever for persons of all ages consists of a single subcutaneous injection of 0.5 ml reconstituted vaccine. Yellow fever immunity following vaccination with 17D strain virus persists for more than 10 years [39]; the International Health Regulation do not require vaccination more often than every 10 years.

Infection with yellow fever vaccine virus poses a theoretical risk to patients with immunosuppression in association with acquired immunodeficiency syndrome (AIDS) or other manifestations of HIV infection; leukemia; lymphoma; generalized malignancy; or with administration of corticosteroids, alkylating drugs, antimetabolites, or radiation. Short-term (less than 2 weeks) corticosteroid therapy or intraarticular, bursal, or tendon injections with corticosteroid should not be immunosuppressive and constitute no increased hazard to recipients of yellow fever vaccine. Persons previously diagnosed as having asymptomatic HIV infections and who cannot avoid potential exposure to yellow fever virus should be immunized. Vaccinees should be monitored for possible adverse effects. Since immunization of such individuals may be less effective than for uninfected persons, the neutralizing antibody response to vaccination may be determined prior to travel. Family members of immunosuppressed persons, who themselves have no contraindication, may receive yellow fever vaccine.

Live yellow fever vaccine is produced in chick embryos and should not be given to persons clearly hypersensitive to eggs; generally persons who are able to eat eggs or egg products may receive the vaccine. If vaccination of an individual with a questionable history of egg hypersensitivity is considered essential because of a high risk of exposure, an intradermal test dose may be administered under close medical supervision. Specific directions for skin testing are found in the package insert.

Reactions to 17D yellow fever vaccine are generally mild. Two to 5% of vaccines have mild headaches, myalgia, low-grade fevers, or other minor symptoms 5–10 days after vaccination. Fewer than 0.2% curtail regular activities. Immediate hypersensitivity reactions, characterized by rash, urticaria, and/or asthma, are extremely uncommon (incidence less than 1/1 000 000) and occur principally in persons with histories of egg allergy. Although more than 34 million doses of vaccines have been distributed, only two cases of encephalitis temporally associated with vaccinations have been reported in the United States; in one fatal case, 17D virus was isolated from the brain.

A prospective study of persons given yellow fever vaccine and 5 ml of commercially available immune globulin revealed no alteration of the immunologic response to yellow fever vaccine when compared with controls [40]. Although chloroquine inhibits replication of yellow fever virus in vitro, it does not adversely affect antibody responses to yellow fever vaccine in humans receiving antimalarial prophylaxis [41].

## Simultaneous Use of Vaccines for Travelers

Experimental evidence and extensive clinical experience have strengthened the scientific basis for giving certain vaccines at the same time. Most of the widely used antigens can safely and effectively be given simultaneously. This knowledge is particularly helpful for international travelers for whom exposure to several infectious diseases may be imminent. In general, inactivated vaccines can be administered simultaneously at separate sites. However, when vaccines commonly associated with local or systemic side effects (such as cholera, parenteral, typhoid, and plague vaccines) are given simultaneously, the side effects can be accentuated. Whenever possible, these vaccines should be given on separate occasions. In general, simultaneous administration (on the same day) of the most widely used live and inactivated vaccines has not resulted in impaired antibody responses or increased rates of adverse reactions.

The safety and efficacy of hepatitis B vaccine, DTP and OPV administered simultaneously is similar to separate administration of the vaccines. Hepatitis B and yellow fever vaccine may be given concurrently [42].

Some data have indicated that persons given yellow fever and cholera vaccines simultaneously or 1–3 weeks apart have had lower-than-normal antibody responses to both vaccines. Unless there are time constraints, cholera and yellow fever vaccines should be administered at a minimal interval of 3 weeks. If the vaccines cannot be administered at least 3 weeks apart, then the vaccines can be given simultaneously or at any time within the 3-week interval.

Determination of whether to administer yellow fever vaccine and other immunobiologics simultaneously should be made on the basis of convenience to the traveler in completing the desired immunizations before travel and on information regarding possible interference. Studies have shown that the serologic response to yellow fever vaccine is not inhibited by administration of certain other vaccines concurrently or at various intervals of a few days to 1 month. Measles and yellow fever vaccines have been administered in combination with full efficacy of each of the components; Bacillus Calmette Guerin (BCG) and yellow fever vaccines have been administered simultaneously without interference. Additionally, severity of reactions to vaccination was not amplified by concurrent administration of yellow fever and other live virus vaccines [43–45]. If live virus vaccines are not given concurrently, 4 weeks should be allowed to elapse between sequential vaccinations. There are no data on possible interference between yellow fever and typhoid, paratyhoid, typhus, plague, rabies, or Japanese encephalitis vaccines.

## Conclusion

The special-use immunobiologics reviewed in this paper are the most powerful tools currently available for preventing specific infectious diseases of travelers. As noted for particular vaccines, there are some concerns for safety, efficacy and availability, but time favors the resolution of these problems with better and more readily available products. Travelers should consider themselves blessed that these disease prevention products are available to them, whereas so many people who live in developing countries, where these diseases are endemic, are not so fortunate.

## References

1. Gangarosa EJ, Barker WH (1974) Cholera: implications for the United States. JAMA 227:170–171
2. Snyder JD, Blake PA (1982) Is cholera a problem for US travelers? JAMA 247:2268–2269
3. Kluge T (1963) Gamma-globulin in the prevention of viral hepatitis: a study on the effect of medium-size doses. Acta Med Scand 174:469–477
4. Mosley JW, Reisler DM, Brachott D, Roth D, Weiser J (1968) Comparison of two lots of immune serum globulin for prophylaxis of infectious hepatitis. Am J Epidemiol 87:539–550
5. Cossar JH, Reid D (1987) Not all travellers need immunoglobulin for hepatitis A. Br Med J 294:1503
6. Larouze B, Gaudebout C, Foulon G, Mercier E, Ancelle JP (1984) Screening for hepatitis A antibody before prescribing standard immunoglobulin for Europeans staying in tropical areas. Lancet I:449–450
7. Palmer J, Caul EO, Roome APCH (1987) Not all travellers need immunoglobulin for hepatitis A. Br Med J 295:554
8. Zajac BA, West DJ, McAleer WJ, Scolnick EM (1986) Overview of clinical studies with hepatitis B vaccine made by recombinant DNA. J Infect [Suppl A]13:39–45
9. Davidson M, Krugman S (1986) Recombinant yeast hepatitis B vaccine compard with plasma-derived vaccine: immunogenicity and effect of a booster dose. J Infect [Suppl A]13:31–38
10. Hadler SC (1988) Are booster doses of hepatitis B vaccine necessary? Ann Intern Med 108(3):457–458
11. Francis DP, Feorino PM, McDougal S et al. (1986) The safety of hepatitis B vaccine: inactivation of the AIDS virus during routine vaccine manufacture. JAMA 256:869–872

12. Hsu TC, Chow LP, Wei HY et al. (1971) A completed field trial for an evaluation of the effectiveness of mouse-brain Japanese encephalitis vaccine. In: Haniman WMD, Kitaoka M, Downs WG (eds) Immunisation for Japanese encephalitis. Igaku Shoin, Tokyo, pp 258–265
13. Kuang CH (1982) Studies of Japanese encephalitis in China. Adv Virus Res 27:71–101
14. WHO (1984) Japanese Encephalitis Surveillance – Report of a WHO Working Group. Weekly Epidemiol Rec 59:21–28
15. McKinney WP, Barnas GP (1987) Japanese encephalitis vaccine: an orphan product in need of adoption. N Engl J Med 318(4):255–256
16. Denning DW, Kaneko Y (1987) Should travellers to Asia be vaccinated against Japanese encephalitis? Lancet I:853–854
17. Griffiss JM, Brandt BL, Altieri PL, Pier GB, Berman SL (1981) Safety and immunogenicity of group Y and group W135 meningococcal capsular polysaccharide vaccines in adults. Infect Immun 34:725–732
18. Greenwood BM, Whittle HC, Bradley AK, Fayet MT, Gilles HM (1980) The duration of the antibody response to meningococcal vaccination in an African village. Trans R Soc Trop Med Hyg 74:756–760
19. Käyhty H, Karanko V, Peltola H, Sarna S, Mäkelä PH (1980) Serum antibodies to capsular polysaccharide vaccine of group A *Neisseria meningitidis* followed for three years in infants and children. J Infect Dis 142:861–868
20. Novelli VM, Lewis RG, Dawood (1987) Epidemic group A meningococcal disease in Haj pilgrims. Lancet II:863
21. McCormick JB, Gusmao HH, Nakamura S et al. (1980) Antibody response to serogroup A and C meningococcal polysaccharide vaccines in infants born of mothers vaccinated during pregnancy. J Clin Invest 65:1141–1144
22. Gold R, Lepow ML, Goldschneider I, Draper TF, Gotschlich EC (1979) Kinetics of antibody production to group A and group C meningococcal polysaccharide vaccines administered during the first six years of life: prospects for routine immunization of infants and children. J Infect Dis 140:690–697
23. Meyer KF (1970) Effectiveness of live or killed plague vaccines in man. Bull WHO 42:653–666
24. Cavanaugh DC, Elisberg BL, Llewellyn CH et al. (1974) Plague immunization. V. Indirect evidence for the efficacy of plague vaccine. J Infect Dis [Suppl] 129:S37–40
25. CDC (1986) Rabies prevention: supplementary statement on the preexposure use of human diploid cell rabies vaccine by the intradermal route. MMWR 35:767–768
26. Bernard KW, Fishbein DB, Miller KD et al. (1985) Pre-exposure rabies immunization and human diploid cell rabies vaccine: decreased antibody responses in persons immunized in developing countries. Am J Trop Med Hyg 34:633–647
27. Pappaioanou M, Fishbein DB, Dreesen DW et al. (1986) Antibody response to preexposure human-diploid cell rabies vaccine given concurrently with chloroquine. N Engl J Med 314:280–284
28. CDC (1984) Systemic allergic reactions following immunization with human diploid cell rabies vaccine. MMWR 33:185–187
29. Dreesen DW, Bernard KW, Parker RA, Deutsch AJ, Brown J (1986) Immune complex-like disease in 23 persons following a booster dose of rabies human diploid cell vaccine. Vaccine 4:45–49
30. Ashcroft MT, Nicholson CC, Balwent S, Ritchie JM, Soryan S, William F (1967) A seven year field trial of two typhoid vaccines in Guyana. Lancet II:1056–1060
31. Edwards EA, Johnson JP, Pierce WE, Peckinpaugh RO (1974) Reactions and serologic response to monovalent acetone-inactivated typhoid vaccine and heat-killed TAB vaccine when given by yet-injection. Bull WHO 51:501–505
32. Wahdan MH, Sere C, Cerisier Y, Sallam S, Germanier R (1982) A controlled field trial of live *Salmonella typhi* strain Ty 21a oral vaccine against typhoid: three year results. J Infect Dis 145:292–295

33. Levine MM, Black RE, Ferreccio C, Germanier R et al. (1987) Large scale field trial of Ty 21a live oral typhoid vaccine in enteric-coated capsule formulation. Lancet 1049–1052
34. Edelman R, Levine MM (1986) Summary of an international workshop on typhoid fever. Rev Infect Dis 8:329–349
35. Taylor DN, Pollard RA, Blake PA (1983) Typhoid in the United States and the risk to the international traveler. J Infect Dis 148:599–602
36. Smithburn KC, Durieux C, Koerber R et al. (1956) Yellow fever vaccination. WHO Monogr Ser 30
37. Wisseman CL Jr, Sweet BH (1962) Immunological studies with group B arthropod-borne viruses. III. Response of human subjects to revaccination with 17D strain yellow fever vaccine. Am J Trop Med 11:570–575
38. Rodhain F, Hannoun C, Jousset FX, Ravisse P (1979) Isolement du virus de la fière jaune à Paris a partir de deux cas humains importés. Bull Soc Pathol Exot 72:411–415
39. Poland JD, Calisher CH, Monath TP, Downs WG, Murphy K (1981) Persistence of neutralizing antibody 30–35 years after immunization with 17D yellow fever vaccine. Bull WHO 59:895–900
40. Kaplan JE, Nelson DB, Schonberger LB et al. (1984) The effect of immune globulin on trivalent oral polio and yellow fever vaccinations. Bull WHO 62:585–590
41. Tsai TF, Bolin RA, Lazuick JS et al. (1986) Chloroquine does not adversely affect the antibody response to yellow fever vaccine. J Infect Dis 154:726
42. Yvonnet B, Coursaget P, Deubel V et al. (1986) Simultaneous administration of hepatitis B and yellow fever vaccines. J Med Virol 19:307–311
43. Tauraso NM, Myers MG, Nau EV et al. (1972) Effect of interval between inoculation of live smallpox and yellow-fever vaccines on antigenicity in man. J Infect Dis 126:363–371
44. Felsenfeld O, Wolf RH, Gyr K et al. (1973) Simultaneous vaccination against cholera and yellow fever. Lancet I:457–458
45. Gateff C (1972) Acquisitions récentes en matière d'associations vaccinales. Bull Soc Pathol Exot 65:784–796

# Variations in Vaccination Recommendations

A. C. Turner

The variations in the recommendations for immunizations, or vaccinations as the World Health Organization (WHO) prefers them to be called, are indeed numerous.

Let us consider first the two which can be considered to be mandatory, namely yellow fever and cholera. The latter should not be so considered but more about that later.

## Yellow Fever

With the definitive lines of yellow fever endemic areas laid down by WHO one would have thought that there was a good chance of unanimity. However, there are variations in endemic and infected areas and urban and rural districts. Nowadays, in general, countries outside the yellow fever endemic areas which demand vaccination only demand it from infected areas and not endemic areas. In February 1988 there were only nine countries in Africa with infected areas and four in South America whilst there are 28 and 10 endemic countries respectively. However, India, Pakistan, Bhutan, Bangladesh and Singapore still require vaccination when travellers arrive from endemic areas. They also consider international airports to be in the endemic areas, which is against WHO recommendations. Some countries in the endemic areas do not demand vaccination for visitors to urban areas but who is to stop the traveller from visiting rural areas once he has entered the country. Mali only demands vaccination if the traveller is staying in the country for 2 weeks or more.

Nearly all countries who require vaccination lay down arrival within 5–6 days after leaving the infected area, but Mauritius states 10 days.

In addition there are 12 countries which demand vaccination even in passengers who are flying through their country and are never leaving the aircraft, if they have been in an infected area within the last 6 days. The United States [1] recommends that infants under 6 months should not be vaccinated because of the increased risk of encephalitis. The United Kingdom states 1 year. However, six countries demand vaccination at 6 months and 25 at any age.

## Cholera

This surely is the most controversial vaccination. It was in December 1970 that Doctor Jesse Steinfeld, Surgeon General of the US Public Health Services, announced that the United States would no longer demand a cholera vaccination certificate from an entrant from any country. In June 1978 the World Health Assembly recommended that this should be a worldwide practice. At the present time there are still about 16 countries demanding vaccination mainly in people who have been in an infected area in the last 6 days. A few demand it of everybody. But the world is improving; it was 29 countries in 1985. No country in the Americas demand vaccination but, surprisingly, Albania and Malta in Europe do. There is an improvement in the system in that one intradermal dose of 0.2 ml of the standard vaccine is sufficient to satisfy the men at the barriers. The old 0.5-ml and a second 1.0-ml subcutaneous injections are no longer required although they still tend to be given worldwide. Regrettably general practitioners in the United Kingdom write certificates on their own letter-headed paper and not on an International Certificate, which is valueless. Cholera vaccination is refused in Canada. Doctors sign the certificate that there is no medical indication for it.

Personally I do not disagree with this opinion, but it does not satisfy a difficult man at the barrier. I have given several Canadians an intradermal injection. They have frequently asked for, and are most grateful to be given, it.

Let us now turn to the medically recommended vaccinations.

## Typhoid

During the last few years monovalent typhoid has replaced typhoid para A and B (TAB) vaccine although certain Western Europe countries still use the latter vaccine.

Wellcome, the producers of vaccine used in the United Kingdom, recommend 0.5 ml H.I. initially followed by 0.1 ml intradermally preferably after 4 weeks and 0.1 ml intradermally as a booster every 3 years. It seems that outside the United Kingdom the intradermal method is not being used. The use of the intradermal method definitely minimizes the side effects. The other problem is that travellers are frequently given only one dose, giving fair protection for 6–8 weeks, whilst the two doses will give cover for up to 3 years. The Centers for Disease Control and the United States Medical Letter [2] recommend immunization of visitors to rural areas of tropical countries and where there are epidemics. Steffen et al. [3] agree with this.

Dr. Robin Leach [4] the world-renowned solo yachtsman, on the other hand, recommends typhoid vaccination anywhere outside northern Europe. The answer must be in between.

In the last few years in Europe there have been epidemics in the Greek Islands and one of the costas of Spain, also at a coastal resort of North Africa. Surely, if typhoid occurs in the rural areas carriers can move into the urban areas. Because of this typhoid vaccination is recommended in the United

Kingdom for all countries including the towns where food or water hygiene is open to doubt.

Vivotif, the oral typhoid vaccine, is used in western Europe. It is not used in the United Kingdom, as it has not yet been approved by the Department of Health. It is not approved in North America or Australasia. Steffen et al. [5] recommends it for all travellers to India as well as those whose stay in other developing countries and endemic areas travel outside the usual tourist areas. Levine et al. [6] carried out an extensive trial in Chile. Then three doses of oral vaccine given within 1 week gave a 67% efficiency for at least 3 years. Increasing the interval between doses to 21 days did not enhance protection. They considered it as effective as the heat/phenol-inactivated whole cell vaccine.

## Poliomyelitis

Sometimes this is the most difficult vaccine to get across to the traveller because, if they live in the developed countries where poliomyelitis has been eradicated, they think vaccination is effective for a lifetime.

Kubli et al. [7] quote 175 cases of paralytic poliomyelitis imported to industrialized nations between 1975 and 1984. Twenty-seven percent were nationals on holiday or business. The highest fatality rate was between 41 and 65 years. Gregory and Spalding [8] quoted two businessmen over 30 years of age confined in respirators for the rest of their lives after brief business trips abroad. It is certain that when poliomyelitis strikes later it strikes harder.

## Meningococcal Meningitis

There are two vaccines available for this serious disease. In France the Pasteur Institute produces Meningococcal meningitis A and C whilst in the United States this vaccine has been replaced by Squibb Connaughts quadrivalent A/C/Y/W-135 vaccine.

In Australia nearly all travellers passing through Asia appear to be given one of these vaccines. In the United States it also seems to be given liberally to visitors to Africa and Asia. In the United Kingdom it has not yet been approved by the Department of Health because a product licence has not been applied for and family doctors in general do not know about it and it is only given in a few special immunization centres. It should be given to visitors to areas known for endemic or epidemic disease, in particular Nepal, northern India and the sub-Saharan countries.

## Rabies

The arrival of Rabies Human Diplococcal Vaccine (HDCV) established pre-exposure vaccination, but regrettably its cost is high. This introduced the possibility of giving a smaller intradermal dose of 0.1 ml instead of the recommended dose of 1.0 ml intramuscular.

In the United States a suitable presentation for the intradermal dose is available. This is not so in the United Kingdom and, as the vaccine is made up at time of use, several people must be immunized at the same time to be economic. Opinions seem to vary as to whether the i.d. dose is as effective as the injection.

Pappaioanou et al. [9] have shown that the taking of chloroquine as a malarial prophylactic at the same time as vaccination interferes with the antibody response to HDCV. The i.m. dose/rate provides a sufficient margin of safety in this setting. In addition if given by the i.d. method the course must be completed at least 30 days before travel. Grandien et al. [10] show i.d. response is less than i.m. response. Because of the method of presentation i.d. is more popular in the United States than in the United Kingdom and Australia.

## Immune Globulins

This surely is the inoculation which has the most patient resistance presumably due to the discomfort it usually causes. The excuses vary from it is not effective, the risk is greater when it is time expired, and also the risk of AIDS.

Pollock and Reid [11] and Woodson and Clinton [12] proved this otherwise. WHO and the US Department of Health state only for travellers to high-risk areas outside ordinary transit routes. In 1970 the Scandinavians [13] recommended it for all travellers to the Mediterranean area. Switzerland [5] recommends it for all visitors to the third world particularly for long stays and when the food conditions and hygiene are poor. In Australia all travellers to the United Kingdom through the East are given immunoglobulin. In the United Kingdom more and more travellers to Africa, Asia and South America are given it. The "overlanding" excursions from London through Africa to Nairobi or through Asia to Nepal demand it. Surely wherever intestinal infections are prevalent it should be considered.

## References

1. US Department of Health and Human Services (1987) Health information for international travel. DHHS, Washington, p 73
2. Anonymous (1987) Advice for travelers. Med Lett Drugs Ther 29:53–56
3. Steffen R, Rickenbach M, Wilhelm U, Helminger A, Schär M (1985) Health problems after travel to developing countries. J Infect Dis 156:84–91
4. Leach RD (1984) Medical aspects of ocean yacht voyages. Travel Traffic Med Int 2:31–35
5. Steffen R, Herzog C, Raeber P, Somaini B, Darioli R, Schrafl C, Schubarth P, Markwalder K (1987) Vaccinations pour les voyages à l'étranger. Annexe to Bulletin de l'Office Fédéral de la Santé Publique, Paris, pp 505–510
6. Levine MM, Black RE, Ferreccio C, Germanier R, Chilean Typhoid Committee (1987) Large scale field trial of Ty 21A live oral typhoid vaccine in enteric-coated capsule formulation. Lancet I:1049–1052
7. Kubli D, Steffen R, Schar M (1987) Importation of poliomyelitis to industrialised nations between 1975 and 1984. Evaluation and conclusion for vaccination recommendations. Br Med J 295:168–171

8. Gregory MC, Spalding JMK (1972) Poliomyelitis in adults (Letter). Lancet I:142–155
9. Pappaioanou M et al. (1986) Antibody response to preexposure human diploid cell rabies vaccine given concurrently with chloroquine. N Engl J Med 314:280–284
10. Grandien M, Fridell E, Kindmark CO (1985) Intradermal immunization with reduced doses of human diploid cell strain rabies vaccine. Evaluation of antibody response by ELISA and mixed hemadsorption test. Scand J Infect Dis 17:173–178
11. Pollock TM, Reid D (1969) Immunoglobulin for the prevention of infectious hepatitis in persons working overseas. Lancet I:28–30
12. Woodson RD, Clinton JJ (1969) Hepatitis prophylaxis abroad. JAMA 209:1053–1058
13. Christenson B (1985) Epidemiological aspects of acute viral hepatitis A in Swedish travellers to endemic areas. Scand J Infect Dis 17:5–10

# Is Vaccination Worthwhile Before Travel?

G. Wiedermann

## Summary

Possible immunizations for travelers to developing countries may be divided into three categories: compulsory, commonly recommended and occasionally recommended immunizations. When trying to judge their beneficial effects we may do so from two points of view: by considering risk and benefit or cost and benefit. Calculations can be done by the introduction of simple mathematical formulas. In the case of risk-benefit calculations the risk-benefit ratio ($Q$) weighs risk of disease against risk of vaccination, which is recommendable if $Q > 1.0$. The risk-benefit difference considers preventable disease or complications. An immunization is recommendable if $D > 0$. Similarly, the cost-benefit ratio ($Q_c$) considers cost-effectiveness and the cost-benefit difference ($D_c$) presents the amount of money saved. Four examples have been chosen for these calculations: vaccination against cholera, tetanus and poliomyelitis and passive immunization against hepatitis A. In the case of cholera $Q_c < 1$, indicating that this vaccination is not cost effective. However, $Q$ is a bit more than 1 and $D$ above 0. Tetanus vaccination of people staying at home or travelling is recommendable and just cost-effective. Costs of OPV are being paid by the Austrian government; $Q$ and $D$ (risk-benefit parameters) are highly positive. Passive immunization against hepatitis A is recommendable and cost-effective for Austrian soldiers on UN mission. For the individual traveler it is cost-effective if the hepatitis risk is $> 1:150$.

Possible immunizations for travelers to developing countries have been divided into three categories by Walker and Williams [12, 13]. These categories include compulsory, commonly recommended and occasionally recommended immunizations. The compulsory immunizations are against yellow fever and cholera. According to the requirements for international travel 1987 and 1988 there are for instance requirements for cholera vaccination in nine countries mostly for travelers immigrating from an infected area [16]. Commonly recommended vaccinations include immunizations against poliomyelitis, tetanus, typhoid fever and passive immunization against hepatitis A. Occasionally recommended vaccinations include immunization against tuberculosis, diphtheria, hepatitis B, meningococcal infections, Japanese encephalitis, and rabies. In some areas of Europe, including certain provinces of Austria, tick-borne encephalitis vaccination might be advisable. In children measles, mumps, and pertussis vaccination status should be up to date.

## Benefit/Risk and Benefit/Cost

Here the above-mentioned question may be raised: Is vaccination worthwhile before travel? The question may be considered from two points of view. That is, we may consider benefit and risk or benefit and cost. Some relatively simple mathematical formulas (and the emphasis really lies on simplicity) for this purpose were developed some years ago [2, 17–19, 21]. For benefit-risk calculations there is the benefit-risk ratio ($Q$) and the benefit-risk difference $D$. The following parameters are used in the formula: the protection rate $p$, the duration of protection in years $t$, the vaccination rate $l$, which tells us about the vaccinated part of a population, the risk of disease $R$ and the risk of vaccination $r$. The risks must of course be comparable and refer to essential complications, which shall be prevented, or death. The risk of disease must, naturally, consider the risk of disease in an unvaccinated population. If this is not known it may be calculated or estimated for instance by means for the formula for a vaccination which does not interrupt the infection chain:

$$R_0 = \frac{R_v}{1-pl}.$$

Thus, if a vaccination with a protection rate of 0.8 and a vaccination rate of 0.9, like the pertussis vaccination, is being abolished in a community, this would mean a fourfold rise in morbidity and complications from disease.

The benefit-risk ratio $Q$ weighs the risks from disease and from vaccination against each other:

$$Q = \frac{Rt}{r+(1-p)Rt}.$$

Thus the risk of disease is compared with the risk of vaccination + vaccination failures during a certain period (namely the duration of protection) and it is easily understandable that the vaccination is beneficial if $Q > 1.0$. The benefit-risk difference designates the annual number of preventable complications from a disease minus those of the vaccination:

$$D = pR - \frac{r}{t}.$$

It is easily understandable that a vaccination is beneficial if $D > 0$.

Another kind of calculation considers the costs of disease risks and of vaccinations. It tells us if money is saved or lost by a vaccination procedure. We have developed similar formulas for the excellently tolerable vaccination against measles under the assumption that nobody will escape infection [19]:

$$Q_c = \frac{C_{Th}}{C_v+(1-p)C_{Th}}.$$

In this equation $C_{Th}$ indicates costs of therapy and $C_v$ indicates costs of vaccination. If this assumption is not the case, this formula may be modified for morbidity and mortality as follows:

$$Q_c = \frac{C_{Th} \cdot R_m}{C_v + (1-p) C_{Th} R_m}$$

or:

$$Q_c = \frac{C_{Th} \cdot R_m + C_L \cdot R_L}{C_v + (1-p) C_{Th} \cdot R_m + (1-p) C_L R_L}$$

respectively. In these formulas $R_m$ indicates disease risk and $R_L$ indicates death rate (mortality) and $C_L$ respective costs.

Four examples of immunization are vaccination against cholera, poliomyelitis, tetanus, and passive immunization against hepatitis A.

## Cholera

Steffen in 1983 provided data for travelers. A risk of disease ($R_m$) of $2 \cdot 10^{-6}$ may be assumed and considering an estimated vaccination rate of 60% (approximately 50% according to Allard [1]) $R_{mo}$ may be accepted as $3 \cdot 10^{-6}$; risk of death $R_L = 0.02 \times R_m$; cost of therapy 5000 Swiss Francs; cost of a death case 1 000 000 Swiss Francs; cost of vaccination, 20 Swiss Francs (1 Swiss Franc = approx. US $0.57). Protection rate ($p$) was about 0.6; if $p = 0.5$ is chosen according to other authors or 0.8 for a two-vaccination schedule, this does not *grosso modo* influence the result significantly.

Inserting all these data into the last-mentioned formula a $Q_c$ is obtained of $3.7 \cdot 10^{-3}$, which means that $Q_c = < 1.0$ and that the vaccination is not cost-effective. This takes care of the benefit-cost calculation. If the benefit-risk calculation is considered, the respective formula for the benefit-risk ratio ($Q$) must be applied. This shows that any vaccination for which $r$ is negligible will produce a value for $Q$ which is greater than 1.0. To obtain a better insight of how many cases can be prevented the risk difference ($D$) must be examined, which is for cholera $= pR$. According to this formula there is, additionally to other measures of exposition prophylaxis, prevention of about one to two caes/1 million travelers with respect to morbidity and three to four cases/100 million travelers to endemic areas with respect to mortality to be expected. This is actually not very much, but $D > 0$ and one has to take into consideration that many people are travelling. So it must finally be left to the consideration of the physician and the traveler if this measure has worth and value for him. And this underlines the conclusions of a WHO article of 1974 about cholera [14], namely that experience over the past decade has shown that spread of vibrios cannot be prevented by the vaccination and, although vaccination is not a barrier against dissemination, it may afford a certain measure of individual protection.

## Poliomyelitis

According to vaccination requirements and the health advice of the WHO in 1987, poliomyelitis has been reported from many countries in Africa, South America, and Asia [16]. Altogether, though, in 1985 only 29 890 cases were reported in 4700 million people (99% of them in developing countries), which corresponds to an incidence of $0.6 \times 10^{-5}$ [15]. Lameness surveys [15] indicate that one should take into account a multiplication factor of four, in some areas even of 100. In developing countries the incidence of paralytic cases is probably $10–30 \cdot 10^{-5}$.

Some years ago in western Europe the benefit-risk ratio and the benefit-risk difference were calculated for oral poliomyelitis vaccination [21]. Among other parameters a rather pessimistic value for risk of vaccination ($r$) was inserted. Our deliberation was as follows: the US Centers for Disease Control reported one paralytic case after vaccination in 3.2 million distributed doses. Since vaccine-related paralytic disease usually occurs only after the first dose and since three doses are usually administered per person, this means one case in 1 million persons. According to our paper [21], 90% of the population had already acquired natural immunity at this time, so that only one in ten was susceptible and the risk of vaccination might thus be $1 \times 10^{-5}$. The $Q$ and $D$ values were high, demonstrating the effectiveness of this vaccination. If we accept similar parameters with a rate of paralytic cases of $20 \times 10^{-5}$ in developing countries we arrive at even higher values for $Q$ and $D$, and figures presented for Brazil in 1984 are far beyond this [4]. $Q$ and $D$ values of travelers lie somewhere in between the values for industrialized and developing countries depending on travel habits and duration of stay (Table 1).

Since vaccination campaigns in the case of poliomyelitis are continuously in operation, there will be practically no additional costs. International travel will only help us to tighten the surveillance.

**Table 1.** Putative benefit-risk ratio and difference after poliomyelitis immunization in industrialized and developing countries

| | |
|---|---|
| $Q_{ind} = 8.6$ | $Q_{dev} = 9.5$ |
| $D_{ind} = 5.4 \times 10^{-5}$ | $D_{dev} = 17.9 \times 10^{-5}$ |

## Tetanus

Tetanus also is a commonly recommended vaccination in Austria. It may be accepted that the protection rate is near 1.0 (100%). Fatal complications after vaccination are negligible and a tetanus-like illness is not known after vaccination. Keeping this in mind it is apparent from the formulas that $Q$ is practically infinite when $r = 0$ and $p = 1$ or at least very high, and the risk difference $D$ de-

**Table 2.** Benefit-cost difference of tetanus

| | | |
|---|---|---|
| $D_c = \sum C_{Th} - \sum C_{Vacc}$ | | |
| $r = 0$ | $R_0 = 305/\text{year}$ | $n_{vacc} = 1$ million vaccinations/year |
| $p = 1.0$ | $C_{Th} = 200\,000$ AS | $C_{vacc} = 30–50$ AS |
| | $\sum C_{Th} = 60$ million AS | $\sum C_{vacc} = 30–50$ million AS |
| $D_c \sim 10–30$ million AS | | |

AS, Austrian schillings

signating preventable disease is practically identical with incidence. When calculating the cost-effectiveness of such a vaccination, it may be stated that the benefit-cost difference $D_c$, i.e., the savings in costs by that vaccination, is equivalent to cost of therapy of tetanus cases in a country minus costs of vaccinating the population (Table 2).

In the years before tetanus vaccination was commonly in use in Austria in 1928–1931, there were on average 305 tetanus cases in the country [2, 7]. The costs of therapy in 1975 when this calculation was done were as high as 200 000 Austrian schillings, which means approximately costs of 60 million Austrian schillings/year (1 Austrian schilling = approx. US $0.07). Costs for vaccination including the doctor's honorarium at this time may be estimated as 30–50 Austrian schillings. If one accepts that 7 million people need about ten vaccinations for lifetime (70 years) protection, this makes 1 million vaccinations/ year, amounting to 30–50 million Austrian schillings for vaccination cases. Thus, $D_c$ would have been equivalent to 10–30 million Austrian schillings/ year. Individual savings would amount in this calculation only to a few schillings, but at least there would be no loss of money. It must be considered, however, that costs of treatment increase much more than vaccination costs and that – most importantly – tetanus incidence in developing countries is often 10–20 times higher than estimated in this calculation. That means that tetanus vaccination is highly beneficial, and on average an investment which means no loss of money at home and when travelling.

## Hepatitis A

Immunization against hepatitis A deserves attention. Our team performed checkups in industrial workers, Peace Corps workers and other travelers before and after stays in tropical countries; among other parameters the incidence of hepatitis antibodies was investigated [5]. There was a seroconversion in hepatitis A antibodies in nearly 15% and in hepatitis B antibodies in 1.6%. This seroconversion usually took place over a period of 1 year. The incidence of the so-called "traveler's hepatitis", which is usually hepatitis A, is different depending on the respective geographical areas, as has been summarized by Steffen [9].

In this paper two kinds of calculations for immunization with immunoglobulin against hepatitis A are presented. The first one was performed by our-

**Table 3.** Hepatitis A immunization of UN military personel for 6 months

| | |
|---|---|
| $Q_c = \frac{R_m C_{Th}}{C_v + (1-p) R_m C_{Th}}$ | $D_c = pR_m C_{Th} - C_v$ |
| $p = 0.94$ | $R_m = 0.021$ |
| $C_{v(I)} = 2 \times 0.05$ ml/kg body wt. $= 558.4$ AS | |
| $C_{Th} =$ (including stay in hospital, loss of income, transportation) | |
| Austria: 82730 AS | UNO + Austria: 198024 AS |
| $Q_c = 2.6$<br>$D_c = 1074.7$ AS | $Q_c = 5.1$<br>$D_c = 3350.6$ AS |

AS., Austrian schillings

selves for Austrian military personnel serving in Cyprus and on the Golan heights in the wake of the United Nations peace-keeping mission [3, 20]. The second one was carried out using data presented by Steffen et al. [10] considering cost-effectiveness of immunoglobulin administration for the average traveler.

The data of the military personnel are shown in Table 3. Before the introduction of immunoglobulin, there was a hepatitis A incidence of 13 out of 611, which corresponds to an incidence of 1:47 ($R_m = 0.021$). After the introduction of immunoglobulin the incidence was 1 out of 744; thus, the protection rate $p = 0.94$ (94%); costs of immunization ($C_v$) including two injections of 0.05 ml/kg body wt. for 6 months were 558.4 Austrian schillings. Costs of therapy ($C_{Th}$) including the stay in foreign and Austrian hospitals, loss in income, and transportation amounted to 82730 Austrian schillings for the Austrian government and 198024 Austrian schillings total costs for Austria+UN per case. Thus, again applying the formula

$$Q_c = \frac{R_m C_{Th}}{C_v + (1-p) R_m C_{Th}}$$

for cost-benefit ratio and $D_c = pR_m C_{Th} - C_v$ for cost-benefit difference, the value for $Q_c$ concerning costs for Austria was 2.6 and $Q_c$ concerning total costs was 5.1. Thus the cost-benefit ratio was greater than 1.0. The cost-benefit difference $D_c$, reflecting saved money, amounted to 1074.7 Austrian schillings per capita for the Austrian government and 3350.60 Austrian schillings total costs per capita. Total savings for 3611 soldiers were 3.88 million Austrian schillings for our government and approximately 12 million Austrian schillings total costs. In this case the hepatitis immunization was a profitable action.

For the average traveller the cost-effectiveness of a hepatitis immunization naturally depends very much on the risk of disease (which is very high in West Africa and Mexico) and of course on costs of immunization and therapy. The following question arises therefore: when costs are known, what is the minimum risk of disease to make immunization cost-effective?

**Table 4.** Cost-effectiveness of hepatitis A immunization for the average traveller

| | | |
|---|---|---|
| $Q_c = \frac{R_m C_{Th}}{C_v + (1-p) R_m C_{Th}}$ | $Q_c = 1$ | $R_m$ = risk of disease for which immunization is just cost-effective |
| | | $R_m = \frac{C_v}{C_{Th} - (1-p) C_{Th}}$ |
| $C_{Th}$ = 8400 Swiss francs | $C_{v(I)}$ = 50 Swiss francs | $R_m = \frac{1}{150}$ |

$P = 0.89$ (average of 0.94 (20) and 0.83 (8))

Expressed in a mathematical formula (Table 4), this means again that:

$$Q_c = \frac{R_m C_{Th}}{C_v + (1-p) R_m C_{Th}}.$$

With the condition of $Q_c = 1.0$, the formula for $R_m$ (risk of hepatitis or hepatitis incidence) is:

$$R_m = \frac{C_v}{C_{Th} - (1-p) C_{Th}}$$

If we insert costs for therapy in Switzerland according to Steffen et al. [10] as 8400 Swiss francs and costs of immunization as 50 Swiss francs (including immunoglobulin and consultation), $R_m = 1:150$, which means that any risk higher than that makes hepatitis immunization cost-effective under the given provisions and cost relations. It is interesting that the risk of disease in our military personnel was 1:47. Again, the benefit-risk ratio (not benefit-cost ratio) will always be positive since $r$ in that formula in the denominator representing risk of immunization is negligible.

The costs of serological testing for hepatitis A may be calculated. If all travelers are to be immunized and if costs for serology are 230 Austrian schillings and average costs for immunization of travelers 366 Austrian schillings, even immunization without serological testing would be cost-effective on average when 63% of travelers are seropositive. According to Kudesia and Follett [6] and Tettmar et al. [11], this may be the case in persons aged between 40 and 55 years.

## References

1. Allard R (1983) Problems in adequately immunizing international travellers. Can Med Assoc J 127:40–41
2. Ambrosch F, Wiedermann G (1975) Mathematische Methoden zur Beurteilung des Nutzens von Schutzimpfungen. Immun Infekt 3:24–31
3. Ambrosch F, Wiedermann G, Wustinger E (1978) Klinische und laborchemische Untersuchungen zur Beurteilung der Gammaglobulinprophylaxe bei Tropenaufenthalten. Wien Med Wochenschr 128:625–627

4. Creese AL (1984) Cost effectiveness of alternative strategies for poliomyelitis immunization in Brazil. Rev Infect Dis [Suppl 2]6:404–407
5. Kollaritsch H, Ambrosch F, Aspöck H, Auer H, Picher O, Stemberger H, Ambrosch F, Wiedermann G (1982) Analyse der Ergebnisse von Tropenrückkehruntersuchungen. Mitt Osterr Ges Tropenmed Parasitol 4:127–134
6. Kudesia G, Follett EAC (1987) Not all travellers need immunoglobulin for hepatitis A. Br Med J 295:118
7. Kunz H (1971) Tetanusprophylaxe – ein Gebot der ärztlichen Vorsorge. Osterr Arzte Z 26:758–763
8. Ohara H, Ebisawa I, Ohtani S (1986) Prophylactic efficacy of immune serum globulin against hepatitis A. Jpn J Exp Med 56:229–233
9. Steffen R (1984) Reisemedizin. Springer, Berlin Heidelberg New York
10. Steffen R, Regli P, Grob PJ (1977) Wie groß ist das Risiko einer Reisehepatitis? Schweiz Med Wochenschr 107:1300–1307
11. Tettmar RE, Masterton RG, Strike RW (1987) Hepatitis A immunity in British adults – an assessment of the need for pre-immunisation screening. J Infect 15:39–43
12. Walker E, Williams G (1983) ABC of healthy travel. Immunisation I. Br Med J 286:629–631
13. Walker E, Williams G (1983) ABC of healthy travel. Immunisation II. Br Med J 286:703–705
14. WHO (1974) Cholera. Weekly Epidemiol Rec 32:269–270
15. WHO (1987) Poliomyelitis in 1985. Part I. WER 37:273–276
16. WHO (1987/1988) Vaccination certificate requirements and health advice for international travel. WHO, Geneva
17. Wiedermann G (1979) Moderne Trends im Impfwesen: Erfassung von Nutzen. Risiko und Kosten von Impfungen. Wien Klin Wochenschr 91:143–150
18. Wiedermann G, Ambrosch F (1974) Probleme von Impfungen. Wien Med Wochenschr 124:161–165
19. Wiedermann G, Ambrosch F (1979) Costs and benefits of immunization against measles and mumps. Bull WHO 57:625–629
20. Wiedermann G, Ambrosch F, Wustinger E, Gnan F (1978) Hepatitisprophylaxe mit Immunglobulin beim österreichischen UNO-Bataillon. Bundesgesundheitsblatt 21:467–471
21. Wiedermann G, Ambrosch F, Kollaritsch H, Kundi M (1984) Risks and benefits of vaccinations. Infect Control 5:438–444

# Observations on Obtaining Immunizations for International Travel and the Need for Routine Immunizations

E. C. Jong and K. Gurung

The records of a travel clinic based at a university medical center in the United States were analyzed retrospectively for patterns in the immunizations received among individuals seeking pre-travel care for international travel. The travelers were referred from community medical practitioners and travel agencies for comprehensive advice on malaria and diarrhea prevention, and travel vaccines. Records for 3253 patients were available for detailed analysis. More than half of the travelers had primary travel destinations in Asia, with Thailand, Nepal, and India being the most popular destinations, respectively. Kenya and Tanzania were the most frequent destinations in Africa; and Brazil and Peru were frequent destinations in South America. Although the patients specifically sought travel-related care, a review of the immunization data showed that many required updating of their routine vaccines in addition to receiving travel vaccines. The data confirm that among adults 20 years of age or older in an urban community, updating of status for common vaccine-preventable illnesses such as tetanus and diphtheria is not being accomplished efficiently through routine channels of adult health care, and that travel clinics can provide an important service in this public health goal.

## Methods

All travelers, regardless of itinerary planned, were routinely questioned about their tetanus/diphtheria, polio, and measles-mumps-rubella status in addition to being assessed for need of travel immunizations. Status with regard to vaccine-preventable diseases was based on written records, verbal history of specific vaccine dates or a physician's diagnosis of the disease in question, or a history of military duty. With regard to an uncertain history of immunity to rubella, measles, mumps, hepatitis A or B, plague and/or rabies, if time before departure allowed, travelers were given the opportunity to have a serum test for immunity before receiving an indicated vaccine. Travel immunizations offered included yellow fever, cholera, typhoid, immune globulin, Japanese encephalitis, plague, rabies and meningococcus. Standard guidelines of the Immunization Practices Advisory Committee (ACIP) and *Health Information for International Travel* of the Centers for Disease Control (CDC) were used to determine the need for primary or booster doses [1, 2].

## Results

During the study period, the first 6 years of the travel clinic, 3253 patients were seen. Of this group, 46.5% were male and 53.5% were female. Ages were available for 3234 (99.4%) and showed that greater than 90% of the clinic population was 20 years old or older. Numbers of travelers receiving routine vaccines are given in Table 1, and numbers of travelers receiving travel vaccines are given in Table 2. Thirty-six percent of travelers were given tetanus/diphtheria vaccine (Td), 45% were given polio vaccine (OPV or IPV), and less than 1% were given measles-mumps-rubella vaccine (MMR). Thirty percent of the travelers received yellow fever (YF) vaccine, 48% got cholera (Chol) vaccine, 62% got typhoid (Typh) vaccine, and 62% got immune globulin (IG) for hepatitis A prophylaxis. During the 3 years included in this study that Japanese encephalitis B vaccine (JEV) was offered, 15% (291 of 2055) of the travelers presented with appropriate indications for JEV and were vaccinated under an investigational protocol sponsored by the CDC. Plague, rabies, and hepatitis B vaccines were needed by less than 1% of the travelers. There was a big increase in the use of meningococcal A, C, Y, W-135 vaccine in 1985–1986 following reports of an outbreak of meningococcal meningitis among trekkers in Nepal.

When the data on the routine vaccines for tetanus/diphtheria and for polio are organized by age stratification, the data suggest that at least one-third

**Table 1.** Travelers receiving routine vaccines

| Year | No. | Tet/dip (%) | Polio (%) |
|---|---|---|---|
| 1980–1981 | 249 | 108 (43) | 151 (61) |
| 1981–1982 | 445 | 175 (39) | 164 (37) |
| 1982–1983 | 604 | 232 (38) | 230 (38) |
| 1983–1984 | 603 | 245 (41) | 268 (44) |
| 1984–1985 | 652 | 235 (36) | 335 (51) |
| 1985–1986 | 700 | 182 (26) | 321 (45) |
| Total | 3253 | 1177 (36) | 1469 (45) |

**Table 2.** Travelers receiving travel vaccines

| Year | Total | YF (%) | Chol (%) | Typh (%) | Ig (%) | JEV (%) |
|---|---|---|---|---|---|---|
| 1980–1981 | 249 | 97 (39) | 172 (69) | 179 (72) | 114 (46) | – |
| 1981–1982 | 445 | 162 (36) | 228 (51) | 228 (51) | 266 (60) | – |
| 1982–1983 | 604 | 202 (33) | 332 (55) | 441 (68) | 359 (59) | – |
| 1983–1984 | 603 | 166 (28) | 254 (42) | 390 (65) | 422 (68) | 66 (11) |
| 1984–1985 | 652 | 278 (27) | 281 (43) | 443 (68) | 456 (70) | 109 (17) |
| 1985–1986 | 700 | 280 (26) | 296 (42) | 361 (52) | 417 (60) | 116 (17) |
| Total | 3253 | 985 (30) | 1563 (48) | 2021 (62) | 2023 (62) | 291 (15[a] |

[a] Total of 2055 patients since 1983–1984 used as denominator

**Table 3.** Routine vaccines received by age group

| Age (years) | No. | Tet/dip (%) | Polio (%) |
|---|---|---|---|
| 0– 9 | 89 | 8 (9.0) | 12 (13.5) |
| 10–19 | 192 | 45 (23.4) | 69 (35.9) |
| 20–29 | 719 | 263 (36.6) | 362 (50.3) |
| 30–39 | 938 | 311 (37.2) | 423 (50.5) |
| 40–49 | 431 | 181 (42.0) | 203 (47.1) |
| 50–59 | 470 | 171 (36.4) | 192 (40.9) |
| 60+ | 496 | 192 (38.7) | 209 (42.1) |
| Unknown | 19 | 6 (31.6) | 7 (36.8) |

(average = 36%) of American travelers over age 20 seeking travel vaccines from our clinic needed updating of tetanus/diphtheria vaccine status, and that more than 40% of these travelers needed updating of polio vaccine status for travel to destinations in developing areas of the world (Table 3).

## Discussion

Immunization against common vaccine-preventable illnesses has been customarily incorporated into the practice of pediatrics in the United States. The private-sector providers of general medical care to the adult population appear to be less familiar with recommended vaccine protocols for adults, and with immunization practices in general. Thus, childhood infections and common vaccine-preventable illnesses have become increasingly diseases of adults who lack immunity. The incidence of tetanus, diphtheria, rubella, measles, and mumps is increasing among persons over age 20 years [3]. In one study, significantly less than 50% of American adults over the age of 60 years who were studied had protective tetanus antitoxin levels, and less than 25% of the entire study group of 183 adults aged 18 to greater than 60 years old had protective levels of diphtheria antitoxin in tests of their serum [4]. CDC statistics [5] show that there is an eightfold increase in the annual incidence rate of reported tetanus cases between persons less than 50 years of age and persons 50 years or older.

Injections for most vaccine-preventable illnesses in adult patients are not consistently covered by private insurance plans or by health maintenance organizations. Medicare only covers the cost of influenza vaccine shots at the present time. In addition to financial concerns, many adults avoid vaccines because of fear of pain. The allure of travel to an exotic place appears to be a strong inducement for adults to seek preventive medical care. Linked to travel vaccine shots which the traveler readily perceives as "necessary" to prevent exotic illnesses, additional shots to bring the status of routine vaccines up-to-date meets with less patient resistance. By recording the administration of routine vaccines on the extra pages provided in the *International Certificates of Vaccination* booklet, the maintenance of routine vaccines becomes part of the "readiness for travel". The record of such vaccines is less likely to be misplaced than other vaccine records, because of the distinctive yellow color of the booklet and the fact that travelers are customarily told to keep their international health record safely along with their passports [6]. In this way, vaccine centers and travel clinics directed toward the needs of international travelers can significantly influence the updating of routine immunizations in this segment of the adult population.

## References

1. Immunization Practices Advisory Committee (1984) Adult immunization: recommendations of the Immunization Practices Advisory Committee. MMWR [Suppl 1]33:1S–68S
2. CDC (1988) Health information for international travel, 1987. CDC, Washington [DHHS publ No (CDC 88-8280)]
3. CDC (1987) Summary of the second national community forum on adult immunization. MMWR 36:677–680
4. Crossley K, Irvine P, Warren JB et al. (1979) Tetanus and diphtheria immunity in urban Minnesota adults. JAMA 242:2298–2300
5. CDC (1987) Tetanus – United States, 1985–1986. MMWR 36:477–481
6. Jong EC (1987) Medical approach to the traveling patient. In: Jong EC (ed) The travel and tropical medicine manual. Saunders, Philadelphia, p 4

# Trends in Vaccination of Travelers over the Last 15 Years and the Future Outlook

G. Lea

The main British Airways Immunization Service in central London, open (since 1946) to any traveler, administers about 100000 vaccinations annually. The total vaccinations given during the 1st week of 1972 and the 1st week of 1987 happen to be virtually identical (see Table 1) but the range of vaccines used was quite different and provides an illustration of the changes over the last 15 years and the likely future trend as a more complete pre-travel medical service is developing.

## Comments

1. 1987: no smallpox (or typhus) vaccinations.
   1972: smallpox = 28% of total vaccinations.
2. Cholera immunizations: number reduced to almost half; have continued to fall rapidly in the year since. (Unlike some countries, cholera vaccine is still widely used in the United Kingdom and the British Airways unit is ahead of the trend.)
3. Typhoid = 78% of optional immunizations in 1972 and is still the most popular (43%), but tetanus, polio and immunoglobulin have all increased markedly (the latter probably one of the most useful pre-travel measures as hepatitis A is one of the most prevalent travel diseases, but non-A hepatitis is on the increase and it is unlikely that immunoglobulin protects). (Tetanus and polio immunizations provide good protection against extremely serious diseases but the incidence of both is very low.)
4. Pre-exposure rabies vaccine used from 1976 (introduction of French human diploid cell vaccine), use of which use has greatly increased for travel to rural developing areas. Recipients are instructed to clean wounds and boost as soon as possible. Postexposure prophylaxis is sometimes also given as few doctors in the United Kingdom are experienced in this field.
5. Meningococcal meningitis A and C vaccine and Japanese encephalitis were used by 1987, but only for known outbreak areas or longer trips to endemic zones.
6. Hepatitis B vaccine usage (introduced in the 1980s, is likely to increase beyond travelers confined to high-risk categories; now a recombinant DNA yeast cell vaccine has allowed a price reduction since the January 1987 figures illustrated above.

**Table 1.** Trends in vaccination of travellers over the last 15 years and the future outlook

| First week of | Smallpox | Yellow fever | Cholera | Typhoid | Tetanus | Polio | 2 ml immuno-globulin | 5 ml immuno-globulin | |
|---|---|---|---|---|---|---|---|---|---|
| 1972 | 542 | 282 | 856 | 203 | 32 | 6 | 11 | – | |
| 1987 | – | 238 | 448 | 526 | 145 | 135 | 204 | 62 | |
| **First week of** | **Pre-exp. rabies** | **Plague** | **Men. meningitis** | **Jap. encephalitis** | **Hepatitis B** | **E. European tick encephalitis** | **Diphteria** | **Typhus** | **Total number given** |
| 1972 | – | 2 | – | – | – | – | – | 4 | 1938 |
| 1987 | 139 | – | 14 | 11 | 10 | – | 4 | – | 1936 |

1972:
- Smallpox, yellow fever and cholera = mandatory vaccinations for certificates = 87%
- Remaining vaccinations = advised = 13%
- Indicative of the pre-occupation with international certificate requirements

1987:
- Only yellow fever and a few of the cholera = mandatory vaccinations for certificates = approx 13%
- Remaining vaccinations = advised = approx 87%
- The proportion of mandatory as compared to advised vaccinations is almost entirely reversed

7. Dilute diphtheria vaccine, only recently available, allows adult use without Schick testing and so use should gradually increase.
8. East European tick encephalitis vaccine has seasonal use so does not appear in the January 1987 figures. Even in spring, few English travelers are aware enough to enquire about its use for walking or camping in risk areas.
9. The number of yellow fever immunizations has remained fairly constant over the years: this is the only example of the table *not* illustrating the general trend.
10. Louse-borne typhus vaccine: this is not of much use and no longer available.
11. The unit does not use BCG (for tuberculosis) or measles vaccine routinely (? may do so in the future).
12. New vaccines which could be developed: hepatitis A, malaria ?, AIDS?.

The unit is designed as a service which should be self-financing and not as a profit-orientated centre. The latter would be difficult to run in the United Kingdom as people are not used to paying for health care at the point of usage and might be unwilling to pay the necessary prices for a (mostly) optional commodity. Travellers pay a small fee per immunization, but are now advised free on prevention of diarrhoea and malaria and can request information about water purification, insect bites, Hep B/AIDS prevention, medical insurance and altitude sickness.

# A Study on Protective Vaccinations in Swiss Long-Distance Travelers

E. Steiger, R. Steffen, and M. Schär

Many recommendations about immunizations for travelers have been published, but there are almost no data available on how well these recommendations are applied in practice. Therefore, we decided to investigate how adequately Swiss travelers to developing countries were immunized according to the recommendations of the WHO and of the Swiss Federal Office of Public Health.

In a cross-sectional study, conducted between August 1986 and February 1988, Swiss citizens were orally interviewed in the departure gates of Zürich Airport immediately prior to boarding their scheduled or charter flight to Africa, Asia, or South America. Personal data, destination, purpose and length of stay abroad, and the vaccination history were recorded. Whenever possible, the vaccination certificates were checked.

A total of 1045 passengers on 82 flights were recruited. Nine (1%) refused the interview. The mean age was $36 \pm 14$ years, and 55% were men. Only 50% had their vaccination certificate with them. The travelers' destination and their vaccination status as reported is shown in Table 1. No significant differences were found between tourists and business travelers, but charter passengers knew less about their vaccination status. Persons living abroad tended to be particularly careless.

**Table 1.** Proportion of travelers reporting to be immunized (%)

| | Total no. | Yellow fever | Cholera | Tetanus | Diphtheria | Polio | Immune globulin | Typhoid |
|---|---|---|---|---|---|---|---|---|
| Africa (excluding South Africa) | 411 | 64 | 14 | 66 | 12 | 55 | 13 | 40 |
| South America (excluding Argentina/Chile) | 268 | 49 | – | 70 | 24 | 68 | 19 | 30 |
| Asia (Middle/Far East) | 366 | – | 3 | 69 | 13 | 71 | 19 | 34 |
| Total | 1045 | – | – | 67 | 15 | 64 | 16 | 35 |

The survey shows that travelers are generally insufficiently protected against tetanus and poliomyelitis, except when they were forced to see a doctor for a compulsory vaccination, e.g., against yellow fever. In another study conducted with Scottish travelers the vaccination discipline seemed to be better [1]. In contrast, German travelers tended to have lower vaccination rates, but that was 10 years ago [2]. Few were certainly immune against diphtheria, as many doctors fear side effects from this vaccination. Poliomyelitis and tetanus are scarcely considered a threat to health by the traveler; this might possibly also explain the low rates of immunization against these infections.

Apparently, Swiss doctors know that there are no cholera endemic regions in South America, and that yellow fever will not be transmitted in Asia. Immune globulin so far is given only to those expected to be traveling under poor hygienic conditions.

Many travelers complained about contradictory vaccination recommendations.

This pilot study shows that interview studies can be conducted at the gates of airports. However, as travelers have many remaining questions, the interviewer should be well acquainted with travel medicine.

## References

1. Grist NR, Cossar JH, Reid D et al. (1985) Illness associated with a package holiday in Romania. Scott Med J 30:156–160
2. Plentz K (1978) Impfschutz im Ferntourismus als Problem des öffentlichen Gesundheitsdienstes. Off Gesundheitswes 40:497–506

# Side Effects of Tetanus Versus Diphtheria-Tetanus Vaccination in Travelers

G. Zürrer and R. Steffen

Diphtheria may, although rarely, threaten international travelers [1, 2]. Comparing this minimal risk and the fact that a combined diphtheria-tetanus vaccine in military and other nontraveling populations has usually caused more side effects than the monovalent tetanus vaccine [3–7], many vaccination centers are hesitant to recommend the combined vaccine, although most experts advise it [8]. In order to compare side effects of the two vaccines and their importance in travelers, a double-blind trial was conducted.

Future travelers presenting themselves at the Zurich University Vaccination Center between August 1985 and December 1986 were invited to participate in the study, if they had received their last doses of tetanus and diphtheria vaccine more than 10 years before and if they were at least 14 years old. Exclusion criteria were acute illness or depature within less than 10 days. The vaccination history was taken in detail. Upon signing informed consent, the volunteers received, according to a weekly randomization scheme, either tetanus toxoid (Te-Anatoxal Berna, 10 Lf) or diphtheria plus tetanus toxoid (dT-Anatoxal Berna, 1 Lf and 10 Lf respectively). Both vaccines were adsorbed to aluminum phosphate and conserved in 0.01% thiomersal. The test vaccine was adminstered intramuscularly into the right deltoid muscle, whereas all other immunizations were injected on the left side. All volunteers were asked to return a questionnaire.

A total of 1750 volunteers were recruited, 1505 (86%) returned their questionnaires, of which 79 (5%) had to be excluded. Evaluations were made is on 773 persons who had received the Te and 653 who had received the dT vaccine. In both groups there were no significant differences with respect to sex (59% women), age (the median age group was 30–39 years old), previous diphtheria and/or tetanus vaccinations, side effects to these vaccinations, or other vaccines given with the test vaccine (yellow fever 42%, typhoid Ty 21a 22%, cholera 3%, meningococcal meningitis 2%, hepatitis B 1%, various <1% each, poliomyelitis not recorded).

The side effects reported are summarized in Table 1. They tended to last longer after dT than after Te vaccination. Less than 3% in each group took some medication to relieve the side effects; three persons in the Te and one in the dT group consulted a doctor. Inability to work occurred in 0.8% of the Te (average 2.0 days) and in 1.7% of the dT (average 1.5 days) group, a nonsignificant difference.

**Table 1.** Side effects associated with the test vaccine

| Test vaccine<br>Side effects | Te<br>(%) | dT<br>(%) | Significance<br>($\chi^2$) |
|---|---|---|---|
| Redness, localized | 12.4 | 19.4 | $P<0.001$ |
| Swelling, localized or arm | 25.0 | 31.8 | $P=0.025$ |
| Pain, heaviness | 58.2 | 63.0 | NS |
| Tiredness | 13.2 | 13.9 | NS |
| Headache | 6.5 | 7.7 | NS |
| Arthralgia | 3.0 | 4.1 | NS |
| Elevated temperature | 4.8 | 5.8 | NS |
| Total with any reaction | 63.4 | 69.7 | $P=0.014$ |

The vast majority of side effects were rated as "slight" or "supportable" by the volunteers. Just 1.8% of all Te and 2.5% of all dT vaccines (NS) rated them as severe.

The smaller number of dT volunteers is due to the fact that randomization allocated dT weeks to weeks with holidays during which less visitors came to the Vaccination Center. This study confirms that dT causes more side effects than Te vaccine [3–7]. However, the vast majority of these reactions were slight and the future travelers tolerated them without being strongly harassed. We therefore conclude that first in view of the small, but not negligible, risk of being infected with diphtheria abroad, second in view of the advantage of protecting a higher proportion of the population living in industrialized countries and third in view of the tolerable increase of side effects, *dT vaccination rather than Te vaccination is to be preferred in travelers.*

## References

1. Begg NT (1988) Imported diphtheria, England and Wales: 1970–1987. Conference on International Travel Medicine, Zurich
2. Höfler W, Heizmann W, Höring E, Kusch G, Weidner F (1989) Three cases of cutaneous diphtheria in travelers to Africa. This volume
3. Macko MB, Powell CE (1985) Comparison of the morbidity of tetanus toxoid boosters with tetanus-diphteria toxoid boosters. Am Emerg Med 14:33–35
4. Ullberg-Olsson K (1979) Vaccinationsreaktioner efter injection av tetanustoxoid med och utan tillsats av difteritoxoid. Lakartidningen 76:2976
5. Ipsen J (1954) Immunization of adults against diphtheria and tetanus. N Engl J Med 251:459–466
6. Deacon SP, Langford DT, Shepherd WM, Knight PA (1982) A comparative clinical study of absorbed tetanus vaccine and adult-type tetanus-diphtheria vaccine. J Hyg 89:513–519
7. Simonsen O, Klaerke M, Klaerke A, Bloch AV, Hansen BR, Hald N, Hau C, Heron I (1986) Revaccination of adults against diphtheria. II. Combined diphtheria and tetanus revaccination with different doses of diphtheria toxoid 20 years after primary vaccination. Acta Pathol Microbiol Immunol Scand [C] 94:219–225
8. WHO (1988) Vaccination certificate requirements and health advice for international travel. World Health Organization, Geneva

# Imported Diphtheria, England and Wales: 1970–1987

N. T. Begg

## Introduction

Diphtheria remains a common disease in many parts of the world. The widespread use of diphtheria toxoid has dramatically reduced the incidence of the disease in developed countries; however, travel to countries where the disease is endemic poses a risk both to the traveller and to his contacts on returning home. This paper reviews travel-related diphtheria in England and Wales from 1970 to 1987.

## Methods

Information on cases and carriers of diphtheria was derived from routine sources, including statutory notifications, death certificates and laboratory reports to the PHLS Communicable Disease Surveillance Centre (CDSC) of toxigenic strains of *Corynebacterium diphtheriae*. Further details, including relevant travel histories, were obtained from the annual reports of the Chief Medical Officer and other published data as well as ad hoc reports by local Medical Officers for Environmental Health (MOsEH) to CDSC.

## Results

Between 1970 and 1987 92 cases were notified, of which 21 (23%) were known to have been acquired overseas or as a result of contact with an imported case or carrier (Fig. 1). In addition, several healthy carriers of toxigenic strains were identified as a result of screening contacts of cases or during the course of a routine medical examination. Thus in the same period, 247 isolates of toxigenic *C. diphtheriae* were reported, of which 50 (20%) were associated with overseas travel.

Most of the importations were associated with the Indian subcontinent, in particular Bangladesh; however, cases were also reported from Africa, Southeast Asia, the Caribbean, Europe and Australia (Table 1).

Two outbreaks following importations were reported during the period of study. The first outbreak affected five children in one family in London who developed diphtheria in September 1975 (Chattophadhay et al. 1977). Four of the children presented with sore throats and recovered uneventfully; a fifth case developed respiratory obstruction and required a tracheostomy. Five

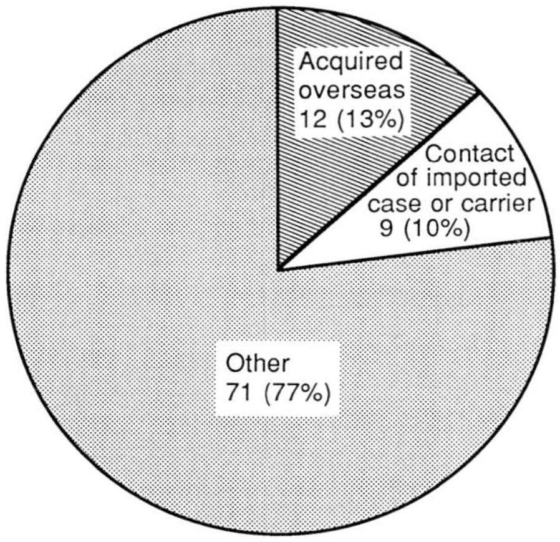


**Fig. 1.** Source of diphteria infection in 92 notified cases, England and Wales 1970–1987

**Table 1.** Imported diphtheria, England and Wales, 1970–1987: countries associated with importations

| Country | Cases | Laboratory reports of toxigenic strains |
|---|---|---|
| Bangladesh | 10 | 30 |
| Pakistan | 4 | 6 |
| India | 4 | 6 |
| Egypt | 1 | 1 |
| Jamaica | 1 | 1 |
| Other[a] | – | 5 |
| Not certain | 1 | 1 |
| Total | 21 | 50 |

[a] Thailand, Vietnam, Zimbabwe, Spain, Australia on each

days before the index patient became unwell the family had moved to London from Birmingham. Subsequent investigation in Birmingham led to the discovery of two pharyngeal diphtheria carriers who were nextdoor neighbours of the affected family and who had arrived from Bangladesh 6 weeks previously. Two secondary subclinical cases occurred in London.

In the second outbreak, a 14-month-old girl developed pharyngeal diphtheria 6 days after arriving in England with her parents and five siblings (PHLS CDSC 1986). A toxigenic strain of *C. diphtheriae* was isolated from a throat swab. The same strain was recovered from three of the siblings, all of whom had sore throats and injected fauces, and from the father, who was asymptomatic.

## Discussion

Almost one-fourth of the cases in this report were associated with overseas travel. In other cases, an imported strain was suspected as the source, although it could not be proved (Simmons et al. 1980; Jones et al. 1984). The true proportion of travel-associated cases was probably much higher. This is supported by the finding that most of the toxigenic strains isolated during the period were non-starch fermenters, a property usually associated with overseas strains. The typing of *C. diphtheriae* has recently been simplified by the use of polyacrylamide gel electrophoresis, a simple technique which produces a high resolution between strains, and should prove a valuable tool in identifying isolates from abroad (Hallas 1988).

Current vaccine coverage (87% in 1987) appears to be sufficient to prevent large-scale diphtheria epidemics. There is, however, some evidence that immunity wanes after childhood immunization (Kjeldson et al. 1985), and 30% of young adults and over 40% of older groups in the United Kingdom are susceptible (Public Health Laboratory Service 1978; Sheffield et al. 1978). It is thus important to boost the immunity of adults who may be exposed to diphtheria.

Low dose (1.5 Lfu) diphtheria toxoid produces a satisfactory immune response in adults, and the incidence of adverse reactions is low (Mortimer et al. 1986). Travellers to areas where diphtheria is endemic could be given a booster dose of 1.5 Lfu toxoid, if more than 10 years have elapsed since the last dose. Adults never previously immunized could be given a full primary course of three doses of low-dose toxoid. Pre-immunization Schick testing is no longer necessary.

## References

1. Chattophadhay B, Fellner IW, Mollison MD, Nicol W, Williams GR (1977) Diphtheria in London and Birmingham, 1975. Public Health 91:169–174
2. Hallas G (1988) The use of SDS-polyacrylamide gel electrophoresis in epidemiological studies of *Corynebacterium diphtheriae*. Epidem Inf 100:83–90
3. Jones SAM, Miller HJ, Rogers TR, Kirk NR, Dulake C, Zamiri I (1984) An experience of diphtheria in Westminster. Public Health 98:3–7
4. Mortimer J, Melville-Smith M, Sheffield F (1986) Diphtheria vaccine for adults. Lancet II:1182–1183
5. Public Health Laboratory Service (1978) Susceptibility to diphtheria. Lancet I:428–430
6. Report from the PHLS CDSC (1986) Br Med J 292:1385–1386
7. Sheffield FW, Ironside AG, Abbott JD (1978) Immunisation of adults against diphteria. Br Med J 1:249–250
8. Simmons LE, Abbott JD, Jones AE, Ironside AG, Mandal BK, Stanbridge TN, Maximescu P (1980) Diphtheria carriers in Manchester: simultaneous infection with toxigenic and nontoxigenic mitis strains. Lancet I:304–305

# Heat Stability of a New 17D Yellow Fever Vaccine

L. Adamowicz, B. Fritzell, and P. Saliou

For more than 50 years, 17D yellow fever vaccines have largely proven to be well tolerated and effective, justifying their recommendations by WHO for the control of yellow fever. Indeed, the quality and the long duration of protection make this vaccine highly effective provided that it contains a sufficient viral amount, 1000 $LD_{50}$ (mice)/dose. The well-known heat sensitivity of classical vaccines, resulting in a rapid loss of the viral titer, constituted a major handicap for its use in endemic areas, as it caused failures of immunization when stored at incorrect temperatures. With this in mind, the development of heat-stable vaccine was considered a priority. Different chemicals were systematically assessed at various concentrations and associations for their protective effect on the virus. A stabilizing medium was consequently defined by Barme and Bronnert [1]. During the preparation procedure of the vaccine, it is added to the viral suspension at the time of freeze drying. An overview of the results of different studies of heat stability and immunogenicity of this new 17D thermostable vaccine is presented.

## Stability Study of the Unreconstituted Vaccine

Nonstabilized and stabilized vaccine prepared from the same five consecutive batches were compared for stability after storage at different temperatures [2].

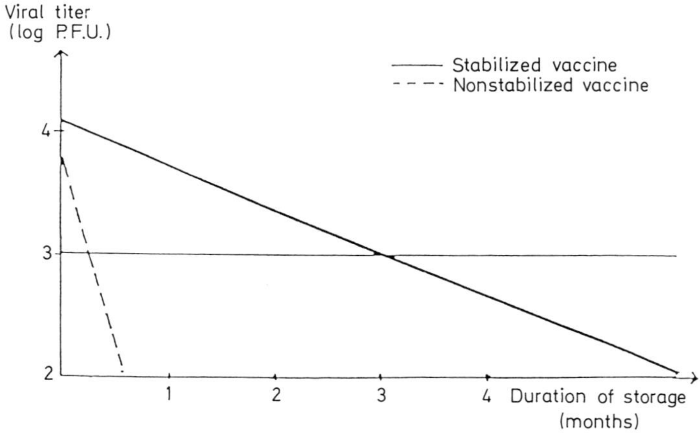


**Fig. 1.** Comparative loss of viral titer after storage at +37 °C

Ampoules of nonstabilized and stabilized preparations of each batch were stored at +4 °C (cold store), +20 °C (room temperature) and +37 °C (immersion in water). Samples were taken at regular intervals, and maintained at −60 °C until titrations were carried out according to the method described by de Madrid and Porterfield [3]. Results were expressed as log PFU per dose and the loss of titer assessed with reference to controls stored at −60 °C for the same duration.

When kept at +4 °C for 3 years, the mean loss of titer was 0.972 and 0.692 log pfu for the nonstabilized and stabilized vaccines respectively. When stored at +20 °C for 6 months, the losses were 1.594 and 0.328 log pfu respectively. The results of this assay at +37 °C are shown in Fig. 1. It is of importance that the mean loss of titer after 2 weeks is only 0.32 log pfu for the stabilized vaccine, which fully meets the WHO requirements on stability for 17D yellow fever vaccines. Overall, this study demonstrated that the loss of titer was significantly lower for the stabilized vaccine.

From the observed values during these assays, the estimated delays to reach the minimum required amount of virus per dose – equivalent to 1000 $LD_{50}$ (mice) – were calculated. Stabilized vaccine was found to reach this limit after 3 months of storage at +37 °C, 24 months at +20 °C, and 160 months at +4 °C. These assays clearly established the heat stability of the vaccine under laboratory conditions. It was then worth assessing it under routine conditions in endemic areas.

Thermostability and efficacy in the field were studied through a 6-month mass immunization campaign in various rural areas of central Africa [4]. Viral titers and potency in children were regularly assessed after prolonged storage at +10 °C, and six successive trips in the field where the vaccine was transported in ice boxes which did not contain ice packs.

Storage for up to 6 months at +10 °C and six trips in the field under tropical conditions resulted in no significant loss of titer (Table 1).

Immunogenicity of the vaccine was evaluated 1 month after vaccination in seronegative children from each rural area of the program. Neutralizing antibodies were found in 94% of the 209 vaccinees.

**Table 1.** Viral titers after different storage conditions and trips in the field

| Storage temperature | No. of months of storage | No. of field trip | Viral titre (log PFU) | Loss of titre (log PFU) |
|---|---|---|---|---|
| −40°C | 6 | 0 | 5.47 | – |
| +10°C | 6 | 0 | 5.46 | 0.01 |
| +22°C | 6 | 0 | 5.14 | 0.33 |
| +10°C[a] | 1 | 1 | 5.48 | 0.00 |
| +10°C[a] | 2 | 2 | 5.40 | 0.07 |
| +10°C[a] | 3 | 3 | 5.31 | 0.16 |
| +10°C[a] | 4 | 4 | 5.45 | 0.02 |
| +10°C[a] | 5 | 5 | 5.32 | 0.15 |
| +10°C[a] | 6 | 6 | 5.47 | 0.02 |

[a] Except when taken out to the field in an ice box which did not contain freeze packs

## Stability Study of the Reconstituted Vaccine

As multidose presentations of yellow fever vaccine are mostly used for mass immunization in endemic areas, it was interesting to study the stability of the vaccine after reconstitution.

Samples of rehydrated vaccine from four batches were stored unexposed to light at three temperatures +20 °C, +37 °C and +45 °C, which may correspond to room temperature in endemic areas.

Viral titer was evaluated, according to the method described by de Madrid and Porterfield [3], at each hour. Results showed that viral titer drops very quickly at +45 °C in less than 1 h and the loss after 4 h at a temperature ranging from +20 °C to +37 °C was compatible with a satisfactory viral amount at the time of immunization.

Heat stability of the reconstituted vaccine was studied by following its potency among children in Cameroun [5]. Ninety children aged 6–8 years were engaged in the study and randomly allocated to three groups A, B and C. Each child received one 0.5 ml dose of Stamaril Pasteur which, after reconstitution, was stored away from light at room temperature (+25 °C to +30 °C) for 1 (group A), 2 (group B) and 3 h (group C). Seroconversion rates 1 month later were 100%, 82% and 67% respectively for the groups A, B and C. The vaccine was at its most effective during the 1st h following reconstitution, but its efficacy was retained even after 2 h.

## Conclusion

All these studies have demonstrated the excellent heat stability of this 17D thermostable vaccine (Stamaril Pasteur). It makes possible its long storage at +4 °C and extenuates the negative effects of breaks in the cold chain. In parallel, its immunogenicity in children was well established. These properties make it particularly suitable for the control of yellow fever in endemic areas.

## References

1. Barme M, Bronnert C (1984) Thermostabilisation du vaccin antiamaril 17D lyophilisé. I. Essai de substances protectrices. J Biol Stand 12:435–442
2. Barme M, Vacher B, Ryhiner ML, Chabannier G (1986) Thermostabilisation du vaccin antiamaril 17D lyophilisé. II. Lots pilotes préparés dans les conditions d'une production industrielle. J Biol Stand 14
3. De Madrid AT, Porterfield JS (1969) A simple microculture method for the study of group B arboviruses. Bull WHO 40:113–121
4. Georges AJ, Tible F, Meunier DMJ, Gonzak JP, Beraud AM, Sissoko-Dybdahl NR et al. (1985) Thermostability and efficacy in the field of a new heat-stabilized yellow fever vaccine. Vaccine 3:313–315
5. Durand JP, Kollo B, Merlin M, le Hesran JY, Josse R, Garrigue GP (1988) Etude de la thermostabilité d'un nouveau vaccin amaril 17D thermostable. J Biol Stand 16:1–7

# Immunogenicity of a New Thermostable 17D Yellow Fever Vaccine

I. Vodopija, N. Djakovic, B. Fritzell, and M. Lhuillier

The vaccine for 17D yellow fever has proved to be very effective and well tolerated, and consequently has been recommended by WHO for travel to countries with yellow fever. A heat-stable preparation was developed to make vaccines suitable for use in endemic areas [1–4], where multidose presentations are mainly used in mass immunization campaigns.

In immunization centers for travelers, this vaccine is usually given at fixed times. This represents a serious limitation and often results in the loss of doses. Therefore, a unidose thermostable 17D yellow fever vaccine was recently developed by Pasteur Vaccins. In the present study we have attempted to assess its tolerance and immunogenicity in healthy volunteers. This was performed in two consecutive open studies.

## Materials and Methods

### Subjects

The vaccinated subjects were all male student volunteers, aged 19–24 years. The vaccinations were carried out at the Tropical Diseases Unit of the Zagreb Institute of Public Health. Excluded from the study were subjects who resided in a yellow fever endemic area, were previously vaccinated against yellow fever, were allergic to egg protein, or had any contraindication to live vaccines.

### Vaccine

The vaccine used was the commercial unidose Stamaril Pasteur, prepared from the 17D strain virus, free from contamination by avian leukosis virus and without neurotropic potential. It is grown in eggs selected from breeding colonies free of specific avian pathogens. Each standard dose (0.5 ml) of reconstituted vaccine contains at least 1000 $LD_{50}$ (mice), in accordance with the WHO recommendations.

### Study Design

In study 1, the standard dose – 0.5 ml – was injected into the deltoid area immediately after rehydration. In the second study, two groups of vaccinees (2A and 2B) received reduced doses, namely, one-fifth and one-tenth of the standard dose, intradermally in the volar side of the forearm. In group 2A the vaccine was reconstituted as recommended to obtain the standard 0.5-ml dose, whereupon 0.1 ml of the preparation was injected intradermally. In group 2B, a double volume – 1.0 ml of diluent – was used to reconstitute a standard dose, followed by intradermal administration of 0.1 ml of the preparation.

## Evaluation Criteria

Serological response and tolerance were the criteria used in the evaluation of the vaccine.

### Serological Response

Two blood specimens were drawn, the first before the injection and the second 30 days after vaccination. The serum was separated and frozen at −20 °C and the specimens were coded for titration at the Pasteuer Institute. Samples were titrated for neutralizing antibodies by the plaque reduction test, using microplaques with the pig kidney cells (PS) with 17D virus as the antigen. A serum was considered positive if it inhibited at least 80% of the plaques and the titer was considered to correspond to the highest positive dilution. The lowest dilution tested was 1 : 5, which is considered protective.

### Tolerance

To assess the tolerance, all vaccinated subjects were given a clinical examination by the same physician 2, 7, 10 and 30 days after the injection. Axillary temperature was noted at each visit.

## Results

One hundred and three subjects were recruited for the two studies, 53 in the first study, 50 in the second. All vaccinees had two blood samples taken and clinical examinations as described in the protocol. In the two studies, none of the subjects had detectable neutralizing antibodies in the specimen drawn before immunization and were eligible for assessment of the serological response. Fifty-three subjects (100%) from the first study had neutralizing antibodies after vaccination, and the distribution of neutralizing antibody titers is shown in Fig. 1. All subjects who received intradermal administration of a reduced dose had neutralizing antibodies after vaccination. The distribution of postimmunization neutralizing antibody titers in recipients of a fifth and tenth of standard dose are presented respectively in Figs. 2 and 3. No fever or systemic reactions were observed. Only local reactions were reported. On day 2, the incidence rates of slight and transient pain at the injection site in the first and second study groups were 24% and 30% respectively. Limited induration – less than 5 mm diameter – was observed more frequently in those who received the vaccine intradermally, and was found in 30%, 22% and 12% of the vaccinees, respectively, at days 2, 7 and 14.

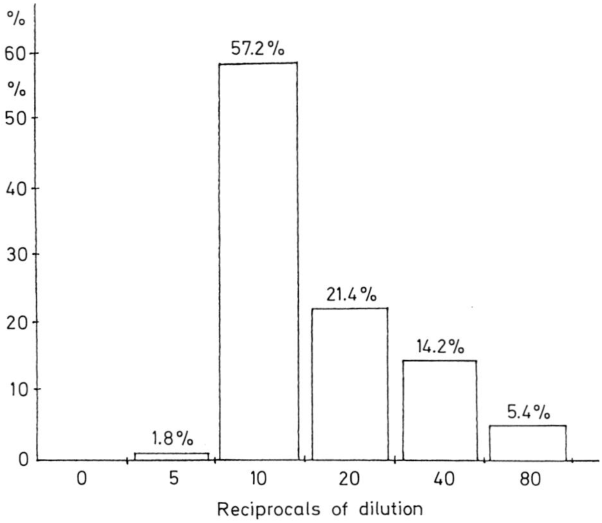


**Fig. 1.** Distribution of neutralizing antibody titers after immunization with a standard 0.5-ml dose

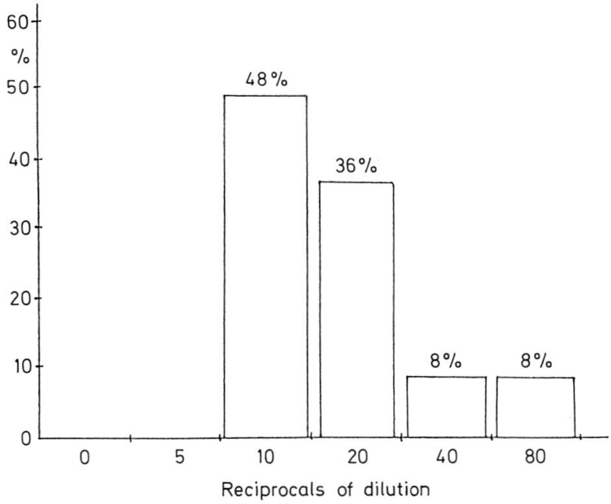


**Fig. 2.** Distribution of neutralizing antibody titers after immunization with one-fifth of the standard dose intradermally injected

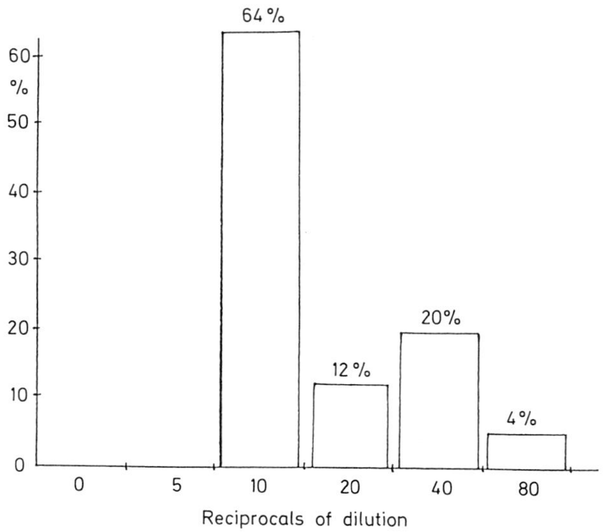


**Fig. 3.** Distribution of neutralizing antibody titers after immunization with one-tenth of the standard dose intradermally injected

## Conclusions

Unidose presentation of 17D yellow fever vaccine was developed by Pasteuer Vaccins to facilitate vaccination in immunization centers for travelers, and to avoid waste of unused reconstituted vaccine. Furthermore, it provides an additional guarantee of potency since the vaccine is used only as and when required for each individual. The present work shows the efficacy of the new 17D thermostable vaccine. All vaccinated subjects developed neutralizing antibodies 1 month after injection. The serological response was comparable to results reported in other studies [3, 5, 6]. An identical serological response was found in subjects who received intradermally a reduced dose (one-fifth and one-tenth of the standard dose). Reactogenicity of the vaccine was limited to mild local pain and small induration following intradermal vaccination, which is the expected reaction to this route of administration. We expect the new unidose thermostable 17D vaccine to represent a significant improvement in the vaccination of travelers against yellow fever.

## References

1. Barme M, Bronnert C (1984) Thermostabilisation du vaccin antiamaril 17D lyophilisé. I. Essai de substances protectrices. J Biol Stand 12:435–442
2. Barme M, Vacher B, Ryhiner ML, Chabannier G (1986) Thermostabilisation du vaccin antiamaril 17D lyophilisé. II. Lots pilotes préparés dans les conditions d'une production industrielle. J Biol Stand 14:67–72

3. Georges AJ, Tible F, Meunier DMJ, Gonzak JP, Beraud AM, Sissoko-Dybdahl NR et al. (1985) Thermostability and efficacy in the field of a new heat stabilized yellow fever vaccine. Vaccine 3:313–315
4. Tomori O, Fabiyi A (1983) Stability of Institut Pasteur 17D yellow fever vaccine. IPP-S-365. Conférence Internationale sur les Vaccins Viraux et Bactériens, Institut Pasteur Production, 12–15 Decembre
5. Durand JP, Kollo B, Merlin M, le Hesran JY, Josse R, Garrigue GP (1988) Etude de la stabilité d'un nouveau vaccin amaril 17D thermostable. J Biol Stand 16:1–7
6. Roche JC, Jouan A, Brisou B, Rodhain R, Fritzell B, Hannoun C (1986) Comparative clinical study of a new 17D thermostable yellow fever vaccine. Vaccine 4:163–165

# Yellow Fever Vaccination and Business Travel

E. R. Waclawski and E. Walker

Holiday travel is usually well planned in advance. Business travel, however, may occur at short notice. This may place the business traveler at increased risk of exotic infection as there may be little time to obtain immunization and commence malaria prophylaxis.

To test this hypothesis a study was performed on travelers attending for yellow fever vaccination. The aim of the study was to identify whether business travelers placed themselves at increased risk by receiving immunization at short notice, compared with holiday travelers.

## Method

A questionnaire was completed by travelers at the time of vaccination at the Yellow Fever Clinic, Glasgow. Information was obtained regarding age, sex, reason for travel (holiday/business/other) and whether the vaccination was a primary dose. Those who were receiving their first dose indicated whether travel was within 10 days of immunization. Statistical analysis was performed by the chi-suare test (with continuity correction).

## Results

Questionnaires were completed by 523 travelers: 481 contained complete information. Two hundred and ninety-three (60.9%) men traveled (mean age $\pm$1 SD:36.8$\pm$14.2 years); 188 (39.1%) women traveled (33.6$\pm$14.2 years). Three hundred and sixty-one travelers received their first yellow fever immunization, of whom 266 were holidaymakers, 109 were business travelers and 26 traveled for other reasons. Of the holidaymakers 24 (10.6%) traveled

**Table 1.** Reasons for travel within 10 days of yellow fever vaccination

| Reason for travel | Travel within 10 days | | |
|---|---|---|---|
| Business | 32 | 77 | 109 |
| Holiday | 24 | 202 | 226 |
| Total | 56 | 279 | 335 |

$\chi_c^2 = 17.244$ ($P < 0.001$)

**Table 2.** Male travellers – Reason versus travel within 10 days

| Reason for travel | Travel with 10 days | | |
|---|---|---|---|
| | Yes | No | Total |
| Business | 28 | 57 | 85 |
| Holiday | 14 | 89 | 103 |
| Total | 42 | 146 | 188 |

$\chi_c^2 = 8.965$ ($P < 0.005$)

within 10 days of vaccination. However, among business travelers 32 (29.4%) travelled within 10 days (Table 1). Analysis by sex of these travelers showed a significant difference between male business and holiday travelers in timing of first yellow fever vaccination (Table 2).

## Conclusion

This study has shown that business travelers are more likely to travel within 10 days of yellow fever vaccination than holidaymakers. This supports the hypothesis that the business traveler may be at increased risk of exotic infection by travelling at short notice. Occupational physicians and company medical advisers who care for businessmen who travel overseas require to ensure that immunization against exotic infection be adequately maintained prior to travel.

# Tolerance and Immunogenicity of a New Combined Meningococcal (A + C)-Yellow Fever Vaccine (Preliminary Results)

G. Soula, P. Gobert, B. Nereli, E. Pichard, I. Ag. Iknane
R. Bandet, M. Lefur, and B. Fritzell

## Introduction

Yellow fever and meningococcal meningitis remain important public health problems in many parts of the world, as clearly demonstrated by the recent outbreaks in Africa. Both may be avoided by mass immunization with the safe and efficacious existing vaccines. A combined meningococcal (A + C)-yellow fever vaccine would increase the benefit of its use for populations at risk in providing protection against both diseases with one injection. The results of a clinical study with such a vaccine are reported.

## Population

After informed consent of their parents and physical examination, 926 children 12–60 months of age were included in the study. The 485 boys and 441 girls represent three consecutive age groups: 191 children were 12–17 months of age, 317 were 18–23 months old and 418 were 24–60 months old, with a mean age of $31 \pm 15$ months. In terms of nutritional status 86% of the children had a weight/height ratio $\geqq 80\%$ of the norm; 11.7% presented slight malnutrition (W/H ratio = 70%–79% of the norm) and 2.2% appeared malnourished. The four groups of children constituted through the randomized protocol were strictly comparable in size, age, sex and nutritional status.

## Tolerance

All children were examined by independent physicians at days 0–2–8. No local reactions were observed in any vaccine group. The mean body temperatures were comparable in the four groups, and their increases at day 2 (mean increase = 0.32°–0.42 °C) slight, although statistically different from day 0. Moderate febrile reactions (t° $\geqq$ 38 °C occurred in 4.4% of the children with high fever ($\geqq$ 39 °C) in 1.3% whatever the vaccine they received. These rates were 3.6% and 0.96% respectively at day 8. A general malaise was observed in 5.1% of the examinees at the 48 h visit and 0.7% at day 8. The other general reactions observed at the 48-h visit were diarrhoea and vomiting in 7 children, fever and vomiting in 12 and conjunctivitis in 3 cases.

## Immunogenicity

The antibody (Ab) response to the vaccines was evaluated blindly on the pairs of sera obtained 6 weeks apart. For the yellow fever Ab we used the neutralization test (PRT), with a protective threshold of $^1/_5$. Preliminary results on 182 pairs of sera (Table 1) indicate that only 7 children (3.8%) had protective Ab titres prior to the vaccination. After immunization 98%–100% of the children seroconverted (≧fourfold increase) and developed high titres of Ab with geometric mean antibody titre (GMT) ranging from 120 to 130. Surprisingly, in the control group (Men A+C) three children moderately increased their Ab levels; this may represent naturally acquired Ab, due to the circulation of the virus, or errors either at the vaccination or at the sampling of the sera. The meningococcal polysaccharide Ab was measured by radioimmunoassay (RIA); an Ab titre of 2 μg/ml represents a protective level. Initial results on 199 pairs of sera (Table 2) demonstrate a high seroprevalence for the A meningococcal serogroup since 98% of the children had protective Ab titres (GMT 4.1 μg/ml) prior to the vaccination. However, after immunization the mean increase of Ab titres is highly significant compared with the control group (YF), with GMT ranging from 6.2 μg/ml for the Men (A+C) group to 7.4 μg/ml for the Men (A+C)+YF group ($P=0.8$). The Ab response seems age dependent,

**Table 1.** Seroprevalence prior to vaccination, seroconversion rates and GMTs to yellow fever vaccine

| Vaccine groups | *n* | Sero + | Seroconversion | | GMT of yellow fever Ab[a] | |
|---|---|---|---|---|---|---|
| | | | *n* | (%) | D0 | D45 |
| Men −YF | 50 | 2 | 48 | (100%) | 1.16 | 130 |
| Men | 31 | – | 3 | (9.7%) | 1 | 1.49 |
| YF | 53 | 4 | 48 | (97.9%) | 1.27 | 119.4 |
| Men +YF | 48 | 1 | 46 | (97.8%) | 1.07 | 131 |

[a] Ab titres are expressed as reciprocal dilutions and seropositivity threshold is 5 with the plage reduction test (PRT)

**Table 2.** Seroprotection rates (Ab≧2 μg/ml) and GMTs to A and C meningococcal polysaccharides

| Vaccine groups | *n* | % with Ab titre ≧2 μg/ml | | | | GMT (μg/ml) | | | |
|---|---|---|---|---|---|---|---|---|---|
| | | Meningo A | | Meningo C | | Meningo A | | Meningo C | |
| | | D0 | D45 | D0 | D45 | D0 | D45 | D0 | D45 |
| Men −YF | 52 | 98 | 100 | 9.6 | 88 | 4 | 6.3 | 1.1 | 5.9 |
| Men | 62 | 98 | 100 | 4.8 | 93.5 | 4 | 6.2 | 1 | 7.1 |
| YF | 32 | 93 | 100 | 9.4 | 12.5 | 4.1 | 4.2 | 1.1 | 1.3 |
| Men +YF | 53 | 100 | 100 | 11.3 | 92.4 | 4.3 | 7.4 | 1.1 | 8.4 |

with a 1.3 mean fold increase in the children 12–17 months old compared with a 2.4-fold increase in the children over 2 years old ($P<0.0001$).

Only 8.5% of the children had significant C meningococcal Ab titres ($\geqq 2$ µg/ml) before the immunization. Six weeks later 88%–93.5% of the children are protected and 87% seroconverted ($\geqq$ twofold increase). The GMTs range from 5.9 µg/ml with the new combined Men (A+C)-YF vaccine to 8.4 µg/ml after simultaneous injection of both single vaccines ($P=0.20$). The Ab response did not significantly differ with the age of the children but was very good, with a mean 11.8-fold increase.

## Conclusion

This study has confirmed that yellow fever and meningococcal vaccines alone, combined or simultaneously administered are very safe. No local reactions were observed and febrile reactions occurred in 5.7% of the vaccinees. These vaccines are highly immunogenic with seroconversion rates of 85% for the C meningococcal polysaccharide vaccine to 100% for the yellow fever vaccine. The new combined meningococcal (A+C)-yellow fever vaccine is a promising association which requires further evaluation. The serological analysis of the overall group will provide such information, particularly on the Ab response according to the age. This study showed a high seroprevalence of the A meningococcal polysaccharide Ab in Mali.

# Prevention of Typhoid Fever by Single-Dose Capsular Polysaccharide Vaccination – 2-Year Results

K. P. Klugman, H. Vosloo, L. Arntzen, and H. J. Koornhof

Typhoid fever is endemic in the tropical areas of Central and South America, Asia and Africa. While the prevalence of disease has been greatly reduced in first world countries [8] largely due to the development of protected water supplies and sewerage disposal systems, the provision of these basic facilities is rare in third world countries, and the prevention of typhoid fever by these means is not an immediate prospect. Typhoid vaccination is therefore an important way to prevent this disease in both travellers to these endemic areas and the local population themselves.

There are problems in the use of whole cell typhoid vaccines. For the traveller, these are the need for two inoculations, separated in time, and the high incidence of local and systemic side effects associated with these vaccines [13, 15]. These problems are compounded when giving whole cell vaccines to endemic populations, as the duration of protection is limited to about 3 years and vaccination is thus needed repeatedly to protect people living in the endemic area [2, 8].

A live-oral suspension of *S. typhi* was shown to give excellent protection for 3 years in an area of low prevalence of endemic typhoid fever [16]. Subsequently, an enteric-coated capsule vaccine, suitable for wide-scale use, was shown to provide adequate, but lesser, protection in an area with moderate endemic prevalence of typhoid fever [12]. The failure of this vaccine in travellers has, however, been documented [6, 7].

A new approach to typhoid vaccination was thus attempted in an area of high endemic typhoid fever prevalence. A single dose of *S. typhi* capsular polysaccharide was administered to 11 284 children in November 1985 in a double-blind study [11]. We present here the results of 2 years of follow-up of this cohort of children.

## Subjects and Methods

Vi capsular polysaccharide was prepared by 1% hexadecyltrimethylammonium bromide extraction [14]. The 25-μg vaccine was prepared and packed in single-dose vials by Institute Merieux, Lyon, France. The control vaccine, prepared in identical vials, was 50 μg meningococcal A+C capsular polysaccharide vaccine. As the peak prevalence of typhoid fever is in children and adolescents, 11 384 children at 36 schools were vaccinated by deltoid intramuscular injection following parental informed consent. The identification of individual vaccines was kept by an independent observer. Approximately equal numbers of children received each vaccine. The 25-μg dose of Vi was chosen on the basis of a previous immunogenicity study in this population [11]. Blood was taken from 26 previously non-immune children 24 months after vaccination for estimation of Vi antibodies using an ELISA assay. Active surveillance consisted of health teams making weekly school visits, visits to clinics three times/week and daily visits to the two hospitals serving this population. Blood cultures were taken on the basis of clinical suspicion of typhoid fever at the clinics and hospitals, and from all pyrexial children traced from schools. A positive blood culture was the sole criterion for case inclusion.

Vaccine efficacy was analyzed as 1 minus (typhoid fever incidence in Vi vaccinates/typhoid fever incidence in control meningococcal vaccinates). Statistical comparisons between these groups were made using the chi-squared test, and those between serological data using Student's *t*-test.

## Results

No severe local or systemic side effects were noted, in keeping with the finding that 25 μg Vi causes minimal side effects [11]. Both ELISA at 6 and 12 months postvaccination and RIA, carried out only at 12 months postvaccination, showed significant increases in Vi antibodies compared with prevaccination levels, in children without pre-existing typhoid immunity [11]. In the subgroup of 26 children from whom blood was taken before vaccination and again 2 years postvaccination there was a significant increase in ELISA OD values at 2 years compared with prevaccination levels in both the typhoid group [15 children (ELISA OD $\pm$95% confidence limits) prevaccination $0.049 \pm 0.015$; 2 years postvaccination $0.132 \pm 0.028$ $P<0.001$] and the meningococcal controls (11 children; prevaccination $0.048 \pm 0.018$; postvaccination $0.136 \pm 0.049$; $P<0.01$).

During 2 years of surveillance, 50 cases of typhoid fever occurred in the control group – an annual incidence of 439/100000 in that group (Table 1). During this period 21 cases of typhoid fever occurred in the Vi vaccinates (184/

**Table 1.** Typhoid fever cases during 2 years following immunization vaccine

| | Vaccine | | Efficacy | *P* value[b] |
|---|---|---|---|---|
| | Vi | Meningo-coccal | | |
| Culture positive, total | 21 | 50 | 58% (30%–75%)[a] | <0.001 |
| Cases >6 weeks after vaccination | 18 | 47 | 62% (34%–78%)[a] | <0.001 |
| Total incidence/$10^5$ | 184.5 | 439.2 | | |

[a] Confidence intervals of 95%
[b] $\chi$-squared test with Yates modification

100 000) representing a vaccine efficacy of 58%. The vaccine efficiency calculated over 2 years from 6 weeks following vaccination is 62% (Table 1).

## Discussion

Capsular polysaccharide vaccines have been shown to be useful vaccines in the prevention of disease caused by encapsulated bacteria [5]. Although *S. typhi* is almost unique amongst the many thousands of salmonella serovars, in that it is surrounded by a capsular polysaccharide, thought to mediate its virulence in both mice [3] and men [4], its previous use as a vaccine preparation was disappointing [10]. It has, however, recently been shown that previous methods of vaccine preparation were associated with a poorly immunogenic product [13] and the rationale for a capsular polysaccharide Vi vaccine was proposed [13].

The side effects of Vi CPS vaccine prepared by detergent extraction [1, 11, 14] are less than those of whole cell vaccines [13, 15], and the single-dose regimen of the Vi capsular polysaccharide vaccine is preferable to the two-dose regimen of whole cell vaccine [8, 15] or the three-dose regimen of live oral vaccine [12].

Vi antibodies as measured in the ELISA assay after 2 years of follow-up showed an increase in antibodies in both groups. In an endemic area the level of antibodies would be expected to increase with age in the control group and the demonstration of a difference between the Vi and controls (or lack thereof) is being investigated by the follow-up of a separate cohort of 346 children from all of whom blood was taken prior to immunization (KPK, personal communiation).

The effectiveness of typhoid vaccination appears to be related to the infectious dose to which the individual is exposed. Volunteers, previously exposed

**Table 2.** Comparison of live-oral and Vi capsular polysaccharide vaccines

| Vaccine | >90% age range in years | No. of doses | Duration of surveillance in months | Mean annual incidence in controls $10^5$ | Efficacy[a] |
|---|---|---|---|---|---|
| Live oral suspension [16] | 6– 7 | 3 | 36 | 49 | 96% (66%–99%)[b] |
| Live oral enteric capsule [12] | 6–19 | 3 | 36 | 103 | 67% (46%–79%)[b] |
| Vi capsular polysaccharide [1] | 5–44 | 1 | 17 | 327 | 72% (41%–87%)[b] |
| Vi capsular polysaccharide (present study) | 5–16 | 1 | 24 | 439 | 58% (30%–75%)[b] |

[a] Blood culture confirmed cases only
[b] Confidence limit of 95%

to typhoid, can be reinfected if the inoculum is sufficiently high [9], and the protection of whole cell vaccine appears to be lower in areas of high infective dose associated with food-borne disease than in areas where water-borne outbreaks occur [15]. Similarly, there appears to be a relation between the efficacy of the two newly available typhoid vaccines and the background prevalence of typhoid fever in that community (Table 2). The live oral vaccine showed 94% protection in Egypt, an area having only 49 blood culture proven cases of typhoid/100 000 population at risk per year [16] compared with 67% protection in Chile, an area with an annual incidence of disease in controls of 103/100 000 [12]. The 58% protection reported here in the eastern Transvaal region of South Africa is in an area of high endemic typhoid fever (incidence 439/100 000/year). Somewhat higher levels of protection (72%) have been noted [1] with the Vi vaccine in another hyperendemic region, Nepal, where the prevalence is more than three times higher than in Chile, yet still 25% lower than that found in South Africa (Table 2).

This study demonstrates the efficacy of a single-dose capsular polysaccharide vaccine for 2 years, without significant side effects, in an area of high prevalence of endemic typhoid fever. No prospective studies have been carried out using this vaccine on travellers, but the immunogenicity of this vaccine in non-immune adults [14], the need for only a single dose, the low incidence of side effects and 2-year efficacy in hyperendemic areas suggest that a vaccine of this kind may be useful to protect travellers from typhoid fever in endemic areas.

## References

1. Acharya IL, Lowe CV, Thapa R et al. (1987) Prevention of typhoid fever in Nepal with the Vi capsular polysaccharide of *Salmonella typhi*. N Engl J Med 317:1101–1104
2. Bodhidatta L, Taylor DN, Thisyakorn V, Echeverria P (1987) Control of typhoid fever in Bangkok, Thailand, by annual immunization of school children with parenteral typhoid vaccine. Rev Infect Dis 9:841–845
3. Felix A, Pitt RM (1934) A new antigen of *B. typhosus*. Its relation to virulence and to active and passive immunization. Lancet II:186–191
4. Felix A, Pitt RM (1951) The pathogenic and immunogenic activities of *Salmonella typhi* in relation to its antigenic constituents. J Hyg 49:92–110
5. Grifiss JM, Apicella MA, Greenwood B, Makela PH (1987) Vaccines against encapsulated bacteria. Rev Infect Dis 9:176–188
6. Hirschel B (1983) Failure with oral typhoid vaccine Ty 21a. Lancet I:817–818
7. Hirschel B, Wüthrich R, Somaini B, Steffen R (1985) Inefficacy of the commercial live oral Ty 21a vaccine in the prevention of typhoid fever. Eur J Clin Microbiol 4:295–298
8. Hornick RB (1985) Selective primary health care: strategies for control of disease in the developing world. X. Typhoid fever. Rev Infect Dis 7:536–546
9. Hornick RB, Woodward TE, McCrumb FR et al. (1967) Typhoid fever vaccine – yes or no? Med Clin North Am 51:617–623
10. Hornick RB, Greisman SE, Woodward TE, DuPont HL, Dawkins AT, Snyder MJ (1970) Typhoid fever: pathogenesis and immunological control. N Engl J Med 283:686–691

11. Klugman KP, Gilbertson IT, Koornhof HJ et al. (1987) Protective activity of Vi capsular polysaccharide vaccine against typhoid fever. Lancet II:1165–1169
12. Levine MM, Ferreccio C, Black RE, Germanier R, Chilean Typhoid Committee (1987) Large scale field trial of Ty 21a live oral typhoid vaccine in enteric-coated capsule formulation. Lancet I:1049–1052
13. Robbins JD, Robbins JB (1984) Re-examination of the protective role of the capsular polysaccharide (Vi antigen) of *Salmonella typhi*. J Infect Dis 150:436–449
14. Tackett CO, Ferreccio C, Robbins JB et al. (1986) Safety and immunogenicity of the *Salmonella typhi* Vi capsular polysaccharide vaccines. J Infect Dis 154:342–345
15. Tapa S, Cvjetanovic B (1975) Controlled field trial on the effectiveness of one and two doses of active acetone-inactivated dried typhoid vaccine. Bull WHO 52:75–80
16. Wahdan MH, Serie C, Cerisier Y, Sallam S, Germanier R (1982) A controlled field trial of live *Salmonella typhi* strain Ty 21a oral vaccine against typhoid: Three-year results. J Infect Dis 145:292–295

# Immunologic Investigations with Oral Live Typhoid Vaccine TY 21A Strain

F. Ambrosch, A. Hirschl, H. Kollaritsch, P. Kremsner, Eva Rappold, and G. Wiedermann

Oral immunization against typhoid fever with the attenuated *S. typhi* strain Ty 21a was introduced a few years ago by Germanier [5–8]. The Ty 21a strain is able to colonize and multiply in the small intestine for a limited period. Due to the defect of the enzyme uridine-diphosphate-galactose-4-epimerase the bacteria are destroyed by bacteriolysis after several generations, thus liberating many immunizing antigens. This in return results in the induction of cell-mediated [11], humoral [9] and local [4] immune response.

As a prerequisite for a successful take of the vaccine a sufficient number of viable bacteria must be transferred into the small intestine without being inactivated by the gastric juice and released there for colonization and multiplication. In order to find out an optimal formulation of the Ty 21a vaccine and an optimal immunization schedule several field trials [10, 12, 13] were conducted (Table 1) as recommended by the WHO [14]. However, these studies are expensive, time consuming and not always conclusive.

This was the reason for us to establish a laboratory method for the evaluation of the individual take of the vaccine measuring the humoral immune response [1–3]. The principle of this method is the determination of the class-specific IgG, IgA and IgM serum antibodies against *S. typhi* LPS before and after immunization of healthy persons with the Ty 21a vaccine compared with a heat-inactivated preparation of the same vaccine formulation.

By means of this method we compared different formulations of the vaccine (Berna, Swiss Serum and Vaccine Institute; Trademarks, Vivotif and Typhoral L) and investigated possible interactions with simultaneously administered antimalarial drugs.

**Table 1.** Efficacy of three doses of Ty 21a vaccine (3 years surveillance)

| Study | Formulation | Protective efficacy |
|---|---|---|
| Egyptian trial<br>Wahdan et al. 1982 | Liquid vaccine with $NaHCO_3$ tablet | 96% |
| Chilean trial<br>Levine et al. 1987 | Gelatine capsules with $NaHCO^3$ | 19%–31% |
| | Enteric-coated capsules | 49%–67% |

# Materials and Methods

## Vaccinces

The investigations were performed in groups of health adults comprising approximately 20 persons each. They had been informed of the aim and the nature of the study and had provided written consent according to the declaration of Helsinki.

## Vaccine

Two formulations of the Ty 21a vaccine were used: a bicarbonate-buffered preparation consisting of two gelatine capsules with 0.4 g $NaHCO_3$ each and one gelatine capsule containing $10^9$ viable organisms of the Ty 21a strain, and an enteric-coated preparation containing $10^9$ viable organisms in capsules resistant to gastric juice. Comparatively, identical but heat-inactivated preparations of each formulation were used. The efficacy of the inactivation procedure had been controlled by culture. The inactivated preparations served as controls to evaluate a possible immune response induced by the ingested bacteria themselves without multiplication.

## Antimalarials

The following antimalarial drugs were investigated: chloroquine (Resochin), containing 150 mg chloroquine base/tablet; pyrimethamine/sulfadoxine (Fansidar), containing 25 mg pyrimethamine and 500 mg sulfadoxine/tablet; and mefloquine (Lariam), containing 250 mg/tablet. The administration of the antimalarials was performed separately and in combination.

**Table 2.** Study groups

| Group | Number of vaccinees | Vaccine | Antimalarial |
|---|---|---|---|
| 1 | 21 | BP | – |
| 2 | 19 | BPI | – |
| 3 | 21 | EC | – |
| 4 | 21 | BP | C |
| 5 | 20 | BP | PS |
| 6 | 19 | BP | C + PS |
| 7 | 21 | EC | C + PS |
| 8 | 23 | EC | – |
| 9 | 21 | EC | M |
| 10 | 21 | EC | M + PS |
| 11 | 20 | ECI | – |

BP, $NaHCO_3$-buffered preparation; BPI, $NaHCO_3$-buffered preparation, inactivated; EC, enteric-coated capsules; ECI, enteric-coated capsules, inactivated; C, chloroquine; PS, pyrimethamine/sulfadoxine; M, mefloquine

## Study Groups

Altogether 11 groups of vaccinees were immunized with different vaccine preparations and treated with different antimalarials (Table 2). The vaccinees were allocated to one of these groups by sequential randomization. In the first three groups the immunological properties of the two different formulations of the Ty 21a vaccine were investigated, in groups 4–11 possible interactions with different antimalarials.

## Administration and Blood Sampling

Administration of the single vaccine doses and the different antimalarials was performed according to the recommended schedules. The administration schedule started with one tablet of the respective antimalarial on day 0 in the evening (only chloroquine was repeated on days 2 and 4), and the vaccine was administered as prescribed on days 1, 3 and 5 in the morning. Blood samples were drawn on days 0 and 14.

## Laboratory Methods

Class-specific antibodies of the IgG, IgM and IgA class against *S. typhi* LPS were determined by means of the ELISA technique. Determination of the $\log_2$ ELISA titers was performed by means of the method of parallel lines [2]. Paired pre- and postimmunization samples were investigated simultaneously, the titration curves plotted and the class-specific titers or the titer increase (TI) at an optical density of 0.3 calculated by a special computer program.

## Statistical Methods

As a measure of the individual immune response the combined class specific titer increase (CTI) was calculated by summing up the class-specific TI values ($CTI = TI_{IgG} + TI_{IgA} + TI_{IgM}$). The mean CTI was used for the comparison of the different groups. The statistical significances were calculated by means of the Mann-Whitney U-test.

# Results

## Immune Response to Different Formulations

In order to evaluate the immune response to different formulations of the Ty 21a vaccine (groups 1–3) the mean values of the class-specific titer increase (TI) as well as of the combined titer increase (CTI) were calculated. Comparing the three vaccine groups there were characteristic and significant differences (Fig. 1).

As expected the inactivated vaccine induced only a small titer increase in the IgG, IgM and IgA class of 0.8, 0.2 and 0.2 $\log_2$ titer steps (mean CTI = 1.2). The immune response in the groups with the $NaHCO_3$-buffered formulation (mean CTI = 2.8) and with the enteric-coated capsules (mean CTI = 5.6) was significantly higher.

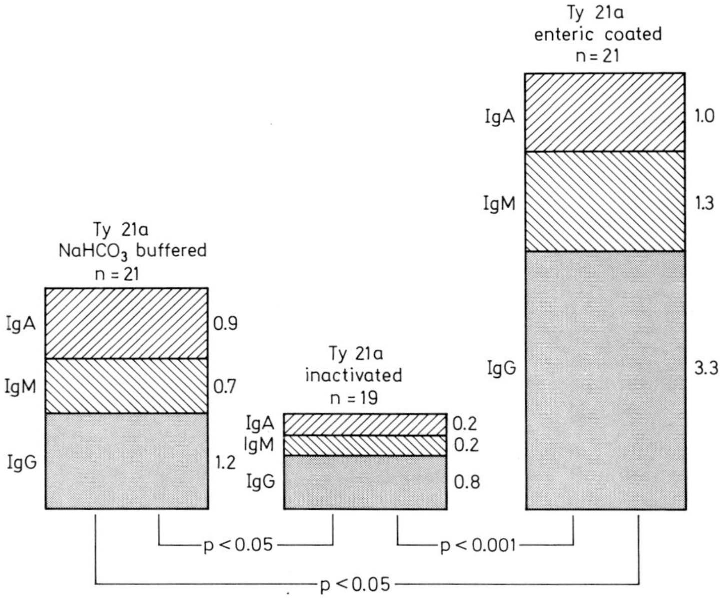


**Fig. 1.** Immune response to different preparations of Ty 21a vaccine mean titer increase of class-specific IgG, IgM and IgA antibodies. Significance calculated by Mann-Whitney U-test

Surprisingly, there was also a significant difference between group 1 (buffered preparation, mean CTI = 2.8) and group 3 (enteric-coated capsules, mean CTI = 5.6) in favor of the enteric-coated capsules. In order to explain this difference we calculated the response rate in the two vaccine groups. An immune response to the Ty 21a vaccine can be defined as a response which is greater than the mean CTI after the administration of the inactivated preparation (group 2). That means that vaccinees with a CTI > 1.2 can be considered responders. The response rates were 68% for the buffered preparation and 86% for the enteric-coated preparation. Additionally, the mean CTI of the responders was 4.0 and 6.8.

These serological results are in good accordance with the results of the Chilean field trial, where protection rates of 19%–31% for the buffered preparation and 49%–67% for the enteric-coated capsules were found.

## Influence of Antimalarial Drugs

In an initial study the possible interactions with chloroquine (Resochin) and pyrimethamine/sulfadoxine (Fansidar) were investigated using the buffered preparation (Table 3). The immune response in the groups with monoprophylaxis and even combined malariaprophylaxis (groups 4, 5, 6) were almost identical and similar to the immune response in the group without malaria prophylaxis (group 1). However, there was a statistically significant difference be-

**Table 3.** Immune response (mean CTI values) after simultaneous administration of Ty 21a vaccine ($NaHCO_3$-buffered formulation) and antimalarials (chloroquine and pyrimethamine/sulfadoxine)

| Group | Vaccine | Antimalarial | Mean CTI |
|---|---|---|---|
| 1 | BP | – | 2.8 |
| 2 | BPI | – | 1.2 |
| 4 | BP | C | 2.6 |
| 5 | BP | PS | 2.6 |
| 6 | BP | C + PS | 3.0 |

BP, $NaHCO_3$-buffered preparation; BPI, $NaHCO_3$-buffered preparation, inactivated; C, chloroquine; PS, pyrimethamine/sulfadoxine

**Table 4.** Immune response (mean CTI values) after simultaneous administration of Ty 21a vaccine (enteric-coated formulation) and mefloquine

| Group | Vaccine | Antimalarial | Mean CTI |
|---|---|---|---|
| 8 | EC | – | 2.5 |
| 9 | EC | M | 1.5 |
| 10 | EC | M + PS | 1.2 |
| 11 | ECI | – | 1.4 |

EC, enteric-coated capsules; ECI, enteric-coated capsules, inactivated; M, mefloquine; PS, pyrimethamine/sulfadoxine

tween these groups and the group 2 having received the inactivated preparation.

This important result, that even combined simultaneous malaria prophylaxis with chloroquine and pyrimethamine/sulfadoxine does not influence the CTI value, could be confirmed by comparing group 3, receiving the enteric-coated formulation, and group 7, receiving both antimalarials. Both groups showed an identical CTI value of 5.6. In a further study the new antimalarial mefloquine (Lariam) was investigated (Table 4). As expected, we again found a difference between group 8, receiving the enteric-coated formulation (CTI = 2.5), and group 11, receiving an inactivated preparation (CTI = 1.4). However, the CTI values of groups 9 and 10, receiving mefloquine and mefloquine plus pyrimethamine/sulfadoxine additionally did not differ from those of group 11, receiving the inactivated vaccine, and were significantly different from group 8 without mefloquine.

## Conclusions

The immunological investigations of two different formulations of the Ty 21a vaccine showed that the preparation using enteric-coated capsules had a better response rate and also a more intense immune response compared with the buffered preparation. However, the response rate even after administration of the enteric-coated capsules was only 86% and should be improved by a better formulation.

Investigation of the influence of simultaneous malaria prophylaxis showed that the antimalarials chloroquine (Resochin) and pyrimethamine/sulfadoxine (Fansidar) do not influence the immune response to the Ty 21a oral live typhoid vaccine and can be administered simultaneously without inhibiting the take of the vaccine. In contrast, the new antimalarial mefloquine (Lariam) actually does affect the immune response strongly and thus the take of the vaccine and should not be administered simultaneously with the Ty 21a vaccine.

## References

1. Ambrosch F, Hirschl A, Kollaritsch H, Kunz C, Stanek G, Wiedermann G (1984) Zur Frage möglicher Interaktionen zwischen oraler Typhus-Lebendimpfung und anderen Maßnahmen der Reiseprophylaxe. Mitt Osterr Ges Tropenmed Parasitol 6:19–24
2. Ambrosch F, Hirschl A, Kremsner P, Kundi M, Kunz C, Rappold E, Wiedermann G (1985) Orale Typhus-Lebendimpfung. MMW 127:775–778
3. Ambrosch F, Hirschl A, Kollaritsch H, Kremsner P, Rappold E, Wiedermann G (1987) Untersuchungen zur Kompatibilität des neuen Malariamittels Mefloquin mit der oralen Typhus-Lebendimpfung. Mitt Osterr Ges Tropenmed Parasitol 9:167–172
4. Cancellieri V, Manzillo G, Fara GM (1985) Demonstration of specific secretory IgA in the faeces of typhoid patients and Ty 21a-immunized healthy volunteers. Ann Sclavo 1–2:149–150
5. Germanier R (1970) Immunity in experimental salmonellosis. I. Protection induced by rough mutants of *Salmonella typhimurium*. Infect Immun 2:309–315
6. Germanier R (1972) Immunity in experimental salmonellosis. III. Comparative immunization with viable and heat-inactivated cells of *Salmonella typhimurium*. Infect Immun 5:792–797
7. Germanier R, Fürer E (1971) Immunity in experimental salmonellosis. II. Basis for the avirulence and protective capacity of gal E mutants of *Salmonella typhimurium*. Infect Immun 4:663–673
8. Germanier R, Fürer E (1975) Isolation and characterization of gal E mutant Ty 21a of *Salmonella typhi*: a candidate strain for a live oral typhoid vaccine. J Infect Dis 131:553–558
9. Kantele A, Arvilommi H, Jokinen I (1986) Specific immunoglobulin-secreting human blood cells after peroral vaccination against *Salmonella typhi*. J Infect Dis 153:1126–1131
10. Levine MM, Black RE, Ferreccio C, Germanier R, Chilean Typhoid Committee (1987) Large-scale field trial of Ty 21a live oral typhoid vaccine in enteric coated capsule formulation. Lancet I:1049–1052
11. Tagliabue A, Nencioni L, Caffarena A, Villa L, Boraschi D, Cazzola G, Cavalieri S (1985) Cellular immunity against *Salmonella typhi* after live oral vaccine. Clin Exp Immunol 62:242–247
12. Wahdan MH, Serie C, Germanier R, Lackany A, Cerisier Y, Guerin N, Sallam S et al. (1980) A controlled field trial of live oral typhoid vaccine Ty 21a. Bull WHO 58:469–474
13. Wahdan MH, Serie C, Cerisier Y, Sallam S, Germanier R (1982) A controlled field trial of live *Salmonella typhi* strain Ty 21a oral vaccine against typhoid: three-year results. J Infect Dis 145:292–295
14. WHO (1983) Live oral typhoid vaccine. Bull WHO 61:251–254

# Relapsing Typhoid Fever with Severe Colitis and Hepatitis

R. Meier, W. Wegmann, and K. Gyr

## Introduction

Relapsing typhoid fever with severe colitis and hepatitis is very rare. We present a patient who simultaneously developed these features.

## Case Report

A 34-year-old man had been hospitalized for sustained fever, headache and nausea in Nepal. Trimethoprim/sulfametoxazol was administered for 3 days, without success. Since typhoid fever was then suspected, therapy was changed to chloramphenicol for 15 days. After initial recovery, fever started again 10 days later and was accompanied by severe bloody diarrhea. The patient returned to Switzerland. On admission the patient was dehydrated, jaundiced and in a bad state of health. Fever was present with a temperature of 40 °C; BP 150/70, PR 92. Mild splenomegaly and general tenderness of the abdomen were found. The stool contained blood. Table 1 shows the laboratory findings.

**Table 1.** Laboratory findings (normal ranges are shown in parentheses)

| Laboratory findings | | Admission day | Peak values | Dismissal day |
|---|---|---|---|---|
| Sodium | (135–149 mmol/liter) | 126 | 124 | 139 |
| Potassium | (3.7–5.3 mmol/liter) | 3.2 | 3.0 | 4.3 |
| Bilirubin total | (5.1–18.8 µmol/liter) | 20 | 130 | 16 |
| Alkaline phosphatase | (60–200 U/liter) | 261 | 1 350 | 504 |
| SGOT | (–20 U/liter) | 37 | 235 | 18 |
| SGPT | (–25 U/liter) | 27 | 160 | 35 |
| LDH | (120–240 U/liter) | 618 | 1 470 | 215 |
| Prothrombin time | (70%–100%) | 80 | 46 | 100 |
| Hemoglobin | (14–18 g/100 ml) | 13 | 9.2 | 10.7 |
| WBC | (4 000–10 000/µl) | 3 600 | 2 500 | 6 600 |
| – Band granulocytes | (3%–8%) | 40 | 40 | 2.5 |
| – Eosinophils | (2%–4%) | – | – | 1.0 |
| Thrombocytes | (150 000–300 000/µl) | 100 000 | 30 000 | 443 000 |

Blood cultures and stool cultures: *Salmonella typhi* (9, 12, Vi: d:–, A); agglutinins for *H. salmonella* antigen 800 (normal <101). Other agents such as *Shigella*, *Yersinia*, *Amoeba*, and *Clostridium difficile* were excluded

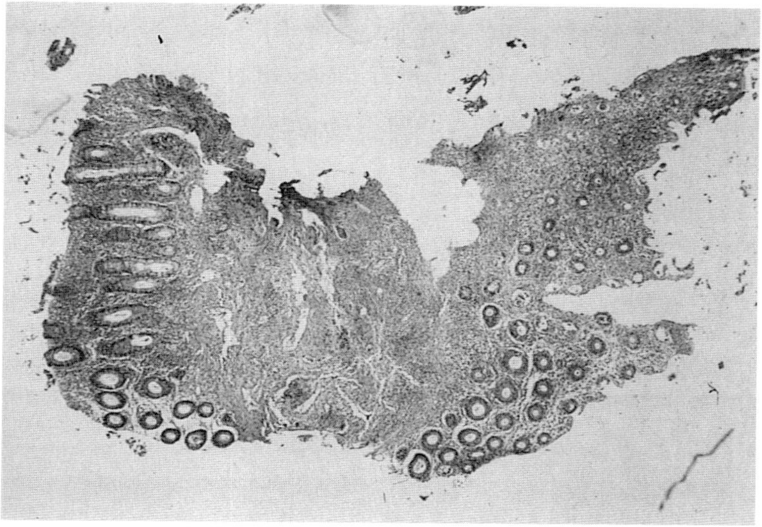

**Fig. 1**

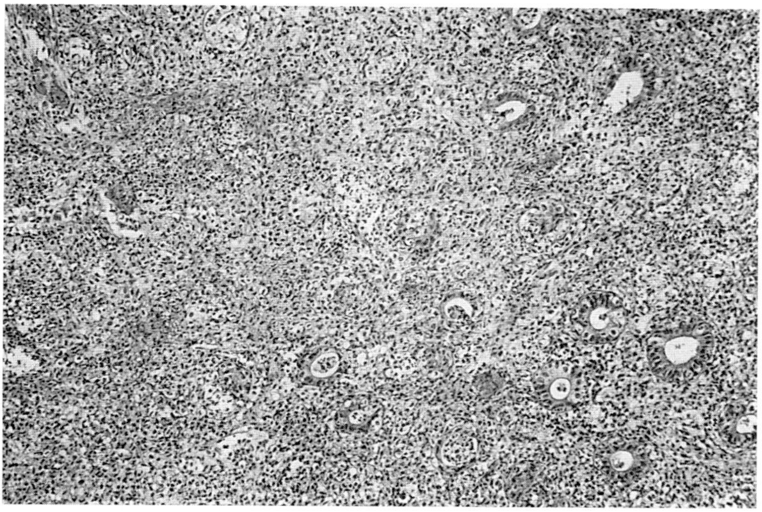

**Fig. 2**

**Fig. 1, 2.** Histological finding of colonoscopy: severe acute erosive and ulcerative inflammation with numerous polymorphonuclear leukocytes and thrombosed capillaries

The colonoscopy on the 2nd day revealed patchy hemorrhages, multiple fibrinous membranes and ulcers from the rectum to the colon transversum. Histologically a severe acute and ulcerative inflammation was found (Figs. 1, 2). After 11 days the treatment with amoxycillin had to be changed to trimethoprim/sulfametoxazol because of a drug reaction. With this management the fever decreased, the stool frequency sank and the patient gained weight. The

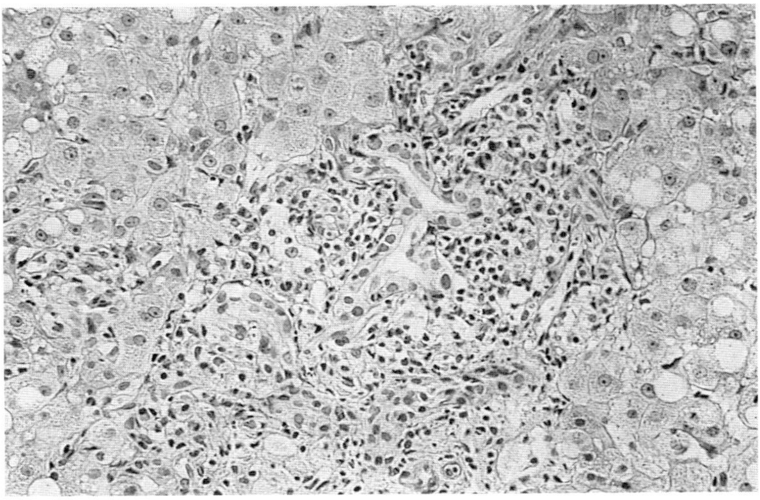

Fig. 3

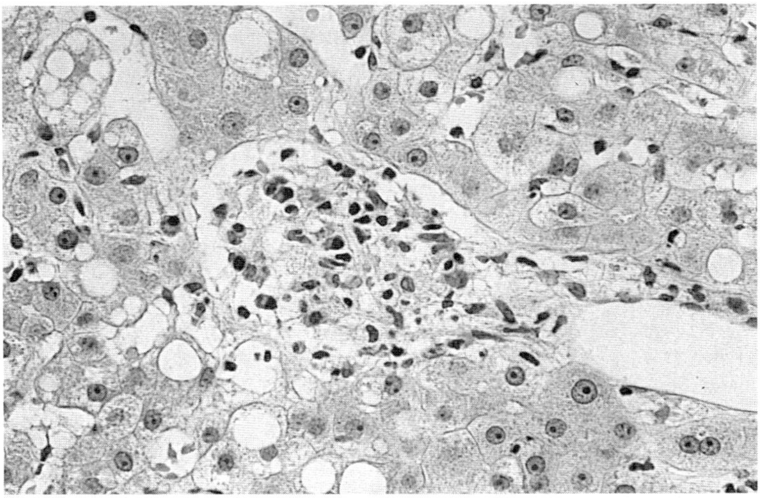

Fig. 4

**Fig. 3, 4.** Liver biopsy: slight edema of the portal tracts with infiltration of mononuclear cells and polymorphonuclear leukocytes, necrosis of single liver cells, regenerating hepatocytes with mitosis, focal proliferation of Kupffer cells, mild cholestasis and steatosis. Small intralobular granulomas consisting of epitheloid cells, large histiocytes, plasma cells and rare lymphocytes

liver function test showed hepatocellular jaundice with cholestasis. After 14 days a granulomatous hepatitis was seen in liver biopsy (Figs. 3, 4). Trimethoprim/sulfametoxazol was given for 3 weeks. At this time colonoscopy control showed normal findings, all stool cultures were negative for *Salmonella typhi* and all laboratory parameters were normalized.

## Discussion

The risk of international travellers contracting typhoid fever is about 1 in 25 000 when visiting tropical areas. For people living in rural areas in India the risk rises to 1 in 1000 (Steffen 1986). Recurrences are observed in 5%–15% of cases after a few weeks (Herzog 1987). The combination of severe ulcerative inflammation of the colon and granulomatous hepatitis with jaundice, markedly elevated liver enzymes and hepatomegaly is uncommon. Colonic involvement is well known for many *Salmonella* species, but rarely observed in *Salmonella typhi* infection (Boyd 1969, 1976; Appelbaum et al. 1976; Mandal and Mani 1976; Kumar et al. 1982; Chikanza et al. 1986; Reyes et al. 1986).

The differentiation between *Salmonella* colitis, ulcerative colitis and ischemic colitis may be difficult, but is important. It is well known that a patient with *Salmonella* in his stool might undergo acute *Salmonella* colitis or active ulcerative colitis with coincident *Salmonella* infection (Mandal and Mani 1976). In such a situation a reliable histological diagnosis should be attempted (Day et al. 1978; McGovern and Slavutin 1979).

The distinction from ischemic colitis is more difficult. The endoscopic and pathological changes are very similar, but crypt abscesses, crypt degeneration and leukocyte infiltration in the wall indicate the inflammatory nature of the disorder. Necrosis of the mucosa, hemorrhages and thrombi, which are occasionally seen, are probably expression of the severe inflammatory damage (McGovern and Slavutin 1979).

About half of the patients show moderately elevated liver enzymes and a slight hepatomegaly (Woodward and Hornick 1980, personal communication). Histologically, hepatic typhoid nodules are found in about one-third of the patients (Nasrallah and Nassar 1978). A real hepatitis "typhosa" with jaundice and markedly elevated liver enzymes is very rare but well documented. The true incidence is not known and may be approximately between 0.4% and 5% (Osler 1905, 1967; Rowland 1961; Faierman et al. 1972; Ayhan et al. 1973; Ramachandran et al. 1974; Rao et al. 1978; Pais 1984). The pathogenesis of typhoid hepatitis is not established yet. Circulating endotoxins and immune complexes are considered to be involved (Zimmermann et al. 1979; Dan et al. 1982). Normally the colonic and the hepatic involvement are fully reversible after successful treatment of the *Salmonella* infection, as in our patient.

The purpose of describing this case is to point to an exceptional combination of rare and dangerous complications in typhoid fever that so far has not been reported.

## References

1. Appelbaum PC, Scragg J, Schonland MM (1976) Colonic involvement in salmonellosis. Lancet II:102
2. Ayhan A, Gokoz A, Karacadag S, Telater H (1973) The liver in typhoid fever. Am J Gastroenterol 59:141
3. Boyd JF (1969) *Salmonella typhimurium,* colitis and pancreatitis. Lancet II:901–902

4. Boyd JF (1976) Colonic involvement in salmonellosis. Lancet I:1415
5. Chikanza IC, Kiire CF, Latif AS, Mason P, Neill P, Okwanga PN, Olweny CL (1986) Typhoid colitis. Cent Afr J Med 32:51–52
6. Dan M, Bar-Meir S, Jedwab M, Shibolet S (1982) Typhoid hepatitis with immunoglobulins and complement deposits in bile canaliculi. Arch Intern Med 142:148–149
7. Day DW, Mandal BK, Morson BC (1978) The rectal biopsy appearances in *Salmonella* colitis. Histopathology 2:117–131
8. Faierman D, Ross FA, Seckler SG (1972) Typhoid fever complicated by hepatitis, nephritis and thrombocytopenia. JAMA 221:60–61
9. Herzog C (1987) Bacterial infections involving the liver. Baillières Clin Gastroenterol 1:231–250
10. Kumar NB, Nostrant TT, Appelman HD (1982) The histopathologic spectrum of acute self-limited colitis (acute infectious-type colitis). Am J Surg Pathol 6:523–529
11. Mandal BK, Mani V (1976) Colonic involvement in salmonellosis. Lancet I:887–888
12. McGovern VJ, Slavutin LJ (1979) Pathology of *Salmonella* colitis. Am J Surg Pathol 3:483–490
13. Nasrallah SM, Nassar VH (1978) Enteric fever: a clinicopathologic study of 104 cases. Am J Gastroenterol 69:63–69
14. Osler W (1905/1967) In: Harvey AM, Ackusick VA (eds) Osler's text book revisited. Appleton-Century-Crofts, New York
15. Pais P (1984) A hepatitis like picture in typhoid fever. Br Med J 289:225–226
16. Ramachandran S, Godfrey JJ, Perera MVF (1974) Typhoid hepatitis. JAMA 230:236–240
17. Reyes E, Hernandes J, Gonzales A (1986) Typhoid colitis with massive lower gastrointestinal bleeding: an unexpected behavior of *Salmonella typhi*. Dis Colon Rectum 29:511–514
18. Rao PN, Bhusnurmath SR, Naik SR (1978) Typhoid fever manifesting with haematemesis, hepatitis and haemolysis. J Trop Med Hyg 81:146–150
19. Rowland MAK (1961) The complications of typhoid fever. J Trop Med Hyg 64:143–152
20. Steffen R (1986) Epidemiologic studies of traveller's diarrhea, severe gastrointestinal infections and cholera. Rev Infect Dis [Suppl 2]8:122–130
21. Zimmerman HJ, Fang M, Utili R, Seeff LB, Hoofnagle J (1979) Jaundice due to bacterial infection. Gastroenterology 77:362–374

# Risk/Benefit Evaluation of Pre-expositional Use of PCEC Rabies Vaccine in Travel Medicine

H. L. Bock, R. Clemens, G. Korger, and U. Quast

Recently, a young women was bitten in India by a stray dog; she died of rabies after returning to the Federal Republic of Germany [6]. In view of the quality of the modern rabies vaccines, there is good reason to ask whether vaccination should be recommended before travel to areas endemic for rabies.

The criteria requiring consideration here are the risks of infection in the country concerned, the manifestation index of the disease, the post-exposure treatment possibilities and their risks, and the prognosis of the manifest disease. In a benefit-to-risk analysis, these must be seen in relation to the safety, seroconversion rate and protection period provided by the new vaccine which can be used for pre-travel immunization.

In absolute as well as relative terms the majority of rabies cases are reported from India, where annually up to 50000 people die of the disease [9] and about 3 million people have to undergo a post-exposure course of rabies vaccination treatment [2, 8]. The incidence of rabies in other developing countries has likewise reached alarming proportions. For example, the official number of post-exposure treatments is 150000 in Brazil, 140000 in Thailand and 19000 in Tunisia [6].

In comparison the incidences of some other important infectious diseases for which vaccines are available are approximately 25000 cases of poliomyelitis, 29000 cases of cholera and 150 cases of yellow fever, worldwide.

The percentage of persons who develop rabies after exposure is estimated to be up to 50% [8]. The incubation period is extraordinarily variable and ranges from 10 days up to 1 year, with a 100% case fatality rate.

The recommended post-exposure treatment consists of local treatment of wounds and immediate administration of both a modern cell culture vaccine and a rabies immunoglobulin. The vaccine has to be injected into the deltoid muscle on days 0, 3, 7, 14, 28 and 90, and for immediate protection has to be accompanied on day 0 by a simultaneous dose of 20 IU/kg body weight of human rabies immunoglobulin (HRIG) or double the dose of antirabies serum (ARS). Up to half of the rabies immunoglobulin should be infiltrated intramuscularly around the wound and the remainder should be applied intragluteally [4]. Since the rabies immunoglobulin has been found to suppress the active induction of antibody formation, the amount administered should not exceed the recommended dosage [3, 4].

The safety record of the vaccine used for immunization is a further important factor with regard to the risks of post-exposure treatment. Here, a distinction must be made between nerve-tissue culture, duck embryo culture and nerve-tissue-free cell culture vaccines. The nerve-tissue-based vaccines are associated with a considerable risk of neurological complications. Beside these complications, there is also a high occurrence of localized and generalized reactions in up to 50% of the cases. Furthermore, compared with the modern cell culture vaccines, the nerve-tissue vaccines possess a far lower level of antigenicity. Consequently there is a relatively high risk of vaccination failures despite a larger number of injections.

The two cell culture rabies vaccines approved in the Federal Republic of Germany, the human diploid cell vaccine (HDCV) and the purified chick embryo cell vaccine (PCECV) have the advantages of high antigenicity, safety and freedom from notable side effects [5]. However, the costs for PCECV are considerably lower.

In the case of pre-exposure vaccination against rabies three doses of a modern cell culture vaccine are administered intramuscularly on days 0, 28 and 56. Alternatively, in a modified schedule, these injections can be given on days 0, 7 and 21, thus enabling active immunization against rabies to be carried out within a relatively short period before the date of travel.

As can be seen in Table 1, showing the geometric mean titres (GMTs) of antibody responses to PCECV pre-exposure regimens, 3 weeks after the second injection high antibody titres were found for both schemes. With the 0-7-21 scheme high titres were seen as early as day 14 [7]. It is generally accepted that protection is achieved at an antibody level of 0.5 IU/ml. This study, as well as others [1, 10, 11], found a 100% seroconversion and titres remaining at a high level for 2 years. A booster injection is recommended after 2–5 years.

The clinical trials and the experience of drug surveillance show that PCECV has a good safety record and is free of significant adverse drug reactions, thus meeting all the requirements necessary for prophylactic use: negligible side effects and reliable protection.

From the practical point of view it is important to know that after exposure those persons who have received a complete course of pre- or post-exposure vaccination require only a booster vaccination as soon as possible in order to achieve a rapid increase in their existing level of specific antibodies, and no immunoglobulin or antiserum has to be administered.

**Table 1.** Geometric mean titres of antibody response to PCECV pre-exposure regimens, i.m. route [7]

| Group | *n* | Schedule (days of vaccination | GMT of rabies neutralizing antibodies (IU/ml) | | | |
|---|---|---|---|---|---|---|
| | | | Day 0 | Day 14 | Day 42/77 | 2 years |
| 1 | 91 | 0, 7, 21 | <0.1 | 5.9 | 8.4 | 3.1 |
| 2 | 28 | 0, 28, 56 | <0.1 | 1.4 | 14.1 | 1.4 |

## References


1. Bijok U (1985) Purified chick embryo cell (PCEC) rabies vaccine. A review of clinical development 1982–1984. In: Vodopija I, Nicholson KG, Smerdel S, Bijok U (eds) Improvements in rabies post-exposure treatment. Zagreb Institute of Public Health, Zagreb
2. Bögel K, Motschwiller E (1986) Incidence of rabies and post-exposure treatment in developing countries. Bull WHO 64:881–887
3. Glück R, Wegmann A, Keller H, Hoskins JM, Germanier R (1987) Human rabies immunoglobulin assayed by the rapid fluorescent focus inhibition test suppresses active rabies immunization. J Biol Stand 15(82):177–183
4. Immunization Practises Advisory Committee (ACIP) (1984) Rabies prevention. MMWR 33:393–402
5. Kuwert E, Triau R, Thraenhardt O (1985) Innocuity and side effects of human diploid cell rabies vaccine: rationale and facts after vaccination of 500000 persons. In: Kuwert E, Merieux C, Koprowski H, Bögel K (eds) Rabies in the tropics. Springer, Berlin Heidelberg New York
6. Neunzig HP, Goossens-Merkt H, Arlt A, Zschocke S, Kunze K, Marcus I (1987) Klinische Manifestation der Tollwut beim Menschen – Kasuistischer Beitrag und Übersicht. Nervenarzt 58:549–556
7. Nicholson KG, Farrow PR, Bijok U, Barth R (1987) Pre-exposure studies with purified chick embryo cell culture rabies vaccine and human diploid cell vaccine: serological and clinical responses in man. Vaccine 5:208–210
8. Scheiermann N, Marcus CI (1987) Tollwut und Tollwutschutzimpfung. In: Impfen nützt – Impfen schützt. Weltgesundheitsthema 1987. Merkur, Troisdorf, pp 87–93
9. Sehgal S, Bhatia R (eds) (1985) Rabies: current status in India. Workshop on Rabies Surveillance and Control, 15–17 October, National Institute of Communicable Diseases, Delhi, pp 10–18
10. Wasi C, Chaiprasithikul P, Chavanich L, Puthavathana P, Thongcharoen P, Trishanananda M (1986) Purfied chick empbryo cell rabies vaccine. Lancet I:40
11. Vodopija I, Sureau P, Lafon M et al. (1986) An evaluation of second generation tissue culture rabies vaccines for use in man: a four-vaccine comparative immunogenicity study using a pre-exposure vaccination schedule and an abbreviated 2-1-1 post-exposure schedule. Vaccine 4:245–248

# Antibody Response to Malaria Sporozoite Vaccine Enhanced by Simultaneous Administration of Alpha-Interferon

M. Just, R. Berger, D. Stürchler, H. Etlinger, M. Fernex, D. Gillessen, H. Matile, R. Pink, F. Sinigaglia, and B. Takacs

*Plasmodium falciparum* malaria is undergoing a worldwide resurgence due to the spread of drug-resistant parasite strains and increasing resistance of mosquitoes to insecticides. Development of an effective malaria vaccine would complement traditional malaria control measures and help to prevent spread of the disease. Unfortunately, so far there is no product available which can be called a malaria vaccine. A few general remarks on the development of a vaccine against the malaria sporozoites follow.

1. Protection was achieved years ago by the groups of Nussenzweig, Clyde and Rieckmann [1–3] immunizing with sporozoites attenuated by radiation.
2. It was shown that antibodies were directed against the circumsporozoite protein (CSP) covering the sporozoite surface [4].
3. The structure of the CSP is similar among various malaria species; the CSP contains multiple tandem repeats of short amino acid sequences [5].
4. Vaccines derived from the circumsporozoite antigen are weakly immunogenic in humans, but nevertheless a challenge study in three humans showed that one of the three volunteers was protected, and two had a delayed infection [6]. A recombinant vaccine also based on the repeat sequence of the CS protein showed a similar protective effect [7].

In an open clinical trial with a few volunteers we have previously shown [8] that a synthetic falciparum sporozoite vaccine in which the dodecapeptide (NANP)3 is conjugated to tetanus toxoid (TT) is safe and well tolerated, but the (NANP)3-TT vaccine was less immunogenic in humans than in the mouse model.

As alpha-interferon has an inducing and enhancing effect on cellular and humoral immune responses in experimental systems, a study was done to explore the immune stimulation of alpha-interferon when simultaneously administered with a low dose of the (NANP)3-TT sporozoite vaccine.

## Methods

For this double-blind, randomized, comparative trial 37 medical students and staff members of the Childrens Hospital, University of Basel, were included. All volunteers received 200 µg (NANP)3-TT on two occasions, 8 weeks apart. One group (placebo) simultaneously received a solution of albumin, one group (low interferon) 0.5 million IU, and one group ("high" interferon) 1.5 million

IU alpha-interferon. Serological tests included enzyme-linked immunosorbent assay using (NANP)50, and tetanus toxoid as antigens, an immune fluorescent antibody test with air-dried sporozoites on slides and lymphocyte proliferation assays: stimulations with (NANP)3, (NANP)50, or TT.

## Results

No vaccine-associated systemic effects were observed. Reactions at the injection site were very mild; the frequency of local events was less after the second than after the first immunization.

Reciprocal IgM antibody titers in ELISA are shown in Fig. 1. Eighty percent of volunteers converted after two immunizations in at least one of the three tests. The geometric mean IgG antibody titer in ELISA was significantly greater in the pooled alpha-interferon groups than in the placebo group.

With respect to the cellular immune response neither the vaccine alone nor its combination with alpha-interferon had a measurable effect on lymphocyte proliferation induced by (NANP)3 or (NANP)50 14 days after the second immunization. The mean stimulation index to TT increased in the alpha-interferon group, while it decreased in the placebo group.

## Discussion

Before a sporozoite vaccine, in combination with adjuvants or without, can be called a candidate vaccine for further clinical trials, it should of course be shown that it not only induces humoral antibodies but gives protection in chal-

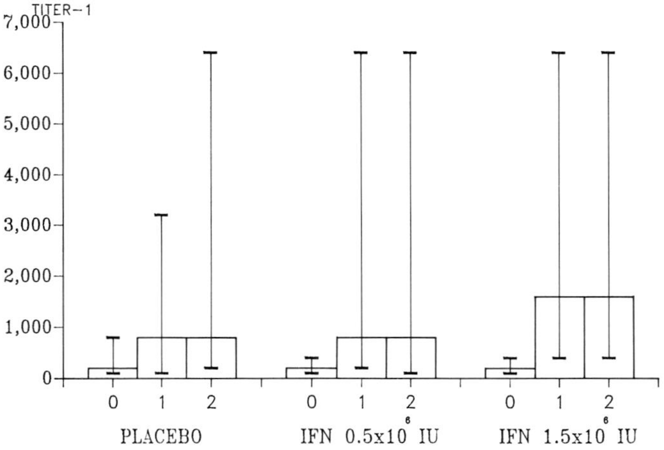


**Fig. 1.** Medians (and range) of IgM antibody titers to $(NANP)_{50}$ in ELISA in three groups of volunteers immunized with two single doses of $(NANP)_3$-TT vaccine and either placebo (*left lane*), a low (*middle lane*), or high (*right lane*) dose of interferon-$\alpha$ (=IFN-$\alpha$). Numbers *0, 1, 2* indicate blood samples taken before, and 4 weeks after, first and second injections respectively

lenge studies. At the moment we are undergoing discussions with ethical committees as to whether we are allowed to perform such experimental challenge studies.

## References

1. Nussenzweig RS, Vanderberg JP, Most H (1969) Protective immunity produced by the injection of X-irradiated sporozoites of *Plasmodium berghei*. IV. Dose response specificity and humoral immunity. Mil Med [Suppl]134:1183–1190
2. Clyde DF, Most H, McCarthy V, Vanderberg JP (1973) Immunization of man against sporozoite-induced falciparum malaria. Am J Med Sci 266:169–174
3. Rieckmann KH, Beaudoin RL, Cassells JS, Sell KW (1979) Use of attenuated sporozoites in the immunization of human volunteers against falciparum malaria. Bull WHO [Suppl 1]57:261
4. Miller LH, Howard RJ, Carter R, Good MF, Nussenzweig V, Nussenzweig RS (1986) Research toward malaria vaccines. Science 234:1349–1356
5. Nussenzweig V, Nussenzweig RS (1985) Circumsporozoite proteins of malaria parasites. Cell 42:401–402
6. Herrington DA, Clyde DF, Losonsky G, Cortesia M, Davis J, Murphy JR, Felix AM et al. (1987) Safety and immunogenicity in man of a synthetic peptide tetanus toxoid conjugate malaria vaccine against *Plasmodium falciparum* sporozoites. Nature 328:257–259
7. Ballou WR, Hoffmann SL, Sherwood JA, Hollingdale MR, Neva FA, Hockmeyer WT, Gordon DM et al. (1987) Safety and efficiency of a recombinant DNA *Plasmodium falciparum* sporozoite vaccine. Lancet I:1277–1281
8. Etlinger H, Felix AM, Gillessen D, Heimer EP, Just M, Pink JRL, Sinigaglia F et al. (1988) Assessment in humans of a synthetic peptide-based vaccine against the sporozoite stage of the human malaria parasite, *P. falciparum*. J Immunol 40:626–633

# Incidence of Antibody to Hepatitis A among Employees of a Multinational Corporation: Implications for Immunoglobulin Prophylaxis

R. McMullen and E. C. Jong

## Summary

As part of a health screening program, serum assays for antibody to hepatitis A (anti-HAV) were performed on 1609 employees of an international hotel and restaurant company. Prevalence of anti-HAV by national groups was as follows: Indonesian 783/816 (96.0%), Filipino 404/421 (96.0%), United States and Canada 76/217 (35.0%), northern European 51/151 (33.8%); the nationality of four persons (0.2%) was undetermined. All persons tested positive for the IgG subclass of antibody except for one person who had the IgM subclass of anti-HAV. Positive results in the North American and European populations demonstrated an age-associated rise: the rate for ages 20–29 in North americans was 20.4% and for Europeans, 10.9%. These increased for ages 30–39 to 40.3% and 30.8% respectively, for ages 40–49 to 56.7% and 50.0%, and for ages 50–59 to 66.7% and 68.0%. The lower incidence of seropositivity in younger age groups is similar to those reported in other studies in developed countries since the end of World War II.

Pre-travel prophylaxis with immune globulin (IG) assumes greater importance as younger travelers from developed countries, who are less likely to have contracted the infection as a child, visit countries where hepatitis A is endemic. There has been some resistance to pre-travel immunization with IG because of patient misunderstanding and fears regarding HIV infection associated with the use of blood products. Travelers to endemic areas should be educated and counseled to receive IG prior to travel.

Epidemics of acute hepatitis A in adults tend to occur in settings where nonimmune persons are exposed to an individual in the infectious prodromal phase of acute hepatitis A. This can result in a large outbreak when persons in a restaurant or institutional setting are exposed to an infectious source; secondarily infected persons may then transmit the infection to others beyond the initial closed environment.

We undertook a serologic screening program for hepatitis A as part of a large multinational hotel and restaurant company's health maintainence program for its employees. A specific concern on the part of corporate management was the risk for disease transmission by employees with frequent contact with guests. Employees of this corporation come from many countries including the United States, Canada, and several nations of northern Europe. However, the majority of food handlers and those engaged in the performance of personal services for the guests are Filipino or Indonesian. This paper reports the findings of this screening study, particularly with regard to the incidence of immunologic evidence of past infection with hepatitis A.

## Methods

Samples of blood were obtained by standard phlebotomy techniques. The serum was separated by centrifugation and aliquots were frozen until serologic testing could be performed. The samples of sera were analyzed for the presence of antibody to hepatitis A (anti-HAV) and also for the IgM immunologic class of anit-HAV using commercially available enzyme immunoassay techniques (HAVAB, HAVAB-M; Abbott Laboratories, North Chicago, Illinois, USA).

Results were reported to patients during individual counseling sessions regarding general health practices. These were conducted by company-employed health care providers.

## Results

A total of 1609 individuals were screened in this program, which represented approximately 95% of those individuals with frequent personal contact with guests. The nationality of all but four of the screened persons was known, and ages were available for 1586 (98.6%). The number of persons from each national group as well as the proportion of males and the average age is shown in Table 1.

Of the 1609 screened, 1315 (81.7%) tested positive for anti-HAV. One person, an Indonesian, was positive for the IgM class of anti-HAV; he had not recently noted symptoms compatible with hepatitis A. There were marked differences in the frequency of anti-HAV among the different national groups represented (see Table 2).

There was no significant difference between the rate of seropositivity for the Indonesians and the Filipinos, and no significant difference between the rate for North Americans and Europeans. However, the difference between the developing and developed countries was highly significant when subjected to chi-square analysis ($P < 0.0001$).

The high rate of seropositivity to hepatitis A among the Filipinos and Indonesians is consistent with the high, often almost universal, incidence of anti-HAV previously reported in populations in developing nations [1, 7]. Lower rates of anti-HAV are usually seen in northern Europeans and North Americans, especially among the young [7, 9], although urban, adult, lower socioeconomic groups may have a high frequency of anti-HAV [6].

When those individuals for whom ages were known were grouped by decades, there was an age-associated rise in prevalence of antibody to hepatitis A among each national group (see Table 3). However, the rise was small in the Filipino and Indonesian groups given the high rate of seropositivity in even the youngest decade group. When controlled for age, there was again no significant difference between the Filipino and Indonesian groups, or between the North American and northern European groups, but the difference between the developing and developed countries was again highly significant ($P < 0.0001$). This finding is consistent with the notion that hepatitis A is primarily a disease of childhood in the developing world.

**Table 1.** Distribution of screened persons according to nationality, sex, and age

| Nationality | Number | Percentage of males | Average age (±SD) |
|---|---|---|---|
| Indonesian | 816 | 100.0 | 33.7± 6.6 |
| Filipino | 421 | 98.3 | 32.4± 7.2 |
| North American | 217 | 61.5 | 33.2±10.2 |
| Northern European | 151 | 90.9 | 35.8±11.2 |
| Total | 1605 | 93.5 | 33.5± 7.9 |

Note: National origin of four persons was unavailable; age data based on 1586 persons with age known

**Table 2.** Frequency of anti-HAV among different national groups

| National group | Number positive for anti-HAV | Number tested | Percentage positive for anti-HAV |
|---|---|---|---|
| Filipino | 783 | 816 | 96.0 |
| Indonesian | 404 | 421 | 96.0 |
| North American | 76 | 217 | 35.0 |
| Northern European | 51 | 151 | 33.8 |

**Table 3.** Increase in seropositivity for anti-HAV among national groups by age in decades

| Decade | North American | European | Indonesian | Filipino |
|---|---|---|---|---|
| 20–29 | 20/98 (20.4) | 6/55 (10.9) | 207/224 (92.4) | 162/175 (92.6) |
| 30–39 | 27/67 (40.3) | 12/39 (30.8) | 415/427 (97.2) | 172/176 (97.7) |
| 40–49 | 17/30 (56.7) | 12/24 (50.0) | 143/146 (97.9) | 59/59 (100.0) |
| 50–59 | 8/12 (66.7) | 17/25 (68.0) | 13/13 (100.0) | 11/11 (100.0) |
| 60+ | 3/5 (60.0) | None | None | None |

## Discussion

It may be postulated that the decreased incidence of anti-HAV in the younger-aged Europeans and North Americans may be due to a cohort effect, as suggested by others [4, 5]. Since the end of World War II, persons in developed countries have grown up in an environment with improved hygiene and sanitation: they might be expected to have lower rates of seropositivity and to remain less likely to convert as they age. However, without a remote comparison study of the persons screened in this study, or a demographically similar group, the existence of a cohort effect cannot be demonstrated by these data alone.

We did find a somewhat higher rate of seropositivity in the younger aged North Americans and Europeans than has been reported in other studies. Our rates may have been influenced by several factors including: (1) relatively low social and economic status of many of the employees as children; (2) that they had worked and lived abroad, in some cases for many years; (3) that some employees were actually immigrants from areas with endemic hepatitis A; and (4) that the preponderance of males in the European and North American groups would result in higher rates from increased exposure to hepatits A due to variables in life-style and sexual preference. Indeed, the percentage of North American and European females positive for anti-HAV (a group which was similar in age distribution to the males) was 24.7, compared with 37.6% for the males.

This study was of interest to the corporation involved because it demonstrated that most of their foodhandlers and other persons with frequent guest contact were already immune to hepatitis A: as long as adequate hygiene is maintained, this group of employees would not appear likely to transmit this disease to guests, who are probably more at risk for hepatitis A infection when consuming food and beverages away from the hotel environment in a developing country.

Another significant aspect of this study is that it reinforces the susceptibility of younger populations from developed countries to hepatitis A. In 1984, international travel within 6 weeks was reported by 7.3% of persons from the United States who contracted hepatitis A; for 5.8%, it was the primary identifiable risk factor [6]. As the world becomes more mobile and people undertake business and pleasure trips to remote or developing areas, prophylaxis with immune globulin (IG), which has been suggested to be highly protective in very suceptible populations [9], may assume even greater significance.

The University of Washington's University Hospital Travel Clinic, among other services, provides pretravel counseling and immunizations. A large proportion of the patients have travel destinations in Africa, Central and South America, the Indian subcontinent, and the Pacific Rim countries; prophylactic IG was deemed appropriate and administered to 2023 of 3253 of patients (62%) seen in recent years. Side effects have been minor and we remain unaware of the development of symptomatic hepatitis A in any of these patients.

There has been reluctance on the part of some patients to accept blood-derived products due to fears regarding HIV infection and newspaper reports of low levels of anti-HIV antibody in lots of immune globulin. However, published studies have failed to show persistence of anti-HIV in persons receiving IG or hepatitis B hyperimmune globulin (HBIG) and the fractionalization process for IG production appears to inactivate the virus. Also, all units of plasma intended for IG production, but which repeatedly test positive for anti-HIV, are now discarded. Thus, IG preparations appear to be safe [2, 8], and most patients with anxieties accept IG after counseling. Pending the development of a reliable vaccine, passive immune prophylaxis and instruction in proper hygiene and food and water precautions represent the best means to prevent acquiring hepatitis A during travel.

## References

1. Burke DS, Snitbhan R, Johnson DE, Scott RN (1981) Age specific prevalence of hepatitis A virus in Thailand. Am J Epidemiol 113:245–249
2. Centers for Disease Control (1986) Safety of therapeutic immune globulin products with respect to transmission of human T-lymphotropic virus type III/lymphadenopathy-associated virus infection. MMWR 35:231–233
3. Centers for Disease Control (1986) Hepatitis Surveillance Report no 50. CDC Atlanta
4. Frösner G, Willers H, Muller R, Schenzle D, Deinhardt F, Hopken W (1978) Decrease in incidence of hepatitis A infections in Germany. Infection 6:259–260
5. Gust ID, Lehmann NI, Lucas CR (1978) Relationship between prevalence of antibody to hepatitis A antigen and age: a cohort effect? J Infect Dis 138:425–426
6. Szmuness W, Dienstag JL, Purcell RH, Harley EJ, Stevens CE, Wong DC (1976) Distribution of antibody to hepatitis A antigen in urban adult populations. N Engl J Med 295:755–759
7. Szmuness W, Dienstag JL, Purcell RH, Stevens CE, Wong DC, Ikram H et al. (1977) The prevalence of antibody to hepatitis A antigen in various parts of the world: a pilot study. Am J Epidemiol 106:392–398
8. Tedder RS, Uttley A, Cheingsong-Popov R (1985) Safety of immunoglobulin preparation containing anti-HTLV-III (Letter. Lancet I:815
9. Weiland O, Berg JVR, Back E, Lundbergh P (1979) Immunoglobulin prophylaxis against hepatitis A among Swedish soldiers in an endemic region. Infection 7:223–225

# Hepatitis B in Canadian Missionaries Serving in Developing Countries

K. L. Gamble, L. Spence, C. R. Smith, and J. S. Keystone

## Introduction

Since hepatitis B vaccine has become available, the question has arisen about who should receive this costly vaccine. Frame, in an unpublished study from New York, quotes a 40% prevalence rate of hepatitis B markers in a missionary population surveyed in West Africa. In view of the high prevalence of hepatitis B markers in the developing world, pressure has been brought to bear on mission organizations to institute the use of the hepatitis B vaccination for their personnel. To assess whether Canadian missionaries serving in developing countries are at greater risk of contracting hepatitis B, a prevalence study of hepatitis B surface antigen (HBSAg) and antibody (HBSAb) was undertaken. In addition, we sought to determine the risk factors associated with the acquisition of the hepatitis B markers in this population.

## Method

Two hundred and two missionaries who were seen consecutively at the Missionary Health Institute and at the Tropical Disease Unit, Toronto General Hospital, were surveyed. Each completed a questionnaire concerning demographic information, previous health as it related to hepatitis, history of blood transfusion and work history. Eight individuals were excluded from the study, either because of incomplete information or because of previous hepatitis B vaccine. A blood sample from each participant was evaluated for HBSAg and HBSAb using standard RIA techniques. The results were analyzed using multiple regression techniques and chi-square analysis.

## Results

The study group consisted of 194 persons, 85 males and 105 females ranging in age from 3 to 72 years. They had served in four major geographic areas (Africa, Americas, Asian subcontinent and Southeast Asia) for a total of 1780 person-years. The mean duration of stay was 9.2 ($\pm$7.8) years. One hundred and fifteen (59.3%) had served in Africa, 32 (16.5%) in the Americas, 8 (4.1%) served in two or more of these geographic regions. Fifty-eight (29%) worked in a rural setting only, 23 (11.9%) in an urban setting, and 113 (58.2%) in both rural and urban environments. The mean age was 37.1 ($\pm$15.1) years. A history of hepatitis of any type was obtained from 21 (10.8%) individuals.

There were 21 individuals (10.8%) who were positive for HBSAb. No participant in the study had serum positive for HBSAg. Only 4 of these 21 individuals had a history of clinical hepatitis. None of the participants had a history of blood transfusion.

To study the factors associated with the risk of seropositivity we analyzed the results of missionaries who worked with blood and blood products and those who did not. Six of the 18 persons (33.3%) whose employment involved handling blood or blood products were positive for HBSAb. All of the infected individuals were female nurses who had served in Africa. Of the 176 individuals who were not in contact with blood or blood products, 15 (8.5%) were seropositive. Thus, contact with blood and blood products was strongly associated with seropositivity ($P<0.001$).

Using chi-square analysis there was lack of statistical correlations with sex and urban versus urban locale. Our sample was too small to demonstrate a correlation with age.

Linear regression analysis failed to demonstrate a significant relationship between hepatitis B risk and length of service abroad. However, when length of stay was considered in a nonparametric manner, comparing career versus noncareer missionaries for various terms, there was a significant difference for career missionaries when length of service was two terms (8 years) or greater ($P<0.05$).

When comparing the prevalence of hepatitis B markers by geographic region, there was no significant difference in the risk of infection when the individuals were grouped according to the four major areas. However, the prevalence of hepatitis B markers was significantly greater in Africa compared with the combined total of the other areas ($P<0.05$). When blood handlers were removed from both groups, the prevalence of hepatitis B markers in Africa was not significantly different from that in other geographic regions. This latter finding suggests that blood handling was the factor which resulted in the high prevalence of hepatitis B markers in Africa as a whole.

Within Africa, however, there was a much higher prevalence of hepatitis B in West Africa when compared with the rest of Africa combined. Of the 30 missionaries who were not blood handlers in West Africa, 12 (26.6%) were seropositive compared with four (2.8%) seropositive cases in the 71 missionaries from other parts of Africa. The length of service was comparable in both groups and this difference remained highly statistically significant ($P\leqq 0.0001$).

## Discussion

As expected, there was a clear relationship between the risk of acquisition of HBSAb and blood-handling activity. A prevalence rate of 33% in the blood handlers in this study compares favorably with the findings of 35% seropositivity in biochemistry technologists in a study of hospital personnel at Toronto General Hospital. Since we did not study hepatitis B core antibody, the overall risk to missionaries in Africa may well be higher than what we determined.

## Conclusion

We conclude that not all missionaries require immunization against hepatitis B. Assuming that the prevalence of hepatitis B markers in Canada is 4%–5%, the overall risk for missionaries to acquire hepatitis B in developing countries is not much greater than for a comparable Canadian population. From our data, there is justification for vaccinating career missionaries and those who are planning to work in West Africa where the risk of contracting hepatitis B appears to be particularly high. Regardless of location, those at risk because of exposure through blood and blood products should be vaccinated.

# Prevention of Hepatitis B in Travelers to Endemic Areas

F. E. André

## Introduction

The latest World Health Organization estimate is that there are about 300 million chronic carriers of hepatitis B virus (HBV) worldwide [1]. Prevalence varies from between less than 1% in western Europe and North America, to 10%–20% in Asia and 7%–15% in parts of Africa [2–5]. Non-immune travellers to countries in areas with a high incidence of hepatitis B who reside in low-incidence countries are therefore at an increased risk of contracting an infection.

Transmission of HBV occurs mainly through close contact with contaminated blood and body fluids, but also through transfusions of unscreened blood or blood-derived products. Injection of only a few microlitres of blood is sufficient to induce infection; the use of contaminated needles (tatooing, acupuncture, drug abuse) can spread HBV. HBV carriers and individuals with acute infections can transmit the hepatitis B virus through body fluids such as saliva, mucosal secretion, semen and vaginal secretions. Hepatitis B is, under some epidemiological circumstances, predominantly a sexually transmitted disease.

About one-third of all individuals who contract acute hepatitis B (HB) have only mild symptoms: headache, malaise, high fever, nausea and abdominal pain. At most 25% of those with acute HB develop jaundice. In rare cases, acute hepatitis develops as fulminant hepatitis, which is almost always fatal within 48 h. HBV infection can also lead to chronic hepatitis and cirrhosis of the liver and probably accounts for up to 80% of all cases of hepatocellular carcinoma. For the milder forms of acute hepatitis B, the duration of symptoms varies widely but may persist for 6 weeks or more. Most infected individuals recover without any long-lasting consequences. However, up to 10% of adults and 90% of newborns will be unable to mount an adequate antibody response and do not clear the virus. The virus remains chronically present in their blood and other body fluids; they become HBV carriers.

## Preventative Measures

Travellers and other at-risk groups of people (e.g. medical personnel, male homosexuals and intravenous drug users) should take preventative measures against hepatitis B. "Safe" sexual behaviour and avoiding close personal contact with infected persons is the easiest way to reduce the chances of infection.

Using condoms and avoiding shared needles also cuts down the risk of acquiring hepatitis B. Another approach is immunization of at risk individuals.

## Passive Immunization

Passive immunization, using hepatitis B immunoglobulins (HBIGs), is especially useful for postexposure prophylaxis; i.e. lessening the severity of HBV infection in individuals recently exposed to HBV. These immunoglobulins are purified from the serum of individuals with high titres of neutralizing anti-HBs antibodies. Although the protection afforded by passive immunization is immediate, it is only temporary. Anti-HBs immunoglobulin should be injected within 24 h after a potential exposure, which is not always recognizable. Immunoglobulin resorption from the injection site is variable. Catabolism of passively acquired antibodies occurs relatively rapidly and, as little as 4 months after injection, circulating antibody levels have fallen to 2% of their maximum value. HBIG is also effective prophylactically but is expensive and provides only short-term protection.

## Vaccination

Active immunization by vaccination is clearly the most practical method of preventing HBV infection and the carrier state. Until recently, only plasma-derived hepatitis B vaccines (PDVs) were available. These vaccines, manufactured from the plasma of chronic HBV carriers, have repeatedly been shown to be efficacious. Although stringent safety tests are performed on each lot of PDV, the fear remains that unidentified pathogenic organisms could escape inactivation during production. Moreover, human albumin present in this vaccine has been shown to cause the formation of auto-antibodies [6]. For these reasons, as well as the limited supply and high cost of PDV, hepatitis B vaccination has until now been restricted. Recombinant DNA vaccines, produced in genetically engineered yeast cells, have recently been developed. This technology permits the manufacture of virtually unlimited quantities of a relatively low-cost vaccine. The primary safety concern with yeast-derived vaccine (YDV), i.e. the possibility of hypersensitivity to yeast proteins, has been shown to be unfounded [7]. Studies in chimpanzees [8] and human trials [9] have shown that the HB surface protein contained in the vaccine elicits an antibody response qualitatively and quantitatively similar to that obtained using a plasma-derived vaccine.

We have carried out, in different countries, vaccination trials with a YDV (Engerix-B, SmithKline Biologicals) involving over 6000 normal, healthy adults as well as approximately 2500 individuals deemed to be at high risk for hepatitis B. Results of two studies in healthy adults, for which data are available up to 3 years after vaccination, are shown in Table 1, as well as immunogenicity of the vaccine in homosexual males and institutionalized patients, two of the high-risk groups in which the protective efficacy of the vaccine was assessed. In every group, vaccination with YDV proved to be highly immuno-

**Table 1.** Anti-HBs response of subjects vaccinated against hepatitis B with a yeast-derived vaccine (Engerix-B)

| Group | Dose[a] regimen (month given) | One month after last injection: seroconversion rate | GMT[b] | At 36 months after first vaccine dose: seroconversion rate | GMT |
|---|---|---|---|---|---|
| Normal adults | 0, 1, 2 | 97% (976/1005) | 145 | | |
| 12 months | + booster at | 99.6% (487/489) | 12956 | 100% (18/18) | 642 |
| | 0, 1, 6 | 99% (833/838) | 981 | 100% (60/60) | 279 |
| Homosexual males | 0, 1, 6 | 96% (175/182) | 732 | | |
| Institutionalized mentally retarded patients | 0, 1, 6 | 97% (215/222) | 1048 | | |

[a] Twenty-microgram
[b] Geometric mean titre (mIU/ml) of anti-HBs in seroconverters

**Table 2.** Protective efficacy of yeast-derived hepatitis B vaccine (Engerix B) in two high-risk groups

| Group | Average annual incidence of hepatitis B | | |
|---|---|---|---|
| | Before immunization[a] | During immunization (0–6 months) | After immunization (6–12 months) |
| Homosexual males | 12% | 2.7% ($n$=223) | 0% ($n$=172) |
| Institutionalized patients | 8.7% | 5.2% ($n$=266) | 0% ($n$=244) |

[a] Immunization consisted of 3 doses of vaccine at 0, 1, and 6 months

genic as nearly all subjects had titres of anti-HBs greater than the accepted protective level of 10 mIU/ml 1 month after completion of the three-dose vaccination schedule. The vaccine was well tolerated; mild soreness at the site of injection was the most common complaint. The protective efficacy of YDV is demonstrated in Table 2. In groups at risk, such as homosexuals and institutionalized mentally retarded patients, the annual incidence of hepatitis B infection decreased during the period of vaccination. No clinical cases of hepatitis B were reported. In the 6 months following vaccination the incidence of hepatitis B infection dropped to 0% in a group of male homosexuals with a historical annual attack rate of 12%. A significant decrease in incidence was also obtained among institutionalized mentally retarded patients. We have also shown that vaccination with YDV can decrease the vertical transmission of HBV in neonates born of $HBeAg^+$ mothers. Without vaccination, 70%–90% of these children become infected and almost all become chronic carriers [10]. In a study comprising 137 children vaccinated before the age of 6 months with the first vaccine dose being given at birth, only 6.5% became HBs antigen positive during the vaccination period, denoting carrier status. No infant has, as yet, become infected after the full course of YDV as all have developed protective antibody levels.

The recommended vaccination schedule of YDV is three injections of 20 µg at 0, 1 and 6 months. As shown in Table 1, this is sufficient to produce high titres of antibodies. A more rapid schedule of injections at 0, 1 and 2 months can also be used, giving lower titres of antibodies. The rapid schedule should therefore be followed by a booster at 12 months. Measurement of antibody titres 3 years after the beginning of the vaccination course shows that all vaccinated individuals have titres above the recommended protective level of 10 mIU/ml (Table 1). Indeed, over 80% of all vaccinees have titres >100 mIU/ml, regardless of the vaccination schedule followed.

Vaccination with YDV is therefore safe, is highly immunogenic and has a marked protective effect. Long-term follow-up studies show that efficacious titres can be maintained for at least 3 years after vaccination. The availability of YDVs should facilitate the routine immunization of travellers against HBV infection.

## References


1. Anonymous (1988) Viral hepatitis. Weekly Epidemiol Rec 63:89–91
2. Sobeslavsky O (1980) Prevalence of markers of hepatitis B virus infection in various countries: a WHO collaborative study. Bull WHO 58:621–628
3. Lingao AL, Domingo EO, West S, Reyes CM, Gasmen S, Viterbo G, Tiu E, Lansang MA (1986) Seroepidemiology of hepatitis B virus in the Philippines. Am J Epidemiol 123:473–480
4. Lok AS-F, Lai C-L, Wu P-C, Wong VC-W, Yeoh E-K, Lin H-J (1987) Hepatitis B virus infection in Chinese families in Hong Kong. Am J Epidemiol 126:492–499
5. Gesemann M, Amazigo U, Marcus I, Dupasquier I, Staugard F, Scheiermann N (1987) Prevalence of hepatitis B virus markers and Delta antibodies in Nigeria and Botswana. Trop Med Parasitol 38:268–269
6. Sansonno DE, Manghisi OG (1987) Auto-antibody to human albumin after vaccination for hepatitis B infection. Ital J Gastroenterol 19:182–183
7. Wiedermann G, Scheiner O, Ambrosch F, Kraft B, Kollaritsch H, Kremsner P, Hauser P et al. (1988) Lack of induction of IgE and IgG antibodies to yeast in humans immunized with recombinant hepatitis B vaccines. Int Arch Allergy Appl Immunol 85:130–132
8. Schellekens H, de Reus A, Peetermans JH, van Eerd PACM (1987) The protection of chimpanzees against hepatitis B viral infection using a recombinant yeast-derived hepatitis B surface antigen. Postgrad Med J 63 [Suppl 2]:93–96
9. André FE, Safary A (1987) Summary of clinical findings on Engerix-B, a genetically engineered yeast-derived hepatitis B vaccine. Postgrad Med J 63[Suppl 2]:169–178
10. Stevens CE; Toy PT, Tong MJ, Taylor PE, Vyas GN, Nair PV, Gudavalli M, Krugman S (1985) Perinatal hepatitis B virus transmission in the United States: prevention by passive-active immunization. JAMA 253:1740–1745

# Safety and Efficacy Aspects of Hepatitis B Vaccination in HIV-Infected Individuals

M. Gesemann, N. Brockmeyer, N. Scheiermann, E. Kreuzfelder, A. Safary, and F. André

Hepatitis B virus infection is a highly prevalent disease in tropical countries; therefore active vaccination has been advised to travelers to these regions. Since human immune deficiency virus (HIV)-infected individuals visit our AIDS counseling hours not only for diagnostic and therapeutic reasons, but also in preparation for long-distance travel, we have developed a limited program to investigate the effects and side effects of hepatitis B vaccination in a small group of infected persons.

The study group consisted of 10 anti-HIV positive and anti-HBc negative persons, 13 anti-HIV and anti-HBc positive persons, and, finally, for control purposes, 19 anti-HIV and anti-HBc negative persons, mostly homosexuals. Hepatitis B recombinant vaccine (Smith Kline-RIT) [4] was administered in 20-μg doses at months 0, 1, and 6 and anti-HBs serum concentrations were measured at months 0, 1, 2, 6, and 7. Once during the study (control group) or at different times before, during and after the study (HIV-infected persons) T-lymphocyte counts and subsets, immunoglobulin and beta-2-microglobulin levels were determined.

Seroconversion rates in HIV-infected persons are shown in Fig. 1. Only four out of ten vaccinees showed anti-HBs antibodies after the complete

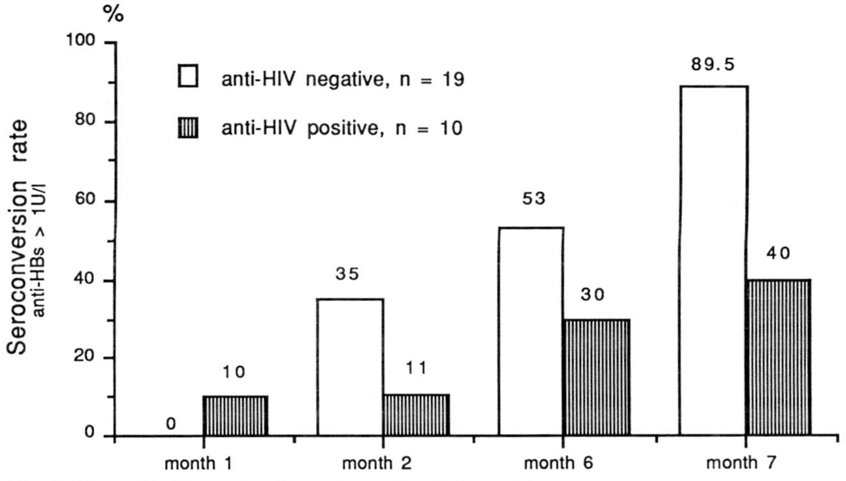


**Fig. 1.** Hepatitis B vaccination at months 0, 1, and 6

**Table 1.** Lymphocyte counts in 23 HIV-infected persons before, during and after hepatitis B vaccination at months 0, 1, and 6

| Lymphocytes | Before | During | After |
|---|---|---|---|
| | vaccination (median) | | |
| Total/µl | 1380 | 1508 | 1800 |
| T3 (%) | 56 | 55 | 59 |
| T4 (%) | 26 | 25 | 27 |
| T8 (%) | 23 | 25 | 23 |
| NK (%) | 10 | 11 | 11 |

course of three vaccinations (40%), whereas in noninfected subjects the seroconversion rate reached 89.5% (17 of 19). The observed difference was significant ($P<0.01$). Anti-HBs measured in geometric mean titer was again significantly lower in HIV-infected persons than in anti-HIV seronegatives after completion of the study (90 U/liter versus 348 U/liter, $P<0.005$). HIV-infected persons with preexisting anti-HBs antibodies showed only a weak antibody booster reaction after three doses of vaccine. The geometric mean titer increased from a level of 161 U/liter to 356 U/liter (factor 2.2). In HIV-infected persons a slight increase in absolute lymphocyte counts during the observation period was noted, but here, as well as for T3, T4, T8 and natural killer lymphocyte subsets, no significant changes occurred ($P>0.05$, Table 1). Furthermore, IgG and beta-2-microglobulin levels were elevated in anti-HIV positive individuals and were considerably higher than in the control group ($P<0.001$). A trend toward an increase of IgG and beta-2-microglobulin values in HIV-infected persons during the observation period was not significant. Clinically, the natural course of infection was not influenced by the administration of three doses of recombinant vaccine.

Hepatitis B vaccination – a vaccination with inactivated, antigenic material – does not seem to represent an immunological hazard for immunocompromised persons such as HIV-infected individuals or dialysis patients. Several vaccinations are officially recommended for HIV-infected children in the United States by Centers for Disease Control [1]. Even yellow fever vaccine – a vaccine containing the highly attenuated 17D strain – poses only low risk to anti-HIV positive persons, as has been recently observed [2]. This statement does not hold true for live vaccine immunization against smallpox [3]. Hepatitis B vaccination with recombinant antigen should be considered early in the possibly long and undulating course of HIV infection, since responsiveness to vaccines is expected to decline with time.

## References

1. Advisory Committee for Immunization Practices (1986) Immunization of children infected with human T-lymphoctropic virus type III/lymphadenopathy-associated virus. MMWR 35:595–606
2. Gürtler L (1987) Anti-HIV-Test vor Impfung gegen Tropenkrankheiten? Dtsch Med Wochenschr 112:1677
3. Redfield RR, Wright DC, James WD, Jones TS, Brown C, Burke DS (1987) Disseminated vaccinia in a military recruit with human immunodeficiency virus (HIV) disease. N Engl J Med 316:673–676
4. Wiedermann G, Scheiermann N, Goubau P, Ambrosch F, Gesemann M, de Bel C, Kremsner P et al. (1987) Multicentre dose range study of a yeast-derived hepatitis B vaccine. Vaccine 5:179–183

# Protection by a Recombinant DNA Vaccine Against Hepatitis B, Preliminary Report

C. Goilav, H. Prinsen, A. Safary, F. E. André, and P. Piot

Between April 1985 and March 1986, 314 gay men, aged 18–64 years, all negative for hepatitis B (HBV) infection, were enrolled into a clinical study to evaluate the immune response and to estimate the protection given by a recombinant DNA vaccine against HBV (Engerix-B, SmithKline Biologicals, Rixensart, Belgium) in a high-risk group. At this time, the vaccine schedule was three doses at months 0, 1 and 6 intramuscularly (deltoid region). Boosters were given if the serum level of anti-HBs was below 100 IU/liter in the follow-up period. Control samples were taken at months −1, 1, 3, 6, 7, 12 and 24. Symptom sheets were collected after each injection. Two doses of vaccine were tested (20 or 40 µg). In the groups available for analysis the seroconversion rate for anti-HBs at month 7 was 98% in both dose ranges and the geometric mean titers (GMTs) of anti-HBs were 1027 ($n=131$) and 2363 IU/liter ($n=66$) respectively. The seroconversion rates and persistence are shown in Table I. Some candidates had a spontaneous rise of their anti-HBs levels (with more

**Table 1.** Seroconversion rates and persistence of anti-HBs levels in homosexual males vaccinated with Engerix-B (vaccine dose 20 µg)

| | Seroconversion rate (%) | Seroconverters with anti-HBs >10 IU/liter (%) | Seroconverters with anti-HBs >100 IU/liter (%) |
|---|---|---|---|
| Month 7 | 142/144 (98.6) | 138/142 (97.2) | 124/142 (87.3) |
| Month 12 | 123/124 (99.2) | 115/123 (93.5) | 88/123 (71.5) |
| Month 24 | 57/57 (100) | 54/57 (94.7) | 9/57 (15.8) |

**Table 2.** Side effects

| Dose | Number of injections | Number of subjects without symptoms | Number of subjects with local and/or general symptoms | Most frequent side effects | | |
|---|---|---|---|---|---|---|
| | | | | General | Local | |
| | | | | Fatigue (%) | Soreness (%) | Induration (%) |
| 20 µg | 466 | 307 | 159 | 12 | 21 | 11 |
| 40 µg | 206 | 142 | 64 | 9 | 20 | 12 |

than two fold increase), suggesting late response to the vaccine or natural contact with the virus.

None of the candidates developed serum markers, suggesting HBV infection after completed vaccination, compared with a 32% prevalence of hepatitis B markers at the initial screening and a 12% incidence of HBV in 1982–1984.

The side effects are shown in Table 2. The study suggests that the schedule of vaccination at months 0, 1, 2 and 12 might be superior to that at months 0, 1 and 6.

Our data suggest that this recombinant DNA vaccine (Engerix-B) induced a good anti-HBs antibody response and that the vaccine induced high protection against infection with the hepatitis B virus.

# Efficacy and Tolerance of Intradermal Versus Intramuscular Hepatitis B Immunization: A Randomized Study

R. Darioli, P. Bovet, P.-A. Raeber, D. Lavanchy, and Ph. Frei

The intradermal route has been successfully used for immunization against several infectious diseases [1–3]. Preliminary trials with small numbers of healthy individuals show that reduced doses of hepatitis B vaccine administered intradermally (i.d.) produce a similar seroconversion rate (83%–100%) to that given by intramuscular (i.m.) injection of 20 μg HBs Ag in seronegative subjects [4–7]. Nevertheless, low doses of i.d. vaccine seem to result in lower anti-HBs levels [5, 8] and several objections are raised concerning the use of the i.d. route for HBV vaccination [9, 10]. The aim of this study was to compare the efficacy and tolerance of the standard dose of 20 μg H-B-VAX inoculated either i.d. or i.m. in healthy subjects.

## Patients and Methods

Seventy-six healthy subjects, 72 males and 4 females aged from 21 to 51 years (mean 32 years), were recruited from employees of the governmental police to participate in the study. Contraindications for participation in the study included known history of viral hepatitis, pregnancy or prior history of hepatitis B vaccination. After obtaining oral informed consent, subjects were randomized and consecutively divided into two groups to receive 20 μg H-B-VAX (Merck, Sharp & Dohme) either i.d. ($n=38$) or i.m. ($n=38$) on days 0, 30 and 180. Intradermal injections were divided into four parts ($4 \times 0.25$ ml) and inoculated with tuberculin syringes in four sites in the area of the omoplates. A visible cutaneous bleb was considered as evidence of i.d. inoculation. Intramuscular injections (1 ml) were administered in the deltoid region. After each inoculation, the participants were asked for adverse experiences. Serum samples were collected 1 month after each scheduled injection for determination of anti-HBs levels by enzyme immunoassay test (Ausab, Abbot). Seroconversion was defined as anti-HBs levels $>1$ mIU/ml. Standard chi-square and logarithm-based Student's $t$-test were used to compare seroconversion rates and geometric mean titres (GMTs).

## Results

We found no significant difference in the seroconversion rate when HBs Ag vaccine was administered i.d. or i.m. (Fig. 1). One month after complete immunization, three participants (8%) in the i.d. group versus five (13%) in the i.m.

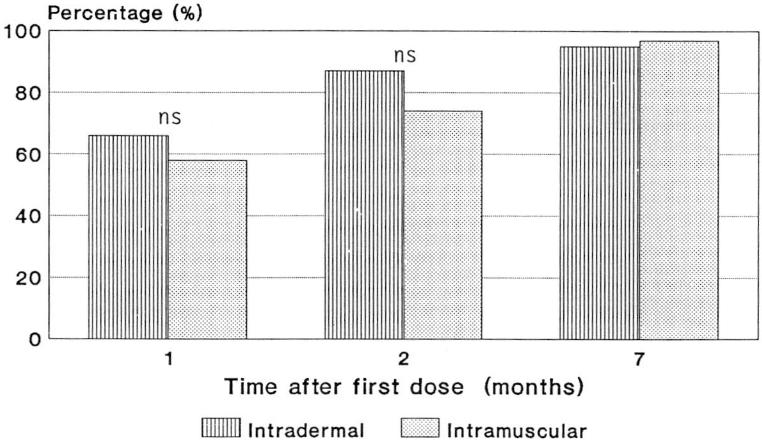


**Fig. 1.** Seroconversion after hepatitis B vaccination

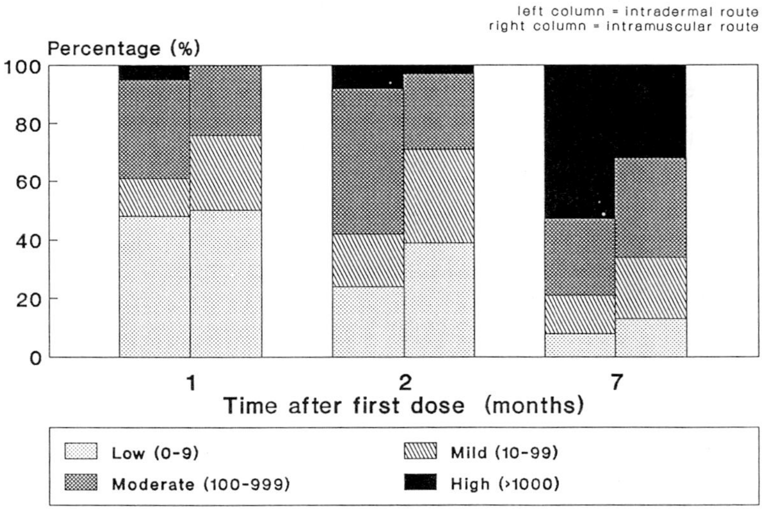


**Fig. 2.** Anti-HBs response after hepatitis B vaccination

group did not obtain protective anti-HBs levels (>10 mIU/ml). The percentage of individuals with anti-HBs > 1000 mIU/ml was higher in the i.d. group (53%) than in the i.m. group (32%; $P<0.06$) (Fig. 2). Intradermal inoculations produce a better ($P<0.03$) immune response when expressed as geometric mean titres (Fig. 3). Adverse reactions are indicated in Table 1. No patients complained of serious side effects.

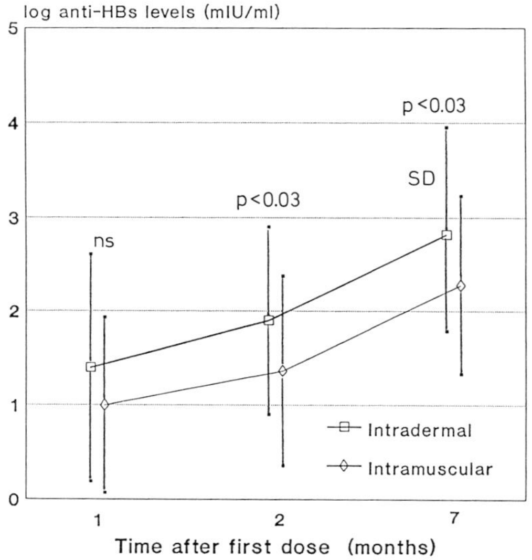


**Fig. 3.** Anti-HBs levels after hepatitis B vaccination

**Table 1.** Adverse reactions

| Types of reaction | First vaccination | | Second vaccination | | Third vaccination | |
|---|---|---|---|---|---|---|
| | Intra-dermal | Intra-muscular | Intra-dermal | Intra-muscular | Intra-dermal | Intra-muscular |
| *Local* | | | | | | |
| Pruritus | 2 | – | 5 | 2 | 2 | 4 |
| Pain | 1 | 3 | – | 2 | – | 2 |
| Subcutaneous nodule | 1 | – | – | – | – | – |
| *Systemic* | | | | | | |
| Fever | – | – | – | – | – | 1 |
| Asthenia | 4 | 1 | 2 | – | – | – |
| Headache | – | – | 1 | – | – | – |
| Nausea | 1 | – | – | – | – | – |

Each number represents the number of patients

## Discussion

Immune response to a vaccine depends on factors such as the antigen dose, the inoculation site and the number and timing of vaccine doses. Intramuscular inoculation of three doses of 20 µg HBs Ag is the recommended dosage and schedule of administration both by the vaccine manufacturer and by the practices advisory committee [11]. However, several studies demonstrated that reduced doses of hepatitis B vaccine administered i.d. over a 4- to 6-month period resulted in higher rates of seroconversion, but lower peak antibody responses were reported than with the standard regimen [4, 5, 12, 13]. There are several objections [10] to the use of the intradermal route for hepatitis B vaccine, including a lack of data on the long-term duration of anti-HBs antibodies, slower seroconversion and frequent adverse reactions after intradermal vaccination. In opposition to Zoulek et al. [6], our study shows that multisite i.d. vaccination with three standard doses (20 µg HBsAg) of hepatitis B vaccine results in rapid and higher immune response than the i.m. route. No serious side effects were observed. Local reactions at site of injection, such as pruritus, were more frequent in the i.d. group but pain was more frequent in the i.m. group. Serum samples will be tested 12 months after complete immunization to confirm the higher efficacy of i.d. hepatitis B vaccination.

In conclusion, intradermal administration of 20 µg H-B-VAX induces significantly higher anti-HBs levels than intramuscular administration. These results suggest that the i.d. vaccine might protect for a longer period. This route of administration is tolerated as well as the intramuscular route.

## References


1. Nicholson KG, Prestage H, Cole PJ, Turner GS, Bauer SP (1981) Multisite intradermal antirabies vaccination. Lancet II:915–917
2. Iwarson S, Larsson P (1980) Intradermal versus subcutaneous immunization with typhoid vaccine. J Hyg 84:11–16
3. Clasener HAL, Bennders BJW (1967) Immunization of man with typhoid and cholera vaccine. Agglutination antibodies after intracutaneous and subcutaneous injection. J Hyg 65:449
4. Miller KD, Gibbs RD, Mulligan MM, Nutmann TB, Francis DP (1983) Intradermal hepatitis B virus vaccine: immunogenicity and side effects in adults. Lancet II:1454–1456
5. Redfield RR, Innis BL, Scott ERM, Cannon HG, Bancroft WH (1985) Clinical evaluation of low-dose intradermally administered hepatitis B virus vaccine. A cost reduction strategy. JAMA 254:3203–3206
6. Zoulek G, Lorbeer B, Jilg W, Deinhardt F (1984) Evaluation of reduced dose of hepatitis B vaccine administered intradermally. J Med Virol 14:27–32
7. Irving WL, Alder M, Kurtz JB, Juel-Jensen B (1986) Intradermal vaccination against hepatitis B. Lancet II:1340
8. Zoulek G, Lorbeer B, Jilg W, Deinhardt F (1984) Persistence of anti-HBs after intradermal inoculation of reduced doses of hepatitis B vaccine. Lancet II:983–984
9. Dienstag JL (1986) Low-dose intradermal hepatitis B vaccine. JAMA 256:351
10. Zuckermann AJ (1987) Appraisal of intradermal immunization against hepatitis B. Lancet I:435
11. Update on hepatitis B prevention (1987). MMWR 36:353–360
12. Gaudeau A, Dubois F, Louq MC, Mozert MC (1984) Immunogenicity of a low-dose (1.25 and 0.31 µg) hepatitis B vaccine. Lancet II:1091–1092
13. Halsey NA, Reppert EJ, Margolis HS, Francis DP, Fields HA (1986) Intradermal hepatitis B vaccination in abbreviated schedule. Vaccine 4:228–232

# Round Table Discussion

# Uniform Recommendations for Vaccinations for Travelers – Utopia?

M. Böttiger (Chairwoman) and R. Steffen (Rapporteur)

*Yellow Fever*. Dr. Vessereau stressed that this vaccination should be the only one required by International Health Regulations. The need for yellow fever vaccination is generally not contested. There are two main reasons for recommending this vaccine: to avoid difficulties with authorities when entering a country which requires proof of vaccination and to avoid the disease. Regardless of international vaccination requirements, travelers should be vaccinated for their own benefit when traveling to an area actively infected with the disease, and additionally when visiting rural regions located in countries within the yellow fever endemic zone. The vaccine is effective and safe.

*Cholera*. Dr. Turner stated that a few countries still required mandatory vaccination, however unnecessary or useless it may be. According to the late world authority Dr. Donald Mackay, a full-dose vaccination, granting 60% protection over 3 months, is only warranted for certain people working in infected areas. Cholera vaccination is generally not recommended for many reasons. It would give limited protection of only one of the many enteric infections, and would additionally provide a false sense of security. Good personal hygiene is a much more effective preventive measure. It does not prevent a person from becoming an asymptomatic carrier. Repeated vaccination cannot be recommended as it may induce a state of serological unresponsiveness or a hypersensitivity reaction. The latter can be avoided with the small intradermal dose. Routine vaccination is unwarranted and WHO has endorsed this. In the new International Vaccination Certificate the page for cholera vaccination has disappeared; cholera vaccination can in future only be declared on the page of other vaccinations. In individual cases with a high risk of exposure, the physician and traveler may nevertheless decide to give a cholera vaccination.

At present (July 1988, source TIM) the following countries still request proof of cholera vaccination: Guinea, Somalia; additionally some embassies (Congo, Mali) apparently request it for issuing a visa and a few countries request proof of vaccination after transiting endemic areas.

*Japanese B Encephalitis*. Dr. Schultz pointed out four issues to be considered. The efficacy of the vaccine used in the United States of America seems to be inferior to the one used in Japan, but this can be overcome by giving three doses instead of two. Side effects were observed in 1%–10%, which shows that tight criteria for this vaccine must be applied. Travelers spending 2 weeks in Beijing in winter certainly need not be immunized; on the other hand travelers staying in rural endemic areas are often unaware of the risk and should be recommended for vaccination. Surveillance is unsatisfactory in many countries and leads to uncertainties with respect to the indication of the vaccination. The vaccine is difficult to obtain in many countries.

*Rabies.* Professor Böttiger observed that only a few countries are free of rabies, e.g. the United Kingdom, Australia, Sweden and Norway. Possibly foxes coming from the Soviet Union have recently imported the disease into Finland. Pre- and postexposure prophylaxis has been described in the vaccine session by Dr. Schultz. This vaccine is recommended primarily for persons staying for a prolonged time in developing countries. Although 100% of healthy persons seroconvert after intradermal injection, this mode of administration is controversial, as resulting titers are lower than after intramuscular application. Postexposure prophylaxis is best advised by experienced specialists; each Swedish Embassy has a small stock of vaccine.

*Meningococcal Meningitis.* Professor Wiedermann described the Sahel zone of Africa, Brazil, Argentina, Mongolia, India and Nepal (where six travelers died in 1985 of the infection) as the main endemic regions. Various mono-, bi- or tetravalent vaccines are available. So far no satisfactory immunization is possible against serotype B, which is predominant in Europe. The vaccine gives a fairly good protection over 3–5 years; in children under the age of 4 years the protection is shortened. Apparently persons with an immune defect are at higher risk of infection. The vaccine is recommended to travelers to traditional endemic countries, particularly if they are going to live under crowded conditions.

*Immune Globulin.* According to Dr. Preblud, several issues need to be reassessed. Recent studies have shown that hepatitis A is not only acquired away from the usual tourist areas, but often in tourist resorts. Some European Mediterranean countries seem to bear a higher risk of infection than the United States. As shown in the subsequent discussion, many questions remain. Should future travelers be screened in order to eliminate persons with hepatitis A antibodies? There is some yet unconfirmed indication that immune globulin offers at least some protection against hepatitis non-A, non-B and hepatitis B. For the same reason the old age cutoff for giving immune globulin may be becoming obsolete. The origin of the immune globulin is important; in some countries only products with a standardized content of hepatitis A antibodies are used. The recommended immune globulin dosage of 0.02 ml/kg (2 ml in adults) is protective over 2 months, and the one of 0.06 ml/kg (5 ml in adults) over 4–6 months.

In summary, the nirvana of unanimity with respect to vaccination recommendations has not been reached, but divergences are limited to details.

# Travelers' Diarrhea

# Travelers' Diarrhea – Its Prevention and Treatment *

H. L. DuPont and C. D. Ericsson

## Summary

Diarrhea continues to be an important problem among persons traveling from low-risk regions to developing areas where enteric infection is hyperendemic in the local population. Persons traveling to these areas should be knowledgeable about how to treat the illness should it occur. For mild to moderate illness (less than six unformed stools per 24 h without disabling cramps and pain) bismuth subsalicylate (4.2 g taken over 4–8 h to be repeated a 2nd day) can be used or loperamide 4 mg initially followed by 2 mg after each unformed bowel movement (not to exceed 8–16 mg/day for 48 h). For severe illness (≧six unformed stools/24 h, when cramps or pain are severe or when there is fever or bloody stools), trimethoprim/sulfamethoxazole (TMP/SMX) can be taken in a dose of 160 mg TMP/800 SMX twice daily for 3 days. Although not entirely effective, exercising care in where and what one eats and drinks is the most practical means of reducing the frequency of illness. Certain preventive medicines are available and effective when taken daily (TMP/SMX and doxycycline). A Consensus Development panel in the United States advised against taking these drugs in this way unless special health problems exist. Recently, the solid form of bismuth subsalicylate was found to be 65% effective in preventing travelers' diarrhea when taken in a dose of 2.1 g/day as two tablets four times a day (with meals and at bedtime). Research is currently being undertaken to develop passive and active immunizing agents against the major cause of illness, enterotoxigenic *Escherichia coli*.

Among persons from highly industrialized areas of northwestern Europe and the United States, acute diarrhea represents the most common medical complaint during travels to developing countries of Africa, Latin America, and southern Asia [21]. The rate of illness varies depending upon regions visited, with an overall frequency of about 40%. The diarrhea rate apparently has not changed over the last 30 years. We began a series of investigations in 1975 designed to determine the cause, epidemiology, therapy and prevention of travelers' diarrhea in United States student populations during short-term stays in Mexico. This report will highlight some of these studies.

* The Studies reported herein were supported by the National Institutes of Health (NIAID) (N01-AI 72534 and R01-AI 23049), by the Environmental Protection Agency (Cr-809331) and by various pharmaceutical sponsors (Norwich Eaton Pharmaceuticals, Burroughs Wellcome Company, Procter and Gamble Co., Miles Pharmaceuticals, Inc.) Ms. Dot Cowan was responsible for word processing.

## Etiology and Source

In studies of acute diarrhea that we have conducted among United States students in Mexico [10], an etiologic agent has been detected in most cases (Table 1). As with studies of such travelers to other Third World settings enterotoxigenic *E. coli* was the most commonly implicated etiologic agent, occurring in approximately 40% of cases [10]. Bacterial agents were found to be responsible for nearly 80% of cases, which explained the remarkable effect of antimicrobial agents when used as therapy or prevention of this form of illness.

Recently we have provided evidence that in 10%–15% of newly arrived United States students with diarrhea a nonenterotoxigenic HEp-2 cell adherent *E. coli* strain could be recovered [18]. Two of these strains of so called enteroadherent *E. coli* have been shown to be pathogenic for humans following volunteer feeding experiments [19], confirming their disease-producing potential. Rotavirus was probably responsible for diarrhea in this population although it was commonly found in students without symptoms [23], casting some doubt on their importance. Bacterial enteropathogens were often found in stools of diarrhea patients in whom rotavirus infection was documented.

In our studies in Mexico, the risk of acquiring diarrhea was clearly related to the place where food was consumed. The greatest risk of acquiring diarrhea was for students who consumed a majority of their meals in the homes of Mexican families; the risk was least for those who prepared most of their meals in their own apartment; the risk was intermediate for those who ate in public restaurants [22, 24]: Those who consumed food more commonly from street vendors also showed a high rate of illness. We performed food microbiologic studies and found high numbers of enteric bacteria in food obtained from Mexican restaurants, and local Mexican homes sponsoring United States students [24]. Further study of these sources demonstrated the common presence of enterotoxigenic *E. coli* and other enteric pathogens. The occurrence of rotavirus infection was not found to correlate with food consumption patterns, suggesting that nonfood sources might be responsible [23]. In studies of water quality we found viable rotaviruses commonly present in tap water samples obtained in Mexico, explaining our epidemiologic observations [3].

**Table 1.** Etiologic agents identified in United States students acquiring diarrhea in Mexico

| Etiologic agent | Percentage of cases |
|---|---|
| Enterotoxigenic *E. coli* | 40% |
| Enteroadherent *E. coli* | 10% |
| *Shigella* | 15% |
| *Salmonella* | 7% |
| *Campylobacter jejuni* | 3% |
| *Aeromonas, plesiomonas* | 2% |
| Rotavirus | 8% |
| *Giardia* | 2% |
| Unknown | 13% |

## Therapy of Travelers' Diarrhea

We have carried out a number of studies of the treatment of travelers' diarrhea in the United States student population under our supervision. These studies have largely established the currently accepted standards for therapy of the disease [2]. Bismuth subsalicylate was shown to reduce the symptoms of diarrhea by approximately 50% when taken in recommended dosage [5]. The intestinal motility-active drug loperamide was found to offer even greater relief of diarrhea symptoms [16]. Antibacterial agents showing in vitro activity against enteric bacterial agents [1] were also found to be effective therapy. Trimethoprim/sulfamethoxazole [7] and ciprofloxacin [13] shortened disease from 3–4 days without treatment to 1 day with the antimicrobial. Drugs which work symptomatically (e.g., loperamide) appeared to work more quickly; yet post-treatment relapses of symptoms were found to be common. Antibacterial agents characteristically were found to be slower to act yet they produced complete cures. A combination of the drugs probably offer the advantages of both [12]. We currently recommend a combination of both types of drugs (loperamide plus TMP/SMX) for the therapy of most cases of moderate to severe travelers' diarrhea.

## Chemoprophylaxis

Our first study of antimicrobial chemoprophylaxis revealed that trimethoprim/sulfamethoxazole (TMP/SMX) would prevent nearly all cases of travelers' diarrhea when subjects were at risk for 2 weeks [8]. Norfloxacin, a quinolone derivative, was also found to be effective in a later study [17]. An occasional side effect of TMP/SMX was skin rash [8] while acquisition of antimicrobial resistant intestinal flora invariably occurred [20]. The major problem with norfloxacin was mild central nervous system stimulation (i.e., insomnia). Since side effects of these drugs do occasionally occur (both trivial and rarely life threatening) and travelers' diarrhea generally is felt to be a nonfatal illness, a Consensus Development panel at the US National Institutes of Health recommended that no one traveling in high-risk areas be encouraged to take antimicrobial chemoprophylaxis [2]. In view of the effectiveness of this class of compounds, and the frequency of illness among certain high-risk travelers, the recommendation probably was overly rigid.

An alternate form of chemoprophylaxis is seen with the chemical compound bismuth subsalicylate (BSS) [6, 9]. Earlier we showed that 60 ml commercial bismuth subsalicylate (Pepto-Bismol), when taken in a four times daily regimen (4.2 g BSS/day), would prevent 62% of cases that would occur without such prophylaxis [6]. Because of convenience, we tested the tablet formulation of BSS in a dose of two tablets given four times daily with meals and at bedtime (2.1 g BSS/day) taken for 3 weeks at risk and found that 65% of cases that would result without treatment were prevented [9]. While not quite as effective as the conventional antibacterial agents, side effects were felt to be inconsequential with BSS chemoprophylaxis (black stools and self-limiting tinnitus). The mechanisms of action of BSS, when used in therapy or in preventing travelers' diarrhea, are not completely understood [4]. Available evidence suggests that the antisecretory effects of the salicylate moiety explain at least a part of the drug's therapeutic value [11]. BSS and the bismuth containing intestinal reaction products have antimicrobial effects [15], which may relate to the prophylactic value of this drug.

## References

1. Carlson JR, Thornton SA, DuPont HL, West AH, Mathewson JJ (1983) Comparative in vitro activities of ten antimicrobial agents against bacterial enteropathogens. Antimicrob Agents Chemother 24:509–513
2. Consensus Conference (1985) Travelers' diarrhea. JAMA 253:2700–2704
3. Deetz TR, Smith EM, Goyal SM, Gerba CP, Vollet JJ III, Tsai L, DuPont HL, Keswick BH (1984) Occurrence of rota- and enteroviruses in drinking and environmental water in a developing nation. Water Res 18:567–571
4. DuPont HL (1987) Bismuth subsalicylate in the treatment and prevention of diarrheal disease. Drug Intell Clin Pharm 21:687–693
5. DuPont HL, Sullivan P, Pickering LH, Haynes G, Ackerman PB (1977) Symptomatic treatment of diarrhea with bismuth subsalicylate among students attending a Mexican University. Gastroenterology 73:715–718
6. DuPont HL, Sullivan P, Evans DG, Pickering LK, Evans DJ Jr, Vollett JJ, Ericsson CD, Ackerman PB, Tjoa WS (1980) Prevention of travelers' diarrhea (emporiatric enteritis): prophylactic administration of subsalicylate bismuth. JAMA 243:237–241
7. DuPont HL, Reves RR, Galindo E, Sullivan PS, Wood LV, Mendiola JG (1982) Treatment of travelers' diarrhea with trimethoprim and with trimethoprim alone. N Engl J Med 307:841–844
8. DuPont HL, Galindo E, Evans DG, Cabada FJ, Sullivan P, Evans DJ Jr (1983) Prevention of travelers' diarrhea with trimethoprim/sulfamethoxazole and trimethoprim alone. Gastroenterology 84:75–80
9. DuPont HL, Ericsson CD, Johnson PC, Bitsura JM, DuPont MW, de la Cabada FJ (1984) Prevention of travelers' diarrhea by the tablet formulation of bismuth subsalicylate. JAMA 257:1347–1350
10. DuPont HL, Ericsson CD, DuPont MW (1985) Emporiatric enteritis: lessons learned from U.S. students in Mexico. Am Clin Climatol Assoc 97:32–42
11. Ericsson CD, Evans DG, DuPont HL, Evans DJ Jr, Pickering LK (1977) Bismuth subsalicylate inhibits activity of crude toxins of *Escherichia coli* and *Vibrio cholerae*. J Infect Dis 136:693–696
12. Ericsson CD, Johnson PC, DuPont HL, Morgan DR (1986) Role of a novel antidiarrheal agent, BW942C, alone or in combination with trimethoprim-sulfamethoxazole in the treatment of travelers' diarrhea. Antimicrob Agents Chemother 29:1040–1046
13. Ericsson CD, Johnson PC, DuPont HL, Morgan DR, Bitsura JM (1987) Ciprofloxacin and trimethoprim/sulfamethoxazole as initial therapy for acute travelers' diarrhea. A placebo-controlled randomized trial. Ann Intern Med 106:216–220
14. Gorbach SL, Kean BH, Evans DG, Evans DJ Jr, Bessudo D (1975) Travelers' diarrhea and toxigenic *Escherichia coli*. N Engl J Med 292:933–936
15. Graham DY, Estes MK, Gentry LO (1983) Double-blind comparison of bismuth subsalicylate and placebo in the prevention and treatment of enterotoxigenic *Escherichia coli*-induced diarrhea in volunteers. Gastroenterology 85:1017–1022
16. Johnson PC, Ericsson CD, DuPont HL, Morgan DR, Bitsura JA, Wood LV (1986) Comparison of loperamide with bismuth subsalicylate for the treatment of acute travelers' diarrhea. JAMA 255:757–760

17. Johnson PC, Ericsson CD, Morgan DR, DuPont HL, Cabada FJ (1986) Lack of emergence of resistant fecal flora during successful prophylaxis of traveler's diarrhea with norfloxacin. Antimicrob Agents Chemother 30:671–674
18. Mathewson JJ, Johnson PC, DuPont HL, Morgan DR, Thornton SA, Ericsson CD (1985) A newly recognized cause of travelers' diarrhea: enteroadherent *Escherichia coli*. J Infect Dis 151:471–475
19. Mathewson JJ, Johnson PC, DuPont HL, Satterwhite TK, Winsor DK (1986) Pathogenicity of enteroadherent *Escherichia coli* in adult volunteers. J Infect Dis 154:524–527
20. Murray BE, Rensimer ER, DuPont HL (1982) Emergence of high-level trimethoprim resistance in fecal *Escherichia coli* during oral administration of trimethoprim and trimethoprim-sulfamethoxazole. N Engl J Med 306:130–135
21. Steffen R, Van der Linde F, Gyr K (1983) Epidemiology of diarrhea in travelers. JAMA 249:1176–1180
22. Tjoa WS, DuPont HL, Sullivan P, Pickering LK, Holguin AH, Olarte J, Evans DG, Evans DJ Jr (1977) Location of food consumption and travelers' diarrhea. Am J Epidemiol 106:61–66
23. Vollet JJ, Ericsson CD, Gibson G, Pickering LK, DuPont HL, Kohl S, Conklin RH (1979) Human rotavirus in an adult population with travelers' diarrhea and its relationship to the location of food consumption. J Med Virol 4:81–87
24. Wood LV, Ferguson LE, Hogan P, Thurman D, DuPont HL, Ericsson CD (1983) Incidence of bacterial enteropathogens in foods from Mexico. Appl Environ Microbiol 46:328–332

# Surveillance of Gastrointestinal Upset in Package Holiday Tourists

R. Y. Cartwright and R. Wheal

Reports of travellers' diarrhoea among British holidaymakers are to be found in the popular press every year during the late summer. The incidence for resorts is often quoted with a degree of certainty not substantiated by any epidemiological evidence. Studies by Reid et al. (1978, 1980) and Cossar et al. (1985) among Scottish tourists have provided evidence that the incidence is not insignificant and that among the package tourists questioned the highest rates were associated with visits to North African countries. Steffen et al. (1983) studied tourists returning to Switzerland and Germany and obtained similar results. All these studies were based on a relatively small number of tourists, were over a short time, did not provide information on differences between individual resorts, and were from the tour operator's position inconclusive. The public hazards of tourists returning with enteropathogenic organisms can be appreciated from laboratory reports of the isolation of such organisms. In England and Wales, these reports are collated by the Public Health Laboratory Service Communicable Disease Surveillance Centre. The reports do not provide data which would enable the incidence of travellers' diarrhoea to be calculated. The responsible tour operator maintains contact with its clients while on holiday and will alert health authorities to serious problems. The need for reliable background information on travellers' diarrhoea which can be continually updated was recognized. Thomson Holidays, who have an active client welfare department, included a simple health question in their client satisfaction questionnaire (CSQ) given to all adult clients during the return flight to the United Kingdom. This paper reports some of the findings of this study and discusses their application in the control of travellers' diarrhoea among package tourists.

## Method

Data were collected during the return flight to the United Kingdom from adult clients of Thomson Holidays. Included in a general CSQ were the questions "Were you ill at any time during your holiday?" and "If 'Yes', please specify illness". The questionnaires were distributed and collected by cabin crew. A sample of questionnaires varying from 1 : 1 to 1 : 4 depending on the resort size were codified for computer entry. The code for travellers' diarrhoea included specified illness of diarrhoea, shits, Tunisian trots, Spanish runs and loose bowels. (The client who signified an excessive alcohol consumption was excluded.) Coding and computer entry was undertaken by a commercial market analysis company. A subset of data including holiday region, resort, hotel, type of catering, age, sex, date of holiday, illness and illness type was written on to magnetic tape then read onto a Prime 9955 computer at the University of Surrey. Analysis of the data was according to the cross tabulation facility of SPSSX (Statistical Package for the Social Sciences).

## Results

In the summer seasons (May–October) 1984–1987 the following number of questionnaires were analysed – 1984, 245264; 1985, 223447; 1986, 199559; 1987, 474526.

The travellers in 1987 had visited 404 resorts and 2094 hotels in Cyprus, Gibraltar, Greek mainland and islands, Italian Rivieras, Sardinia, Malta, Morocco, Portugal, Mediterranean Spain, four Balearics, Canaries, Tunisia and Yugoslavia. The incidence of diarrhoea rose during each season, reaching a peak in August and September of between 13% and 15% (Fig. 1). The seasonal variation was similar for each region but differences between regions were apparent (Table 1). The greatest differences were observed during August. The Italian Rivieras were associated with a low incidence (3%–8%) in contrast to Tunisia (33%–41%) and Morocco (34%–48%). For individual regions year to year differences were generally not large. The high level in the Algarve in 1984 compared with successive years was related to an outbreak of gastroenteritis in the resort of Albufeira.

The incidence in resorts was usually similar to that for the appropriate region unless and outbreak occurred. The events in Albufeira in 1984 were apparent from a comparison with the other Portuguese resorts (Table 2). Apart from resorts in Tunisia, Morocco and Costa Blanca the resort incidence was usually less than 20%.

Calculation of individual hotel incidence was undertaken when an increase of travellers' diarrhoea was reported by the tour operators in resort representatives or if an unexpected increase in resort incidence was observed from this

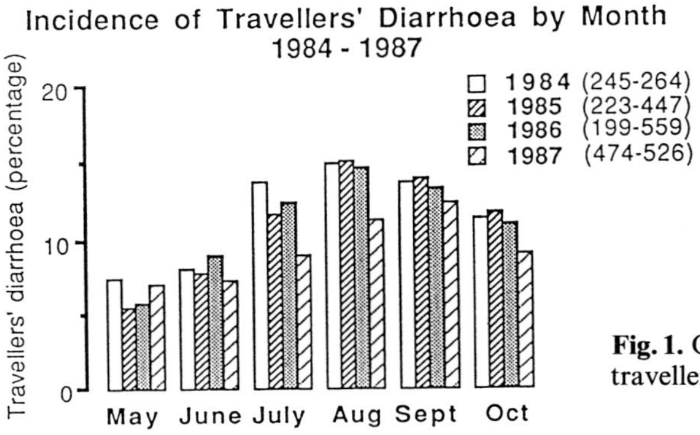


**Fig. 1.** Overall monthly incidence of travellers' diarrhoea, 1984–1987

**Table 1.** Incidence (percentage of visitors) of gastrointestinal symptoms in August by region

| | 1984 | 1985 | 1986 | 1987 |
|---|---|---|---|---|
| Spain | | | | |
| Costa Brava | 20 | 19 | 16 | 13 |
| Costa Blanca | 30 | 30 | 37 | 31 |
| Costa del Sol | 17 | 18 | 18 | 16 |
| Majorca | 10 | 10 | 9 | 7 |
| Ibiza | 16 | 14 | 13 | 11 |
| Minorca | 12 | 11 | 8 | 11 |
| Formentera | 15 | 15 | 30 | 22 |
| Portugal | | | | |
| Algarve | 34 | 17 | 10 | 14 |
| Estoril coast | 15 | 19 | 14 | 12 |
| Madeira | 26 | 21 | 21 | 24 |
| Italy | | | | |
| Adriatic Riviera | 4 | 4 | 4 | 4 |
| Venetian Riviera | 5 | 4 | 3 | 4 |
| Neopolitan Riviera | 8 | 8 | 6 | 5 |
| Sardinia | 9 | 8 | 3 | 7 |
| Greece | | | | |
| Aegian Islands | 7 | 11 | 8 | 10 |
| Greece Mainland | 10 | 6 | 7 | 8 |
| Corfu | 23 | 19 | 12 | 11 |
| Crete | 10 | 12 | 9 | 7 |
| Rhodes | – | 9 | 7 | 7 |
| Malta | 15 | 13 | 31 | 19 |
| Tunisia | 41 | 36 | 33 | 33 |
| Morocco | 45 | 48 | 41 | 34 |
| Yugoslavia | 12 | 12 | 9 | 10 |

**Table 2.** Incidence (percentage of tourists) with travellers' diarrhoea by resort for Portugal in August 1984 and Tenerife in September 1985

| | | | |
|---|---|---|---|
| Portugal | | Tenerife | |
| Albufeira | 53 | Playa de las Americas | 22 |
| Lagos | 12 | Puerto de la Cruz | 18 |
| Carcavelos | 24 | Los Cristianos | 21 |
| Cascais | 12 | Los Gigantes | 39 |
| Estoril | 13 | Puerto de Santiago | 14 |
| Alvor | 21 | | |
| Praid de Rocha | 15 | | |

study. In September 1985, the representatives in Puerto de la Cruz reported increased numbers of clients with diarrhoea. In resort investigation suggested an association with one hotel, which was confirmed by incidence for that hotel being 73% whereas the incidence in other hotels in the resort was between 4% and 21%. The resort incidence was 18%. In Albufeira in 1984, the incidence for all hotels was raised to 30%–80%, suggesting a cause involving all the resort. Investigations revealed faecal contamination of both potable and recreational waters.

## Discussion

The epidemiological data from this study has many imperfections. It only reflects illness among adults, is totally subjective, relates only to illness occurring during the holiday, is retrospective as the results are not available until 6–8 weeks after data collection and only covers those resorts used by one tour operator. The symptoms included under the heading travellers' diarrhoea may also be caused by excessive alcohol intake and dietary indiscretions.

The data are, however, relatively easy to collect, provide a denominator enabling incidence rates to be calculated, are ongoing; and results correlate well with confirmed outbreaks of gastroenteritis. The low incidence in some resorts suggests that factors such as alcohol intake and dietary changes are not in themselves very important in the aetiology of travellers' diarrhoea.

The results have confirmed previous observations (Steffen et al. 1983) that North African resorts are associated with a high incidence of travellers' diarrhoea. The outbreaks in Albufeira and Puerto de la Cruz have not only validated the study but have also demonstrated that the results can be used to monitor remedial actions. The information has been used by United Kingdom health officials, resorts authorities and the tour operator. The observed high incidence in some regions and resorts has resulted in approaches to health authorities in the countries concerned to discuss further investigations, so that action can be taken to safeguard the tourist's health.

The results of this study should be taken as indicators of the incidence of travellers' diarrhoea in a region, resort or hotel. Unexpected findings are an indication for further investigation. This study is not of value for the early recognition of outbreaks which will continue to rely on the vigilance of tour operators' resort representatives or laboratory isolations from returning tourists. It is of value, however, in providing background information, for monitoring general changes in regions and resorts; and by presenting to resort management the tour operator results pertaining to their area, greater awareness ensues and contributes to this vigilance.

## Conclusion

Information on the incidence of travellers' diarrhoea in holiday regions, resorts and hotels has been obtained by the inclusion of a health question in a tour operator's client satisfaction questionnaire. The results correlate well with known outbreaks of gastroenteritis and have been of value to the tourist industry, resort health authorities and the British health authorities in taking action to reduce the health risks to tourists.

## References

1. Cossar JH, Reid D, Grist NR, Dewar RD, Fallon RJ, Riding MH, Bell EJ (1985) Illness associated with travel. Travel Med Int 3:13–18
2. Reid D, Grist NR, Najera R (1978) Illness associated with "package tours": a combined Spanish-Scottish study. Bull WHO 56:117–122
3. Steffen R, van der Linde F, Gyr K, Schär M (1983) Epidemiology of diarrhoea in travellers. JAMA 249:1176–1180

# Problems in the Investigation of Food Poisoning Associated with In-flight Catering

T. M. S. Reid and L. D. Ritchie

## Introduction

Food poisoning outbreaks are increasingly being reported on land (Palmer and Rowe 1986), at sea on cruise liners (Merson et al. 1976; Centres for Disease Control 1986) and on offshore installations (Forbes et al. 1986) and in the air associated with in-flight catering (Beers and Mohler 1985; Steffen et al. 1985; Tauxe et al. 1987). Recently the management of outbreaks of food poisoning and communicable disease has come under increasing scrutiny and health authorities have been encouraged to produce contingency plans clearly outlining the objectives, responsibilities and lines of communication should a public health problem arise (Report 1986). Equally, in the offshore oil industry, guidelines for the investigation and control of food poisoning and communicable disease have been issued to all oil companies (United Kingdom Offshore Operators Association 1987).

We believe that airline outbreaks by their very nature would benefit from such an approach and to this end we describe a recent outbreak of food poisoning associated with in-flight catering and attempt to draw some useful lessons from the problems encountered.

## The Outbreak

On Tuesday 15 May 1984, 88 passengers on a charter flight arrived back in Aberdeen following a 14-day holiday in Tenerife. Ten days later, on Friday 25 May, the Regional Laboratory, City Hospital, Aberdeen, isolated *Salmonella enteritidis* (subsequently typed as phage type 4) from faecal samples sent in by local primary care physicians. The community medicine specialist was informed that day and he immediately made contact with the local airport handling agency for the airline, requesting a complete passenger manifest (including names and addresses). Preliminary enquiries revealed that all of the passengers with positive cultures had stayed at different hotels, had not eaten at the airport prior to departure and had all been taken ill within 48 h of arriving back in Aberdeen. In view of this it was reasonable to assume the most likely source was food consumed on the plane itself. Accordingly, the local handling agents were asked to telex the airline of our suspicions and to ask them to embark on a local investigation at their food preparation station in Tenerife. It became clear that three other flights from the same airline had departed ex Tenerife for the United Kingdom on the same day bound for Glasgow, Cardiff and Belfast. All this information was immediately communicated to the Communicable Diseases (Scotland) Unit in Glasgow in order that the relevant health authorities could be informed of the possibility of further cases.

Of the 88 passengers on the flight, 17 had booked under travel company A, who telexed a list of passengers and addresses on the same day (Friday 25th). In spite of repeated requests, travel company B failed to provide us with the requisite information until some 5 days later, when a list of names only, together with a list of booking agencies was provided. As a result, local environmental health officers from Aberdeen District Council had to be deployed on a "gumshoe" exercise round the relevant travel agencies to ascertain further particulars. Despite this, all 88 passengers were contacted with a letter of explanation, interviewed and asked to submit a stool specimen. Eighty-two submitted stool specimens; the remaining six, who had not had any symptoms, declined to comply. On enquiry, 70% of the passengers admitted to being symptomatic. Thirty patients had positive cultures (27 *Salmonella enteritidis* type 4, 1 *Salmonella heidelberg*, 1 *Salmonella ohio* and 1 *Salmonella typhimurium* type 10).

## Discussion

The potential for food poisoning associated with in-flight catering is well established (Beers and Mohler 1985; Steffen et al. 1985), and is illustrated once again by this outbreak occurring as it did soon after a large outbreak of salmonellosis on transatlantic flights (Tauxe et al. 1987).

With the speed of modern air travel, the incubation period, e.g. for salmonellosis, invariably exceeds the duration of the flight. Consequently, in the event of an outbreak, those at risk are already widely scattered, posing considerable problems in tracing individuals. Equally, such are the pressures of the airline business that the aircraft with its crew complement and remaining in-flight meals have long since departed. Under these circumstances the onus for the prompt recognition of such outbreaks frequently falls on primary care physicians. It is essential that they make specific enquiry for any history of recent travel when first encountering the patient, and, most importantly, that they request that a stool specimen be taken during the acute phase of the illness. Given appropriate samples, the microbiology laboratory, which will often serve a large area or population, may be able to verify the existence of an outbreak by correlating the results of tests performed on apparently unrelated patients from different practices. Where a history of recent travel is not immediately apparent on the request form, preliminary confirmation can be obtained when the positive report is telephoned to the practice. Simultaneously, the consultant microbiologist, by contacting the community medicine specialist (Communicable Disease Control) is able to trigger a public health investigation involving health visitors, environmental health officers and their counterparts in other health regions. Finally, the Communicable Diseases Surveillance Unit is informed and in so doing the knowledge can be rapidly disseminated nationally and internationally as in this case where the additional flights to other destinations in the United Kingdom were immediately put under suspicion. Using this communication network, it was possible, despite the limitations of the passenger data, to trace all the passengers, to have them interviewed by staff experienced in epidemiology and to arrange submission of stool samples to the laboratory.

However, several shortcomings in current airline practice were identified which hampered the investigation, notably the apparent lack of an accurate passenger manifest, the delays in providing such information as was available and the lack of a designated individual with responsibility for such matters within the airlines, to whom questions could be addressed. When confronted with similar deficiencies in the management of an outbreak of food poisoning associated with hospital catering, a committee of enquiry recently urged health authorities to review their current procedures for managing a major outbreak, be it food poisoning or other communicable disease, and to produce a written model contingency plan if not already available which could be activated at short notice (Report 1986). It is arguable that without such a plan most health authorities, and indeed airlines, would be unable to deal effectively and efficiently with future outbreaks of in-flight food poisoning.

We would suggest that the preparation of a model contingency outbreak plan or code of practice for investigating and managing outbreaks associated with in-flight catering should be given a high priority. The code might initially be introduced on a voluntary basis but there would be scope for extending the arrangement to include all major international airlines both scheduled and charter operators. From our experience in investigating this outbreak, we would counsel that any such code of practice should include the following recommendations.

1. Airlines should cooperate with public health personnel and render all reasonable assistance when requested to do so. Regrettably in this outbreak, levels of cooperation were minimal and no feedback was received from the airline or handling agent.
2. Airlines should nominate an individual or department with defined responsibility to represent the airline in matters of outbreak management, who can be contacted by community medicine specialists in the event of public health problems.
3. The full passenger manifest including names and addresses should be retained for at least 1 month after the flight and be readily accessible when required. In the United Kingdom there is currently no requirment for the addresses of passengers to be recorded. Where a booking number is available it will be possible to contact the agency who issued the tickets and ascertain indirectly from invoices or credit card details the passengers' addresses. The inadequacy of passenger information held by airlines has recently been responsible for difficulties and delays in tracing contacts of a case of meningococcal meningitis (Department of Social Services and Community Health Government of Alberta 1987). The experience of the airline

involved is that contact telephone numbers and addresses can only be obtained for 50% of those for whom it holds reservations.

## Conclusion

The investigation and control of an outbreak of food poisoning associated with in-flight catering requires speedy and concerted action by all members of the Communicable Disease "team" working in close association with the airline(s) concerned. Given the shortcomings of existing procedures and the lack of guidelines there would appear to be a strong case for establishing a Code of Practice including a model contingency plan for management of such outbreaks which could be activated at short notice in the event of food poisoning or communicable disease problems.

## References

1. Beers KN, Mohler SR (1985) Food poisoning as an in-flight safety hazard. Aviat Space Environ Med 56:594–597
2. Centres for Disease Control (1986) Gastroenteritis outbreaks on two Caribbean cruise ships. MMWR 35:383–384
3. Department of Social Services and Community Health, Government of Alberta (1987) Meningitis on an aircraft, Alberta, Canada. Epidemiol Notes Rep Communic Dis Control Epidemiol 11:60–62
4. Forbes GI, Sharp JCM, Collier PW, Reilly WJ (1986) Foodborne infections recorded in Scotland associated with the offshore oil industry 1976–1985. Communic Disease Scotland Weekly Rep 20(28):5–7
5. Merson MH, Hughes JM, Lawrence DN, Wells JG, d'Agnese JJ, Yashuk JC (1976) Food and waterborne disease outbreaks on passenger cruise vessels and aircraft. J Milk Food Technol 39:285–288
6. Palmer SR, Rowe B (1986) Trends in salmonella infections. PHLS Microbiol Digest 3(2):2–5
7. Report (1986) of the Committee of Inquiry into an outbreak of food poisoning at Stanley Royd Hospital. HMSO, London
8. Steffen R, Somaini B, Gubser A (1985) Incidents of epidemiological significance at intercontinental airports. Travel Med Int 3:9–12
9. Tauxe RV, Tormey MP, Mascola L, Hargrett-Bean NT, Blake PA (1987) Salmonellosis outbreak on transatlantic flights; foodborne illness on aircraft: 1947–1984. Am J Epidemiol 125:150–157
10. United Kingdom Offshore Operators Association (1987) Environmental health guidelines for offshore installations-UK continental shelf. UKOOA

# Microorganisms in Faeces of Patients with Diarrhoea

A. Kansouzidou, V. Kiosses, M. Labropoulou, B. Gatzoflia, A. Sofianidou, and B. D. Danielides

Northern Greece is a developing tourist area. It has a permanent population of three million, with more than two million tourists coming from all over the world every year. Diarrhoea as a clinical entity has been recorded since the beginnings of our civilization. It affects mainly children and is found in both developing and developed countries [1].

The clinical symptoms of diarrhoea seldom point to an aetiological agent. Therefore an attempt to isolate the enteropathogenic agent is advisable. In this study 642 patients (529 children and 113 adults) suffering from acute diarrhoea syndrome were examined. They all were inpatients of the Infectious Diseases Hospital, Thessaloniki, during 1986. One or more samples of each patient's faeces were examined. However, in this paper only the first isolation of enteropathogenic agent is mentioned. In every sample, the "older" enteropathogenic agents (*Salmonellae* spp. and *Shigellae* spp.) were looked for, as well as the more recently recognized ones, i.e. *Campylobacter, Yersinia* spp., *Aeromonas* spp. and *Cryptosporidium*. In children less than 2 years old, an additional search for rotavirus antigens was made. The methodology of this study followed a protocol based on a previous paper of our laboratory [2].

From the distribution of the patients with diarrhoea according to their age, was found that the newborn babies and infants under 1 year of age exceeded 40% of the total.

In 324 out of 642 patients with diarrhoea (50.5%) one or more enteropathogenic agents were found; the percentages were 51.2% for the 529 children and 46.9% for the 113 adults . In 25 patients, more than one enteropathogenic agent was isolated, mainly rotavirus, with some other agent.

The distribution of the various enteropathogenic agents in the various age groups can be seen in Fig. 1, and their monthly distribution is shown in Fig. 2. The commonest serotypes of the isolated *Salmonellae* were *S. enteritidis, S. typhimurium* and *S. goldcoast*. *Shigella* strains were *S. sonnei* (24 strains) and *S. flexneri* (10 strains). *Campylobacter* strains were *C. jejuni*. Among them 87% were of biotype 1 and 13% of biotype 2 of Skirrow and Benjamin. The majority of *Yersinia enterocolitica* strains were of the type 4/03/VIII. All isolated *Aeromonas* were *A. hydrophila*. *Cryptosporidium* cysts were found in 11 children and 2 adults, all of them without having any immunological disturbances or taking any immunosuppressive medication. Rotavirus was found in 45% of children examined.

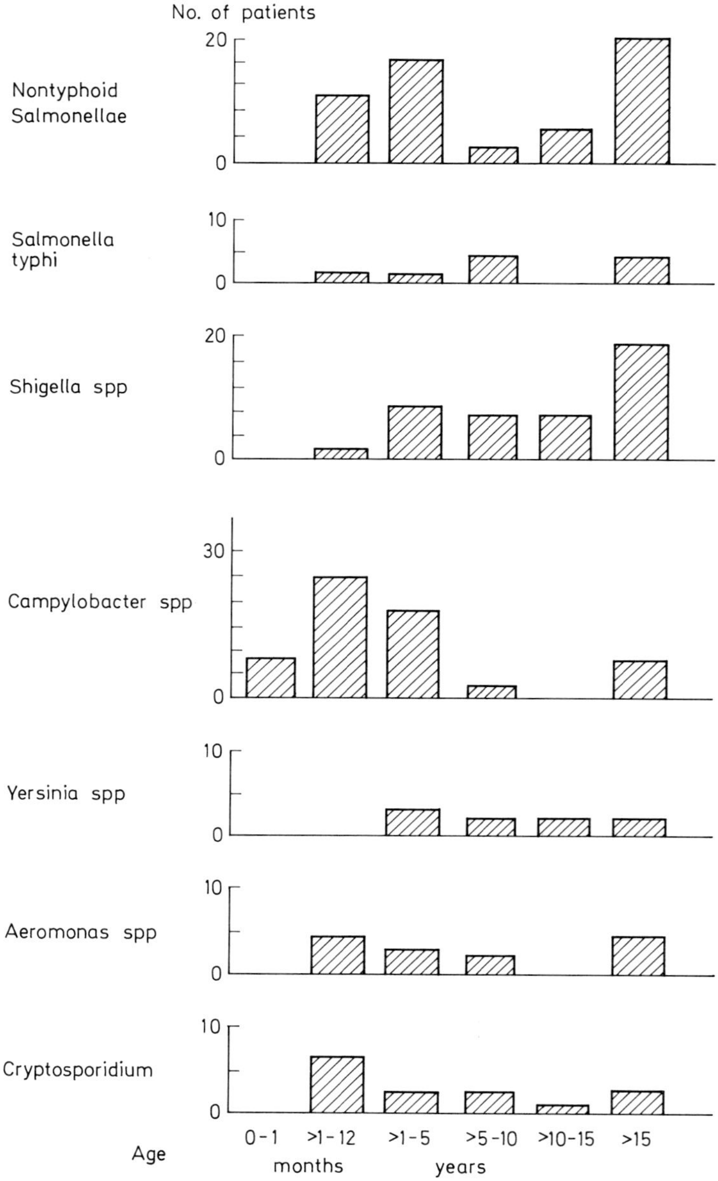


**Fig. 1.** Distribution of enteropathogenic agents apart from rotavirus in various ages

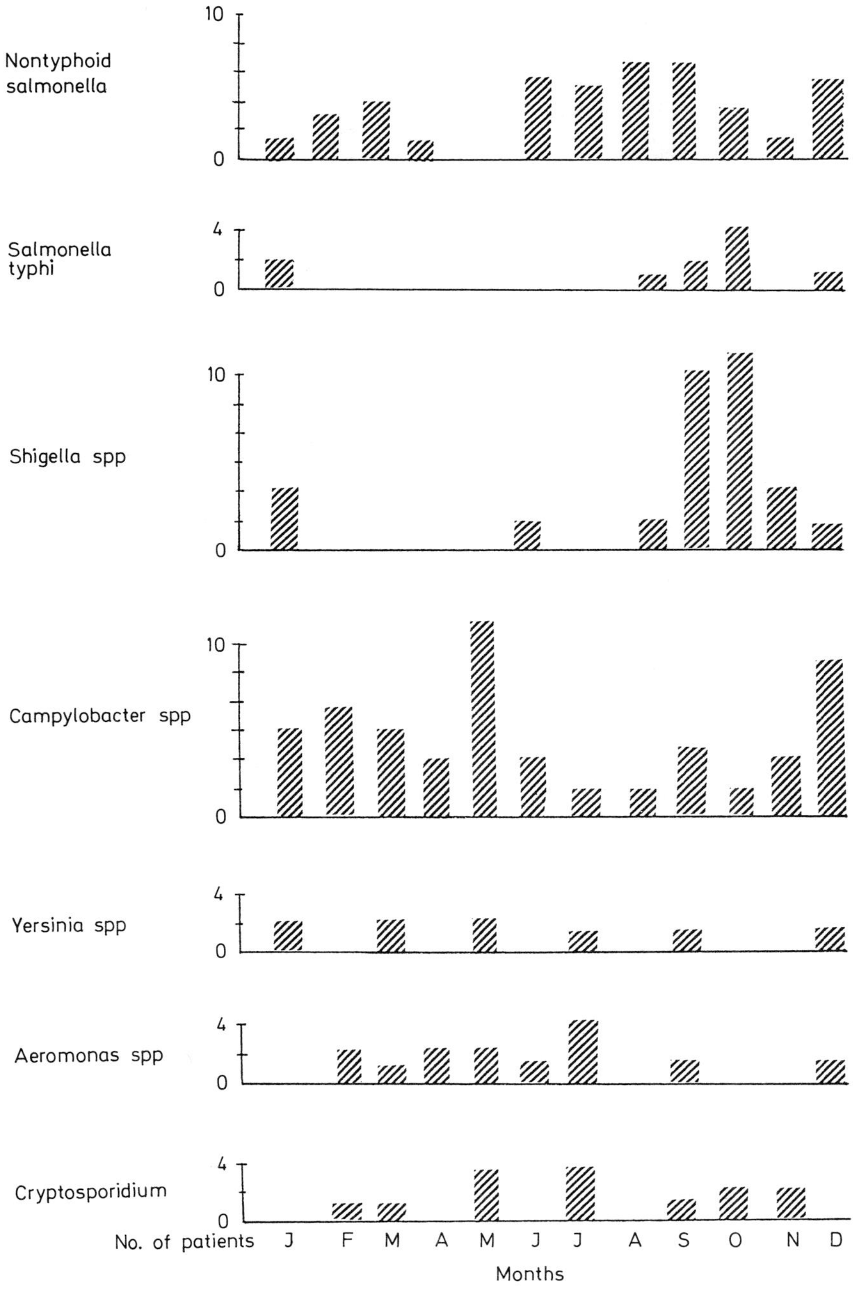


**Fig. 2.** Monthly distribution of various enteropathogenic agents

A great increase of *Campylobacters* as a cause of acute diarrhoea, mainly in children, is observed. The presence of the other "new" enteropathogenic agents (*Yersinia* spp., *Aeromonas* spp. and *Cryptosporium*), especially in children, is low; however it is necessary to search for them.

Furthermore there has been a change in the serotypes of *Salmonellae* isolated, that, instead of the classical *S. typhimurium, S. enteritidis* predominated. A change in the species of *Shigella* has also been observed; thus *S. flexneri*, which prevailed previously, is now replaced by *S. sonnei*.

The results of this study are similar to the results found in other countries [3–5], as well as in previous studies from Greece [6, 7].

The incidence of enteric infection in the population and tourists of the area studied illustrate the low risk of traveller's diarrhoea in northern Greece.

## References

1. Guerrant RL, Shields DS, Thorson SM (1985) Evaluation and diagnosis of acute infectious diarrhoea. Am J Med 78:91–98
2. Kansouzidou-Kanakoudi A, Danielides BD (1986) Diagnosis and investigation of gastroenteritis. Microbiolog Chron 2:3–19
3. Velasco AC, Mateos ML, Mas G, Pedraza A, Diez M, Guttierrez A (1984) Three-year prospective study of intestinal pathogens in Madrid, Spain. J Clin Microbiol 20:290–292
4. Feldam RA, Riley LW (1985) Epidemiology of *Salmonella* and *Shigella* infections in the United States. In: Takeda Y, Miwatani T (eds) Bacterial diarrheal diseases. Nijhoff, Bonston, pp 103–116
5. Uhnoo I, Wadell G, Svensson L, Olding-Stenkvist E, Ekwall E, Molby R (1986) Aetiology and epidemiology of acute gastro-enteritis in Swedish children. J Infect 13:73–89
6. Arseni A, Malamou-Ladas H, Koustia-Karousou C, Charisiadou A (1986) Isolation rate of old and new enteropathogens from stool specimens of children with diarrhoea. Iatriki 50:361–364
7. Trikka E, Foundouli K, Arseni A (1986) Enteropathogenic bacteria in the faeces of diarrhoeic children during 1983–1984. Acta Microbiol Hell 31:56–65

# Etiology of Diarrheal Disease Among Travelers and Foreign Residents in Nepal

D. N. Taylor, R. Houston, D. R. Shlim, P. Echeverria, M. Bhaibulaya, and B. L. P. Ungar

Diarrheal disease affects as many as one-third of travelers to developing countries [3]. Previous studies on travelers' diarrhea have focused on the acute illness of the short-term traveler and have not determined the cause of diarrhea in westerners who reside for long periods in developing countries or in persons with persistent diarrhea [4]. Although prophylactic antibiotics have been shown to prevent diarrheal disease in short-term travelers, their use is impractical in foreign residents and long-term travelers. The aim of this study was to determine the etiology of diarrhea among foreigners in Nepal so that appropriate recommendations can be given to persons traveling in remote areas and to assist physicians who see returning travelers.

## Materials and Methods

From February 1986 to January 1987 we studied the first two patients who presented at the US Peace Corps Medical Clinic or the CIWEC Clinic for evaluation of gastrointestinal symptoms. Patients were accepted for study if they could produce a liquid stool specimen at the clinic.

Stools were also inoculated onto MacConkey and Hektoen agar media. After overnight incubation at 37 °C, lactose-positive and lactose-negative colonies were picked from these plates, inoculated onto nutrient agar slants, incubated at 37 °C overnight, and refrigerated at 4 °C along with the original plates until they could be transported to Bangkok, where they were processed for enteric pathogens as previously described [6]. *Campylobacter* species were isolated using the membrane filter technique on nonselective medium under microaerobic conditions [2]. Specimens of stool were also frozen and sent to Bangkok on dry ice to be processed for rotavirus. Rotavirus was detected using a monoclonal enzyme-linked immunoassay (Pathfinder, Kallestad Laboratories, Austin, Texas). To detect intestinal parasites, a direct smear and formalin-ether concentration of stool was examined microscopically in Kathmandu. Stool specimens were also examined by enzyme immunoassay (ELISA) for *Entamoeba histolytica* antigen [7].

## Results

Among 328 expatriate patients with diarrhea seen at two medical clinics in Nepal, a bacterial pathogen was isolated from 47% of patients.

Enterotoxigenic *Escherichia coli (24%), Shigella* (14%), and *Campylobacter* species (9%) were the most frequent bacterial pathogens isolated. *Giardia lamblia* was detected in 12% of patients, rotavirus in 8%, *Cryptosporidium* and *E. histolytica* in 5% each. *Blastocystis hominis* was present in 33% of patients. Eleven percent of patients had more than one bacterial or viral pathogen, and 17% had both bacterial and protozoal pathogens present. Patients with prolonged symptoms (for more than 2 weeks) were more likely to have giardiasis (27%) and less likely to have shigellosis (5%) than patients with acute symptoms, $P=0.02$ and $P=0.05$, respectively. The isolation rates of bacterial pathogens decreased with length of stay in Nepal, but bacterial pathogens remained the most common finding, even among long-term foreign residents.

## Discussion

Travelers' diarrhea is a syndrome caused by a number of enteric pathogens, either singly or in combination. Bacteria account for approximately 50% of the diarrheal disease; however, *Shigella* or enteroinvasive *E. coli* (15%) and *Campylobacter* (10%) taken together were as commonly isolated as enterotoxigenic *E. coli*. Rotavirus, detected in 8% of patients, was most commonly detected during the winter and spring. Protozoal pathogens, (Giardia, *E. histolytica*, and *Cryptosporidium*) were detected in 22% of patients, and in 41% of patients the etiology was unknown. The abrupt onset of severe diarrhea, regardless of length of time in Nepal, was associated more often with a bacterial pathogen. Protozoa were detected more often among patients who had been in Nepal for greater than 3 months, or whose diarrhea had persisted for more than 2 weeks before seeking treatment.

The ELISA was a useful method for detecting *E. histolytica*. A bacterial pathogen was also present in 9 of 16 patients with *E. histolytica* identified by ELISA, and the overall detection rate of only 5% of persons with diarrhea suggests that it was an infrequent cause of diarrheal disease in foreigners in Nepal. The role of *B. hominis* as a cause of diarrheal disease has not been established. When other pathogens were isolated, it is likely that *B. hominis* was not the principle cause of diarrhea. If it is a cause of diarrhea it appears to be self-limited and may not require treatment [1].

This is the first comprehensive study of diarrhea in foreigners in Nepal. It confirms previous studies in Thailand that found travelers' diarrhea to be a polymicrobial illness [5]. In Thailand, *Salmonella* was a sprevalent as enterotoxigenic *E. coli*, while in Nepal *Shigella* and *Campylobacter* were more common. Awareness of regional differences in the etiology of diarrheal disease as well as the effects of length of time abroad and duration of symptoms are important considerations in the diagnosis of diarrheal disease in travelers.

## References


1. Markell EK, Udkow MP (1986) *Blastocystis hominis*: pathogen or fellow traveler? Am J Trop Med Hyg 35:1023–1026
2. Steele TW, McDermottz SN (1984) The use of membrane filters applied directly to the surface of agar plates for the isolation of *Campylobacter jejuni* from feces. Pathology 16:263–265
3. Steffen R, van der Linde F, Gyr K, Schär M (1983) Epidemiology of diarrhea in travelers. JAMA 249:1176–1180
4. Taylor DN, Echeverria P (1986) Etiology and epidemiology of travelers' diarrhea in Asia. Rev Infect Dis 8:S136–S141
5. Taylor DN, Echeverria P, Blaser MJ, Pitarangsi C, Blacklow NR, Cross JH, Weniger B (1985) Polymicrobial aetiology of travellers' diarrhoea. Lancet 1:381–383
6. Taylor DN, Echeverria P, Pal T, Sethabutr O, Wankijtcharoen S, Sricharmorn S, Rowe B, Cross J (1986) The role of *Shigella* spp., enteroinvasive *E. coli*, and other enteropathogens as causes of childhood dysentery in Thailand. J Infect Dis 153:1132–1138
7. Ungar BLP, Yolken RH, Quinn TC (1985) Use of a monoclonal antibody in an enzyme immunoassay for the detection of *Entamoeba histolytica* in fecal specimens. Am J Trop Med Hyg 34:465–472

# An Investigation into Gastrointestinal Upsets Among Package Holidaymakers in a Spanish Resort

R. Y. Cartwright

Results of a study on the resort incidence of travelers' diarrhoea among clients of Thomson Holidays showed an above average value for Benidorm Spain. In August of 1984 and 1985 the incidence was 30% and 31% respectively. In the regions of Costa Brava and Costa del Sol the corresponding rates were 17% –19%. The values were calculated from the answers to two health questions in a tour operator's general client satisfaction questionnaire (CSQ). The definition of travelers' diarrhoea was crude, including all tourists who indicated that they had diarrhoea during their holiday irrespective of severity or duration.

In July and August 1986, a comprehensive questionnaire survey was undertaken among tourists during the journey from Benidorm to Alicante airport at the end of their holiday. Information was sought on the personal details, accommodation, water and food consumed, recreational waters used and details of any illness. The data was coded and analysed on a Prime 9955 computer using SPSSX (Statistical Package for the Social Sciences).

The aim of the study was to assess whether the travelers' diarrhoea described in CSQ was a significant illness, whether there was any association with tap water consumption, whether there was any association with the use of recreational water and whether there was any association with a particular food or type of food outlet.

For the purpose of this study travelers' diarrhoea was defined as "diarrhoea plus fever, rigor, nausea, vomiting colic or headache lasting for 3 or more days."

A total of 2153 questionnaires were completed sufficiently for analysis. The medium age of the respondents was 35 years. The overall incidence of travelers' diarrhoea was 23% but in those aged under 35 years was 29% compared with 20% in those over 35 years ($P < 1 \times 10^{-5}$).

Overall a significant association was found with the use of ice in drinks ($P = 0.0079$), cleaning teeth in tap water ($P = 0.023$), consumption of gassy drinks ($P = 0.007$), use of the hotel swimming pool ($P = 0.002$), eating meals in cafes ($P = 0.001$) and using the Poniente Beach ($P = 0.012$).

The difference between hotels ranged from 10% to 45%, with seven hotels having an incidence above 30%. These top seven hotels also had an above average number of clients under the age of 35 years. The incidence in the younger age group staying in these hotels was significantly greater than those above 35 years ($P = 0.001$). Using Cochran's test, however, the hotel and age were found to be risks independent of each other (both $P \times < 0.05$). The clients staying in the top seven hotels were studied in greater detail and there was a highly significant risk associated with eating ice cream ($P = 0.0048$), eating in cafes ($P = 0.014$) and using the hotel pool ($P = 0.03$). No association could be demonstrated with cleaning teeth in tap water, using ice in drinks, the consumption of gassy drinks or the use of a particular beach. The significant risks were tested for independence using Cochran's test – age was found to be an independent risk factor from ice cream consumption and ice cram consumption independent from age. The same was true for ice cream consumption and eating in cafes. Eating ice cream was an independent risk from pool use but not the reverse. Staying in one of the "top seven" hotels was not independent of eating ice cream nor was eating ice cream independent of staying in one of those hotels.

The majority of tourists classified as having travelers' diarrhoea from the CSQ had a significant illness suggestive of an infectious origin. Those who were under the age of 35 years, ate ice cream, ate in unspecified cafes or stayed in one of seven hotels were more likely to develop travelers' diarrhoea. This study does not implicate either potable water or recreational water as significant sources of infection.

Further studies into the cause of travelers' diarrhoea in tourist visiting Benidorm should concentrate on the eating habits of those under 35 years, staying in hotels of known high risk. The ice-cream consumed should be investigated and the hygiene of the cafes used. In order to obtain further information on possible sources of infection it will be necessary to combine further questionnaires with the microbiological examination of faeces from infected tourists and relevant foodstuffs.

*Acknowledgements.* This study could not have been undertaken without the assistance of the staff of Thomson Holidays, the cooperation of the Benidorm municipality and the statistical analysis undertaken by the staff of the Communicable Disease Surveillance Centre of the Public Health Laboratory Service.

# Intestinal Infections in Swedish Travelers

M. Böttiger and Y. Andersson

In Sweden, 2–3 million people out of 8.4 million go abroad every year. Swedish tourists travel particularly to the south of Europe and to other countries around the Mediterranean. Spain and Italy are important receivers of Swedish holidaymakers as well as France, Greece and Yugoslavia. Remote charter flight destinations are Sri Lanka, Kenya and the Gambia. The most common illness contracted abroad is gastrointestinal infection, but pneumonia, sexually transmitted diseases and hepatitis are also frequent.

From 1930 to 1950 about 300–1000 salmonella cases were registered/year. In the mid-1950s, when the number of travelers abroad increased, the number of salmonellosis and shigellosis cases also grew and new serotypes were seen. During the last 10 years, between 2850 and 5000 cases of salmonellosis and between 600 and 1000 cases of shigellosis were reported every year.

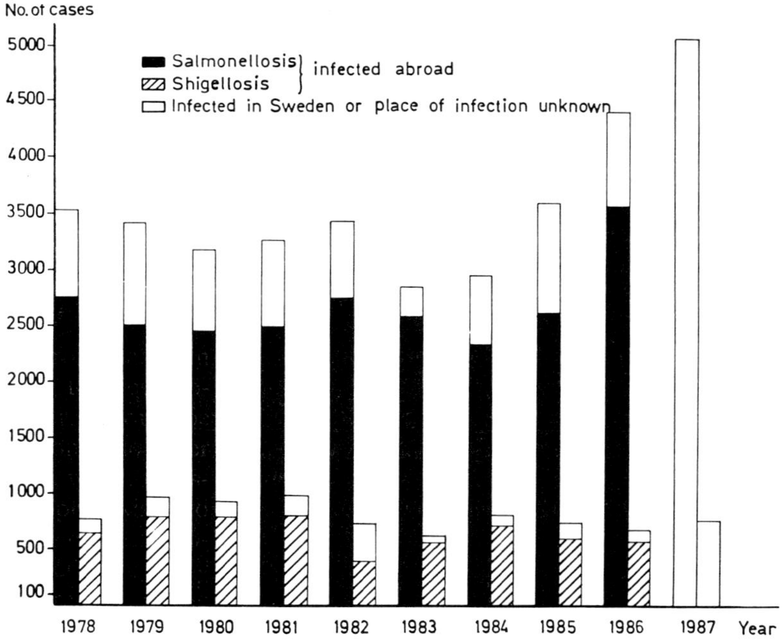


**Fig. 1.** Salmonellosis and shigellosis cases per year. The figures for 1987 are not yet finalized

The number of travelers to different countries was investigated by collecting various official statistics such as travel by air, car, boat or charter. The figures for salmonellosis and shigellosis were collected from the national statistics for communicable diseases in Sweden. About 80% of the 2800–5000 cases of salmonellosis and 600–1000 cases of shigellosis reported annually in Sweden are infected abroad. Between 500 and 800 cases of salmonellosis/year are of domestic or unknown origin. In 1986, at least 3553 travelers of 4344 registered cases contracted salmonellosis and 564 of 663 shigellosis (Fig. 1).

Salmonellosis dominates in isolations from persons visiting Spain, Portugal, Cyprus and Tunisia. Shigellosis dominates in tourists returning from Turkey, but is also common from India and Israel. The serotypes differ in different countries. In Sri Lanka, *S. krefeld, S. typhimurium* and *S. paratyphi B variety java* dominate. In India *S. sonnei* and *S. flexneri* dominate and among the salmonella types *S. typhimurium, S. mbandaka* and *S. virchow* are most common. In tourists from the Gambia we see a quite different pattern. *S. virchow, S. flexneri, S. typhimurium* and *S. tyresoe* dominate. *S. tyresoe* especially is very unusual from other countries. In Spain, including the Canary Islands, 600–1100 travelers/year contract salmonellosis/shigellosis. There the pattern is quite different, *S. enteritidis* being the most common serotype. The risk of contracting salmonellosis or shigellosis is higher in remote countries such as Sri Lanka, India, the Gambia and in the Mediterranean area, Morocco, Tunisia and Egypt (Fig. 2). The incidence of salmonellosis has increased during recent years among Swedish travelers to Majorca, Madeira and also to a lesser extent the Canary Islands. The dominating type in the southwest of Europe is *S. enteritidis*. Most cases appear as single cases.

The practice of using salmonellosis and shigellosis as monitors of diarrhoeal diseases may be discussed. The information provides useful background knowledge for the hygienic advice given to travelers. It also permits the changes in communicable diseases in different countries to be followed. This investigation has resulted in fruitful cooperation with tourist and public health organizations in other countries, for which we are very grateful.

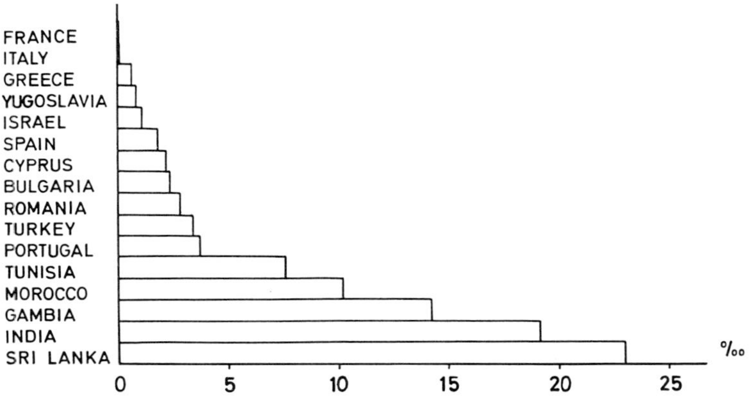


**Fig. 2.** Number of reported salmonellosis and shigellosis cases for 1986 per thousand travelers to some selected countries

# Enteric Pathogens in Finnish Travelers

H. Kyrönseppä and H. Peltola

In the Clinic for Tropical Diseases in Finland, where about 1500 Finnish nationals from tropical and other southern regions are examined annually, intestinal findings were analysed in order to get an idea about the risks of contracting enteric infections, in various areas, in relation to time spent in endemic areas, and how intestinal findings compare with abdominal symptoms.

## Patients and Methods

In the decade 1977–1986, 14605 Finnish nationals were examined for enteric infections. The majority were asymptomatic, and were routinely checked after having worked or stayed a lengthy period in the tropics (67% over 6 months). Short-term visitors (less than 1 month) made up 16%. Examinees were missionaries (18%), employees of the Finnish Foreign Office and some UN organizations (40%), tourists (11%), and various experts, advisers, technicians and the like. They were grouped into nine categories according to the geographical area visited, of which the biggest were East Africa (37%), Southeast Asia (14%), Indian subcontinent (9%), Near East (12%), and South America (8%). All patients had a number of routine tests performed, which included two stool samples for parasitology, examined with the modified formalin-ether concentration technique, and for culture of salmonellae and shigellae. Other bacteria were cultured only when considered necessary.

## Results

In all, 2539 faecal pathogens were found in 15% of examinees. In the group of enteric bacteria, symptoms were common (in 48%), in the group of protozoa less common (28%), and in helminthic infections infrequent (16%).

A small portion of the total (6%) had abdominal symptoms, mostly diarrhoea. Table 1 shows all the enteric findings, Table 2 their relation to time and Fig. 1 their relation to different geographical areas.

## Conclusions

The yield of enteric pathogens in people coming from the tropics was so high that we conclude that such people should have their stools examined for parasites and bacteria, particularly those with present or recent abdominal symp-

**Table 1.** Intestinal findings

| | *n* | % |
|---|---|---|
| Total no. of examinees | 14605 | 100 |
| Examinees with positive findings | 3905 | 26.7 |
| Pathogenic protozoa | 1002 | 6.9 |
| – *Giardia lamblia* | | 4.4 |
| – *Entamoeba histolytica* | | 2.3 |
| – *Cryptosporidium* (1985–1986) | | 0.1 |
| Helminths | 599 | 4.1 |
| – Hookworm | | 0.3 |
| – *Strongyloides* | | 0.1 |
| – *Ascaris* | | 1.3 |
| – *Trichuris* | | 1.8 |
| – *Taenia* sp. | | 0.1 |
| – *Schistosoma (mansoni)* | | 0.2 |
| – Other | | 0.4 |
| Bacteria | 938 | 6.4 |
| – Salmonellae | | 4.1 |
| – Shigellae | | 1.1 |
| – *Campylobacter* | | 1.1 |
| – *Clostridium difficile* | | 0.1 |
| Total no. of pathogenic findings | 2539 | 17.4 |
| Apathogenic protozoa, including *Entamoeba coli, Endolimax nana, Iodamoeba bütschlii* | 2381 | 16.3 |

**Table 2.** Relation to time spent in endemic areas

| | <1 month | 1–6 months | >6 months |
|---|---|---|---|
| *n* | 2334 | 2456 | 9815 |
| % | 16 | 17 | 67 |
| Helminths | | | |
| Hookworm | 0.1 | 0.4 | 0.3 |
| *Trichuris* | 0.6 | 0.9 | 2.3 |
| *Ascaris* | 0.2 | 0.8 | 1.7 |
| Protozoa | | | |
| *Giardia lamblia* | 4.1 | 6.2 | 4.3 |
| *Entamoeba histolytica* | 1.3 | 2.1 | 2.7 |
| Bacteria | | | |
| *Salmonellae* | 9.0 | 5.7 | 2.6 |
| *Shigellae* | 2.1 | 1.8 | 0.7 |
| *Campylobacter* | 4.1 | 1.7 | 0.3 |

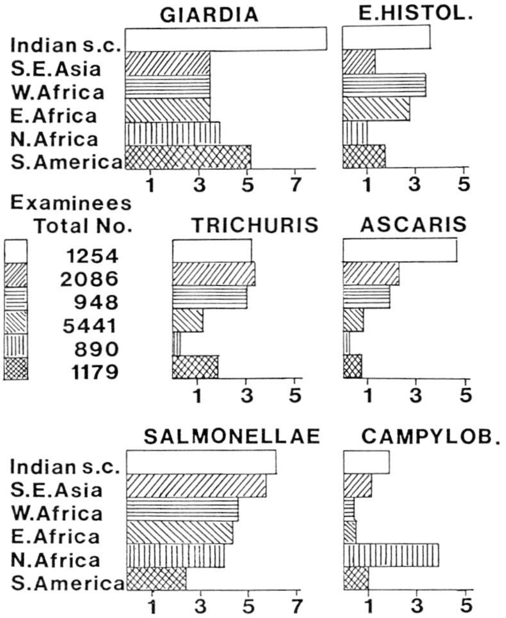


**Fig. 1.** Enteric pathogens according to region (% infected)

toms. This could be beneficial for individuals, and also epidemiologically in the situation which prevails in Finland, where there are practically no endemic intestinal parasites, and where most *Salmonella, Shigella* and *Campylobacter* infections are imported.

# Intestinal Parasite Infestation Risks in Temporary Residents in Warm Climates

J. Jedlička, V. Tolarová, and E. Švandová

Intestinal parasites remain an important agent responsible for morbidity, especially in countries with warm climates [4]. The purpose of the present study was to ascertain life-habit risk factors that might influence the infestation level in temporary residents in these areas.

A total of 525 adult returnees from warm climates in Africa, Latin America and Asia were interviewed in order to ascertain data concerning life habits during their stay. For coprologic examinations, two concentration methods (Faust's and AMS III) and trichrome-stained smears were used, two to three samples being collected every other day. For the purpose of detecting the total incidence of parasitoses, results of the parasitological investigations carried out by local laboratories were included.

The incidence of infestation by intestinal parasites during on average a 16-month stay in the risk area is summarized in Table 1. Total incidence, dependent on the area visited, varied from 6.8% (East Asia) to 30% (Central Africa). The impact of particular risk factors on the incidence rate is summarized in Table 2.

We confirmed the health risks of some well-known habits: consumption of unboiled water from local municipal supplies, consumption of fruits and vegetables of unknown cleanliness and taking community meals in facilities provided by local personnel, thereby completely confirming an old British statement "boil it, peel it, cook it or forget it" [2]. Rinsing fruits and vegetables in disinfectant solutions (Pantocit, Javel) failed as a preventive measure against the overall infestation by intestinal parasites. Commonly used chlorination of

**Table 1.** Incidence of infestation by intestinal parasites in 525 returnees

| Parasites species | Incidence (%) |
|---|---|
| *Entamoeba histolytica* (cysts) | 3.8 |
| *Giardia intestinalis* | 2.1 |
| Helminthiases *(Ascaris lumbricoides, Trichuris trichiura, Enterobius vermicularis)* | 2.1 |
| Nonpathogenic protozoa *(Entamoeba coli, Ent. hartmanni, Endolimax nana, Dientamoeba fragilis, Chilomastix mesnili, Iodamoeba bütschlii)* | 8.2 |
| Total | 14.1 |

**Table 2.** Risk factors influencing the infestation level

| Risk factor | Persons infected (%) Risk factor | | Statistical significance ($\chi^2$-test) |
|---|---|---|---|
| | Present | Absent | |
| Consumption of unboiled water from municipal supplies | 20.7% | 11.0% | $P<0.01$ |
| Community meals in facilities with local personnel | 15.6% | 7.4% | $P<0.05$ |
| Consumption of fruits and vegetables of unknown cleanliness | 23.9% | 12.5% | $P<0.05$ |
| Rinsing fruits and vegetables in disinfectant solutions | 21.4% | 12.3% | $P<0.05$ |
| Repeated stay in the risk area | 18.1% | 11.7% | $P<0.05$ |

drinking water (containing 0.2–0.5 mg $Cl^-$/liter) has been proved to be ineffective in killing *Entamoeba histolytica* cysts [3]. Previous visits to the same region showed reduced incidence of "travelers' diarrhea" [1] in distinction from intestinal parasitoses in the present group, although the route of infection was identical in both cases. Explanation of the latter fact is probably travelers' declining caution and not the persistence of infection.

Summarizing, behavior does influence the infestation level by intestinal parasites, which is especially important in the situation when other types of prophylaxis are lacking.

## References

1. Steffen R, Gsell O (1981) Prophylaxis of travelers' diarrhoea. J Trop Med Hyg 84:239–242
2. Steffen R, Stransky M, Kozicki M (1984) Vorbeugende Maßnahmen gegen Reisediarrhoe. Schweiz Med Wochenschr [Suppl]17:35–38
3. WHO (1969) Amoebiasis. WHO Tech Rep Ser 421
4. WHO (1987) Prevention and control of intestinal parasitic infections. WHO Tech Rep Ser 749

# Amoebiasis Risk Group Delimitation in Returnees from the Tropics and Subtropics

J. Jedlička, V. Tolarová, J. Prokopeč, and E. Švandová

Amoebiasis is the tropical infection which seems to be most frequently imported by returnees from the tropics and subtropics [2]. The diagnosis of intestinal amoebiasis represents a problem in coprologic detection because of the need for multiple stool sampling. Six samples, taken on consecutive days and each subjected to both concentration technique and a stained smear, are required for 90% diagnosis of positive cases of intestinal amebiasis [3]. Sometimes ten samples are required for a diagnosis [1], which is inapplicable in all returnees. The purpose of the present study was the attempt to delimitate the risk group as concerns the presence of *Entamoeba histolytica* in returnees from its endemic areas.

A total of 525 adults were examined after their return from the tropics and subtropics, as represented by 50 states in Asia, Africa and Latin America. For routine coprologic examinations Faust's concentration method and trichrome-stained smears were prepared; two to three samples from each person collected every other day were needed.

Parasitological findings of particular intestinal protozoa and mixed infections of *Entamoeba histolytica* with other intestinal protozoa are summarized in Tables 1 and 2, respectively. The 1% prevalence of mixed infections was significantly higher than the expected one ($P < 0.01$). Graphic presentation of the prevalence of *Entamoeba histolytica* in returnees is demonstrated in Fig. 1.

**Table 1.** Prevalence of intestinal protozoal infections in 525 returnees

| Protozoal species | Persons infected | |
|---|---|---|
| | Absolute number | Percentage |
| *Entamoeba histolytica* | 10 | 1.9 |
| *Entamoeba coli* | 28 | 5.3 |
| *Endolimax nana* | 25 | 4.8 |
| *Giardia intestinalis* | 10 | 1.9 |
| *Entamoeba hartmanni* | 3 | 0.6 |
| *Dientamoeba fragilis* | 1 | 0.2 |
| *Chilomastix mesnili* | 1 | 0.2 |
| *Iodamoeba bütschlii* | 1 | 0.2 |
| Total | 62 | 11.8 |

**Table 2.** Prevalence of mixed infections by *Entamoeba histolytica* and other intestinal protozoa in 525 returnees

| Mixed infection of *Entamoeba histolytica* and | Persons infected (%) | |
|---|---|---|
| | Ascertained value | Expected value[a] |
| *Entamoeba coli* | 0.4 | $1.0 \cdot 10^{-1}$ |
| *Endolimax nana* | 0.2 | $9.0 \cdot 10^{-2}$ |
| *Giardia intestinalis* | 0.2 | $3.6 \cdot 10^{-2}$ |
| *Entamoeba hartmanni* | 0 | $1.1 \cdot 10^{-2}$ |
| *Dientamoeba fragilis* | 0.2 | $3.6 \cdot 10^{-3}$ |
| *Chilomastix mesnili* | 0 | $3.6 \cdot 10^{-3}$ |
| *Iodamoeba bütschlii* | 0 | $3.6 \cdot 10^{-3}$ |
| Total | 1.0 | $2.5 \cdot 10^{-1}$ |

[a] Prevalence $= P$

$P_{\text{mixed infection}} = P_{\textit{Entamoeba histolytica}} \times P_{\text{particular protozoal species}}$

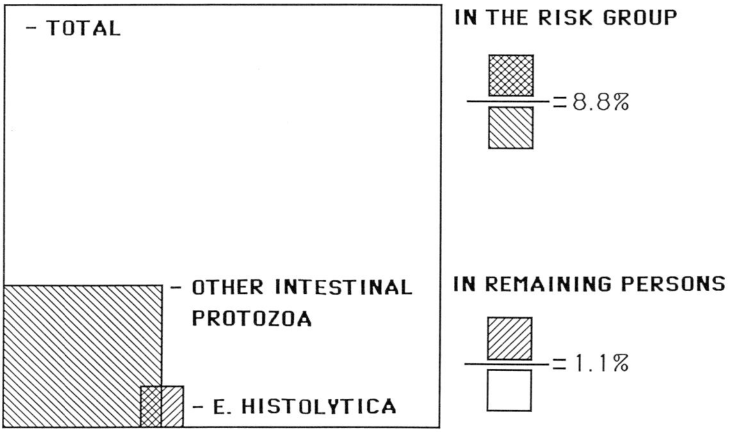


**Fig. 1.** Graphic presentation of prevalence of *Entamoeba histolytica* in returnees from the tropics and subtropics

Based on the fact that the occurrence of intestinal protozoa should be regarded as indicating microscopic coprophagia, it was reasonable to define the risk group as those in whom *Entamoeba histolytica* was present. Persons infected by nonpathogenic protozoa should be considered as being the risk group. Hence the risk group thus defined represented 9.9% of returnees from the tropics and subtropics. In this group the prevalence of *Entamoeba histolytica* reached 8.8%, i.e., eight times higher than in the other returnees.

It is therefore recommended that in the risk group the following examinations are carried out:

1. Prolonged and repeated coprologic examinations or, if available, an immunoassay test for detection of *Entamoeba histolytica* antigen in the feces;
2. Serological tests to disclose the possible extraintestinal involvement; it is known that in more than half of the patients suffering from extraintestinal amoebiasis coproprotozoological tests yield negative results [4].

## References

1. Degrémont A (1977) Diagnostic biologique de la malaria et de l'amibiase. Schweiz Med Wochenschr 107:641–642
2. Despommier DD (1981) The laboratory diagnosis of *Entamoeba histolytica*. Bull NY Acad Med 57:212–216
3. Granz W (1983) Klinik und Therapie der Amöbiasis. Z Gesamte Inn Med 38:63–70
4. Ockert G (1987) Results of amoebiasis – IFAR using a simple prepared *E. histolytica* antigen. 6th Symposium on immunodiagnosis of tropical parasitoses and actual problems of tropical medicine, 14–16 Sept, Liblice

# Drug Susceptibility and Virulence of Different *Entamoeba histolytica* Strains

G. D. Burchard and Mirelman

## Introduction

According to the WHO definition, amoebiasis is defined as a condition in which the body harbours *Entamoeba histolytica* irrespective of the presence of symptoms. *E. histolytica* is frequently imported to Europe by travellers from tropical countries. In a screening investigation in Hamburg *E. histolytica* was detected in stool specimens in 4% of travelers returning from tropical countries. Only a small percentage of these patients develop clinical manifestations. Amoeba from carriers have not been studied in detail. It is not known whether the expression of virulence in these strains may depend on the microenvironmental conditions of the host intestine. We therefore characterized these strains more closely and also tested the drug susceptibility.

## Material and Methods

Four E. histolytica isolates from asymptomatic carriers were compared with characterized, well-known strains of patients suffering from invasive amoebiasis. These strains were grown in TYSGM 9 medium.

The destruction of tissue culture monolayers was taken as a semiquantitative assay for the virulence of trophozoites in vitro. Baby hamster kidney cells are cultured in tissue culture plates and are exposed to the amoeba for 1–2 h. The uptake of a dye (methylene blue) by the remaining intact cells is taken as a measure of the damage of the monolayer.

The capability of the different *E. histolytica* strains to phagocytize red blood cells was also determined because virulent *E. histolytica* are known to show a high rate of phagocytic activity.

The behaviour of *E. histolytica* isolates in animal models can be taken as a semiquantitative measure of disease-causing potential. We tested the virulence in the hamster liver and devised a model for intestinal infections in rats. A cecal loop is prepared by a ligature of the cecum distal to the cecal-colonic valve without affecting the blood supply. The trophozoites are then inoculated into the loop. The animals survive 1 week, and controls without amoeba did not show mucosal damage.

As isoenzyme patterns of hexokinase and phosphoglucomutase have been used as markers to distinguish between pathogenic and nonpathogenic strains, we also determined the mobility patterns of these isoenzymes in thin-layer agarose mini-gel electrophoresis.

In vitro drug testing was performed with emetine and metronidazole. For characterization of the drug effects, the 50% inhibitory concentration defined as concentration in which the number of living parasites was 50% of the control was used.

## Results

All four *E. histolytica* strains originating from asymptomatic carriers electrophoretically exhibited a so-called nonpathogenic isoenzyme pattern with a reduced electromobility of the hexokinase and of the phosphoglucomutase as compared with the pathogenic zymodeme group II of the pathogenic strain HM : 1. In the virulence test on monolayer tissue cultures, two of the four isolates from asymptomatic carriers showed a high grade of monolayer destruction; the two other strains were less cytolytic. The bacterial flora alone from the carrier strains did not result in a tissue layer destruction. On measuring the rate of erythrophagocytosis, the strains from the asymptomatic carriers cultivated in xenic medium showed a lower activity than the axenic strains. However, all of the strains were able to phagocytize red blood cells. The lower rate of phagocytosis in the xenically grown strains could be related to the fact that these trophozoites still contained rice starch granula. In the animal studies, the number of amoeba producing an abscess in more than 50% of the hamsters was taken for comparison. Only when live amoeba could be detected were the abscesses considered as amoebic. Two carrier strains exhibited a high virulence in this model. The bacterial flora alone did not produce abscesses. The same carrier strains that did cause liver abscesses in hamsters sometimes also produced mucosal damage in the rat cecal loop.

Drug testing showed that the four carrier strains had a comparable susceptibility to emetine, as the standard strain HM-1 : IMSS; the same was true for metronidazole.

## Discussion

A series of experiments have been developed to investigate the pathogenic potential of different *E. histolyca* strains in vitro and in vivo. The models used by us, i.e. tissue culture monolayer destruction and erythrophagocytosis, can be taken as semiquantitative markers of virulence and as an indication for pathogenicity. Also the ability of *E. histolytica* trophozoites to induce the formation of hepatic lesions in hamsters and cecal ulcerations in rodents correlates with the disease-causing potential. Comparative virulence studies have been performed hitherto predominantly with axenically grown pathogenic strains. Our results show that also strains from asymptomatic carriers with a nonpathogenic isoenzyme pattern obviously may have a disease-causing potential.

# Cryptosporidiosis in a Group of Travelers to Puerto Vallarta, Mexico, 1986

S. Waterman, W. Keene, J. Meade, C. Sterling, and C. Ruiz-Matus

A group of 30 tennis-playing tourists visited Puerto Vallarta, a popular seaport resort on the west coast of Mexico, from 14 May to 18 May 1986. Two of the tourists, one of whom was hospitalized, developed stool-confirmed cryptosporidiosis upon return to Los Angeles, California, and were reported to the Los Angeles County Health Department. We conducted an epidemiologic investigation to determine whether other group members had been infected with *Cryptosporidium* and to identify, if possible, a transmission source. Questionnaires were administered and blood and stool samples were collected several weeks after the tourists' return. In addition to routine testing for bacterial and parasitic pathogens, stools were examined for *Cryptosporidium* by rotamine/auramine, modified acid fast, and safranin/methylene blue staining and sucrose flotation. Blood samples were tested for *Cryptosporidium* antibodies by Western blot and IFA assays. Filtered water samples taken in October 1986 were also tested by direct FA using monoclonal antibodies to *Cryptosporidium*.

Two additional shedders of *Cryptosporidium* oocysts were identified. Serologic testing by Western blot was positive in 22/22 (100%) of tourists tested and in 5/19 (26%) of control sera ($P < 0.01$). The mean duration of symptoms was 8.9 days (range of 1–25 days), and the median incubation period was 6 days. Watery diarrhea, abdominal cramps, loss of appetite, and increased gas were experienced by the majority of patients. Six (30%) of 20 laboratory-positive patients saw a physician because of their symptoms. Persons with moderate to severe diarrhea were significantly more likely to have an underlying medical condition than those well or mildly ill. Comparison of moderate to severely ill tourists with mildly ill or well persons revealed no significant differences in exposure to uncooked or unpasteurized foods, amount of water drunk, restaurants visited, swimming or animal contact. The only universal exposure in the travelers was water and/or ice. All water sampling was negative for *Cryptosporidium*. However, technical difficulties with the filters possibly diminished the sensitivity of the procedure.

This investigation indicates that an outbreak of cryptosporidiosis occurred among a group of tourists visiting Puerto Vallarta, Mexico. Supportive evidence includes stool confirmation in four persons and a highly significant difference in serologic positivity in travelers compared with controls. Also, clinical findings, an incubation period of about 6 days with watery diarrhea lasting somewhat longer than typical traveler's diarrhea, and illness associated with underlying medical conditions were consistent with cryptosporidiosis. We were unable to demonstrate a common source of infection in this outbreak. Multiple sources of infection may have existed. Alternatively, a lack of uninfected controls and interviews performed several weeks after exposure may have limited our analysis. Despite negative water sampling, the high attack rate in this group of tourists and the paucity of other common exposures suggests a ubiquitous source such as water [1, 2]. This report reemphasizes that cryptosporidiosis should be considered in persons with traveler's diarrhea [3–8].

## References

1. D'Antonio RG, Winn RE, Taylor JP, Gustafson TL, Current WL, Rhodes MM, Gary GW, Zajac RA (1985) A waterborne outbreak of cryptosporidiosis in normal hosts. Ann Intern Med 103:886–888
2. CDC (1987) Cryptosporidiosis – New Mexico, 1986. MMWR 36:561–563
3. Jokipii L, Pohjola S, Jokipii AMM (1983) *Cryptosporidium*: a frequent finding in patients with gastrointestinal symptoms. Lancet I:358–361
4. Holten-Andersen W, Gerstoft J, Henriksen SA, Pedersen NS (1984) Prevalence of *Cryptosporidium* among patients with acute enteric infection. J Infect 9:277–282
5. Soave R, Ma P (1985) Cryptosporidiosis – traveler's diarrhea in two families. Arch Intern Med 145:70–72
6. Isaacs D, Hunt GH, Phillips AD, Price EH, Raafat F, Walker-Smith JA (1985) Cryptosporidiosis in immunocompetent children. J Clin Pathol 38:76–81
7. Ma P, Kaufman DL, Helmick CG, d'Souza AJ, Navin TR (1985) Cryptosporidiosis in tourists returning from the Caribbean. N Engl J Med 312:647–648
8. Sterling CR, Seegar K, Sinclair NA (1986) *Cryptosporidium* as a causative agent of travelers' diarrhea. J Infect Dis 153:380–381

# Prevention of Traveler's Diarrhea: A Double-Blind Randomized Trial with *Saccharomyces cerevisiae* Hansen CBS 5926

H. H. Kollaritsch and G. Wiedermann

"Travel broadens the mind and loosens the bowels." This metaphor of Sherwood L. Gorbach outlines the problem of traveler's diarrhea in modern tourism. With an attack rate of 25%–50% diarrheal illness may affect more than four million visitors from industrialized countries annually, of whom 30% are ill enough to be confined to bed and 40% have to alter their scheduled activities [1].

Thus, extensive efforts have been undertaken to find an effective and well-tolerated prophylactic compound to prevent gastrointestinal disorders during short-term stays in warm climate countries. Antibiotics have proved to be useful to prevent diarrhea, but at the price of side effects [2]. At present, following the results of an international consensus conference in 1986, use of antibiotics to prevent episodes of traveler's diarrhea is not recommended [3]. Several nonantibiotic substances, such as halogenated hydroxyquinolines, lactobacilli, ethacridine, nonspecific antidiarrheal agents like activated charcoal, and enteral vaccines, have been tested for their prophylactic value. With the exception of bismuth subsalicylate none of these preparations reduced significantly the attack rates or influenced the clinical course of traveler's diarrhea [4]. This failure, however, may be due to the heterogeneity of the etiological agents causing diarrheal illness. Different patients have been reported to be infected with distinct pathogenic microorganisms, but mixed enteric infections can also frequently be found in a single patient [5, 6]. In addition, seasonal influences on etiology were reported recently [5]. Nevertheless, enterotoxigenic *E. coli* (ETEC) is thought to be the most common cause of diarrhea, although regional differences in prevalence are reported.

We performed a randomized, double-blind and placebo-controlled trial to evaluate the efficacy of viable, lyophilized *Saccharomyces cerevisiae* Hansen CBS 5926 *(ScH CBS 5926)* to prevent traveler's diarrhea independent of etiology.

The participants were 1231 healthy Austrian volunteers during a stay in a warm climate country. They were advised to take – according to random allocation – placebo capsules, $2 \times 125$ mg *ScH CBS 5926*, or $2 \times 250$ mg ScH CBS 5926, corresponding to $5 \times 10^9$ or $1 \times 10^{10}$ viable germs/day, respectively. Intake had to begin 5 days before departure and continued during the whole stay abroad. Prophylaxis had to be continued also in the case of diarrhea. Data recording was performed individually by use of a detailed questionnaire. For statistical evaluation only completed reports of volunteers who took their regimen regularly were included.

**Table 1.** Prophylactic efficacy of *Saccharomyces cerevisiae*

| Group | No. of subjects | Traveler's diarrhea | | Incidence | Protection rate (%) |
|---|---|---|---|---|---|
| | | Developed | Not developed | | |
| Placebo | 406 (33%) | 173 | 233 | 42.6% | |
| Group 1 (2 × 125 mg) | 426 (34.5%) | 143 | 283 | 33.6% | 21.2%* |
| Group 2 (2 × 250 mg) | 399 (32.5%) | 127 | 272 | 31.8% | 25.4%* |

* $P < 0.01$

The used questionnaires had been found to be useful in previous studies. Information about age, sex, body weight, previous travel history, actual destination, duration of stay, accomodation, environmental conditions of travel, dietary hygiene, and compliance with respect to regular intake of medication was requested. In addition, participants were requested to describe intercurrent episodes of diarrhea in detail: day of onset of disease, duration of illness, mean frequency of stools during acute illness, quality of stools, and concomitant clinical symptoms such as abdominal cramps, nausea, vomiting and fever. Travelers who reported additional use of other drugs to treat acute diarrhea, e.g. loperamide, diphenoxylate or antibiotics, were excluded. Also excluded were volunteers who reported an acute gastrointestinal disorder within the last 3 weeks before departure or patients suffering from colitis or Crohn's disease.

The three groups were nearly identical with respect to number of participants. Demographic data were similar and did not differ in any respect. The mean duration of stay was 19 days, independent of destination.

Use of *ScH CBS 5926* reduced the attack rates of traveler's diarrhea (Table 1). Whereas 42.6% of the volunteers in the placebo group reported an episode of traveler's diarrhea, the volunteers who received *Saccharomyces* had attack rates of 33.6% and 31.8%. The incidence was reduced by 21.2% in group 1 and 25.4% in group 2 compared with the placebo ($P < 0.007$ and $P < 0.002$, respectively). The difference between group 1, receiving 250 mg *ScH CBS 5926*daily, and group 2, with a daily dose of 500 mg *ScH CBS 5926*, may suggest dose dependency, but this difference was not significant statistically. Comparing our results with those of recent studies by DuPont and coworkers on the prophylactic efficacy of bismuth subsalicylate, it appears that *ScH CBS 5926* provides less protection. DuPont found a dose-dependent incidence reduction of approximately 40% with the highest dose used in his studies [7].

However, because *ScH CBS 5926* is easily administrated and lacks any side effects in normal, healthy hosts, our results should be sufficiently encouraging to evaluate whether higher numbers of organisms may further enhance the prophylactic efficiency. It should be noted that *ScH CBS 5926* did not cause any clinical improvement in nonpreventable cases of diarrhea. When compar-

**Table 2.** Risk of diarrhea in different geographical regions and protective efficacy of *Saccharomyces cerevisiae*

| Region | Total subjects | Placebo | Group 1 2 × 250 mg SMC | R [a] | Group 2 2 × 250 mg SMC | R [a] | Group 1+2 | R [a] | Significance [b] |
|---|---|---|---|---|---|---|---|---|---|
| Northern Africa | 208 | 50.7% (33/65) | 30.1% (22/73) | 41% | 21.4% (15/70) | 58% | 25.9% (37/143) | 49% | $P<0.0025$ |
| | | | | $P<0.01$ | | $P<0.001$ | | | |
| Western Africa | 51 | 52.6% (10/9) | 33.3% (6/18) | 37% | 21.4% (3/14) | 59% | 28.1% (9/32) | 47% | $P<0.01$ |
| Eastern Africa | 251 | 48.6% (34/70) | 35.7% (35/98) | 27% | 36.1% (30/83) | 26% | 35.9% (65/181) | 26% | NS |
| | | | | $P<0.05$ | | $P<0.1$ | | | |
| South Africa and Near East not evaluated [c] | | | | | | | | | |
| Middle East | 85 | 66.6% [d] (14/21) | 68.8% (22/32) | 0 | 65.6% (21/32) | 0 | 67.2% (43/64) | 0 | NS |
| Far East | 228 | 31.4% [e] (27/86) | 25.9% (18/72) | 20% | 30.0% (21/70) | 5% | 27.5% (39/72) | 13% | NS |
| Middle East (Isles) | 123 | 40.0% (18/45) | 28.9% (13/45) | 28% | 24.2% (8/33) | 40% | 25.6% (20/78) | 36% | $P<0.05$ |
| | | | | $P<0.1$ | | $P<0.05$ | | | |
| Middle America | 76 | 31.3% (10/32) | 38.9% (7/18) | 0 | 30.7% (8/26) | 0 | 34.0% (15/44) | 0 | NS |
| South America | 97 | 50.0% (19/38) | 33.3% (8/24) | 33% | 37.1% (13/35) | 26% | 35.6% (21/59) | 29% | NS |
| Worldwide tours | 34 | 50.0% (6/12) | 25% (3/12) | 50% | 40.0% (4/10) | 20% | 31.8% (7/22) | 36% | NS |

[a] Reduction of risk versus placebo/significance
[b] Significance of protection versus overall risk reduction (group 2, Table 1)
[c] According to small numbers of subjects traveling to these regions, risk reduction was not evaluated
[d] Risk of diarrhea significantly *higher* ($P<0.05$) than overall incidence in the placebo group
[e] Risk of diarrhea significantly *lower* ($P<0.05$) than overall incidence in the placebo group

ing time of onset, mean duration of disease, frequency and quality of stools, and incidence and severity of concomitant symptoms such as abdominal cramps, nausea, vomiting and fever, no significant clinical or statistical differences could be found. Thus, protection by *ScH CBS 5926* seems to follow an "all-or-nothing" principle.

The most intriguing results of our study were found when assessing the prophylactic efficacy of *ScH CBS 5926* in different geographic regions (Table 2). To evaluate the risk of diarrhea for tourists in different regions, countries of destination were divided into 11 geographic regions. The incidence of diarrhea in the placebo group ranges between 31.3% in the "Far East" region to 66% in India and Nepal. Compared with an overall risk of 42.6%, the risk of acquiring traveler's diarrhea is significantly lower in the Far East ($P<0.05$) and significantly higher in Middle Eastern countries ($P<0.05$). The reduction of the incidence of diarrhea in groups 1 and 2 versus the placebo group ranged between 0% and 59% in different geographic areas. The protection rates in northern Africa, western Africa and in the Islands of the Indian Ocean (Sri Lanka, Seychelles, Maldives, Mauritius) were 58%, 59% and 40%, respectively, in group 2 and were significantly higher than the overall risk reduction rate of 25.4% in group 2 (Table 1). The reduction could not be statistically evaluated in other regions due to the small numbers of travelers. In the countries of the Middle East, India and Nepal, and in Middle America, particularly Mexico, we found no protective efficacy of *ScH CBS 5926*. These results may indicate a selective mode of action of *ScH CBS 5926*, as the demographic data of our volunteers did not differ with respect to destination.

Travel conditions such as duration of stay, accomodation, and personal dietary hygiene during stay did not vary with destination (not shown).

This possible selectivity cannot be explained because the mode of action of *ScH CBS 5926* is not fully understood. *Saccharomyces cerevisiae* produces in vitro as well as in vivo all B vitamins, approximately 20 amino acids, 30 different enyzmes, has interfering effects in mixed cultures with enteropathogenic bacteria, and inhibits adherence of pathogenic microbial agents to enterocytes. Furthermore, possible interactions of *ScH CBS 5926* with defense mechanisms of the host are described, such as complement activation, stimulation of phagocytic activity and respiratory burst of phagocytic cells as well as increase of lysozyme level [8–11]. These observations may help to understand the observed prophlactic efficacy, although the exact mode of action of *ScH CBS 5926* in diarrheal illness remains to be clarified.

In summary, the *Saccharomyces* preparation seems to be a valuable tool in the development of a new non antibiotic preparation for prevention of traveler's diarrhea. Lack of side effects and easy administration enhance the value of this preparation, and negligible toxicity permits an increase of the daily regimen, which may increase the protection capacity.

## References


1. Gorbach SL (1987) Bacterial diarrhea and its treatment. Lancet II:1378–1382
2. DuPont HL, Ericsson CD, Johnson PCJ (1985) Chemotherapy and chemoprophylaxis of traveller's diarrhea. Ann Intern Med 102(2):260–261
3. Consensus Development Conference Statement (1986) Rev Inf Dis [Suppl 2]8:S227–S233
4. Steffen R, Heusser R, DuPont HL (1986) Prevention of traveller's diarrhea by nonantibiotic drugs. Rev Infect Dis [Suppl 2]8:S151–S159
5. Adkins HJ, Escamilla J, Santiago LT, Ranoa C, Echeverria P, Cross JH (1987) Two-year survey of etiologic agents of diarrheal diseases at San Lazaro Hospital, Manila, Rep. of Philippines. J Clin Microbiol 25(7):1143–1147
6. Taylor DN, Echeverria P, Blaser MI, Pitarangsi C, Blacklow N, Cross I (1985) Polymicrobial aetiology of traveller's diarrhea. Lancet I:381–383
7. DuPont HL, Sullivan P, Evans EG, Pickering LK, Evans DJ, Vollet J, Ericsson CD et al. (1980) Prevention of traveller's diarrhea (emporiatric enteritis): prophylactic administration of subsalicylate bismuth. JAMA 243:237–241
8. Cotte J (1967) Expertise biologique concernant l'activité saccarisique de *Saccharomyces boulardii* 17 lyophilisée. Verdict
9. Brugier S, Patte F (1975) Antagonisme in vitro entre l'ultralevure et different germs bacteriens. Med Paris 45:3–8
10. Riggi SI, di Luzio NR (1961) Identification of a reticuloendothelial stimulating agent in zymosan. Am J Physiol 200:297–300
11. Petzold K, Müller E (1986) Animal experimental and cell biological studies on the effect of *Saccharomyces cerevisiae* Hansen CBS 5926 on the unspecific enhancement of the resistance to infection. Drug Res 36[2]:1085–1088

# Prophylactic Efficacy of Lactobacilli on Traveler's Diarrhea

F. T. Black, P. L. Andersen, J. Ørskov, F. Ørskov, K. Gaarslev, and S. Laulund

It is well established in double-blind controlled studies that travelers' diarrhea to a great extent can be prevented by prophylactic intake of antimicrobial chemotherapeutics [1, 2, 4]. Doxycycline; the combination of sulfamethoxazole/trimethoprim and trimethoprim alone; mecillinam; and recently norfloxacin and ciprofloxacin have shown protection rates of 60%–95%. However, the use of these agents may cause adverse reactions and may lead to emergence of resistant strains of enteric pathogens.

Studies of the efficacy of nonantibiotic prophylaxis have also been performed, bismuth subsalicylate being the most effective, showing a protection rate between 35% and 65% [3, 5].

In a prospective double-blind controlled study we have applied the concept of probiotics by using lactobacilli as prophylaxis against travelers' diarrhea, in spite of the fact that previous studies of lactobacilli as prophylaxis have come out with negative results [5].

The study group comprised 94 Danish tourists participating in a 2-week round trip to Egypt in the autumn 1986. The participants were randomized into two groups, one receiving capsules containing lactobacilli, the other receiving placebo capsules. The mean age in group one was 51 years, in group two 49 years. Sex distribution was comparable in the two groups.

Each lactobacillus capsule contained a mixture of approximately $3 \times 10^9$ live lyophilized organisms of four different human species: *Lactobacillus acidophilus, Bifidobacteria bifidum, Lactobacillus bulgaricus* and *Streptococcus thermophilus*. The first two species constituted 90% of the mixture. The four species have the following characteristics in common: high production of acids, high bile tolerance, and metabolically active at low pH values (acid tolerance). The mixture showed a 99.3% inhibition of ETEC in liquid medium. The dose regimen was one capsule three times daily, starting 2 days prior to departure, ending on the last day of travel.

Each participant completed a diarrhea diary recording the number of daily bowel moments, characteristics of the stools (normal, loose, watery), and presence of accompanying symptoms such as fever, nausea, vomiting and abdominal cramps. All subjects with diarrhea were examined by the accompanying physician. Moderate and severe cases of diarrhea were given a short course of loperamide capsules.

Travelers' diarrhea was defined as either three or more watery stools/24 h, or one watery stool with at least one of the accompanying symptoms. Recur-

**Table 1.** Travelers' diarrhea in Danish tourists in Egypt

| | Prophylaxis | |
|---|---|---|
| | Lactobacilli | Placebo |
| No. of subjects | 40 | 41 |
| No. with diarrhea (%) | 17 (43%) | 29 (71%)* |
| Duration of diarrhea in days (mean) | 1–6 (1.9) | 1–7 (2.2) |

* $P=0.019$

**Table 2.** Pathogens isolated from subjects with diarrhea

| | Prophylaxis | |
|---|---|---|
| | Lactobacilli | Placebo |
| No. with diarrhea | 17 | 29 |
| No. of stools examined | 16 | 20 |
| No. with ETEC-associated diarrhea | 5 | 10 |
| Heat-labile enterotoxin | 3 | 6 |
| Heat-stable enterotoxin | 2 | 5 |
| Other bacteria isolated | 0 | 0 |
| Rotavirus demonstrated | 0 | 0 |

rent diarrhea was defined as episodes separated by two or more asymptomatic days.

Thirteen subjects were excluded from the study, seven in the lactobacillus group and six in the placebo group. Four in each group were excluded, because of treatment with antacids. All eight developed diarrhea.

Stool samples from participants with diarrhea were collected with cotton swabs, which were then covered with liquid paraffin in a test tube and stored in a container with liquid nitrogen until microbiological examination could be performed in Copenhagen.

Prophylaxis with lactobacilli significantly reduced the frequency of diarrhea from 71% to 43% in travelers in Egypt ($P=0.019$). The protection rate was calculated to be 39.4%. The mean duration of the diarrheal episodes was similar in the two groups (1.9 vs. 2.2 days). The majority of cases occurred around day 6 in both groups. Seven persons in each group developed diarrhea within 1 week after returning home. In a similar study conducted in 1987 the capsules were administered 1 week before and continued until 4 days after return, resulting in no cases of diarrhea in the lactobacillus group after return and six cases in the placebo group. No adverse effects were recorded in any of the two groups.

Stool samples were obtained from 16 out of 17 cases of diarrhea in the group receiving lactobacilli and from 20 out of 29 cases in the placebo group. ETEC were isolated from 5/16 (31%) and 10/20 (50%) in the two groups, respectively. The difference is not statistically significant. No other bacterial pathogens or rotavirus were demonstrated.

## Conclusion

The concept of probiotics seems to work as prevention of travelers' diarrhea. One capsule containing a lyophilized mixture of *Lactobacillus acidophilus, Bifidobacteria bifidum, Lactobacillus bulgaricus* and *Streptococcus thermophilus* administered three times daily gives a protection rate of 39.4% against travelers' diarrhea in Egypt. The regimen can without risk of adverse effects be recommended to all travelers except those belonging to the "high-risk groups," where the more effective antimicrobial chemotherapeutics should be recommended. In the future more effective species or combinations of species of lactobacilli should be looked for.

## References

1. Black FT, Gaarslev K, Ørskov F, Ørskov J, Stenderup A, Stenderup J, Christensen O (1983) Mecillinam, a new prophlactic for travellers' diarrhoea. Scand J Infect Dis 15:189–193
2. DuPont HL, Ericsson CD, Johnson PC, Cabada FJ (1986) Antimicrobial agents in the prevention of travelers' diarrhea. Rev Infect Dis [Suppl 2]8:167–171
3. DuPont HL, Ericsson CD, Johnson PC, Bilsura JAM, DuPont MW, Cabada FJ (1987) Prevention of travelers' diarrhea by the tablet formulation of bismuth subsalicylate. JAMA 257:1347–1350
4. Sack RB (1986) Antimicrobial prophylaxis of travelers' diarrhea: a selected summary. Rev Infect Dis [Suppl 2]8:160–166
5. Steffen R, Heusser R, DuPont HL (1986) Prevention of travelers' diarrhea by nonantibiotic drugs. Rev Infect Dis [Suppl 2]8:151–159
6. Wiström J, Norrby SR, Burman LG, Lundholm R, Jellheden B, Englund G (1987) Norfloxacin versus placebo for prophylaxis against travellers' diarrhoea. J Antimicrob Chemother 20:563–574

# A Portable Device To Obtain Bacteriologically Safe Water

I. Ebisawa, H. Ohara, and M. Takayanagi

Diarrhea is a common problem for international travelers, and it is not always easy to pinpoint its source. However, drinking water is frequently incriminated as a source of diarrhea, because tube water in many tropical countries is not adequately processed for drinking. We report here a simple portable device which can effectively remove enteropathogenic bacteria from drinking water.

## Materials and Methods

### Structure of the Device[1]

This device weighs 370 g, and measures 10 × 10 × 25 cm. Its filter element consists of a column of silver-activated carbon particles (8 × 3 × 3 cm) and about 950 hollow polyethylene fibers, which are 18 cm long and hang in the upper part of the element. The upper ends of the fibers penetrate a plastic disk, and are fixed so well and tightly that water can reach the exit only through the hollow of the fibers. The water to be filtered is pumped manually upward through the carbon particles and enters into the fibers from outside, and ultimately exits the device through an outlet at the top. The arrows in Fig. 1 indicate the direction of water flow.

The inner diameter of the polyethylene fibers is 260 μm, with a wall thickness of 55 μm. There are many irregularly shaped clefts (about 1000 × 250 nm) in the fiber walls. The device is sterilized using ethylene oxide gas. When the water in the device is contaminated by bacteria, i.e., by *E. coli*, they are trapped outside of the fibers (Fig. 2). Figure 2 shows many clefts in the fiber walls, and more than 20 bacteria which are trapped at its surface.

### Bacterial Strains and Culture Mediums

Six bacterial strains were used in the experiment. They were: *Salmonella typhi*, 0901/w, *Serratia marcescence*, 181, *Vibrio cholerae*, NCTC 4715, *Shigella sonnei*, I, *Salmonella typhimurium*, TMS-2, and *Escherichia coli*, NIH JC-2.

Heart infusion broth and ordinary agar medium (Eiken Co., Tokyo) and Endo's medium (MF-Endo broth, Millipore Co.) were used for preincubation and quantification of these bacteria, respectively.

[1] The device is a product of Mitsubishi Rayon Co., Ltd. and is commercially available under the name "Mashimizu" from Nihon Chemifa Co., Ltd. Tokyo, Japan.

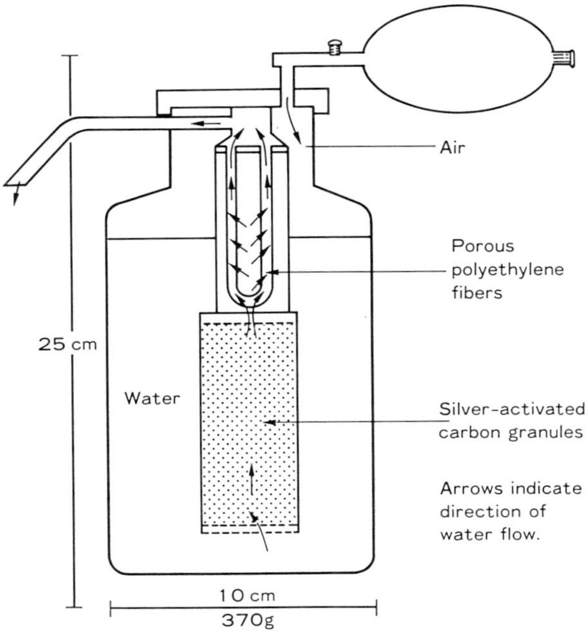


**Fig. 1.** Portable water sterilizer. About 950 porous polyethylene fibers hang in the upper part of the filter element

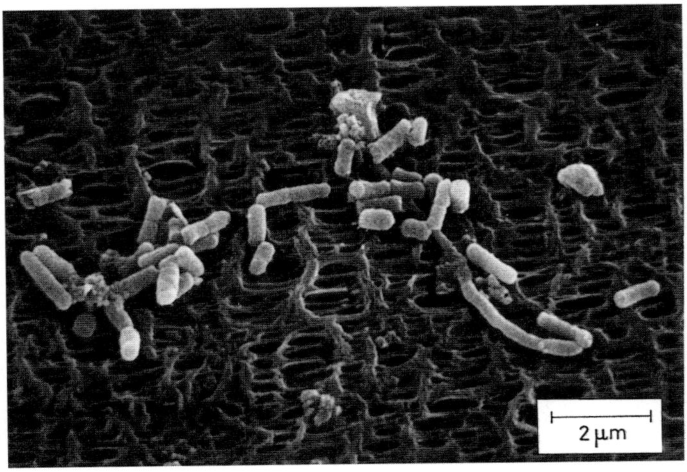


**Fig. 2.** *Escherichia coli* trapped at the surface of a porous polyethylene fiber. A *bar* in the figure indicates 2 μm

A loopful of each bacterial strain was preincubated at 35 °C overnight in heart infusion broth; 1 ml of the broth was diluted in 1 liter sterile water and was used immediately for the experiment. The water was passed through this filter, collected in an Ehrenmeyer flask, and then passed through a millipore filter (Bacteriological Analysis Monitor, 0.45 μm, Millipore Co.). Endo's agar medium was poured onto the millipore filter and the trapped bacteria were counted.

## Results

*Experiment 1. Salmonella typhi, Ser. marcescence, V. cholerae, Sh. sonnei, S. typhimurium* and *E. coli* at densities of 85–720 million colony-forming units/liter water were passed through this device. The filtrate was found to be completely free from all bacterial species (Table 1).

*Experiment 2.* The same experiments were repeated after 50 liter of tap water had been passed through the filter and the device left on a desk for a week. The same six bacterial species, at densities of 80–640 million colony-forming units/liter water, were passed through the filter. The filtrate was again completely bacteria-free.

*Experiment 3.* Fifteen liters of river water was passed through the filter and the device was left standing for a week on a desk. Water containing *E. coli* and *Ser. marcescence*, at densities of 550 and 660 million colony-forming units/liter, was passed through the filter. The filtrate was again completely bacteria-free.

*Experiment 4.* The oral polio vaccine virus was found to pass freely through this filter. Therefore, hepatitis A virus may likewise pass through this filter. However, polio can be prevented by prior administration of either oral or inactivated vaccine, and hepatitis A can be prevented by the administration of human immune globulin. A chemical procedure to remove enteroviruses from the contaminated water is now under study.

**Table 1.** Viable count of bacteria/liter water before and after passage through the water sterilizer

| Bacterial species | Before | After |
|---|---|---|
| *Escherichia coli* | $5.4 \times 10^8$ | 0 |
| *Serratia marcescens* | $7.2 \times 10^8$ | 0 |
| *Salmonella typhi* | $3.5 \times 10^8$ | 0 |
| *Vibrio cholerae* | $8.5 \times 10^7$ | 0 |
| *Shigella sonnei* | $6.2 \times 10^8$ | 0 |
| *Salmonella typhimurium* | $4.0 \times 10^8$ | 0 |

## Conclusion

Although there are limitations to the usefulness of this device, it may help to prevent travelers' diarrhea when safe tube water or boiled water is not available during trips to developing countries.

## Reference

1. Ohara H, Ebisawa I, Takayanagi M (1987) Water-sterilizing capacity of a filter equipped with multi-porous hollow fibers and silver-activated carbon particles (in Japanese). Nettai 20(2):47–54

# Self-Treatment of Uncomplicated Diarrhoea and of Dysentery in Travelers: A Controlled Study

R. Steffen, R. Heusser, A. Tschopp, and H. L. DuPont

Many agents are propagated for self-treatment of travelers' diarrhoea [1–3]. In various previous studies never more than two agents have been compared at one time, and this was usually done only in Mexico. It is, therefore, unknown which agent offers the fastest cure, causes the least side effects, and is effective in all developing countries.

## Methods

A total of 2580 volunteers, ranging in age from 16 to 70 years, travelling to Africa, Asia or Latin America between July 1984 and December 1986, were randomly assigned in double-blind fashion to take bismuth subsalicylate (525 mg every ½ h up to 8 doses/24 h), doxycycline (100 mg twice/24 h), loperamide (2 mg, two capsules initially, plus one after each liquid stool, up to 8 capsules/24 h), mecillinam (400 mg three times/24 h), *Streptococcus faecium* ($75 \times 10^6$ SF 68 three times/24 h), or trimethoprim/sulfamethoxazole (160/800 mg twice/24 h). Each participant was instructed to complete a questionnaire and to take the study medication for 48 h as soon as diarrhoea occurred. Stools were not collected for aetiological assessment.

## Results

The questionnaires of 2098 travelers with a mean gage of $36 \pm 12$ years and an average duration of stay abroad of $19 \pm 7$ days were evaluated. The remaining 422 travelers were excluded, because they cancelled their journey, failed to reply, or their medication was lost, stolen, or given to other travelers. Most travelers experienced no diarrhoea. The trial medication was used by 654 volunteers (31.2%), but 112 were excluded for poor compliance, for taking an additional agent during the trial period, or for contradicting answers. An additional nine volunteers dropped out from the efficacy evaluation, as they ceased to take medication due to side effects. Comparison of the various treatment groups revealed no differences in age, number of previous journeys to the tropics, or characteristics of places where the meals were taken. The countries visited did not differ except for trimethoprim/sulfamethoxazole, which was not given to travelers using pyrimethamine/sulfadoxine for malaria prophylaxis.

**Table 1.** Objective assessment of the proportion of patients (%) cured

| Therapeutic agent | *n* | Time from start of medication to disappearance of all symptoms | | | | Significance to placebo |
|---|---|---|---|---|---|---|
| | | 4 h | 8 h | 24 h | 48 h | |
| Bismuth subsalicylate | 58 | 19.0 | 46.6 | 62.1 | 75.9 | 0.002 |
| Doxycycline | 85 | 11.8 | 29.4 | 63.5 | 87.1 | 0.0001 |
| Loperamide | 94 | 41.5* | 48.9 | 69.1 | 76.6 | 0.0001 |
| Mecillinam | 81 | 11.1 | 29.6 | 60.5 | 80.2 | 0.003 |
| SF 68 | 79 | 12.7 | 25.3 | 43.0 | 67.1 | 0.24 |
| TMP/SMX | 40 | 22.5 | 45.0 | 67.5 | 82.5 | 0.0006 |
| Placebo | 93 | 11.8 | 18.3 | 39.8 | 54.8 | |
| Total | 530 | | | | | |

* $P<0.0001$ compared with the other active agents or placebo

The overall subjective and objective assessment until the resolution of all symptoms gave almost identical results. Loperamide was the fastest-acting agent (Table 1), but by 48 h each of the active test medications had cured about 80% of the patients, with the exception of SF 68, which showed no significant benefit compared with the placebo. In the first 24 h of treatment placebo volunteers voided 4.6 stools, as compared with 3.5 with loperamide ($P<0.01$) and 3.8 with bismuth subsalicylate ($P<0.05$). In the second 24 h each of the active agents except SF 68 significantly reduced the number of stools in comparison with the placebo (1.4–1.7 vs. 2.8 stools, $P\leqq 0.05$).

Dysenteric cases ($n=94$), marked by fever over 37.0 °C and/or bloody stools, were cured after 48 h by any of the three antimicrobial agents in 70%–75% ($n=9$–16), whereas this rate was 53% for loperamide ($n=15$) and 44% each for bismuth subsalicylate ($n=9$) or the placebo ($n=16$) ($P=0.08$ for the sum of all antimicrobials vs. placebo). In the second 24 h of treatment all active agents had a smaller number of unformed stools (range 1.5–2.9) than the placebo (4.0) but this was significant ($P<0.05$) only for any antimicrobial vs. placebo. Side effects were reported in 2.5%–5.5% of the various active treatment groups and in 4.1% of the placebo group. Within the nine patients who ceased to take medication, six claimed that the bad taste of bismuth subsalicylate made them stop. No severe adverse reactions were reported.

## Discussion and Conclusions

Loperamide, bismuth subsalicylate and antimicrobial agents were all significantly superior to the placebo in stopping diarrhoea and accompanying symptoms, mainly abdominal cramps. Loperamide showed a faster action, which was due to its effect in the non-dysenteric cases (82% of all cases); however, in dysenteric cases, loperamide appeared to be less effective than antimicrobial agents, although the numbers here were too small to be significant. Otherwise no significant difference was observed between the agents compared. None of the test medications resulted in severe or more frequent side effects than the placebo. As some 20% of the patients in each group remained sick after 48 h of treatment, further evaluation is necessary in order to assess the cause of the delay and the outcome of these patients.

In view of potential adverse reactions due to antimicrobial agents, loperamide is the first choice for self-treatment of uncomplicated travelers' diarrhoea. In dysenteric cases self-therapy with antimicrobial agents may be considered, as antimotility agents may increase the symptoms [4, 5]. Bismuth subsalicylate, although being less effective, may be considered for self-therapy in both non-dysenteric and dysenteric illness, if one prefers to include only one drug in the travel kit.

## References

1. Ericsson CD, DuPont HL, Johnson PC (1986) Nonantibiotic therapy for travelers' diarrhea. Rev Infect Dis [Suppl 2]8:S202–S206
2. DuPont HL, Ericsson CD, Reves RR, Galindo E (1986) Antimicrobial therapy for travelers' diarrhea. Rev Infect Dis [Suppl 2]8:S217–S222
3. Johnson PC, Ericsson CD, DuPont HL, Morgan DR, Bitsura JAM, Wood LV (1986) Comparison of loperamide with bismuth subsalicylate for the treatment of acute travelers' diarrhea. JAMA 255:757–760
4. Steffen R, Stransky M, Kozicki M (1984) Vorbeugende Maßnahmen gegen Reisediarrhöe. Schweiz Med Wochenschr [Suppl 17]114:35–38
5. DuPont HL, Hornick RB (1973) Adverse effect of lomotil therapy in shigellosis. JAMA 226:1525–1528

# Round Table Discussion

## Future Prospects for the Prevention of Travelers' Diarrhea

H. L. DuPont (Chairman and Rapporteur)

The first speaker was Dr. Klaus Gyr, who spoke on "Future Prevention Concepts and Definition of Risk Population and Miscellaneous Classification of Drugs." Dr. Gyr indicated that a number of populations could be defined which would benefit by receiving chemoprophylaxis to prevent travelers' diarrhea during periods at high risk. Specific entities included those with immunodeficiency syndromes (AIDS), those with low levels of gastric hydrochloric acid (including those taking $H_2$ receptor antagonist), and individuals with disturbed intestinal motility, pancreatic insufficiency and ulcerative colitis. Drugs which have been used to prevent travelers' diarrhea include lactobacillus preparations, bismuth subsalicylate and antimicrobial agents. Drugs which enhance small intestinal motility might well be studied for their favorable effect on gut homeostasis by decreasing the potential for intestinal colonization by pathogens.

Dr. Klaus Plentz discussed "Diet, Food and Beverage as Sources of Travelers' Diarrhea." Dr. Plentz indicated that water supplies in developing countries are often contaminated, either in the ground or in on-premise reservoirs. Food hygiene standards are suboptimal and supervision of kitchen activities is not routinely carried out. The immediate solution for the larger hotels and clubs is to have the tour operators exert influence on these institutions to require adequate hygienic standards following implementation of an educational program. Ultimately, to deal with the difficulty, governments will need to become involved in the control of sanitation and hygiene. In the meantime, the traveler will need to select where and what he eats with care.

Dr. R. Bradley Sack gave a discussion of "Immunoprophylaxis in Travelers' Diarrhea." One of the major arguments supporting the development of vaccines in populations of travelers is that these measures should be effective in controlling endemic disease in the natural population. The other justification is that the attack rate is extremely high in travelers, which translates to great economic costs. The major thrust in immunoprophylaxis is to prevent disease due to enterotoxigenic *E. coli* and strains of *Shigella*. Enterotoxigenic *E. coli* (ETEC) show common toxins; however, the serotypes vary widely, as do the colonization factor antigens important in rendering the strains adherent to intestinal cells. Currently, attempts are being undertaken to use the colonization factor antigens or the binding subunit of the ETEC strains or related cholera antigens as an immunogen. A separate approach is to use passive immunization techniques whereby cow's milk obtained from cattle immunized with ETEC antigens is administered several times a day. This latter approach may not be practical considering the frequency of administration and cost of preparation.

# Sexually Transmitted Diseases, AIDS

# Sexually Transmitted Diseases and Travel

P. Piot

## Summary

Historically, travel has always been associated with casual sexual contacts, and nowadays tourism may be explicitly directed at sexual encounters. This results in an increased risk for various sexually transmitted diseases (STDs), the onset of which may occur after return to the country of residence of the traveler. STDs are associated with considerable morbidity and sequelae such as pelvic inflammatory disease and infertility. Travelers returning from some geographical areas may present with STDs which are unusual in Europe or North America such as chancroid or lymphogranuloma venereum, and may be infected with bacterial strains which are resistant to antimicrobial agents routinely used for treating STDs in the country of residence (i.e., penicillinase-resistant *Neisseria gonorrhoeae*). Travelers should be informed about the risks of acquiring HIV infection and other STDs, and the use of condoms should be recommended to those who may engage in sexual encounters while traveling.

## Introduction

Historically, sexually transmitted diseases (STDs) have been associated with population movements and individual travel. This is even reflected in the terminology of syphilis in the sixteenth century (*"mala franzos ..."*), when continuous unrest and wars undoubtedly contributed to the spread of all kinds of infectious diseases. It is also striking to note that in virtually all nations there has been a continuing tendency to blame the public health problem of STD on foreigners and foreign countries – as if a country's own population were sexually monogamous or abstinent. Immigration laws in many countries include compulsory screening for STDs in candidate immigrants, and STD treatment centers in all seaports have been organized by an international convention.

## Epidemiology

Migrant labor, tourists and businessmen and women nowadays represent high-risk groups for STD. Travel for sex has even become socially acceptable for many parts of the population in Europe and North America, and some destinations are notorious for heterosexual or homosexual sex tourism. However, published data on sexual activity during travel and on the incidence of STD are virtually not available. Among European men working in Central Africa seronegative for the human immunodeficiency virus, 51% and 31% reported extramarital sex with a local woman or with a prostitute, respectively. In the same study, 23% reported an STD during the previous 2 years [2]. Among travelers to developing countries, Steffen et al. [6] reported a 0.7% incidence of genital discharge or ulcer, and an incidence of 330 cases of gonorrhea/100 000 travelers for a stay of 1 month in a developing country. In this study, STD ranked seventh as a health problem after a visit to a developing country.

Travel is not only associated with a higher level of sexual activity, but sexual encounters are also more likely to occur with individuals who are themselves at increased risk for STD or who belong to populations with a high prevalence of STD [3]. In addition, some STDs, such as chancroid, occur mainly in the developing world, and European or North American physicians may not be familiar with their diagnosis and treatment. Finally, bacterial STD agents such as *Neisseria gonorrhoeae* and *Haemophilus ducreyi* more frequently exhibit antimicrobial resistance in many parts of the tropics, as compared with the industrialized world, again complicating patient management.

## Diseases Spectrum and Management

For a detailed discussion of STD, the reader is referred to some recently published books [1, 4, 5]. In general, genital ulcerations are more common in the tropics than in the Western world. In contrast to Europe and North America, where herpes is common, chancroid and syphilis are the leading causes of genital ulcer disease in the tropics.

Patients with genital ulcerations after returning from abroad should be thoroughly investigated for the main known causes, including syphilis, herpes, chancroid and lymphogranuloma venereum (LVG) (Table 1). This may require referral to a specialized centre for STD. Antimicrobial therapy of chancroid has been well evaluated, and single-dose treatment regimens have been developed (Table 2). Tetracycline and sulfonamides are not effective for these indications.

Treatment of gonorrhea acquired in most developing countries should be directed at multiresistant strains of *N. gonorrhoeae*. Indeed, approximately 50% of all gonococcal strains in Africa and Southeast Asia are now penicillinase producing, and a substantial proportion are chromosomally resistant to penicillin or tetracycline or both. Recommended regimens for the treatment of uncomplicated urogenital gonococcal infections acquired in such areas are given in Table 3.

## Prevention

Avoiding casual sex during travel is the most certain way to prevent acquisition of an STD. Though antimicrobial prophylaxis is effective for the prevention of gonorrhea, it is not recommended because of the emergence of antimicrobial resistance among *N. gonorrhoeae* strains. In any case, the magic drug protecting against all the STDs listed in Table 1 does not exist. Condoms, if correctly used, offer protection against STDs, and should be part of the travel

**Table 1.** The most important sexually transmitted pathogens and the diseases they cause

| Agent | Disease or syndrome |
|---|---|
| Bacterial agents | |
| *Neisseria gonorrhoeae* | Urethritis, epididymitis, cervicitis, procties, pharyngitis, conjunctivitis, endometritis, perihepatitis, Barthlinitis, amniotic infection syndrome, disseminated gonococcal infection. Premature delivery and premature rupture of membranes. Salpingitis and related sequelae (infertility, ectopic pregnancy, recurrent salpingitis) |
| *Chlamydia trachomatis* | Urethritis, epididymitis, cervicitis, proctitis, inclusion conjunctivitis, infant pneumonia, otitis media, trachoma and lymphogranuloma venereum, perihepatitis, Bartholinitis, Reiter's syndrome, salpingitis and related sequelae |
| *Mycoplasma hominis* | Postpartum fever, salpingitis |
| *Ureaplasma urealyticum* | Urethritis, low birth weight? Chorioamnionitis |
| *Treponema pallidum* | Syphilis |
| *Gardnerella vaginalis* | Vaginitis |
| *Haemophilus ducreyi* | Chancroid |
| *Calymmatobacterium granulomatis* | Donovanosis |
| *Shigella* species | Shigellosis (sexually transmitted among homosexual men) |
| Group B streptococcus | Neonatal sepsis, neonatal meningitis |
| Viral agents | |
| Herpes simplex virus | Primary and recurrent genital herpes, aseptic meningitis, neonatal herpes with associated mortality of neurological sequelae, spontaneous abortion and premature delivery |
| Hepatitis B virus | Acute, chronic and fulminant hepatitis, with associated immune complex phenomena |
| Cytomegalovirus | Congenital infection: gross birth defects and infant mortality, cognitive impairment, heterophile-negative infectious mononucleosis, protean manifestations in the immunosuppressed host |
| Human papilloma virus | Condyloma acuminata, laryngeal papilloma in infants, cervical cancer |
| Molluscum contagiosum virus | Genital molluscum contagiosum |
| Human immunodeficiency virus | AIDS and related conditions |
| Protozoan agents | |
| *Trichomonas vaginalis* | Vaginitis, urethritis, balanitis |
| *Entamoeba histolytica* | Amebiasis (sexually transmitted especially among homosexual men) |
| *Giardia lamblia* | Giardiasis (sexually transmitted especially among homosexual men) |
| Fungal agents | |
| *Candida albicans* | Vulvovaginitis, balanitis and balanoposthitis |
| Ectoparasites | |
| *Phthirus pubis* | Pubic lice infestation |
| *Sarcoptis scabies* | Scabies |

**Table 2.** Single-dose therapy of chancroid

| |
|---|
| Trimethoprim (160 mg)/sulfamethoxazole (800 mg) four tablets by mouth |
| Ceftriaxone, 250 mg intramuscularly |
| Spectinomycin, 2 g intramuscularly |
| Ciprofloxacin, 200 mg by mouth |

**Table 3.** Treatment regimens for urogenital gonorrhea due to penicillin-resistant strains

| |
|---|
| Spectinomycin, 2 g intramuscularly |
| Ceftriaxone, 250 mg intramuscularly |
| Cefoxitin, 2 g intramuscularly with 1 g probenecid by mouth |
| Cefuroxime, 2 g intramuscularly with 1 g probenecid by mouth |
| Norfloxacine, 800 mg by mouth |

kit of those who may have sexual encounters during their trip. Pre-travel counseling should include information in a nonmoralizing way about STDs and AIDS, about safer sexual practices, and about condom use. Travel agencies, airlines and vaccination centers should actively provide this information to their clients.

## References

1. Arya P, Osoba AO, Bennet J (1987) Tropical venereology. Livingstone, London
2. Bonneux L, van der Stuyft P, Taelman H, Cornet P, Goilav C, van der Groen G, Piot P (1988) Risk factors for HIV infections among European expatriates in Africa. (Submitted for publication)
3. D'Costa LJ, Plummer FA; Bowmer I, Fransen L, Piot P, Ronald AR, Nzanze H (1985) Prostitutes are a major reservoir of sexually transmitted diseases in Nairobi, Kenya. Sex Transm Dis 12:64–67
4. Holmes KK, Märdh PA, Sparling PF, Wiesner PJ (eds) (1988) Sexually transmitted diseases, 2nd edn. McGraw-Hill, New York
5. Osoba AO (ed) (1987) Sexually transmitted diseases in the tropics. Ballière-Tindall, London
6. Steffen R, Rickenbach M, Wilhelm U, Helminger A, Schär M (1987) Health problems after travel to developing countries. J Infect Dis 156:84–91

# International Travel and AIDS

J. M. Mann

## Summary

The global scope of HIV has an impact on international travel. International travelers may be exposed to HIV in three general ways: through sexual contact with an infected person; through receiving blood transfusions; or through receiving injections or other invasive procedures with a contaminated needle/syringe or other skin-piercing instrument. The risk of sexual exposure for travelers may be enhanced by: ignorance about the global epidemiology of HIV or routes of HIV transmission, the escapist psychology of travel, or participation in frank sexual tourism. Specific measures to reduce risks of sexual and parenteral exposure to HIV during travel will be discussed. HIV-Infected persons should be informed about theoretical risks of travel related to immune system activation (infections) or to the immunological impacts of medication, or the fatigue and stress of travel. While these risks are theoretical, they should be considered as part of an individualized programme for health protection of HIV-infected prospective travelers. Travel has certainly contributed in a general manner to the global spread of HIV. However, this is a truism, for excepting transmission through imported blood and blood products, HIV is transmitted directly (sexually) from person-to-person. Fears of travelling, like most fears related to HIV infection, usually result from exaggerated or distorted information about risks of exposure. Sexual contact, the major route of HIV spread worldwide, is under the traveler's personal control. Blood transfusions are rarely needed and HIV-screened blood is increasingly available in developing countries. "Emergency injections" are virtually never required; the time needed to ensure sterilization before injection (usually by boiling) is almost always available. As HIV is not transmitted by casual contact, food, water, or insects, no additional precautions are required. Finally, many governments have considered imposing restrictions on short-term travelers based on HIV status, but most have agreed with WHO's opposition to such measures, as such programmes would, at best and at great cost, slow only briefly the spread of HIV into and within countries. Physicians and others dealing with international travelers have an obligation to ensure that travelers are informed and educated about AIDS, that HIV-infected persons are carefully counselled, and to help ensure that coercive measures to prevent international HIV transmission, of deceptive simplicity and dubious value, are not adopted.

The global scope of infection with the human immunodeficiency virus (HIV) has an important impact on international travel. International travelers may be exposed to HIV infection, travelers have been blamed for international transmission of HIV, and HIV-infected travelers require special counselling. For these reasons, medical and public health practitioners must be aware of the global epidemiology of HIV, of precautions to be recommended to international travelers, and of the social and political dimensions of HIV worldwide.

## Global Epidemiology of HIV

Throughout the world, HIV is transmitted in the same basic ways: through sex or blood and from mother to child. While variations exist regarding, for example, the dominant mode of sexual spread (heterosexual or homosexual), or the principal route of blood transmission (sharing of needles among intravenous drug users or reuse of contaminated needles for medical injections), the fundamental unity of HIV transmission wordwide must be emphasized. In addition, despite intense international scientific scrutiny, no other modes of HIV transmission have been documented and no evidence has emerged to suggest any change in modes of HIV transmission. Finally, there is no evidence to support any inherent racial or ethnic resistance to HIV infection or to the pathogenic effects of the virus.

The pandemic of HIV infection appears to have started during the mid-1970s. The World Health Organization estimates that five to ten million persons have thus far been infected with HIV worldwide.

As of 1 April 1988, a total of 85273 AIDS cases have been officially reported to WHO from 137 countries around the world. Of all reported cases, 73% (62536) are from 42 countries in the Americas, 13% (10995) are from 43 African countries, 13% (10677) are from 27 European countries, and the remaining 1% (1065) are from 25 countries in Asia and Oceania. Fifty countries have each reported more than 50 AIDS cases to WHO, including 18 countries from the Americas, 14 from Europe, 15 from Africa and 3 from Asia/Oceania.

The HIV epidemic is worldwide, yet the current stage of the epidemic is not the same everywhere. Three distinct epidemiological patterns can be described; these patterns appear to reflect the period when HIV may have been introduced or began to spread extensively, the relative importance of the three modes of HIV transmission in the population, and details of sexual and other social risk behaviours.

The first pattern (pattern I) involves western Europe, North America, Australia, New Zealand and some areas in Central and South America. In pattern I, homosexual and bisexual men and intravenous drug users are the major affected groups. Sexual transmission is predominantly homosexual. While heterosexual transmission is occurring and is increasing, it currently accounts for a much smaller portion of sexually acquired HIV infections than homosexual transmission. In pattern I areas, transmission through blood principally involves intravenous drug users. HIV spread through blood or blood products is not a continuing problem, due to screening of blood for transfusion and appropriate treatment of blood products. In pattern I areas, perinatal transmission is uncommon, but is increasing as the number of HIV-infected women rises.

Pattern II areas include most of sub-Saharan Africa and parts of the Caribbean. In these areas, sexual transmission is predominantly heterosexual and therefore the sex ratio for HIV infection is approximately equal. In some urban areas, up to 20%–25% of the 20- to 40-year-old group may be HIV-infected, although substantial intracountry and intercountry variations are observed. Further, up to 90% of female prostitutes in some pattern II areas may be HIV-infected. In pattern II, transfusion of HIV-infected blood remains a problem, as does reuse of non-sterile needles, syringes and other skin-piercing instruments. Finally, as a reflection of heterosexual spread, perinatal transmission is a substantial problem; in some urban areas, 5%–15% or more of pregnant women may be HIV-infected.

Pattern III areas include Asia, most of the Pacific region, the Middle East, North Africa and eastern Europe. In these areas, HIV seems to have appeared more recently, in the early-to-mid 1980s. Most AIDS cases in pattern III areas involve homosexual or heterosexual contact or receipt of imported blood or blood products. In pattern III areas, the prevalence of HIV infection in high-risk behaviour groups, such as male or female prostitutes, is generally very low. However, increasing infection amoung intravenous drug users and prostitutes has recently been documented. Thus, while HIV has not yet penetrated into the general population of pattern III countries, the virus is present and evidence of within-country HIV transmission in increasing.

## Recommendations for International Travellers

In March 1987, the World Health Organization's Global Programme on AIDS (GPA) organized an expert consultation on "International Travel and HIV Infection." The report of this meeting (WHO/SPA/GLO/87.1) stated:

The routes of HIV transmission have been documented to be the same throughout the world. Therefore, the behaviours that put individuals at risk of acquiring HIV are similar worldwide. Preventive measures against HIV are also the same worldwide, regardless of whether the individual is a traveler or a resident of a given country. Educational material should be made available for international travelers to increase awareness of how HIV is transmitted and how it can be prevented ... Such educational material should indicate specific preventive measures, in clear, easily understood language ... it is essential to discuss these sensitive issues openly to protect the international traveler.

In accordance with this recommendation, GPA has produced an informational brochure, "AIDS – Information for Travelers" in conjunction with the World Tourism Organization. This brochure has been distributed to travel agencies, transport companies and national authorities worldwide.

The basic message of this brochure is that no matter where people live or travel, they need to know about AIDS. Sexual contact is the most common route of HIV transmission worldwide. The risk of sexual exposure for international travelers may be enhanced by ignorance about the global scope of HIV infection, the escapist psychology of travel, or participation in frank sexual tourism. However, people can easily protect themselves during their travels by following some simple rules:

1. Do not have sex with prostitutes (male or female) or casual acquaintances, even in countries that may claim there is no AIDS problem. You cannot tell by appearances if someone is HIV infected.

2. If you are going to have sexual relations with someone who might be HIV-infected: remember that vaginal, anal or oral sex can spread AIDS; men should always use a condom, each time, from start to finish and women should make sure their partner uses one; and reducing the number of your sexual partners will lower the risk of exposure to HIV.

The only other route of HIV transmission relevant to international travelers is parenteral. Specifically, exposure could occur through sharing of contaminated needles (self-injecting drug behaviour), receiving a medical injection with a contaminated needle or syringe, having an invasive procedure (surgery, dental) with a contaminated instrument, or receiving an HIV-containing blood transfusion.

The prevention of HIV transmission through self-injecting drug behaviour is the same regardless of geographical location. However, other possible parenteral exposures are directly related to the health care system in each country.

Injections and other skin-piercing practices (tattooing, acupuncture, ear-piercing, dentists' tools) should not create a risk for HIV infection if the following guidelines are followed:

1. Avoid injection and all skin-piercing procedures unless absolutely necessary. Emergency injections are almost never required – the time needed to sterilize the injection equipment can nearly always be taken. Travelers should also realize that most injections are probably not necessary and that other routes of administration, especially oral, may be just as effective.
2. If an injection is needed, make sure either that both the needle and syringe either come directly from a sterile package or that proper sterilizing practices have been observed. A needle and syringe that have been cleaned and then boiled for 20 min are ready for re-use. In general, for skin-piercing instruments, sterilization or high-level disinfection with heat (steam sterilization, dry heat, or boiling) is recommended. Avoid exposure to needles, syringes or skin-piercing instruments that have only been immersed in a chemical disinfectant, as this method is not reliable in field situations.
3. Do not carry your own needles and syringes with you unless you have a doctor's authorization; this is to avoid misunderstandings and legal complications.

Blood transfusions can transmit HIV. While increasingly, blood for transfusion is being screened for HIV contamination throughout the world, screened blood may not be widely available in some areas. The risk of HIV infection through blood transfusion is reduced by taking precautions to prevent serious injury. Most injuries requiring blood involve motor vehicles, so that use of a seat belt, defensive driving and avoiding driving under the influence of alcohol are important precautions. In addition, the need for blood rather than for a volume expander (colloid, crystalloid) must be clearly established. Finally, however, in some situations a blood transfusion may be needed. In this case, screened blood should be sought; today, in most cities worldwide, at least one location providing HIV-screened blood should be available.

## Travelers and International Spread of HIV

In a general manner, travel has certainly contributed to the spread of HIV infections worldwide. Yet this is a truism, for except for transmission through imported blood and blood products, HIV is transmitted directly (sexually, needle-sharing) from person-to-person.

During 1987, many governments considered imposing restrictions on short-term international travelers based on HIV status. The WHO expert consultation on "International Travel and HIV Infection" addressed this question and concluded:

No screening programme of international travelers can prevent the introduction and spread of HIV infection. Therefore ... HIV screening programmes for international travelers would, at best and at great cost, retard only briefly the dissemination of HIV both globally and with respect to any particular country.

During 1987, only one country imposed a requirement for HIV screening for short-term international travelers. However, screening requirements have been developed in some countries for long-term (usually 1 year or longer) visitors, including students, and for immigrants. Finally, some countries restrict the entry of persons ill with AIDS, as they restrict persons with other serious illnesses.

## Travel of HIV-Infected Persons

The expert consultation on "International Travel and HIV Infection" concluded that:

Use of any public conveyance (e.g., train, bus, airplane, boat) by persons infected with HIV does not create a risk of infection for others sharing the same conveyance ... Therefore, there is no specific reason to limit the use of pubic conveyances by HIV-infected persons.

However, the HIV-infected person should be counselled carefully regarding proposed international travel. International travel is stressful (including disturbances of circadian rhythm), involves considerable fatigue, may result in exposure to unfamiliar pathogens, and may require immunizations for health protection and legislative purposes. Finally, clinically ill persons may not be permitted entry into many countries.

## Responsibilities of Health Providers

Physicians and others dealing with the health of international travelers should ensure that travelers are informed and educated about AIDS. The escapist phenomenon associated with international travel must be recognized, for travelers may behave differently during travels compared with their behaviour at home. Fears of traveling related to AIDS usually result from exaggerated or distorted information about risks or routes of potential HIV exposure. Virtually all persons who have become infected during travel have been infected through sexual contact, which is under the control of each traveler.

Finally, it is in the interests of all that coercive measures to prevent international HIV transmission, of deceptive simplicity and extremely dubious value, are not adopted. Health providers dealing with the health of international travelers share the responsibility to prevent such policies from being adopted.

# Tourism and AIDS – The Mauritian Experience

C. Chan Kam

Mauritius is a small island of less than 2000 $km^2$, lying about 1000 km off Madagascar in the Indian Ocean. With a population of one million it is one of the most densely populated countries in the world. Since the mid-1970s, Mauritius has started a love affair with tourism which shows no signs of turning sour. Apart from a few uneasy moments in the early 1980s, the affair has been passionate, with the number of tourist arrivals having steadily increased in the last 5 years and accelerated over the last 2 years. 1987 saw well over 210000 visitors flocking to Mauritius. The forecasts at a seminar on tourism 3 weeks ago were optimistic, with the number expected to top 300000 by 1992.

In economic terms the tourist industry is now the third main source of foreign exchange earnings – over 120 million dollars yearly – after the traditional sugar industry and that other behemoth, the manufacturing industry. A look at the countries which bring us most of our visitors shows that the great majority are from france, Reunion Island (a neighbouring French "departement"), and South Africa. There are increasingly large groups from western Europe, viz. the United Kingdom, Italy, Germany, Switzerland, and a sprinkling from the Far East, Australia, United States, Kenya and Zimbabwe.

Until recently there were no dissenting voices when it came to promoting tourism. An aggressive marketing strategy abroad was accompanied by the rapid development of infrastructures at home. Promoters feel we are still well below the threshold of tolerance as far as accomodation of tourists is concerned. But in the last year or so cautionary, if not dissenting, voices have been heard as the effects of this rapid development have become more tangible, both on our natural environment and socioculturally. Indeed the sociocultural upheavals of the last decade resulting from the changes linked not just to tourism, but specially to the manufacturing industry, have yet to be fathomed.

In the midst of all this we now have AIDS. That many Mauritians now equate the threat of AIDS with tourists or foreigners is increasingly obvious. This simplistic view is fuelled by the official statistics – one case of AIDS and three seropositives. The case of AIDS was a Mauritian, but on the other hand all seropositives identified to date have been visiting foreigners. This public perception of AIDS is also reflected in the stance of some policymakers who are advocating the screening of certain foreign nationals or even all visitors likely to stay more than 1 year. The situation regarding a legal/administrative framework for AIDS is, as in most countries, very fluid and there is as yet no official policy. Needless to say there are some very sound economic reasons why the authorities are handling the matter carefully and it is the unstated unofficial policy not to recommend the screening of international travellers.

But, economy and finance aside, Mauritius has, I feel, deep-rooted commitments to the maintenance of the ideal of individual liberties above all else, and it is this particular attachment, more than the need for pragmatism or realism, which will, I hope, govern future policies. When in addition the cold facts and figures also underline the futility of mass screening and of restrictive or coercive measures I can only conclude that our current approach to tourism and HIV is not only practical but also sound public health policy.

Since the initiation of the official AIDS Prevention Programme a little over 6 months ago we have concentrated our efforts on information and education of OUR population at all levels. We have been careful in not targetting groups but rather in emphasizing the need to avoid high-risk behaviour. This is where the cookie crumbles and where we face our most difficult challenge. I have talked about the social upheavals of the last 10 years and it is quite clear to all of us involved in Health Promotion that, when it comes to sexual behaviour, in particular the gap between information and a change of behaviour and attitudes is enormous. The tourist industry has no doubt played its part in those changes of attitudes and behaviour. We firmly believe, however, that there is no better alternative to continuing and continuous education and information of our population to minimize the impact of HIV through appropriate low-risk behaviour.

In this context we have had awareness sessions with hotel managers, personnel managers and health officers in the tourist industry and we are reinforcing our programme in the hotel sector as well as the general public with the help of trainers in AIDS education whom we trained over the last 4 months. We are also developing our own audiovisual support – videos, radiocassettes, mobile exhibitions, posters, TV spots, and other publicity material. We are also organizing meetings with the media and with elected parliamentarians so as to gain their necessary support in sensitizing public opinion. Indeed the success of our prevention programme will not be measured by the number of AIDS cases or of seropositives but by the changes in attitudes vis-à-vis our visitors and HIV carriers.

Besides information, repeated serosurveys to gauge the prevalence of HIV infection are carried out and hotel employees are regularly included in those, on a voluntary, informed consent basis. The tourism industry has so far been fairly cooperative and, in many cases, hotel management have instituted awareness programmes on AIDS and other STDs for their staff and have made condoms more readily available.

While we believe in relying especially on the informed low-risk behaviour of our nationals at home and in preparing guidance for Mauritians travelling abroad to minimize the spread of HIV, we are also aware that control can only be achieved through *global* cooperation and that similar measures should be taken worldwide. We are preparing material targetted very discreetly at tourists and visitors where we shall seek to emphasize the POSITIVE aspects of HIV in Mauritius, notably the low prevalence.

We are cautiously optimistic, but nonetheless aware, of the very volatile situation. We are therefore prepared to adapt our messages, our policies, our activities to the demands of a changing situation. It is fashionable and necessary these days to talk of ecology and that fragile relationship between man and his environment. Similarly, one can look at tourism and my country. My hope – indeed my sincere belief – is that we can build on the very virtues of the only weapons we have so far against AIDS – tolerance, information and education, responsible behaviour – to strengthen that relationship for the mutual benefit of the tourist and Mauritius. We therefore wholeheartedly support the WHO philosophy and policy about international travel – and, I repeat, not just for selfish economic reasons but because it is also sound public health strategy.

# Prevention of Sexually Transmitted Diseases

R. O. Babalola

Sexually transmitted diseases (STDs) are among the most frequent and widespread infectious diseases despite advances in diagnostic techniques and the availibility of drugs to treat most of the STDs. The STDs include syphilis, gonorrhoea, chancroid, lymphogranuloma venereum, granuloma inguinale, and AIDS.

Many patients with an STD may concurrently have non-specific urethritis, trichomoniasis, genital candidosis, scabies, and pubic infestations.

## Prevention and Control

Prevention and control requires sustained intensive and coordinated efforts from all sectors of society, medical personnel, social agencies, and researchers. Emphasis needs to be placed on prevention, health education, and treatment. Women may effectively be reached through prenatal and family planning clinics. Health education needs to be targeted at high-risk population groups of all ages.

# Heterosexual Transmission of HIV in Northern Italy: Its Incidence Among Travelers

G. Barbarini, T. Gola, G. Trespi, D. Scevola, A. Maccabruni, A. Chiesa, and W. Calderon

Human immunodeficiency virus (HIV) is transmitted primarily during homosexual or heterosexual contact. In fact HIV has been recovered in the semen of AIDS-affected men [4], and semen of healthy carriers of HIV has been shown to transmit HIV infection to female recipients of artificial insemination [6]. HIV has been isolated also from cervical and vaginal secretions of female HIV carriers [7, 8]. Many well-documented examples of heterosexually transmitted HIV infections were presented to WHO by many countries all over the world. The data of WHO demonstrate that heterosexual transmission is the commonest way of transmission of HIV in Africa [5]; in Europe the infection has been clearly established and can be expected to spread. The extent of heterosexually acquired infection can be monitored by detecting HIV prevalence in subjects with known heterosexual contact with persons at risk. Today the real extent of HIV among heterosexual active subjects in Italy is unknown; so it is necessary to pursue systematic epidemiological research and to develop adapted information programmes.

Screening for HIV infection was begun in outpatients attending the Clinic of Infectious Diseases at the S. Matteo Polyclinic, University of Pavia, in April 1985, and is being continued. Two different tests are used: ELISA simultaneously and seropositivity is always confirmed by Western blot. From June 1985 to June 1987 we tested for HIV, to evaluate the patterns of heterosexual risk behaviour, 28 female prostitutes, 96 partners of HIV-positive patients (74 females and 22 males), 155 men who had related their many heterosexual contacts with prostitutes, and 48 travellers coming from countries with a high incidence of seropositivity, with an anamnesis of multiple heterosexual contacts. In the Magenta Hospital (near Milan), as a non-risk population, 3451 blood donors (donors for at least 2 years) were tested for HIV. All the examined subjects were volunteers; so every group may not be a representative standard of the relative population.

HIV seropositivity was found in only one of the 26 prostitutes who had spontaneously come to the day hospital; they were generally middle-aged women (aged 28–43 years) who had been selling themselves for at least 15 years; the social origin of these women was low but they had never used drugs. Of the two young prostitutes, both drug addicts, one was seropositive. Prevalence of seropositivity among heterosexual partners of HIV-positive subjects was 22% among the 74 female partners (mean age 24 years) of infected men and 9% among 22 male partners (mean age 29 years) of infected women. Only

**Table 1.** Blood donors (for at least 2 years) tested in Magenta Hospital

| | Subjects | HIV positive | % positive |
|---|---|---|---|
| Men | 2374 | 2 | 0.08% |
| Women | 1077 | 0 | 0% |
| Total | 3451 | 2 | 0.05% |

1 subject who declared sporadic heterosexual contacts with prostitutes was HIV positive; his contacts were with a Brazilian. Among 3451 blood donors tested in Magenta Hospital we found two seropositive men; they asserted that the only way of transmission of HIV was by heterosexual intercourse (Table 1). We tested 48 male travellers (aged 32–54 years) coming from highly endemic countries, obtaining a positive history for many heterosexual intercourses; the incidence of seropositivity was 8%. Four patients were seropositive for HIV; they came from: the Caribbean (two subjects), Brazil (one subject), and London (one subject). All patients reported sexual intercourse only with coloured women.

Prevalence of seropositivity verified among heterosexual partners of HIV-positive subjects (20%) confirm what has already been reported in the international literature [3]. In Northern Italy, female prostitutes who are not also intravenous drug addicts are not at increased risk for HIV infection. Apart from the seropositive men among travellers reported above, a further three cases have been detected between October 1987 and March 1988. In the absence of effective vaccines or therapeutic agents, the extent of spread of HIV will be determined by the effectiveness of changing the risk behaviour. To obtain this effectiveness will require specially adapted programs of adult education; addiction prevention centers where individuals can find information should be instituted for travellers going to highly endemic countries [1]. Finally it is important to give public policymakers essential information about the approaches to social practices such as prostitution and the condom (an effective barrier against sexual transmission of HIV) which should be recommended to sexually active travellers going to highly endemic countries [2].

## References

1. CDC (1986) Additional recommendations to reduce sexual and drug abuse-related transmission of HTLV III/LAV. MMWR 35:152–155
2. Conant M, Hardy D, Sernatinger J et al. (1986) Condoms prevent transmission of AIDS-associated retrovirus. JAMA 225:1706–1709
3. Fisch MA, Dikinson GM, Scott GB et al. (1987) Evaluation of heterosexual partners, children and house contacts of adults with AIDS. JAMA 275:640–645
4. Peterman TA, Dortman DP, Curren JW (1985) Epidemiology of the acquired immunodeficiency syndrome. Epidemiol Rev 7:1–21
5. Piot P, Plummer FA, Mhalu FS et al. (1988) AIDS: an international perspective. Science 1239:573–579

6. Stewart GJ, Tyler JPP, Cunningham AL et al. (1985) Transmission of human T-cell lymphotropic virus Type III (HTLV III) by artificial insemination by donor. Lancet II:581–585
7. Vogt MW, Witt DJ, Craven DE et al. (1986) Isolation of HTLV III/LAV from cervical secretions of women at risk for AIDS. Lancet I:525–527
8. Wofsy CB, Cohen JB, Haver LB et al. (1986) Isolation of AIDS associated retrovirus from genital secretions of women with antibodies to the virus. Lancet I:527–529

# Prevalence of HIV, HBV, HDV and HAV Markers in Pregnant Women in Indonesia

R. Vranckx, A. Alisjahbana, W. Devillé, W. Ngantung, E. Sugita, A. Sukadi, A. Usman, and A. Meheus

Hepatitis B virus (HBV) infections are still a public health problem in Southeast Asia. Despite improvements in hygiene, hepatitis A virus (HAV) infections still prevail in the most densely populated areas of the developing world [4]. Little is known about the spread of HIV infections in Asia. Only a number of isolated cases of AIDS have been reported from Thailand, Japan and some islands of the South Pacific [8]. In order to evaluate the prevalence of antibodies to these infections in Indonesia, we tested sera from pregnant women living in the Bandung area. Additionally, in the HBsAg-positive sera, anti-hepatitis Delta virus was assessed.

## Material and Methods

*Population.* Almost 2000 sera were collected in 1986 and 1987 during a prevalence study of HBV markers in pregnant woman at two hospitals in Bandung.

*Laboratory Tests.* HBsAg, anti-HBS and anti-HBc was determined by RIA (Abbott). Anti-HBe, HBeAg and anti-HBc/IgM was determined by RIA (Medgenix). Samples for anti-HD testing were selected on the basis of HBsAg positivity. Anti-HD was determined by RIA (Medgenix). The screening for anti-HA (total) was determined by EIA (Abbott). The sera positive for anti-HA (total) were tested for anti-HA/IgM by EIA (Abbott). Anti-HIV screening was determined by EIA (Medgenix), and positive results were confirmed by EIA Envacore (Abbott) and W. B. (Medgenix).

## Results

*HBV Markers.* The mean age of 300 pregnant women screened for HBV markers was 26 years, with a range of 17–42 years. Prevalence of HBV markers was 4.7% for HBsAg, 26.0% for anti-HBs (with or without anti-HBc) and 9.7% for anti-HBc alone. Two women were positive for all three markers. Almost 60% (59.7%) was seronegative for HBV markers. The prevalence of HBV markers increased from 19.1% in the 15- to 19-year-old group to 52.9% in the group of women aged 35 and over. HBeAg was found in 64.3% of HBsAg-positive women and anti-HBe in 35.7%. Anti-HBc/IgM was present in 2 out of the 14 HBsAg positive sera.

*HDV Markers.* One hundred and thirty HBsAg-positive sera were screened for anti-HD; all the results were negative. Most of these HBsAg-positive women were chronic carriers (anti-HBc/IgM negative).

*HAV Markers.* We tested 331 sera for anti-HA (IgG and IgM) and anti-HA (IgM); 376 (98.4%) were positive for anti-HA (IgG and IgM), and none was positive for anti-HA (IgM).

*HIV Markers.* We screened 1918 sera from pregnant women. Thirty-seven were positive in the screening but they were all false positive because none of these positive results could be confirmed by the confirmation tests.

## Discussion

The results of HBV serology found in this study are intermediate to higher for the Southeast Asian region. Much higher rates have been reported in Taiwan [2] and in some parts of Indonesia [6]. Similar HBsAg prevalences in pregnant women have been observed in other parts of Indonesia [1] and in nearby Singapore [3]. In our survey HBV marker prevalence increased with age. This might be explained by two convergent tendencies. HBV infection could be decreasing in younger generations because of improving hygienic conditions [4]. On the other hand, there might be an increasing risk with age; this would imply important parenteral and nonparenteral transmission mechanisms in adulthood.

Knowledge of the epidemiology of the HDV infection is very scarce in many parts of the world. Despite the high prevalence of HBV infection in Southeast Asia, HDV infection does not appear to be a significant problem in this area of the world. Markers of HDV infection are in some regions very frequent (e.g., parts of China); in other regions they are almost absent (e.g., Taiwan) [5, 7]. Although HBsAg is frequent in Bandung we could not find any anti-HD positive results. From these data it can be concluded that HDV infection has not yet been introduced in that densely populated area of Indonesia.

Seroepidemiological data provide meaningful indices of the worldwide distribution and specific epidemiological characteristics of HAV infections. The age patterns of anti-HAV prevalence clearly depend on the level of endemicity and on the degree and rate of change in prevailing socioeconomic, hygienic and housing conditions during recent decades [4]. Our data on anti-HA prevalence (98.4%) in a young adult population strongly indicate that HAV infection is predominantly a childhood disease in Indonesia.

The absence of anti-HIV among 1918 controlled sera from pregnant women strongly indicates that HIV infection has not yet been introduced into the general population of West Java, Indonesia. But a surveillance system for the infection should be started immediately, in order to be able to implement control measures.

## References

1. Bandaso R, Nielsen AL, Ury F (1985) The prevalence of HBsAg among pregnant women in Ugung Pandang Indonesia. Acta Med 15:231–134
2. Beasley RP, Trepo C, Stevens CE, Szmuness W (1977) The e antigen and vertical transmission of hepatitis B singore antigen. Am J Epidemiol 105:94–98
3. Chan SH, Tan KL, Goh KT, Tsakok M, Oon CJ, Ratnam SS (1988) Material – child hepatitis B virus transmission in Singapore. Int J Epidemiol 14:173–177
4. Papaevangelou GJ (1987) Epidemiology of hepatitis A and B. Infection 15:221–227
5. Rizetto M, Gerin JL, Purcell RH (1987) The hepatitis delta virus and its infection. Prog Clin Biol Res 234
6. Van der Veen J, Padmodiwirgo S, Basuki L, en Jansz S (1973) Hepatitis B (Australië) – antigen bij gezonde personen in Indonesië. Ned T Geneeskd 117:1961–1964
7. Wang DQ, Cheng HH, Minuk GY, Anand CM, Stowe TC, Wang HX, Ying DC et al. (1987) Delta hepatitis virus infection in China. Int J Epidemiol 16:79–83
8. (1987) Acquired immunodeficiency syndrome (AIDS): global data. Weekly Epidemiol Rec 19:137

# Round Table Discussion

# AIDS – Do Travelers Need Specific Recommendations?

B. Somaini (Chairman and Rapporteur)

Tourism is not going to change dramatically because of AIDS. Suddenly confronted with the AIDS problems, short sporadic outbursts of tourists changing their plans have occurred with tourists perceiving of natives as special risks and natives looking at incoming tourists as being hazardous to their health. Only consistent, clear and direct information worldwide can lead to a solution: information, education, tolerance and responsible behavior are keywords also with respect to tourism.

The way AIDS is transmitted is the same the world over. Therefore, appropriate behavior at home should also be observed abroad. Most infections result from sexual contact. Therefore, AIDS information to travelers is necessary, for every casual sex partner can be dangerous. If one cannot abstain from sexual encounters then the use of a good reliable condom can minimize the risk. This applies especially to volunteers working in developing countries. Experience shows that the HIV infection is rather frequent in this group. It has been established that the overwhelming majority of these cases result from heterosexual contact with a number of unknown partners in the foreign country. In the case of Belgian volunteer workers no infections have been found among their children even though these children spent extended periods in high HIV areas and had extensive contact with native children. All volunteer workers have to be informed clearly about the ways this infection is transmitted and about protective measures.

When drug addicts travel abroad they should never exchange syringes. If they carry a supply of sterile equipment with them this of course can lead to problems during security checks. So it may be advisable to tell such people they should procure their supplies locally. HIV has spread throughout the world mainly through sexual contact and through the use of contaminated injection material.

Many travelers are disturbed about the prospect of acquiring AIDS through a blood transfusion. When discussing this problem, it is necessary to pay attention to the fact that any transfusion which is not really necessary should be avoided. It is possible today even in Third World countries to find alternatives to blood transfusions. The ultimate goal is to provide noncontaminated blood not only for tourists, but also for the indigenous population. In various countries where blood transfusions are systematically screened this goal has almost been reached within the last 2 or 3 years. In the larger cities worldwide all blood is being tested for HIV before being used.

Accidental contact with someone else's blood also worries many travelers. Statistics show that accidental injuries to medical personnel with HIV-contaminated blood poses a very small infection risk (0.1%–1%). Although such accidental contact cannot be theoretically be excluded, the chances of infection are incredibly small. All personnel dealing with blood on a regular basis, e.g., volunteer health workers, should observe the same hygienic standards that apply in industrialized countries. Whether or not to undergo surgery or childbirth in a foreign country has to be decided personally. The HIV situation is only one element in such a decision. People who reside abroad for long periods are able to learn about the health care in their particular host country and make their decision based on this information. In emergency cases, however, there may be little choice. The same incidently is true for dental treatment, which may be undertaken if standards of hygiene are observed. In many cases consumer pressure has turned out to be more effective than theoretical information, that is to say the patient himself insists on the correct use of hygiene.

In principle, there are no justifiable travel restrictions for health reasons for HIV-positive people. There are speculations about which cofactors cause AIDS to progress. Infections are naturally in the foreground. Therefore HIV-infected travelers should avoid infectious diseases like malaria, diarrhea and parasitical illnesses. Prophylactic medication should be recommended according to individual cases. As of now there are not enough epidemiological data to confirm such speculations. Preliminary studies in Africa show that vaccinations do not have more side effects with HIV-positive patients than with HIV-negative ones. A vaccination should therefore be administered if the individual risk situation allows it.

Restrictive measures by an entire country cannot therefore be based on epidemiological reasons. Why should not an AIDS-infected son be able to reenter the country in which his father is working? However, certain restrictions are already in force in several countries. While they contribute little to containing the spread of AIDS, they lead to enormous problems, for example, compulsory screening at the border. Who should be tested and how often? Should commuters be tested daily on their way home from work each day? Who would store the data and the names of the tested people? Neither the testing nor the screening is inherently bad, it is the way they are used.

At this congress a lot of time was spent discussing why people are traveling more. AIDS will hardly change this situation "People want to get loose and free of the normal social pressure – freedom of the normal constraints!" Fun and Well-being – those are the buzz words. To assure that wellbeing health advisors, such as doctors and medical consultants, are called responsible. We must advise people so that well being can be maintained even in this age of AIDS.

# Various Infections and Intoxications

# Pilot Study of the Potential Benefit of Tocainide in the Management of Ciguatera Toxicity *

W. R. Lange and S. D. Kreider

Ciguatera is a variety of food poisoning associated with the consumption of contaminated marine fish. It is the most common foodborne illness due to a chemical toxin and is characterized by a rather distinctive complex of gastrointestinal, neurologic, and cardiovascular symptoms [1]. The neurologic manifestations of the syndrome tend to occur in the majority of symptomatic individuals, and they invariably are the most bothersome [2–4]. In protracted cases, paresthesias may persist for months, or even years.

Ciguatera is a complex ecological problem, and one of appreciable public health and economic importance in many areas of the world. It has actually been a factor in limiting economic development in some areas of the Third World [5]. The condition exists in a broad circumglobal belt extending from 35° north to 35° south latitude and is endemic throughout most of the Caribbean and Indo-Pacific islands [1]. Toxicity occurs on occasion in the United States; the annual incidence in Miami is estimated to be at least 5 cases/10000 resident population [6]. A small epidemic occurred in Vermont in late 1985 as a result of contaminated fish shipped from Florida [7]. The condition is not reportable, and it is vastly underdiagnosed and frequently misdiagnosed. Even though the syndrome is a greater health threat to the indigenous population residing in high-risk regions of the world, it is periodically a cause of illness in tourists and other international travelers.

Treatment of ciguatera has always been symptomatic, supportive, and, for the most part, unsatisfactory. Recently, amitriptyline has been suggested as a remedy [8], but its benefit has been inconsistent.

The responsible agent, ciguatoxin (CTX), is a lipid-soluble, heat-resistant, acid-stable toxin produced by a single-celled, free-swimming marine dinoflaggelate, *Gambierdicus toxicus*. This organism appears to proliferate in response to natural and man-made damage to tropical and near-tropical reefs. CTX has been shown to be a novel type of $Na^+$ channel toxin [9] which opens voltage-dependent sodium channels in the cell membrane, notably within nerve and muscle tissue. Local anesthetics such as lidocaine work in a manner opposite that of CTX. They block conduction by decreasing or preventing the large transient increase in the permeability of the membrane to sodium ions [10]. This would suggest that lidocaine-like drugs might be efficacious in the management of ciguatera toxicity. Lidocaine has been effective in countering some

* Parts of this paper originally appeared in the *American Journal of Medicine*

**Table 1.** Case reports

| Case | Patient | Primary symptoms[a] | Duration of symptoms | Suspected | | Clinical response to | |
|---|---|---|---|---|---|---|---|
| | | | | Fish | Location | Amitriptyline | Tocainide |
| 1 | 45 y/o WF | 1, 2, 3, 5, 6, 8 stable | 4.0 years | Red snapper | Tortola | No benefit | Improvement |
| 2 | 44 y/o WM | 1, 2, 3, 5, 6, 9 stable | 2 months | Grouper or pompano | Bahamas | No benefit | Improvement |
| 3 | 41 y/o WM | 2, 3, 4, 5 stable | 15 months | Red snapper | Miami or Haiti | Not used | No definite improvement |
| 4 | 38 y/o BM | 2, 3, 5, 8 improving | 5 months | Grouper or red snapper | Southwest United States | Moderate relief with high dose | Improvement continued, no apparent benefit |
| 5 | 53 y/o WM | 2, 4, 5, 7 improving | 6 months | Red snapper or sea bass | Dominican Republic | No benefit | Improvement continued at faster pace |

[a] Symptoms: 1. Chronic GI distress; 2. Paresthesias, lower extremity; 3. Paresthesias, circumoral; 4. Pruritis; 5. Hot to cold temperature dysesthesia; 6. Weakness; 7. Joint, muscle pain; 8. Headache/dizziness; 9. Chills

of the cardiovascular effects of CTX [11], and we investigated the potential benefit of tocainide, an orally effective lidocaine analogue, in attenuating the protracted neurologic symptoms in five patients with chronic toxicity.

## Case Reports

Five cases of ciguatera toxicity, three of which were health care providers, volunteered to participate in an open-label pilot study intended to assess the potential efficiency of tocainide in reducing symptoms. The drug was administered 400 mg, three times daily with meals, and symptoms were reassessed after 2 weeks. Four of the patients were male and one was female (Table 1), and all had paresthesias as a principal complaint. All had hot-to-cold temperature dyesthesias, which many regard as being pathognomonic of ciguatera toxicity. In addition, three participants reported that their symptoms worsened following alcohol ingestion, and this is another hallmark of the disorder.

The duration of symptoms ranged from 2 months to 4 years. One case was contracted in the southwest United States, likely the result of the transcontinental shipment of contaminated fish, and the rest were most likely contracted during travel to the Caribbean. Red snapper and grouper were most often the fish incriminated. These tend to be the predominant vectors in the Caribbean, whereas amberjack is reported to be the most common cause in Hawaii [1].

Amitriptyline was not reported to be efficacious at the dose generally recommended, 25 mg twice daily [8]; however, tocainide appeared to attenuate the symptoms in three of the five cases. The drug was well tolerated with no apparent side effects. Two subjects whose condition was stable reported improvement on tocainide; another stable patient reported no benefit. Of two subjects with gradually improving symptoms, one felt that rate of improvement increased, the other did not.

## Discussion

In this open-label uncontrolled trial, tocainide was well tolerated and appeared to alleviate symptoms of ciguatera in the majority of participants without any apparent side effects. The cases in this report were not randomly selected, and both they and their physicians went into the trial in an unblinded and potentially biased fashion. Consequently, there could have been a strong placebo or Hawthorne effect.

The therapy, which does not appear to have been previously tested, appears specific and warrants further investigation. Nevertheless, in spite of the potential benefit, widespread use of this treatment modality may be limited because of the potential side effects that have been associated with tocainide therapy [12]. We conclude that tocainide may effect a diminution of the neurologic symptoms in select patients with ciguatera toxicity.

## References


1. Lange WR (1987) Ciguatera toxicity. Am Fam Physician 35(4):177–182
2. Bagnis R, Kuberski T, Laugier S (1979) Clinical observations on 3900 cases of ciguatera (fish poisoning) in the South Pacific. Am J Trop Med Hyg 28:1067–1073
3. Morris JG, Lewin P, Hargrett NT, Smith W, Blake PA, Schneider R (1982) Clinical features of ciguatera fish poisoning. A study of the disease in the US Virgin Islands. Arch Intern Med 142:1090–1092
4. Gillespie NC, Lewis RJ, Pearn JH et al. (1986) Ciguatera in Australia. Occurrence, clinical features, pathophysiology, and management. Med J Aust 145:584–590
5. Lewis ND (1986) Disease and development: ciguatera fish poisoning. Soc Sci Med 23:983–993
6. Lawrence DN, Enriquez MB, Lumish RM, Maceo A (1980) Ciguatera fish poisoning in Miami. JAMA 244:254–258
7. CDC (1986) Ciguatera fish poisoning – Vermont. MMWR 35:254–264
8. Davis RT, Villar LA (1986) Symptomatic improvement with amitriptyline in ciguatera fish poisoning. N Engl J Med 315:65
9. Bidard JN, Vijverberg HPM, Frelin C et al. (1984) Ciguatoxin is a novel type of $Na^+$ channel toxin. J Biol Chem 259:8353–8357
10. Ritchie JM; Greene NM (1980) Local anesthetics. In: Gilman AG, Goodman LS, Gilman A (eds) The pharmacological basis of therapeutics, 6th edn. MacMillan, New York, p 301
11. Legrand AM, Lotte C, Bagnis R (1985) Respiratory and cardiovascular effects of ciguatoxin in cats; antagonistic action of hexamethonium, atropine, propranolol, phentolamine, yohimbine, prazosin, verapamil, calcium, and lidocaine. In: Gabrie C, Salvat B (eds) Proceedings of the Fifth International Coral Reef Conference, Tahiti, vol 4. Antenne Museum-ephe, Moorea, pp 463–466
12. Arrowsmith JB, Creamer JI, Bosco L (1987) Severe dermatologic reactions reported after treatment with tocainide. Ann Intern Med 107:393–396

# Brucellosis in Travelers and Brucella That Travels

E. J. Young

Zoonoses are diseases of animals that are transmissible to humans. Of the more than 250 communicable diseases affecting man, more than 80% are zoonoses. Worldwide, brucellosis ranks high among serious zoonotic diseases, and in some countries, especially in developing nations, the incidence of human brucellosis has reached epidemic proportions [1].

Brucellosis occurs in both wild and domestic animals, but the majority of human infections are the result of direct contact with domestic or semidomestic animals raised for meat or milk.

The genus *Brucella* consists of six recognized species and their biovars; of which four species (*B. abortus, B. melitensis, B. suis* and *B. canis*) are known to be pathogenic for man. Brucellosis is transmitted by direct contact with diseased animals, their secretions and carcasses, or via the ingestion of unpasteurized dairy products from infected animals. Humans are always accidental hosts, playing no role in maintaining the disease in nature.

The skin is the most common route by which brucellosis is transmitted to man, with organisms gaining entry through small cuts and abrasions contaminated with the blood or secretions of infected animals. Other less common routes of transmission include the conjunctival sac, the upper respiratory tract and the mucosa of the gastrointestinal tract.

Persons whose occupation or avocations place them in close contact with animals are at greatest risk of contracting brucellosis. This includes farmers, abattoir workers, veterinarians, meat inspectors and laboratory personnel. In contrast to direct contact with diseased animals, brucellosis acquired from the ingestion of contamined foods (principally dairy products) is generally not occupation related and often involves women and children who have no contact with animals. In addition, food-borne brucellosis can occur in travelers to brucella-endemic areas, especially if they partake of local delicacies, and in persons residing in brucella-free areas from imported foods, such as fresh cheeses [2].

*Brucella* can survive in milk products for varying periods of time and survival in cheese is dependent upon such factors as the type of cheese, its moisture content, salt content, pH, temperature, the age of the cheese and the biochemial effects of other saprophytic microorganisms that may be present (Table 1) [3]. Since the low pH of human gastric juice provides some protection against ingested microorganisms, persons taking antacids or histamine-blocking drugs such as cimetidine appear to be at increased risk of contracting brucellosis by the oral route [4, 5].

**Table 1.** Survival of *Brucella* in cheeses

| Cheese | Species | Survival time |
|---|---|---|
| Various types | *B. abortus* | 6–57 days |
| Feta | *B. melitensis* | 15–100 days |
| Pecorino | *B. melitensis* | 4–16 days |
| Roquefort | *B. abortus* | 60 days |
| Eritrean | *B. melitensis* | 44 days |
| White | *B. melitensis* | 1–8 weeks |

**Table 2.** Goat cheese associated human brucellosis in Texas

| Year | No. cases/annual total | Location |
|---|---|---|
| 1968 | 6/unknown | El Paso |
| 1973 | 15/34 (44%) | El Paso |
| 1983 | 29/84 (35%) | Houston |
| 1985 | 9/47 (20%) | Laredo |

**Table 3.** Human brucellosis cases 1983–1987

| | |
|---|---|
| Total cases confirmed | 57 |
| *Brucella* species | |
| *Brucella melitensis* | 25 |
| *Brucella abortus* | 6 |
| *Brucella suis* | 4 |
| *Brucella canis* | 1 |
| Unidentified | 21 |
| Travel to brucella-endemic country | 15 (26%) |
| Goat cheese ingestion during travel | 9 (60%) |
| Total with goat cheese exposure | 22 (38%) |
| Goat cheese ingestion without foreign travel | 13 (59%) |

*Brucella melitensis* was eliminated from native animals in the United States in 1972; yet there have been at least four outbreaks of human brucellosis caused by this species in the state of Texas since 1968 (Table 2). Although three of these outbreaks occurred in cities on the Texas/Mexico border (northern Mexico is known to be an endemic area for brucellosis in goats), the outbreak that occurred in 1983 involved patients in Houston, a city some 450 miles from the border. These outbreaks were all linked to unpasteurized goat's milk cheese obtained either during travel to Mexico, or imported illegally into the United States [6–8].

Between 1983 and 1987 we studied the sera of more than 250 patients suspected to be suffering from brucellosis in addition to the patients involved in the 1983 and 1985 outbreaks. On the basis of epidemiologic, clinical and laboratory data the diagnosis of brucellosis was confirmed in 75 cases (Table 3). Twenty-five cases had positive cultures for *B. melitensis* and 15 patients gave a history of travel to a brucella-endemic area (primarily Mexico) shortly before the onset of symptoms. Of these 15 travelers, 9 admitted to consuming locally produced goat's milk cheese (queso blanco). In all, 22 patients gave a history of goat cheese consumption, of whom 13 (59%) denied foreign travel. In these cases, like those from previous outbreaks, cheese was imported from a brucella-endemic area.

The risk for travelers of infections such as diarrhea, malaria, hepatitis, typhoid fever, and sexually transmitted diseases is well recognized and widely publicized [9, 10]. The risk of contracting brucellosis is perhaps lower, but nonetheless serious [11]. As the incidence of animal brucellosis increases in many countries, the risk of infection to humans increases. In addition, *Brucella* contaminating apparently fresh cheese can travel to areas where brucellosis is rare, presenting an increasing challenge to clinicians everywhere.

## References

1. Mousa ARM, Elhag KM, Khogali M, Marafie AA (1988) The nature of human brucellosis in Kuwait: study of 379 cases. Rev Infect Dis 10:211–217
2. Young EJ (1983) Human brucellosis. Rev Infect Dis 5:821–842
3. Stiles GW (1945) Brucellosis in goats. Rocky Mt Med J 42:18–25
4. Steffen R (1977) Antacids – a risk in travelers brucellosis? Scand J Infect Dis 9:311–312
5. Editorial (1978) Antacids and brucellosis. Br Med J 1:739–741
6. Seyffert WA, Bernard JA (1969) Brucellosis: report of six cases. Tex Med 65:47–52
7. Young EJ, Suvannoparrat U (1975) Brucellosis outbreak attributed to ingestion of unpasteurized goat cheese. Arch Intern Med 135:240–243
8. Thapar MK, Young EJ (1986) Urban outbreak of goat cheese brucellosis. Pediatr Infect Dis 5:640–643
9. Steffen R, Rickenbach M, Wilhelm U, Helminger A, Schar M (1987) Health problems after travel to developing countries. J Infect Dis 156:84–91
10. Anonymous (1987) Advice for travelers. Med Lett 29:53–56
11. Arnow PM, Smaron M, Ormiste V (1984) Brucellosis in a group of travelers to Spain. JAMA 251:505–507

# Kala-azar Imported to the Federal Republic of Germany 1943–1980

E. Vanek and L. Knaus

Kala-azar is the visceral form of leishmaniasis caused by the protozoon *Leishmania donovani*, endemic in several parts of the tropics and subtropics. There are three main foci where tourists from central Europe may contract this disease, which is fatal for non-immunes: India and East Africa, but also the Mediterranean (Fig. 1), where kala-azar is a significant, but not predominant, disease with about 500 cases/year among the indigenous population (Stürchler 1981). The infection occurs there only in places suitable as biotopes for sandflies of the genus *Phlebotomus*, which transmit the infecting agent from its main reservoir – dogs and foxes – to man. The sandfly prefers dark and moist breeding habitats, such as old masonry and caves, and being unable to fly over longer distances it sticks to these places, flying only near the ground. Unfortunately many of our tourists prefer to spend their holidays in old farmhouses, bungalows, camping places and tents. It takes only a few hours by plane, or a day's journey by car, to reach the beaches of the Mediterranean Sea in Italy or Yugoslavia. The automobile – favoured by families with children and/or dogs – also allows tourists to choose their own camping site. Many of them prefer to stay in houses offered for rent, in their own caravan or even in tents on camping places – in any case as near as possible to the ground. In 1976/1977 more Germans spent their holidays abroad than in their own country: 19.7 mil-

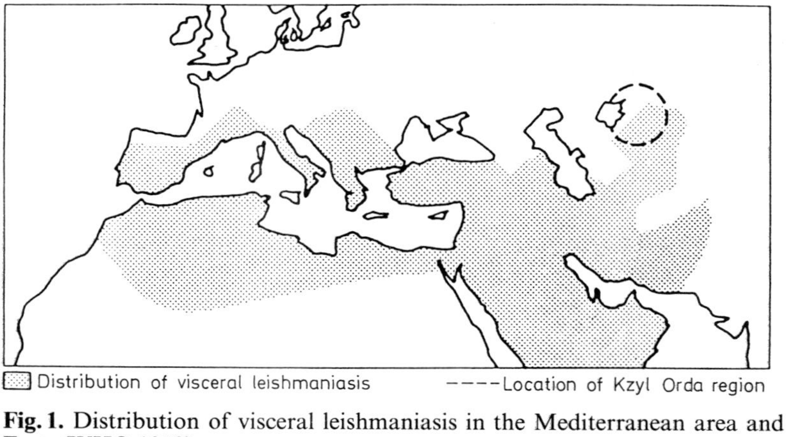


**Fig. 1.** Distribution of visceral leishmaniasis in the Mediterranean area and the Near East. (WHO 1979)

lion vs. 16.41 million. Seventy percent of these almost 20 million went to the Mediterranean region of Europe and Africa. One-third of the tourists were children under 14 years of age (Reeb 1978).

In 1976/1977 we were confronted with three cases of kala-azar in the space of 2 years. The clinic of the university of Ulm covers a rather rural area with a population of about a million. This raised the question of why kala-azar is not seen more often in hospitals in the larger towns of our country. During the 38 years between 1943 and 1980 no more than 53 cases of kala-azar were discovered in the Federal Republic of Germany and 42 of them were evaluated by Knaus (1985), with the following results: 34 of the 42 evaluable patients were of German nationality, 2 were Austrians, 1 was a Greek working in Germany and infected during vacations in his homeland, 5 were children of foreign labourers coming from Mediterranean countries and infected during a visit in their homeland: Italy, Yugoslavia and Spain. *Outcome:* Five of the 42 died; in 3 of them kala-azar was diagnosed postmortem, in two others shortly *ante finem*. Thirty-four were males, 8 were females.

There were two peaks in the *age distribution:* the under fives and adults between 20 and 30. *Reason of travel:* 3 of the 42 were soldiers or prisoners of World War II in southern France, northern Africa or Albany. After the war there is a gap of 2 decades. The new wave of tourism started in the mid-sixties with the arising prosperity (*Wirtschaftswunder*). Twenty-six out of 29 were tourists.

The infections were acquired throughout the whole of the Mediterranean. Benidorm on the Costa Brava in Spain and the island of Elba are the only places with a cluster of four and seven cases, respectively. The *exposure* lasted 2–4 weeks in 16 out of 32 cases, the shortest being 3 days in a child. The shortest *incubation period* lasted less than 3 weeks, the longest more than 2 years, there being no correlation between incubation period and the age of the patient. *Initial symptoms* of the 42 analysed cases: Fever and hepatosplenomegaly were the major signs of kala-azar. In 5 of the 42 cases the full-blown picture developed under immunosuppressive treatment with corticosteroids.

## Laboratory Findings

The sedimentation rate reached 50–100 mm (Westergreen) in the 2nd hour in 90% of all cases. In 95% there was anemia, in 87% leukopenia, and in 100% thrombozytopenia. The total globulin level in the serum was normal or elevated in 21 out of 25 of our cases. Electrophoresis showed a pronounced dysproteinemia: low albumin level, highly increased immunglobulins chiefly the alpha-1- and the gamma-globulins, and in these the IgG more than the IgM globulins. These antibodies are imperfect, non-protective and therefore unable to eliminate the parasite and other infecting agents – which finally succeed and cause the patient to die. The effective immune response in kala-azar is cell mediated, and impeded by the *L. donovani* proliferating in the immunoreactive tissues as the disease proceeds. The *diagnosis* of kala-azar was established by demonstration of the *L. donovani* in 32 out of the 42 cases (76%), in 28 of them ante- and in 4 postmortem. Serological findings were positive in 27 cases (64%).

## Conclusions

Kala-azar is endemic in the Mediterranean area, and it is unknown to most physicians in central Europe. The indigenous population acquires an immunity during childhood, kala-azar being mainly a disease of children in this area. Tourists spending their holidays there are not immune and are therefore susceptible to this infection. It runs a fatal course in most if not diagnosed and treated.

Kala-azar should be taken into consideration in any case of long-lasting, remittent or periodic fever and a history of travelling in the Mediterranean during the preceding 2 years, irrespective of season. The incubation period may even be longer than that, and as short as 10 days.

Modern serological methods allow a preliminary diagnosis, which should be confirmed by the isolation or demonstration of the infecting *L. donovani* in specimens of bone marrow or in biopsies of the liver or spleen. Only experienced laboratories, i.e. those of tropical institutes, should be used for the diagnostic procedures, not the lab around the corner.

## References

Knaus L (1984) Importierte Kala Azar in Deutschland. Thesis, University of Ulm

Leupold DM Wild M, Vanek E, Kleihauer E, Fabel U, Kosenow W (1979) Leishmaniosis visceralis (Kala azar). Padiatr Prax 21:643–652

Reeb A (1978) Urlaubs- und Erholungsreisen 1976/1977. Bundesgesundheitsblatt 18:225–232

Stürchler D (1981) Endemiegebiete tropischer Infektionskrankheiten. Huber, Bern

WHO (1979) Receptivity to malaria and other parasitic diseases. Report on a WHO-Working Group, 11–15 Sept 1978, Izmir. WHO Regional Office for Europe, Copenhagen EURO reports and studies no 15

# Acute Schistosomiasis in *Schistosoma haematobium* Infection

P. C. Stuiver

As an imported disease acute schistosomiasis (Katayama fever) is typically a condition of the uninformed, inexperienced traveller [1] or the more adventurous type taking part in certain expeditions [2]. With the enormous increase of people travelling to the tropics it was to be expected that the number of patients with acute schistosomiasis would rise accordingly [1]. Since the first experience with this syndrome in our hospital in 1982, twenty patients have been recognized, all them infected with *Schistosoma mansoni*. It has been stated that this syndrome is seldomly [3–5) if ever [2, 6, 7] seen in primary infection with the species *S. haematobium*. However, recently we have observed six patients with severe acute schistosomiasis caused by *S. haematobium*.

## Patients and Methods

Criteria for the diagnosis of acute schistosomiasis were: a history of first exposure to contaminated water; symptoms and signs consistent with the clinical picture of the disease [1]; laboratory confirmation, including positive serology (IFA > 1 : 16, ELISA > 1 : 32); and the demonstration of living eggs of *S. haematobium* in urine, stools or rectal mucosa. Other infectious diseases with a similar clinical picture were excluded by appropriate laboratory investigations.

## Results

An outbreak of acute schistosomiasis occurred among a group of 17 Dutch travellers who had made a trip on *fellukka* sailing boats on the river Nile. On 23 July 1985, 15 of the 17 participants swam in the Nile at Luxor. Several months later ten swimmers (66%) appeared to have been infected with a *Schistosoma* species according to a positive schistosomal serology. Five were also parasitologically positive. In the latter cases exclusively *S. haematobium* eggs were found. Four patients (three excreting numerous eggs of *S. haematobium* and one only serologically positive) suffered from Katayama fever. In addition we have seen two patients with acute schistosomiasis due to *S. haematobium* who contracted the disease after they had joined the local people swimming in a river in Benin.

The incubation time varied from 14 to 50 days, the length of illness from 14 to 119 days. There was no distinction as to manifestations, clinical variety or severity between these six patients with acute schistosomiasis due to *S. haematobium* and our patients with this syndrome caused by *S. mansoni*.

## Discussion

Acute schistosomiasis is an exotic disease of increasing importance in travellers. Although the clinical manifestations may vary considerably from general malaise to a very protean and severe illness, the most constant and conspicious feature is eosinophilia. A history of travel to Africa or to another endemic area in a patient with an obscure illness should alert the clinician to the possibility of an acute helminthic infection in general and that of acute schistosomiasis in particular. Eosinophilia is an important characteristic and should be the clue to a correct diagnosis. In the prepatent period before eggs are being excreted schistosomal serology is diagnostic, but these tests are not generally available.

Our observations prove that the syndrome of acute schistosomiasis also occurs in *S. haematobium* infections and that the clinical picture is similar to that of the other *Schistosoma* species. Most impressive in our series of six patients were the long-lasting fevers, persistent unproductive cough, lassitude, exhaustion and loss of body weight.

While safe and effective schistosomicidal drugs are available, they lack evaluation in acute schistosomiasis. Arguably, these drugs should be given with caution during that period, because of the possible sudden release of antigens that are believed to induce the acute syndrome. Occasional observations have reported a beneficial effect of corticosteroids on the severe toxaemic phenomena and the clinical deterioration after chemotherapy [8, 9].

Travellers to the tropics must be aware of the dangers of water-based diseases such as schistosomiasis, which is prevalent where defective sanitation is combined with the presence of fresh water weed and the snail vector. In this age of mass tourism tour operators bear a special responsibility. They should not play down the risk of swimming at the local beauty spot. On the contrary it is their duty to prevent schistosomiasis by appropriate information of their clients.

In order to ensure the health of travellers it is necessary to develop international policies and regulations for the most optimal information about exotic diseases to be provided for by travel agencies.

## References

1. Stuiver PC (1984) Acute schistosomiasis (Katayama fever). Br Med J 228:221–222
2. Istre GR, Fontaine RE, Tarr J, Hopkins RS (1984) Rafting the Omo River, Ethiopia. JAMA 251:508–510
3. Ritchken J, Gelfand M (1954) Katayama disease, early toxaemic stage of bilharziasis. Br Med J 2:1419–1420
4. Parasitic disease surveillance (1983). Weekly Epidemiol Rec 2:9–11
5. Rollinson D, Simpson AJG (eds) (1987) The biology of schistosomes. Academic Press, New York, p 202

6. Case records of the Massachusetts General Hospital (1985). N Engl J Med 312:1376–1383
7. Manson-Bahr PEC, Bell DR (1987) Manson's tropical diseases. Baillière-Tindall, London, p 458
8. Monson MH (1987) Praziquantel in acute schistosomiasis. Trans R Soc Trop Med Hyg 81:777
9. Farid Z, Mansour N, Kamal K et al. (1987) The diagnosis and treatment of acute toxaemic schistosomiasis in children. Trans R Soc Trop Med Hyg 81:959

# African Trypanosomiasis in American Travelers: A 20-Year Review

R. T. Bryan, H. A. Waskin, F. O. Richards, T. M. Bailey, and D. D. Juranek

African trypanosomiasis, commonly known as African sleeping sickness, results from blood and tissue invasion by protozoal parasites of the genus *Trypanosoma*. Transmitted by the bite of the tsetse fly, the disease is endemic to certain areas of sub-Saharan Africa. Two forms of this disease are classically described and both progress from an early or hemolymphatic stage to a later stage with central nervous system invasion. Gambian or West African trypanosomiasis is a chronic infection that exists primarily in riverine areas of west and central Africa. It tends to occur in residents of riverside villages and is rarely a threat to travelers. In contrast, the Rhodesian or East African form is an acute and fulminant febrile illness. It occurs in scattered foci throughout the savannas of eastern and southern Africa [1–3]. As tsetse flies are common in the game parks of these regions, game-viewing travelers may be at risk for this serious and potentially fatal condition [1, 4, 5].

## Materials and Methods

In the United States, medications used in the treatment of trypanosomiasis are distributed by the Parasitic Disease Branch of the Centers for Disease Control (CDC). Consequently, cases treated in the United States are usually known to our branch and ten of the cases reported here were attended at the bedside by branch physicians. Case information was obtained from the following sources: hospital records, CDC case investigation records, and published case reports.

## Results

### Epidemiology/Risks

From 1967 through 1987, 15 American travelers were treated in the United States for East African trypanosomiasis [6–14]. Ages ranged from 19 to 74 years (mean = 49 years). Males outnumber females by a ratio of 2 : 1. Although patients' backgrounds and occupations were diverse, most (11 of 15) were participating in organized photographic or hunting safaris.

Compared with malaria and diarrheal illnesses, African trypanosomiasis appears to occur rarely in American travelers [15, 16]. Limited game park visitation data, however, make accurrate risk assessment difficult. Nevertheless,

**Table 1.** Risk factors

| Duration of exposure | Month of exposure | Country of exposure |
|---|---|---|
| Range: 2–28 days | Jan (2) | Kenya (1) |
| Mean: 14 days | Mar (2) | Malawi (1) |
| | May (1) | Sudan (1) |
| | Jun (1) | Zambia (1) |
| | Jul (2) | Zimbabwe (1) |
| | Aug (3) | Botswana (3) |
| | Sep (2) | Rwanda (3) |
| | Nov (2) | Tanzania (4) |

estimates indicate that travel to East African destinations has increased dramatically. For example, in 1979, 31 000 Americans departed Nairobi. By 1986, that figure had almost doubled to approximately 60 000 [Economic Survey, Central Bureau of Statistics, Kenya]. The increasing popularity of adventure-oriented African tours supports the assumption that many of these Americans are visiting game parks. It is not surprising, therefore, that the number of trypanosomiasis cases treated in the United States has doubled from the five cases seen from 1967 through 1977 to ten cases seen in the past decade.

For our 15 cases, risk factors other than exposure to tsetse flies were not identified (Table 1). Duration of travel was not a risk factor as the time spent within endemic areas was often minimal. Likewise, illness developed throughout the calendar year and no specific month or season was associated with an increased liklihood of infection. Finally, although Rwanda, Tanzania, and Botswana were most frequently identified as sites of tsetse exposure, data reflecting the total numbers of travelers to these areas are unavailable. We must conclude, therefore, that the risk for human trypanosomiasis is likely to exist in all tsetse endemic foci regardless of the duration of travel or the time of year that travel takes place. Limited data make accurate quantification of that risk impossible.

## Clinical Characteristics

Estimated incubation periods ranged from 6 to 28 days, with 12 patients (80%) noting symptom onset within 14 days of a memorable tsetse bite. Among presenting signs and symptoms, fever was universal and cutaneous manifestations were common (Table 2). Ten patients had lesions consistent with a trypanosomal chancre. Although not invariably present, the chancre is often the earliest clinical sign of this disease and has been observed in 50%–90% of reported cases [3, 19]. Typically, the chancre first appears as an area of tender, erythematous induration. The lesion then subsides over a period of 2–3 weeks during which time crusting and desquamation develop [1, 11].

Rashes were noted in seven patients. The trypanosomal rash tends to be a nonpruritic, erythematous, macular eruption. Although sometimes circinate in character, the rash can be evanescent and difficult to appreciate [11, 18].

**Table 2.** Presenting signs and symptoms

| Sign/symptom | Number (%) |
|---|---|
| Fever | 15 (100%) |
| Rash/skin lesions | 12 (80%) |
| Lethargy/malaise | 10 (67%) |
| Headache | 7 (47%) |
| Gastrointestinal complaints | 7 (47%) |
| Confusion/personality changes | 6 (40%) |
| Myalgias | 5 (33%) |

The gastrointestinal symptoms noted here were nonspecific, but prominent presenting complaints. The 47% frequency was unusually high as compared with other published reports in which these symptoms are rarely mentioned [6, 13].

Although six patients exhibited changes in mental status, only two had documented trypanosomal invasion of the central nervous system. These findings suggest that confusion and personality changes can occur early and that such symptoms do not necessarily reflect progression to the later or central nervous system stage of this disease [18].

Within 7 days of symptom onset, 14 patients (93%) had seen a physician. Time required for correct diagnosis ranged from 2 to 15 days. In all cases, diagnosis was confirmed by the demonstration of trypanosomes in Wright-stained peripheral blood smears and/or cerebrospinal fluid. Hemolymphatic disease was diagnosed in 13 cases. Diagnostic delays of 10 and 15 days in two patients were associated with central nervous system involvement. This observation is consistent with previous reports and suggests that diagnostic delays may result in the unnecessary progression to central nervous system invasion [14, 18, 19].

Treatment with suramin resulted in clearing of parasitemia and defervescence in all patients. Adverse reactions were minimal. One patient, however, developed urticaria, dizziness, hypotension, and bradycardia. Successful management with hydrocortisone allowed subsequent doses of suramin to be administered uneventfully. The two patients with central nervous system involvement required treatment with the arsenical compound melarsoprol. One patient did well, but the other developed ataxia, increased weakness, and tremor – symptoms consistent with reactive encephalopathy. Treatment was stopped and symptoms resolved.

Overall, adverse reactions to therapy were outweighed by the serious morbidity of the disease itself. Lengths of hospitalizations ranged from 6 to 32 days and intensive care unit support was often required. Transient elevations of hepatic transaminases were common (ten patients or 67%) as was thrombocytopenia (ten patients or 67%). Two patients developed disseminated intravascular coagulation. Coagulation abnormalities eventually resolved and rapid treatment of the underlying parasitemia appeared to be the most effective means of reversing the sometimes severe coagulopathy [7].

Nine (60%) patients exhibited some form of renal dysfunction. Renal impairment, however, also resolved with antitrypanosomal therapy. The fact that renal function improved during treatment with suramin is an important point in that this medication is considered to be nephrotoxic [1]. Our experience suggests that suramin can be given with the expectation that renal impairment will resolve rather than worsen during the course of therapy.

Other significant clinical findings included anemia (nine patients), leukopenia (seven patients), and hyponatremia (three patients). Also of note were two patients who developed cardiac decompensation and hypoxia. Cardiopulmonary complications may arise prior to central nervous system involvement and are the most frequent cause of death in patients with East African trypanosomiasis [4].

Despite these complications, all 15 patients reported here recovered from their acute illness and no relapses occurred. No fatal cases have been reported in patients treated in the United States in the past 20 years. There is little doubt that rapid diagnosis and prompt therapy have contributed to the absence of fatalities in these patients because, if not recognized and treated, this disease is almost invariably fatal [4, 19].

## Prevention

Safe and effective chemoprophylaxis for East African trypanosomiasis is not available [1]. Hence, the best protection for travelers would be to avoid tsetse fly habitats. This may be difficult, however, for those persons who have, at considerable expense, traveled to Africa to view or hunt wild game. For these travelers, knowledge of tsetse fly behavior may help in the implementation of personal protective measures.

Tsetses are large, gray-brown flies that are active only during daylight hours. Visually, they are attracted to bright or contrasting colors [1]. Furthermore, the heat, dust, and motion of vehicles such as Land Rovers and vans appear to be strong attractants to the savanna species. Many travelers have reported being bitten repeatedly while riding in such vehicles [CDC, unpublished data]. Tsetses are also known to bite despite the presence of insect repellant and their sturdy proboscis often enables them to bite through clothing. Nevertheless, personal protective measures may be helpful. Dull-colored, ankle and wrist length clothing made of heavier weight fabric is recommended as is the liberal use of insect repellant. Questioning local inhabitants about how best to avoid known tsetse-infested areas and encouraging tour operators to install air-conditioning or window screens in their vehicles may also be helpful.

Finally, visitors to endemic areas should be educated as to the early symptoms of African trypanosomiasis and be encouraged to seek medical attention promptly should symptoms develop. Furthermore, patients should always inform their physicians of their travel histories and exposure to tsetse flies.

## References

1. World Health Organization (1986) The African trypanosomiases. WHO Tech Rep Ser 739
2. Baker JR (1982) African trypanosomiasis. In: Steele J (ed) Parasitic zoonoses, vol 1. CRC Press, Boca Raton, p 121 (CRC handbook series in zoonoses)
3. Willett KC (1974) African human trypanosomiasis. In: Woodruff AW (ed) Medicine in the tropics. Livingston, London
4. Eyckmans L (1985) *Trypanosoma* species (African sleeping sickness). In: Mandell G, Douglas J, Bennett J (eds) Principles and practice of infectious diseases. Wiley Medical; New York, p 1537
5. Spencer HC (1984) African trypanosomiasis. In: Strickland GT (ed) Hunter's tropical medicine. Saunders, Philadelphia, p 553
6. Spencer HC, Gibson JJ, Brodsky RE, Schultz MG (1975) Imported African trypansosmiasis in the United States. Ann Intern Med 82:633–638
7. Barrett-Connor E, Ugoretz RJ, Braude AI (1973) Disseminated intravascular coagulation in trypanosomiasis. Arch Intern Med 131:574–577
8. Centers for Disease Control (1969) An outbreak of African sleeping sickness among Americans on safari – United States. MMWR 18(44):385–386
9. Centers for Disease Control (1970) African trypanosomiasis – California. MMWR 19:233–234
10. Centers for Disease Control (1983) African trypanosomiasis. MMWR 32(8):112–113
11. Cochran R, Rosen T (1983) African trypanosomiasis in the United States. Arch Dermatol 119:670–674
12. Perera D, Donovan DL, Stroud GM, Schultz MG (1969) Imported African sleeping sickness. JAMA 209:270
13. Ginsberg R, Ackley A, Stoner E, Lee L (1986) African sleeping sickness presenting in an American emergency department. Ann Emerg Med 15:86–88
14. Quinn TC, Hill CD (1983) African trypanosomiasis in an American hunter in East Africa. Arch Intern Med 143:1021–1023
15. Lobel HO, Roberts JM, Somaini B, Steffen R (1987) Efficacy of malaria prophylaxis in American and Swiss travelers to Kenya. J Infect Dis 155:1205–1209
16. Black RE (1986) Pathogens that cause travelers' diarrhea in Latin America and Africa. Rev Infect Dis [Suppl 2]8:S131–S135
17. Gelfand M (1966) The early clinical features of Rhodesian trypanosomiasis with special reference to the "chancre" (local reaction). Trans R Soc Trop Med Hyg 60:376–379
18. Duggan AJ, Hutchinson MP (1966) Sleeping sickness in Europeans: a review of 109 cases. J Trop Med Hyg 69:124–131
19. Gear JHS, Miller GB (1986) The clinical manifestations of Rhodesian trypanosomiasis: an account of cases contracted in the Okavango swamps of Botswana. Am J Trop Med Hyg 35:1146–1152

# Three Cases of Cutaneous Diphtheria in Travelers to Africa

W. Höfler, W. Heizmann, E. Höring, C. Junga, G. Kusch, and F. Weidner

Skin lesions caused or secondarily invaded by *Corynebacterium diphtheriae* are common in children in tropical countries, being a major reservoir of the organism and leading to early acquisition of immunity. Therefore, travelers living in close contact with the indigenous population are at risk of contracting the disease.

As far as is known from publications and an inquiry addressed to 21 countries, 24 cases of skin diphtheria have been observed in Europe during the years 1964–1986, at least 14 of them being imported from tropical countries. These figures may be an underestimate since many physicians are not familiar with the disease. In this context, it may be justified to report three clustered cases we have seen in October 1987.

## Case Reports

Three young males on a trekking tour in northwest Africa (Algeria, Burkina Faso, Algeria) suffered from skin ulcers beginning about 5 weeks before their return to Germany. They had frequently stayed overnight in the houses of indigenous people. The first patient was seen on 15 October 1987 at the Institute of Tropical Medicine in Tübingen. He was also the first of the group to develop ulcers on his feet and hands. He remembered that a few days before he noticed his ulcerations, he had treated children in Mali for similar lesions with a topical disinfectant. At the examination he showed two small residual ulcers, originally 2 cm in diameter, on the proximal joints of his big toes with dirty secretion, several smaller ones on both hands, and on the back of his left hand a scabbed scratch mark with a livid, infiltrated centre. Blood sedimentation rate and other laboratory findings were normal. A direct smear stained with methylene blue showed besides other bacteria clubbed rods suggesting *Corynebacteria*. The clinical suspicion was confirmed by the isolation of *Corynebacterium diphtheriae* type mitis together with $\beta$-haemolysing streptococci. Toxin could be demonstrated by ELEK-agargel precipitation. The second patient was admitted 4 days later. On both his feet near the ankles were ulcers 1 cm in diameter with dirty discharge and slightly undermined and partially inverted margins, and an older scar nearby with a depressed centre and several smaller, nearly healed lesions. *Corynebacterium diphtheriae* was isolated together with *Staphylococcus aureus*, but toxin could not be demonstrated. BSR was 15/33; other laboratory findings were inconspicious.

The third patient was traced by the health authorities. He showed several healing wounds covered with scurf on his lower legs, an oval ulcer measuring 3 by 1 cm with raised, partially inverted margins over the right tibia and three just healed lesions on both thumbs. *Staphylococcus aureus* and toxinogenic *Corynebacterium diphtheriae* were isolated. BSR was 13/38; other laboratory findings normal.

On the advice of the health authorities, the three patients were isolated in two different hospitals. According to the antibiogram they were treated for 6–8 days with 8–12 mg penicillin; the two patients with *Staphylococcus aureus* additionally received flucloxacillin and cefotaxim, respectively. Gentian violet was applied topically.

Although there are contradictory opinions on the indication for antitoxin treatment, we decided on the application of antitoxin since the possibility of toxic complications, although rare in primary cutaneous diphtheria, cannot be excluded. In the case of the first patient Diphuman Berna was available. With this human immunoglobulin lower doses (1200–20000 IU) are needed and the duration of protection (3–4 weeks) is longer than with heterologous serum.

All ascertained contacts received two doses of toxoid vaccine. The patients were discharged after 10–14 days, the lesions being completely or largely healed and wound, throat and nasal swabs negative for *C. diphtheriae*.

## Conclusions

Slowly healing ulcers in travellers under primitive living conditions should arouse the suspicion of skin diphtheria. The main differential diagnosis is ecthyma streptogenes: punched out lesions without raised or inverted margins. A preliminary diagnosis can be made by a direct smear but has to be confirmed by culture. It is advisable that travellers planning a journey with probable close contact with the indigenous population receive a diphtheria toxoid vaccination which is readily compatible with all other vaccinations. It should be realized, however, that the vaccination does not prevent *Corynebacterium diphtheriae* from invading wounds and that such an infection may be a source of transmission.

## References

1. Belsey MA, Leblanc DR (1975) Skin infections and the epidemiology of diphtheria: acquisition and persistence of *C. diphtheriae* infections. Am J Epidemiol 102:179–184
2. Fleischer K, Köhler B, Pöllath M, Hof H, Kraus A (1987) Hautdiphtherie aus Afrika. Dtsch Med Wochenschr 112:884–886
3. Gunatillake PDP, Taylor G (1968) The role of cutaneous diphtheria in the acquisition of immunity. J Hyg 66:83–88
4. Kwantes W (1984) Diphtheria in Europe. J Hyg 93:433–437

# Screening for Pulmonary Tuberculosis Among the Expatriates Entering the Socialist People's Libyan Arab Jamahiriya

M. T. Elghul and S. S. Abounaja

Tuberculosis is still one of the major public health problems in the developing countries. The first attempt to assess the magnitude of the problem of pulmonary tuberculosis in Libya was made in 1959 with WHO assistance in one of the eastern provinces of Libyan Arab Jamahiriya. The survey revealed the prevalence of bacteriologically confirmed cases of pulmonary tuberculosis to be 1.83% [4]. Subsequently, in 1976–1977, a National Tuberculosis Prevalence Survey was undertaken with technical support from WHO. The findings of this study revealed the prevalence of X-ray positives to be 2.5% and prevalence of bacteriologically confirmed cases to be 1.6/1000. It also noted that 22% of the total newly diagnosed cases were from immigrants [4].

Due to the massive influx of immigrants there is always a risk of importing the infection for the native population. Thus, in order to reduce the pool of tuberculosis infections and to protect the home population from the disease carried by immigrants, all foreigners are subject to prospective screening for pulmonary tuberculosis. This includes mandatory investigation of chest X-rays and among the X-ray positives further bacteriological examination of sputum (microscopy and culture). It is only after this screening that a foreigner is issued a residence visa. In order to check further transmission of the disease those found to be positive for pulmonary tuberculosis are sent back to their respective countries for necessary treatment. Therefore the present study was undertaken with the limited objective of assessing the magnitude of the problem of pulmonary tuberculosis among the expatriates entering Libya.

The records of Gurji Chest Clinics, Tripoli, constituted the material for the present study. In all, the screening tests performed on 20 336 expatriates during the period January to October 1987 were analyzed.

The majority of expatriates entering Libya who were screened for pulmonary tuberculosis in the study clinic were from Europe (37.29%), Africa (34.53%) and Asia (27.54%) and very few from America Australia (Table 1). The overall prevalence of X-ray positive shadows suspected to be of pulmonary tuberculosis was 0.99%, 0.91% and 0.77% among the immigrants from Europe, Africa and Asia respectively.

These X-ray positives, numbering 182, were further subjected to sputum smear microscopy and sputum culture. The results showed (Table 1) that the overall infectious pool, i.e., sputum positivity rate, was 0.19%, and continent-wise breakdown of sputum bacteriology revealed that the prevalence of sputum positivity was highest in African entrants (0.47%) compared with Asians (0.07%) and Europeans (0.03%).

**Table 1.** Distribution of expatriates screened for pulmonary tuberculosis according to different continents (January–October 1987)

| Continents | Expatriates examined | | X-ray positives | | Sputum positives | |
|---|---|---|---|---|---|---|
| | No. | % | No. | % prevalence | No. | % prevalence |
| Africa | 7023 | 34.53 | 64 | 0.91 | 33 | 0.47 |
| Asia | 5601 | 27.54 | 43 | 0.77 | 4 | 0.07 |
| Europe | 7584 | 37.29 | 75 | 0.99 | 2 | 0.03 |
| America | 125 | 0.61 | – | – | – | – |
| Australia | 3 | 0.01 | – | – | – | – |
| Total | 20336 | 100 | 182 | 0.89 | 39 | 0.19 |

**Table 2.** Distribution of phage types of *M. tuberculosis* isolates from pulmonary tuberculosis patients of Libya

| Phage type | Batch I | Batch II |
|---|---|---|
| A | 84% | 53% |
| I | 11% | 25% |
| B | 3% | 21% |

The sex-wise distribution of sputum positives showed that there were 31 males (79.5%) and 8 females (20.5%). Furthermore the records of the chest clinics were also examined for nonpulmonary tuberculosis. It was thus observed that out of 235 nonpulmonary tuberculosis cases reported in the year 1987, 213 (90.6%) were Libyans as compared with 22 (9.4%) expatriates.

In previous studies [1–3] the susceptibility of *Mycobacterium tuberculosis* to lytic activity of mycobacteriophage was used as a constant criterion for epidermiological study of strain variation in *M. tuberculosis* isolates from pulmonary cases of Libyan patients. In reporting the differences in major types (Table 2), it became apparent that alterations had taken place during the 3-year time interval during batch 1 period (September 1976–June 1977) and that of batch II (January–June 1979). There was an increase in phage type "B" and "I", whereas phage type "A" showed considerable decline. The bacteriophage pattern of *M. tuberculosis* isolates from pulmonary cases of expatriates during 1979 demonstrated that phage types "I" and "B" were in contrast in certain nationalities; in Asians three out of four strains were type "I", whereas in Egyptians three out of four strains were type "I", whereas in Egyptians three out of four strains were type "B". Taking these together the influence of expatriates upon the native populations might suggest the hinderance to a certain extent of the control program for tuberculosis.

## References

1. Elghul MT, Grant J (1981) Mycobacteria phage typing techniques applicable to Libyan *M. tuberculosis* isolates. IRCS Med Sci 9:1098–1099
2. Elghul MT, Grant J (1981) Phage pattern variations in Libyan *M. tuberculosis* isolates, residence and expatriates. IRCS Med Sci 9:1158–1159
3. Grant J, Elghul MT (1981) Variation in lytic mycobacteriophage susceptibility among *M. tuberculosis* isolates of Libyan origin. IRCS Med Sci 9:1100–1101
4. Park JE, Zaheer M, Aly HK (1982) A short text book on community medicine. McDougall, Edinburgh, p 94–95

# Primary Amebic Meningoencephalitis

J. G. Gustavo dos Santos Neto

Primary amebic meningoencephalitis is a rare disease, 139 cases having been described worldwide so far. The chances that a traveler acquire it are remote; yet the organism is thermophilic, and the use of thermal baths (this was the source of infection of the New Zealand cases) may present a threat.

The author witnessed 11 of the 16 cases described in Richmond, Virginia. Four cases were uncovered during a retrospective autopsy survey. The disease mimics bacterial meningitis and this diagnosis is favored. Gram-stained smears as well as culture of cerebrospinal fluid are negative for bacteria. Antibacterial therapy fails. Although seeing the movement of the "Naegleria" amoeba and the culture of the same, which is the sine qua non, are the procedures of choice, the unfamiliarity of most physicians with the disease leads to these procedures not being performed.

Yet cerebrospinal fluid smears manually prepared for differential white cell count stained with Wright's stain (Fig. 1) or preferably Giemsa stain (Fig. 2) reveal the organism clearly even retrospectively.

At autopsy the brain reveals a hemorrhagic component which is greater than the inflammatory component. Numerous amebas are usually seen in nests in the perivascular spaces yet occasionally (our cases 5 and 9) they are scarce.

The infection is acquired by aspirating hot contaminated water into the nose during swimming and diving, placing the head under water faucets or simply aspirating hot contaminated water.

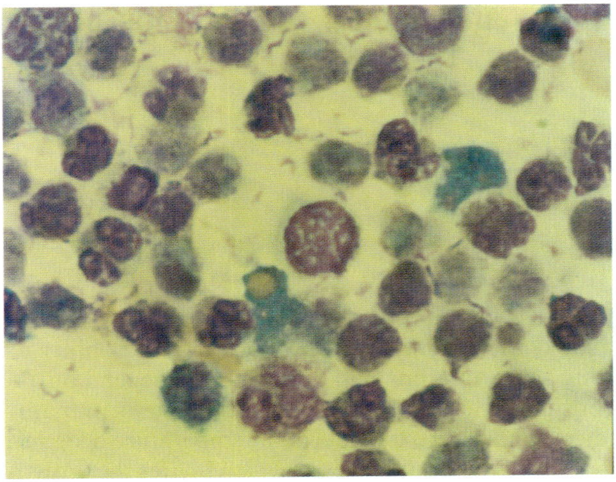

**Fig. 1.** Cerebrospinal fluid sediment stained with Wright's stain. Two amebas easily seen among inflammatory cells (oil immersion, ×1000)

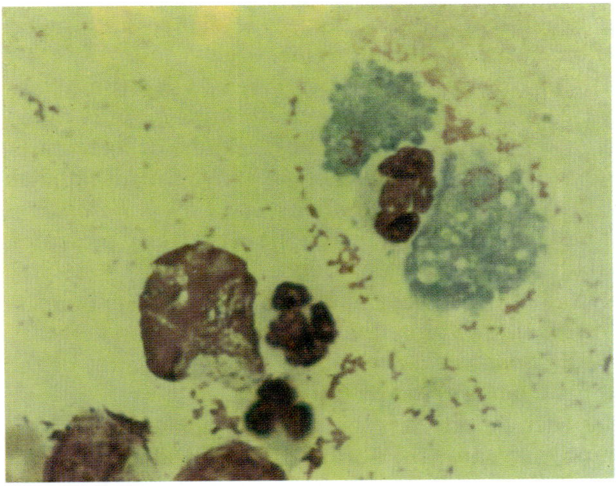

**Fig. 2.** Cerebrospinal fluid sediment stained with Giemsa stain. The amebas with their sky blue cytoplasm and delicate nuclei are easily distinguished from the inflammatory cells (oil immersion, ×1000)

# Digestive Interactions and Clues to the Diagnostic Dilemmas of Travelers

M. E. Gordon

There is an old Bantu saying "He who never travels thinks mother is the only cook." Obviously sundry cooks are encountered during travel. Our ability to elicit the cause of devastating acute vomiting and diarrhea may depend on assessing not only what is consumed but the variable conditions in its preparation and serving. Cooked rice standing too long at room temperature becomes replete with *Bacillus cereus* as does some soft cheeses, which invites the growth of *Listeria monocytogenes*. Chopped garlic "preserved" in bottled soybean oil produces botulism weeks later. Contaminated water sprays used by some merchants to "freshen" their produce may produce the colitis or liver abscess of amoebiasis. Cobalt sulfate used by brewers in the past to improve the "head" on beer may produce cardiac failure. Forty-two percent of all illnesses suffered by man are food borne and are usually difficult to identify.

The many cruise ships that pass through our ports may be a short-lived luxurious home for some, but 22 of 55 international cruise ships recently failed to pass sanitary inspection in United States ports, one reason being bilge water was found to flow through some ship's freshwater lines! We are all familiar with the mini-epidemics of *Staphylococcus, Salmonella, Vibrio Parahemolyticus*. Norwalk virus, and others originating from these elegantly presented but perishable canapes, salads, and seafood delicacies.

The expansion of today's catering services makes the frequent flyer increasingly more vulnerable. You recall that more than 600 passengers and crew of a major airline were felled by *Salmonella enteritides* – a contaminant of the aspic powder used in the hors d'oeuvres served inflight.

Other inflight problems such as travelers with sudden sickle cell crisis or basilar pulmonary infarction may cause the abrupt onset of abdominal pain, mimiking an acute surgical abdomen. The persistence of bowel sounds should aid in the correct assessment. Crucial to any diagnosis is extracting the traveler's prior medical history. However, the use of triazolam (Halcion) to avoid jet lag can produce transient global amnesia which may hamper the ability to give an accurate history.

Ocean depths contribute their "own grand rounds" during the flight. There are over 3 million scuba divers in the United States alone and the hypnotic allure of the coral's panorama may invite the risk of nitrogen disassociation when in the air if the flight's departure occurs less than 12 h after that "last dive." The abdominal symptoms and the substernal burning sensation may be a sobering reminder of Boyles's law.

During descent, traveler's are encouraged to chew gum inflight to prevent barotrauma. Few of us will correlate the subsequent pseudoappendicitis signs with that prior use of sugarless gum containing the culprit, sorbitol.

After landing, many immediately race to their adventure travel, often described as "inconvenience, well considered." Hang gliding has been known before and like trekking, high mountain climbing, ballooning, and skiing above 3000 m, presents subtle hazards. Few recognize its role in the nausea, projectile vomiting, headache, and malaise masqueradings as an acute "GI upset." In fact, it often signals the onset of mountain altitude sickness with the potentially serious pulmonary and cerebral edema occasionally followed by paralysis, coma, and death.

Other travelers immediately proceed to their "dine around," overindulging in the market place "treats," oblivious of its perils, be it the ultimate temptress, the pork sausage replete with *Trichina* or *Yersinia*, the steak tartar with the *Taenia saginata* gloating at the gluttony, the sampled tonka beans that contain coumarins, producing GI or menstrual bleeding, or using the folk herbal teas, especially Gordo-Lobo-Yerba tea, often given for diarrhea and cough, which can invoke venoocclusive liver disease.

The widespread consumption of Asian sushi or scandinavian raw herring may produce severe abdominal pain that is instantly relieved if the embedded larva of *Anisakis* is endoscopically removed from the gastric musosal phlegmon. The onset of the B12 deficiency anemia of *Diphyllibothyrium latum* infestation or the pancreatitis, cholangitis and liver disease of clonorchiasis may appear later. The treachery of raw fish is place and culturally oriented, e.g., in Korea, raw fish is often masked by a coating of a hot bean paste. The thai festive raw fish dish "koi-pla" is probably responsible for the extensive liver infection found in many villages. When a traveler to Asia becomes ill with jaundice, hepatomegaly, and a peculiar hot abdominal sensation, it is often characteristic of *Opisthorchis viverrini* infection. The subsequent association with liver cholangiocarcinoma has been demonstrated.

The scuba diver's earlier kaleidoscopic underwater spectacle may be matched by the subsequent ingestion of these same barracuda, red snapper, grouper, and amberjack, causing *Ciguatera* poisoning. The initial GI symptoms of abdominal pain, vomiting, and diarrhea become overshadowed by the rash, fever, distressing dysthesias of the mouth (hot tastes cold and cold tastes hot) and in some cases, paralysis. The toxin concentrates in the viscera and flesh of various fish, undetectable by taste, odor, and sight. Similarly, improperly stored fish, releasing histamine, can produce the flushing, headache, and abdominal distress of scombroid poisoning.

How many travelers recognize that most oysters and clams can filter and concentrate over 15 liters of estuary water daily, replete with the adjacent sew age organisms and viruses? The shipment labels destined for elegant restaurants can hardly insure an uncontaminated delicacy.

The traveler to Oceania should be warned that the pig roasts may cause "Pigbell" – a devastating necrotizing jejunitis due to the toxins of *Clostridium perfringens*. On-site skilled use of our olfactory senses may alert us to the unmistakable "pig-pen odor" of balantidiasis, the baked brown bread odor of typhoid, the butcher-shop scent of yellow fever, or the rotten-apple odor of *Clostridium* gas gangrene.

Our pre-trip briefing emphasizing the need to consume well-done meat, especially for our pregnant patients, can avoid a potential *E. coli* verotoxin hemolytic-uremic syndrome or a *Toxoplasmosis gondii* fetal infection. Rabbit meat can also convey this organism. The hunter's temptation to consume the prepared meat of his freshly killed bear invites trichinosis. Prolonged diarrhea for weeks, along with nausea, occasional vomiting, and abdominal pain, may also be the presenting symptoms in arctic trichinosis, due to the infected native walrus meat.

Our most common exposure to the subtlties of parasitic diseases probably relate to the irritable colon syndrome. The so-called "typical" syndrome can fool many clinicians if adequate diagnostic searches are not pursued. The amoeboma may mimic a cecal carcinoma. Trichuria or hookworm infestations may cause the "tolerant" type of chronic anemia, suggesting malignancy. The *strongyloides* larvae may produce radiographic signs of peptic ulcer and chronic inflammatory bowel disease as well as intractable skin rashes. The explosive dissemination of these larva in the immunosuppressed patient is often life threatening, yet can be easily diagnosed by an enterocapsule or duodenal drainage. Occasionally we endoscopists may "fish" for larger nematodes and snare an ascarid from the ampulla of Vater.

*Cryptosporidia*, now a more readily recognized hazard to the African and Indonesian traveler, can implant on the small bowel, producing a secretory diarrhea exceeding 17 liters/day. Cryptosporidiosis is being reported more frequently in homosexual populations as well as the day care nurseries of the world. Less well recognized is its association with AIDS – producing symptoms of typical biliary colic, abnormal liver function tests and X-rays suggesting sclerosing cholangitis. ERCP drainage is often positive for the organism, frequently attached to the gallbladder mucosa.

The vulnerability of the trekker and the skier to the life habits of the beaver, ultimately infecting the mountain streams with *Giardia*, has been well described. There have now been 90 recorded outbreaks of giardiasis in United States municipalities with chlorinated water supply systems that do not use ancillary sand-filtering tanks. Other mysterious modes of *Giardia* infection may relate to swimming in the hotel pools where infants are being taught the skills of swimming before mastering the art of fecal control!

Water immersion is another entrapment for the hapless traveler. It can initiate havoc, be it swimming near the "expeditious" sewage systems of some hastily built hotels, the Nile river, or cooling off in a seemingly pristine lake. The subsequent conjunctival suffusion with scleral icterus immediately suggests the diagnosis of leptospiral disease.

The schistosomal cercariae have but a short time limit to penetrate the skin of the unfortunate white water rafter, yet the resulting Katayama fever a few weeks later can produce not only fever, hepatosplenomegaly, lymphadenopathy, and eosinophilia, but transverse myelitis. Overlooking the prior exposure of the patient with this colonoscopic findings can misdiagnose these schistosomal inflammatory polyps.

Increasing our own daily awareness of global etiologic agents reminds us that gastrectomized traveling patients may have increased vulnerability to enteropathic *E. coli, Giardia lamblia. Vibrio cholera*, tubercle bacillus, and *C. botulism*. Prophylactic antibiotics in this high-risk group are probably warranted.

Consideration of some vector-transmitted arboviruses are often omitted in our daily vexing decisions. When jaundice, toxicity and disseminated intravascular coagulopathy appear after a trip in the sub-Sahara, what seems like viral hepatitis with subacute necrosis may, in fact, be Rift Valley fever, clued by its characteristic retinopathy.

Hantaan virus outbreaks are now evident in NE France and Greece. Its hemorrhagic fever with renal syndrome, like its Korean prototype, may require urgent renal dialysis.

The category of vector bites and contact is no less hazardous to our beseiged traveler or native. The onset of malaria in children frequently does not display the usual fever periodicity, but presents with symptoms which mimic "gastroenteritis." The avid competition for plasma glucose by the parasite causes depleted glycogen stores with ensuing hypoglycemic symptoms, associated with hypotension, disseminated intravascular coagulopathy, and the like.

The lyme tick will be the instigator of a series of puzzling problems seeking correlation by many specialties: the gastroenterologist, for the hepatomegaly and abdominal pain at its onset, the dermatologist (erythema chronicum migrans), the rheumatologist (arthritis), the cardiologist (myocardiopathy), and the neurologist (Bell's palsy).

Another recently emphasized disease caused by a vector bite, the dog tick, produces Mediterranean spotted fever or Boutonnese fever, now reported in Belgium, the Mediterranean, as well as Africa. This black spot found at the site of the bite on the extremities is characteristic along with a flu-like syndrome and rash (like Rocky Mountain spotted fever). The abnormal liver functions are due to hepatocellular necrosis. The vasculitites may involve the pancreatic septa. Mediterranean spotted fever and Lyme disease both respond to proper antibiotics.

The kissing bug, *Triatoma infestans*, may have a future bearing on our traveler's subsequent achalasia or megacolon, wrought by the chagasian *Trypanosoma*, also producing anginoid symptoms, tachyarrythmias, and congestive heart failure. The cardiomyopathies of trichinosis and toxoplasmosis are both similar to Chagas' disease, and like toxoplasmosis, can also be conveyed by blood transfusions.

The treacherous *Aedes albopictus* mosquito is now spreading throughout the Caribbean, transmitting dengue with its nausea and vomiting, often preceding the more familiar distressing myalgia, back pain, blanching rash, and saddleback fever.

Whether the "local witch doctor" or the board certified, we members of the healing arts can prevent regrettable illnesses, empasizing the the necessary pretravel precautions and immunization requirements. In doing so, it will reinforce the dictum that dire consequences need not "come with the territory." Should illness occur, the diverse digestive interactions offer clues to the solving of many diagnostic dilemmas of travelers.

# Unfamiliar Infectious Diseases Acquired During Travel in the United States

M. E. Wilson

In South Carolina in the summer of 1983, a previously healthy 13-year-old girl visited her physician because of sore throat and high fever. She was treated with oral penicillin. She worsened. Three days later she was admitted to a hospital where she died of plague. Two days before onset of her illness she had handled a wild chipmunk in new Mexico, a plague-endemic area, more than a thousand miles away (CDC 1983).

Travelers and physicians are becoming more knowledgeable about infectious disease risks in tropical and developing countries. There is less awareness that infections that are unfamiliar to most physicians in the world can also be acquired during travel in developed countries.

Outdoor activities such as hiking, camping, and archeological digging yield physical and intellectual challenges and satisfactions. Occasionally they provide the setting for contact with unexpected pathogens. In this paper I will discuss eight infections that may be acquired during outdoor activities in the United States (Table 1).

The infections included are unlikely to be suspected because they are uncommon or absent in most other areas of the world. The emphasis will be on infections with geographically focal distributions, often determined by soil characteristics or capacity of an area to support a specific arthropod vector or

**Table 1.** Infections acquired during travel in the United States

| Infection | Frequency | Geographic distribution |
|---|---|---|
| Rocky Mountain spotted fever | 700–1 200 reported/year | Esp. SE states, E coast |
| Plague *(Yersinia pestis)* | 10–40 reported/year | West, esp. New Mexico |
| Colorado tick fever | 200–300 reported/year est. >2000/year | Western mountains, esp. Colorado |
| Tick-borne relapsing fever | 20–40 reported/year | Western mountains |
| Lyme disease | 1 000–1 500 reported/year | NE coastal states, northern MW, far NW |
| Babesiosis | 10–20 reported/year | NE coast; rare MW |
| Coccidioidomycosis *(Coccidioides immitis)* | Est. 35 000 infections (new) in California/year | Arid SW (California to Texas) |
| Histoplasmosis *(Histoplasma capsulatum)* | Est. 1/2 million new infections/year | Central, SE states, esp. Mississippi and Ohio river valleys |

animal host. All can be acquired during a brief exposure and are treatable or transmissible, or both. These are infections acquired by entering an environment; the event that allows transmission is often inapparent to the host. One night and one bite may be sufficient. Not included are infections acquired by sexual exposures.

Tick-transmitted Rocky Mountain spotted fever, caused by *Rickettsia rickettsii*, is a severe, systemic, infection characterized by high fever, headache, myalgias and rash. It is lethal in 15%–20% of patients in the absence of timely, specific therapy, usually tetracycline or chloramphenicol. In 1983 4% of the more than 1000 reported cases in the United States died of the infection. The name Rocky Mountain spotted fever is misleading on two counts: infection is infrequent in the Rocky Mountains and the spots, the rash, may be absent in more than 10%, or delayed in onset. Fewer than one-half of patients have a rash during the first 3 days of illness (Helmick et al. 1984). Although cases are reported from all regions of the United States except Alaska and Hawaii, 85% of the cases in 1986 were from 15 states (CDC 1987), primarily in a band stretching from Oklahoma to the eastern seaboard. Typically no eschar is present at the site of the tick bite. A history of activities in woody, bushy rural areas within the previous 2 weeks may be the only reminder to consider the diagnosis.

Plague persists in fleas and rodents in focal areas of almost a dozen western states. Humans are occasionally caught up in the cycle, leading to 10 to more than 40 reported cases of plague per year in the United States, the largest number from New Mexico (CDC 1987). Awareness of the infection is high in endemic areas where patients often present with fever and tender lymphadenopathy. Although the overall mortality is about 18%, mortality was 56% in the group of patients between 1957 and 1983 who sought medical attention outside of the state where infection was acquired (CDC 1983).

Colorado tick fever, caused by a red blood cell-associated RNA virus, is included for two reasons: (1) illness may be prolonged, lasting 3 weeks or longer in the majority of adults and (2) the virus which persists in RBCs for 4 months or longer, even after the patient is asymptomatic, can be transmitted by blood transfusions. Illness begins abruptly with fever, headache, and myalgias. Figure 1 shows the estimated distribution of the hard tick vector, found in areas covered with grass and low shrubs, at altitudes between 1200 and 3000 m (Eklund et al. 1955). In some areas up to 40% of the ticks carry the virus in the springtime (Goodpasture et al. 1978). The estimated risk of infection in Rocky Mountain National Park in Colorado is one per 400 camper-days.

Tick-borne relapsing fever, caused by *Borrelia* species, is found in some of the same western mountain areas but is diagnosed infrequently. The soft tick vector is found in cabins in the mountains, around wood piles, and in animal hides. Usually active only after dark, it feeds for 10–20 min without causing pain and then drops off, usually unnoticed. Prolonged and relapsing fevers can be interrupted with tetracycline, chloramphenicol, or penicillin (Horton and Blaser 1985). The states with the largest number of reported cases are Califor-

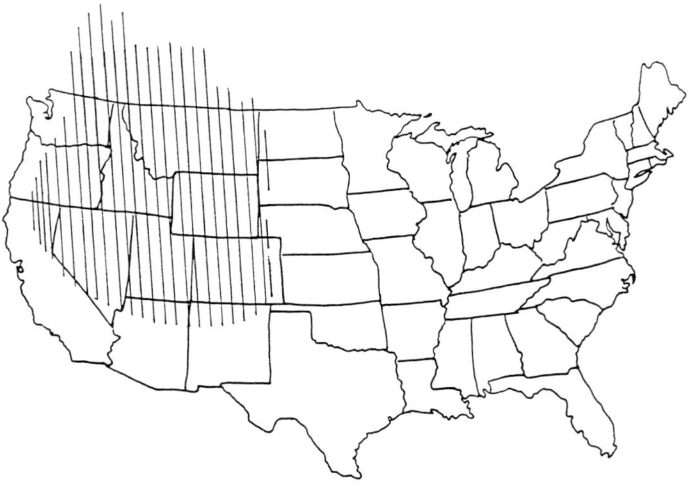

**Fig. 1.** Colorado tick fever: distribution of tick vector, *Dermacentor andersoni*. (Eklund et al. 1955)

nia, Arizona, Colorado, and Oregon. As with the other diseases discussed, infection can be acquired only in focal areas of each state.

The most common reportable tick-borne infection in the United States is Lyme disease, named after Old Lyme, Connecticut, and caused by the spirochete, *Borrelia burgdorferi*. Although not unique to the United States, having been diagnosed in Europe, Asia, Africa, and Australia, the greatest concentration of reported cases is in the U.S. (Schmid 1985). In 1986 infection was documented serologically in more than 1200 persons in Connecticut alone (CDC 1988), a state less than one-third the size of Switzerland. In some areas of New York state up to 100% of the ticks collected are infected with the spirochete (Burgdorfer et al. 1985). Although infection has now been reported from more than 30 states, three foci still account for over 90% of the cases: the coastal Northeast (especially Connecticut, New York, New Jersey, Massachusetts, Rhode Island), the northern Midwest, in Wisconsin and Minnesota, and the far Northwest (California, Oregon, Nevada).

Lyme disease causes skin changes, carditis, neurologic abnormalities, and arthritis, alone or in combination. Lyme disease is especially important for travelers because: (1) it is common in vacation spots, easily reached by travelers; (2) the tick, usually the nymphal stage, that transmits infection is very small (1–2 mm) and the bite often not noticed; (3) the characteristic skin lesion, erythema chronicum migrans, is often absent or not recognized [In one study in Connecticut 79% of patients with arthritis did not report antecedent erythema chronicum migrans (CDC 1988).] (4) signs and symptoms may first appear months or more than a year after acquisition of infection; and (5) antimicrobials, such as penicillin, may be beneficial even if started months after onset of infection.

An unrelated infection, caused by the protozoan *Babesia microti*, that infects RBCs, is transmitted by the same tick and is found in some of the same, but much more limited, geographic areas. Babesiosis is sometimes confused with malaria because of persistent fevers, splenomegaly, and intraerythrocytic parasites visible on blood smears. Infection may be severe, even fatal in asplenic patients who should avoid endemic areas where more than 5% of persons may become infected during one summer season (Filstein et al. 1980).

Soil-associated fungi cause acute, subacute, and chronic infection after being inhaled. Coccidioidomycosis is found only in arid areas of the Southwest in a belt from Texas to California. Although most infections are mild or self-limited, disseminated and sometimes lethal disease occurs with increased frequency in pregnant women (Drutz and Catanzaro 1978).

Histoplasmosis is extremely common, especially in areas near the Mississippi and Ohio River valleys. A study of skin test reactivity of Navy recruits to histoplasmin found more than 80% of lifetime residents from many counties in the central part of the country had evidence of prior infection with histoplasma (Edwards et al. 1969). Erythema nodosum and eosinophilia may be prominent features of primary infection with both fungal infections (Goodwin et al. 1981). Immunocompromised patients, including persons infected with the human immunodeficiency virus, are more likely to develop disseminated disease.

Unfamiliar infections associated with outdoor activities may be acquired during travel in the United States. In general, the overall risk of infection is low and immunizations and prophylaxis are not available or are not indicated for the usual traveler. Because some infections, such as histoplasmosis, coccidioidomycosis, and babesiosis may be disseminated or lethal in patients with certain underlying conditions, physicians should review anticipated itineraries and activities prior to travel for patients who are immunocompromised, pregnant, or asplenic.

Types of infectious diseases and probability of acquiring infection are vastly different depending on destination. I propose that area-specific risk assessment, amplified by activity- and host-specific history, should become an integral part of medical evaluation before and after travel to some areas of developed countries as well as to tropical and developing areas of the world.

## References

Burgdorfer W, Lane RS, Barbour AG, Gresbrink RA, Anderson JR (1985) The western black-legged tick, *Ixodes pacificus*: a vector of *Borrelia burgdorferi*. Am J Trop Med Hyg 34:925–930

Centers for Disease Control (1983) Plague – South Carolina. MMWR 32:417–418

Centers for Disease Control (1985) Update: lyme disease occurring during pregnancy – United States. MMWR 34:376–378, 383–384

Centers for Disease Control (1987) Summary of notifiable diseases United States, 1986. MMWR 35:4–9, 46,51

Centers for Disease Control (1988) Lyme disease – Connecticut. MMWR 37:1–3

Dammin GJ (1978) Babesiosis. In: Weinstein L, Fields BN (eds) Seminars in infectious diseases. Grune and Stratton, New York, pp 169–199

Drutz DJ, Catanzaro A (1978) Coccidioidomycosis. Am Rev Resp Dis 117:559–585, 727–771
Edwards LB, Acquaviva FA, Livesay VT, Cross RW, Palmer CD (1969) An atlas of sensitivity to tuberculin, PPD-B, and histoplasmin in the United States. Am Rev Resp Dis 99 [Suppl]:1–132
Eklund CM, Kohls GM, Brennan JM (1955) Distribution of Colorado tick fever and virus-carrying ticks. JAMA 157:335–337
Filstein MR, Benach JL, White DJ, Brody BA, Goldman WD, Bakal CW, Schwartz RS (1980) Serosurvey for human babesiosis in New York. J Infect Dis 141:518–521
Goodpasture HC, Poland JD, Francy B, Bowen GS, Horn KA (1978) Colorado tick fever: clinical, epidemiological, and laboratory aspects of 228 cases in Colorado in 1973–1974. Ann Intern Med 88:303–310
Goodwin RA, Loyd JE, Des Prez RM (1981) Histoplasmosis in normal hosts. Am Rev Respir Dis 60:231–266
Helmick CG, Bernard KW, D'Angelo LJ (1984) Rocky Mountain spotted fever: clinical, laboratory, and epidemiological features of 262 cases. J Infect Dis 150:480–488
Horton JM, Blaser JM (1985) The spectrum of relapsing fever in the Rocky Mountains. Arch Intern Med 145:871–875
Schmid GP (1985) The global distribution of Lyme disease. Rev Infect Dis 7:41–50

# Risks of Zoonotic Diseases to Travellers in West Africa

D.O. Alonge

Travellers in West Africa are open to yellow fever, Lassa Fever, rabies and African sleeping sickness, four most important zoonotic diseases. Between 1974 and 1986, a total of 70991 confirmed yellow fever cases resulting in 3762 deaths were reported from Sierra Leone, Gambia, Senegal, Ivory Coast, Burkina Fasso and Nigeria. In 1969 and 1970, 7 out of 29 cases died of Lassa fever while a range of 0.2%–22.4% prevalence has been reported among the inhabitants of West Africa. In Ghana, between 1977 and 1981, 102 human rabies were officially reported. In Nigeria, an average of 18 cases of rabies with a range of 8–28 cases have been reported since 1962. All cases were fatal. Though alarming epidemics of sleeping sickness (African trypanosomiasis) have been controlled across Africa, at least 8000 cases were reported yearly in Nigeria and from Uganda.

## Rabies

Exposure potential for dog handlers, pet owners, veterinarians, research scientists employing dogs and other susceptible animals in research and pathology technologists is higher than all other groups in the population. Travellers to West Africa with dogs already vaccinated must revaccinate their dogs, as cases of rabies in vaccinated dogs have been reported. Rodents and bats are not reserviors of rabies in West Africa (Okoh 1982).

## Yellow Fever

Three transmission cycles are recognized. The enzootic forest cycle is limited to the rain forest zone with monkey – monkey transmission and no human infection, and the jungle yellow fever cycle of monkey-mosquito-man is restricted to the equitorial tropical belts of Africa. Human infection follows exposure during forest clearing and wood-cutting activities. Researchers and travellers going through the tropical rain forest of Africa are open to this disease. The third cycle is the epidemic urban yellow fever which is purely man–man with *Aedes aegypti* serving as the main vector. Travellers to West Africa must take the yellow fever vaccination at least 2 weeks prior to date of arrival. The 17D vaccine confers long-lasting immunity in about 99% of vaccinated persons (Tomori and Nasidi 1987).

## Lassa Fever

A viral disease transmitted from the rodent reservoir – *Mastomys natalensis* – from the aerosolized infectious rodent urine. Travellers in West Africa must note that outbreaks occur in January–February, coinciding with the post-harvest and post-bush burning period during which the rodent reserviors invade houses in large numbers (McCormick and Johnson 1978).

## African Human Trypanosomiasis (Sleeping Sickness)

This condition is restricted to some areas of West, Central and East Africa. In West Africa, riverine tsetse flies of the genus *Glossina* are mainly responsible for transmission. People fishin, drawing water or washing near rivers and lake shores and forest officers are more at risk. An unusual route of infection is by consumption of raw meat, whereby trypanosomes penetrate into the bloodstream via sores and abrasions in the mouth (Gibson 1984).

## References

Gibson EC (1984) Epidemiology and control of African trypanosomiasis. Postgrad Doctor Afr, April 1984:108–115

McCormick JB, Johnson KM (1978) Lassa fever. Historical review and contemporary investigation. In: Pathyn SH (ed) Ebola virus haemorrhagic fever. Elsevier, Amsterdam

Okoh AEJ (1982) Canine rabies in Nigeria 1970–1980. Reported cases. Int Zoon 9(2):118–119

Tomori O, Nasidi AY (1987) Yellow fever and the Nigerian situation (1913–1987). A report. Federal Ministry of Health, Lagos

# Environmental and In-Flight Problems

# Stresses of Families Abroad

E. F. Rigamer

## Summary

By becoming aware of the more common adjustment reactions to relocation and adaptation to other cultures, the physician is in an ideal position to assist the traveler to adjust to short- or long-term stays abroad. For the short-term traveler, symptoms of extreme fatigue, confusion, faulty judgment and occasionally frank suspiciousness are not uncommon and are often complicated by alcohol or self-administered tranquilizing or hypnotic medications.

The various stages of cross-cultural adaptation are experienced by all those who remain abroad for more than a few weeks. After an initial period of excitement and sense of well-being, it is not uncommon for one to go through a period of disillusionment with the host country as well as the work. Rarely is this acknowledged for what it is; more often the individual presents with somatic complaints that may or may not have an organic basis. Other presenting symptoms can include apathy, lethargy, and sleep disturbances. A smaller number of patients may voice extreme negativism about the culture, reconsider their decision to remain abroad and show some signs of paranoid ideation.

Treatment of these problems is usually very successful. Recognition of the symptoms for what they are and explaining their causes to the patient are important aspects of treatment. Predeparture orientation programs that include culture familiarization and language training pay handsome rewards in the prevention area.

## Introduction

"What is it like to live over there?" "Do you really like it?" "Life there sounds so exotic while things here are so humdrum." These questions, familiar to the expatriate visiting home, reflect the widely held view of life overseas. While living abroad has many attractions and is certainly not humdrum, it has stresses which are seldom apparent to others. For the professional caring for people who live abroad, there are probably few other occasions when it is more important to evaluate a presenting problem in the context of the individual's life circumstances. This article will describe some of the psychological stresses faced by families who change their countries of residence every 3–4 years.

## The Move

A stress common to all who live abroad is the one due to the move. This constitutes a significant event in one's life and, for those moving to another country, there are special changes of language, customs and culture, in addition to the usual ones of forming friendships and settling into a new neighborhood. It is now recognized that several major changes within a year increase the susceptibility to physical and psychological problems. A move to another country ranks high in this category.

In adults the responses to the stress of relocation are determined by the period in the individual's life when the move takes place. It does not necessarily follow that the more one moves the easier it becomes to adapt. A move when one is 20 years of age and single or newly married and beginning a new career may present few problems, even if it may be to a difficult post in the Third World, as usually happens to newly assigned foreign service officers. A move later in life, for example when one is 45 years old, has more ramifications. High-school age children may not want to leave their friends. If the wife has not been an employee of the organization she may be reluctant to move once again, now that she is in the midst of creating a career for herself as her responsibilities for the children decrease. There is a stage in life where one's own parents are elderly and other members of the family may feel it is time that obligations to them be equally shared. These issues complicate the move and become significant factors in how one adapts, regardless of how appealing the city or the assignment may be. Very often these personal factors are more significant in determining the success of settling into another culture than the objective realities of the culture itself.

## Family Stress

Families sometimes overlook the stresses caused by this change. A father who as the principal employee represents the reason for the family's being abroad may find it expedient to minimize the dissatisfactions expressed by the mother and children. Dealing with the objections head on and only with logic, he may attempt to talk his family out of any ill-feeling by reminding them of all the advantages which come with living abroad by comparing their present life more favorably with the one they had at home. Usually the responses to the stress are not recognized as coming from the change, probably because they often are not new expressions of malaise but rather a reappearance of old psychological symptoms and conflicts. Marital problems, hitherto quiescent, flare up; depressive symptoms may reappear; exacerbations of psychophysiological disorders may dominate the clinical picture and lead the individual into focusing only on physical complaints.

In a new environment there is a tendency to project the cause of distress onto the outside, especially when the culture is unfamiliar or inhospitable. It is helpful to realize the role that change by itself has in generating this malaise. In seeing the outside as the sole cause of the distress, and perhaps unconsciously waiting for it to alter, the feeling of being able to do something for oneself is lost and a sense of depressing passivity sets in. In sorting out the reason for a depression following a move, most people are easily helped to distinguish between the contribution made by long-standing personal conflicts, previously under control and now exacerbated, and those factors which come from the unfamiliarity of the new environment which will improve over time.

The move stirs the pot, and understanding the repertoire of one's psychological reactions to it is essential in managing the associated stress.

## Children

Some children regress in response to a move. Younger ones, although able to verbalize some feelings of unhappiness, more frequently show distress by the temporary loss of recently achieved behavioral milestones. Toddlers may become more clinging and object to being left with babysitters. An elementary school age child may lose academic skills and go into a slump at school. A shy adolescent may spend several months being depressed before becoming reestablished in a peer group. The effects of change are especially noticeable in the group who are described as "slow to warm up" by Chess and Thomas in their New York University longitudinal study in 1977 of temperament and behavior disorders in children. These children are slow to adapt to change and may show signs of behavioral disturbance for as long as a year after a move.

As children are usually regarded as happy movers and eager for change (which is untrue, for they are notoriously conservative) they are sometimes judged as misbehaving when in fact they are as distressed as the adult members of the family. Anxiety and depression are often disguised by behavior in this age group, and recognizing this helps parents and teachers to modify their approaches accordingly.

## Adaptation

After the move is negotiated, adapting to the country is usually next in the order of business. There are as many styles of relating to a foreign culture as there are individuals. In some Third World countries expatriates may choose to live in compounds and socialize in clubs which are transplants from home. Their contact with the culture is formal and usually perfunctory, while friendships are primarily with others of their background. Then there are those – missionaries or Peace Corps volunteers, for example – who live in close contact with citizens of the host country and are at ease in surroundings where there are few features or conveniences similar to those at home. The majority live at virtually every possible point on the continuum between these two extremes. The best method of adapting to a culture is the one which is most compatible with the individual's temperament and sensitivities.

Whichever style of settling-in is followed, it is important that at least the salient features of the country's history, culture and customs are learned, ideally from the beginning.

Not everyone has the opportunity to acquire the language but whenever this is possible it should be done. The more that is known, the less strange the new environment becomes and the sooner a sense of location and belonging sets in. A sense of alienation lasting more than a few months usually comes from failing to understand or misinterpreting the myriad of gestures, behaviors and mannerisms of the inhabitants of the host country. This is especially true when the culture is radically different from one's own.

## Terrorism

Nowadays, another significant stress comes from the threat of terrorism. While most people are not in positions that endanger them personally, there is the possibility for anyone to be a target, merely as a representative of his or her country, or to be accidentally hit while visiting an Embassy or a high-risk area. Personal security has become a major issue of concern and therefore one that must be dealt with by both the sponsoring agencies and the individuals. This is a complex problem and there are many approaches to it. As a minimum, one must learn and observe the basic security precautions. An awareness of one's own psychological responses to the threat, and how these affect behavior, can be helpful in managing anxiety. Two maladaptive responses are denial, leading to carelessness, and exaggerated concern, which becomes preoccupying and limiting.

## The Physician

The physician treats best when he treats the patient in the context of his or her life. He plays an especially important part in the care of those who move often and live outside their home country. One of the first things a family does after a move is to establish a relationship with a doctor and to learn where to go in a medical emergency. In the early phases of settling in, a person may voice physical complaints while he is acutally seeking an opportunity to work through the anxieties of dislocation.

In the initial contacts with the new patient, a part of the consultation could be profitably spent discussing change and eliciting the patient's descriptions of his or her own responses to it. In doing so, the physician is presenting himself as someone who knows about this process, is willing to listen, and is able to sort out and take care of the gamut of complaints. During a move or resettlement even the most independent, highly functioning adult has dependency needs which are reawakened and prompt a desire to be taken care of. If the physician responds to these needs in the early contacts, he establishes a relationship which becomes an important part of the healing process.

## The Psychiatrist

Although there are no statistics to demonstrate it, the incidence of psychiatric disorders among expatriates does not appear to be greater than that of the general population. What does seem different, however, is the length of time such disorders go untreated considering the economic and social background of the population. This is not surprising. There is usually some resistance in everyone when it comes to acknowledging the need for help. The lack of common language, the reluctance to be treated by someone of a different background, and the ever-present wish that the situation will improve with the next move all provide legitimate rationalizations to postpone a decision to address the problem. The result is that in many instances the morbidity of the disorder is greater than it would have been had the person been living at home and had not had these factors to reinforce his resistance.

The delay in diagnosing and treating psychological and educational problems is especially disadvantageous in the life of a child. Optimum development of the young personality requires specific tasks to be met in each stage of development in order to go forward and complete successfully those of the next stage. Later remedial measures, though not impossible, are more difficult. A child who has a reading problem, for example, should have the disorder diagnosed as soon as possible and then begun on a program which can be followed over a length of time, usually 1–4 years. What too often occurs in a population on the move is that the teacher in first grade may delay and not recommend much more than a "watch and wait" attitude. The family moves to a new assignment in another country and the second grade teacher advises the parents to wait and see how the youngster is after he settles into the new setting. Perhaps by January of the school year the diagnosis of a reading disorder is agreed by all, but the school may not have special educational facilities.

To carry the worst case scenario further, a definitive evaluation may not be possible until summer leave, and then the family is faced with the decision on how to address the issue given the facilities available to them in post. The early diagnosis of this type of problem is important and sometimes the strong urging of the family physician is required in order to cut through rationalizations and set priorities.

## Prevention

One important aspect of the U.S. State Department's Mental Health Program for its diplomats is primary prevention. Many aspects of the stresses can be handled by educating individuals as to what they are and developing an awareness of one's own responses to them. In the area of child rearing, educational tapes, seminars and discussion groups on raising children abroad have helped parents to understand and manage the problems unique to children who move and live in a series of different cultures.

## Conclusion

With more people living abroad and with new complicating circumstances such as the security issue, we are becoming aware of the many associated stresses which this life-style entails.

In most instances the stresses do not overshadow the many advantages and opportunities which come from living in different cultures. However, there is no circumstance where they are not present and, if improperly managed, they detract considerably from the pleasures of such experiences. Orientation and educational programs about the psychological and physiological aspects of relocation and cross-cultural living do enhance one's ability to manage the stresses effectively.

# Mental Stress as International Hazard

L. Heber

"Stress, like beauty, is in the eye of the beholder. What matters is the way people perceive and react to every disastrous experience around them." (Jenkins 1985)

## Introduction

According to Hoff (1984), stress is defined as the discomfort, pain, or troubled feeling arising from emotional, social, or physical sources resulting in the need to relax, to be treated, or to seek relief.

Selye (1956) refers to stress as a specific syndrome that is non-specifically induced. Ramsey (1982) states that stress has an indefinite meaning and symbolizes different things to people from various disciplines.

There are two types of grouping of stress (Hoff 1984):

- Acute stress is brief in duration, in which predictable manifestations of symptoms and results may lead to crisis.
- Insiduous stress is of longer duration, of weeks, months, and years, with less awareness by the individual experiencing it. As time goes on this may lead to burnout or disease due to its cumulative effect.

This paper presents some physiological, psychological, cultural and spiritual factors of air travel stress and may provide a means for identifying behavioural changes of the air traveler.

## Types of Stress Experiences

### Physiological Stress

Air travel experience may result in physiological stress manifested as apprehension or anxious behaviour. One can identify apprehensive or anxious passengers by exhibited or non-exhibited symptoms. Exhibited symptoms include restless behaviour and nausea. Non-exhibited symptoms include palpitations, rapid pulse, and increased blood pressure. Physiological symptoms may be relieved by medications, pre-flight counselling, and emotional support.

### Psychological Stress

Psychological stress may be more complex and difficult to identify than physiological symptoms. Psychological stress includes symptoms of tension, worry,

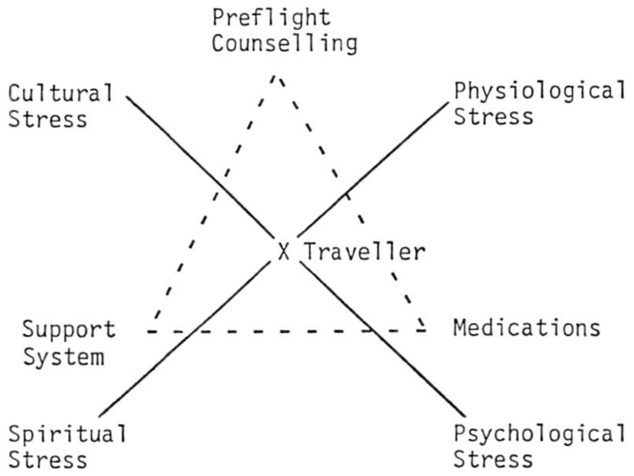


**Fig. 1.** Travel stress and preventive measures

anxiety, apprehension, loss of appetite, insomnia, sadness, crying or indecisiveness. Many of these symptoms may be expressed by a passenger several days or weeks before a flight and can be observed by family members and friends as unusual behaviour, or by family physician as possible anxiety related to air travel.

## Cultural Stress

Air travel may bring about stress due to cultural disorientation which is the first stage of culture shock. Culture disorientation is a psychological response to an unfamiliar cultural milieu, characterized by anxiety and depression. The individual traveler suffering from cultural disorientation is faced with the need for rapid and frequent responses to the new situation. Rapid response is most difficult when conditions are constantly changing with little time for adjustment. The result may be disorientation that lasts throughout the flight or travel experience. The consequence of travel anxiety and cultural disorientation may be far reaching and bizarre as experienced by an Ojibway Indian family from northern Ontario in Canada. The practice of Ojibway Indians is to carry their infant in a cradle-board or "Tikinagan". A security guard at the Winnipeg International Airport passed the cradle-board, with the baby inside, through a hand luggage X-ray machine. A contributing factor to this unfortunate incident may have been the parents' unfamiliarity with airport procedure and cultural disorientation.

## Spiritual Stress

Spiritual stress for air travelers involves anticipated accidents or misadventures occurring in a situation where the individual has no control over their destiny. A spiritual response may be employed to relieve anxiety or other stressors. Spiritual stress may take the form of meditation or self-preoccupation. Meditation may involve the use of spiritual aids such as prayer books and prayer beads. Self-preoccupation may involve the use of fetish objects such as lucky charms employed in an attempt to maintain control over the situation. Through the use of spiritual aids, levels of anxiety may be controlled or reduced. It is noted by Jenkins (1985) that "people who regularly practice meditation or relaxation techniques produce measurable body changes, including slower heart rate, decline in blood pressure and slower metabolism as well as increased feelings of calmness and well-being."

## Conclusion

Air travel contributes to mental stress that may lead to emotional turmoil and unhappy travel experiences. Through increased awareness of symptomatic behaviour, travelers, aircrew, and medical professionals may intervene to reduce emotional stress and promote happy trips.

Overall, preventive measures such as meditation and introspective practices during air travel provides self-relief from travel stress. Insiduous group type of stress can be identified by initial assessment of the various factors of air travel stress.

## References

1. Andrews M, Ludwig P (eds) (1984) Nursing practice in a kaleidoscope of cultures. College of Nursing, University of Utah, Salt Lake City
2. Bankowski Z, Gutteridge F (1987) Health, ethics and human values. World Health, pp 9–11
3. Davies R (1987) Be a health traveler. World Health 8–9
4. Dawood R (1987) Traveller's health. World Health 3–5
5. Jenkins D (1985) Life crisis. World Health 10–12
6. Hamburg D (1987) Habits for health. World Health Forum 8:9–12
7. Hoff L (1984) People in crisis. Addison-Wesley, Don Mills
8. Lachman V (1983) Stress management. Grune and Stratton, Toronto
9. Mangen S (1982) Sociology and mental health. Curchill Livingstone, New York
10. Ramsey JM (1982) Basic pathophysiology: modern stress and the disease process. Addison-Wesley, Menlo-Park
11. Selye H (1956) The stress of life. McGraw-Hill, New York
12. Sparacino J (1982) Blood pressure, stress and mental health. Nurs Res 31:2

# Dehydration and Thermoregulatory Mechanisms Affecting the Traveler

C. Karpilow

Since the human body depends on numerous heat-sensitive enzymatic and chemical reactions, life is possible only within a very narrow range of body temperatures. Nevertheless, man is capable of living and traveling in very hot environmental temperatures. However, this can only be achieved successfully if the body's fluid balance is maintained at adequate levels. Thermoregulatory systems and hydration are vital aspects of the well-being of the traveling patient.

If one accustoms oneself to increasing activity and exposure to warmer climates, the sweat glands will be trained to produce more, to start more quickly and continue longer, producing fluid longer and at the same time retaining more salt in the body. The body trains itself to absorb more fluid from that which is consumed in the gastrointestinal tract, and to transport it to the sweat glands in the skin, where it is evaporated for cooling the body.

Travelers who are not in excellent health are potential victims of dehydration from many causes. One common cause is diarrhea. This increase in fecal water results from an increase in intestinal secretion of fluid from the plasma into the intestinal lumen. A diarrheal disease will alter the normal fluid absorption.

Unlike some mammals, humans have a delay in rehydration (involuntary dehydration) after fluid loss. There are two factors that probably contribute to involuntary dehydration in humans: (1) our upright posture and (2) extracellular fluid and electrolyte loss by sweating from exercise and heat exposure. Increased plasma renin activity appears to be the key factor in the upright postural changes. Heat exposure has the least inhibitory effect on voluntary water intake versus exercise as the greatest inhibiting factor. The rate of voluntary fluid intake, after fluid depletion, is slow in man as compared with most other mammals.

## Methods

A comparative study was made between two groups of tourists in Agra, India. These two groups consisted of American and British nationals on a tour of Agra, emanating from New Delhi. Both groups consisted of 40 individuals, ranging in age from 8 years to 63 years. The mean age of group 1 was 43; the mean age of group 2 was 46. The itinerary of both groups on the 1-day tour was identical in non-airconditioned buses. Ambient temperature in the two cities was a maximum of between 40 °C and 42 °C and a minimum of 36 °C.

Participants were tested with a pre-test questionnaire, measurement of body temperature, pulse, blood pressure, weight and psychological tests. General observations were also made.

Participants in group 1 were allowed to drink fluids only during specified times of the day. They were given choice of tea, coffee or bottled water at breakfast, lunch, afternoon rest time and dinner. Other food intake was identical with group 2. Group 2 was offered the same fluids at any time during the day it was desired.

## Results

Group 1 averaged 2458 ml fluid consumption during the test period in comparison with group 2, who averaged 5503 ml. Group 1 averaged 73% positive responses to post-test questionnaires regarding headache, nausea, thirst and strong smell of urine versus only 17% positive responses in group 2.

As far as performance testing in completion of Serial 7's and crossword puzzles, group 1 averaged 7 errors out of 15 in Serial 7's versus group 2, who had only 3 errors per 15. In the crossword puzzle, group 1 took an average of 6.8 min versus group 2, who took 5.6 min on average. Physiologic parameters are summarized in Table 1.

**Table 1.** Average physiologic parameters measured in two groups of tourists

| | Group 1 | Group 2 |
|---|---|---|
| Pulse | 84 | 78.3 |
| Oral temperature | 38.1 °C | 37.2 °C |
| Blood pressure | 140/82 | 143/79 |
| Weight | | |
| Before | 84.09 kg | 82.76 kg |
| After | 82.326 kg | 82.01 kg |

## Conclusion

This study demonstrated how humans have a delay in rehydration. It showed how this voluntary dehydration can be incapacitating to the traveler. It decreased their endurance and mental performance. These could be devastating effects if those travelers were negotiating international treaties, multimillion dollar business transactions, or acting as educators. As Travel Medicine specialists, one must diligently manage the hydration of your traveling patient so that effectiveness and well-being is maintained.

## References

1. Bar-Or et al. (1980) Voluntary hypohydration in ten to twelve year old boys. J Appl Physiol 48:104–108
2. Candy BC (1984) Diarrhea, dehydration and drugs (Editorial). Br Med J 289(6454):1245–1246
3. Melville KEM (1984) Stay alive in the desert. Lascelles, Glendon
4. Shepard RJ (1982) Exercise physiology and biochemistry. Praeger, New York

# Effect of Transmeridian Flights: Objective and Subjective Sleep Parameters

A. Buck, I. Tobler, and A. A. Borbély

## Summary

Present-day aircraft operating around northern and southern latitudes cross time zones almost at the same rate as the earth rotates. Journeys between continents can be completed within a few hours, and a shift of the day or night is experienced. After a daytime westward flight the day will appear to have lengthened and after a night-time eastward flight the night will appear to have been shortened and several hours rest will have been lost. Clearly it is in the interests of the intercontinental traveler to avoid or minimize disturbance of sleep during the journey, but even if sleep loss is avoided during the journey there is still the adaptation to the new time zone.

Motion sickness is a condition which occurs when man is exposed to real or apparent motion with which he is unfamiliar and so unadapted. It is a generic term and includes air sickness and there are very considerable differences in the susceptibility of individuals to the condition. The incidence of air sickness is only a fraction of 1% in large civil transport aircraft, but in trainee pilots perhaps about two-thirds suffer from the condition.

In this paper the nature of the disturbances associated with jet lag and motion sickness are discussed as well as their prevention and treatment.

Transmeridian flights are known to disrupt the sleep-waking cycle. This effect has recently been investigated in aircrew members in an extensive multinational study [3–8]. The major objective of the present study was to investigate the effect of long-haul flights over different numbers of time zones on objective and subjective sleep parameters of aircrew members.

## Materials and Methods

*Abbreviations.* ANC, Anchorage; BOM, Bombay; BKK, Bankok; HKG, Hongkong; KHI, Karachi; NBO, Nairobi; NRT, Tokyo; ZRH, Zurich

*Investigated Flights.* Three flights were compared with each other. *Flight 1* (6 days): ZRH–NBO (NBO; +1 h), 5 nights in NBO, NBO-ZRH. *Flight 2* (11 days): ZRH–ANC (ANC, −10 h), 2 nights in ANC, ANC–NRT (NRT, −17 h), 5 nights in NRT, NRT–ANC, 2 nights in ANC, ANC–ZRH. *Flight 3* (8 days): ZRH–BOM (BOM, +4.5 h), 1 night in BOM, BOM–HKG (HKG, +7 h), 2 nights in HKG, HKG–BKK (BKK, +6 h), 1 night in BKK, BKK–KHI (KHI, +4 h), 2 nights in KHI, KHI–ZRH.

*Subjects.* The same 16 subjects (mean age, 37.5 years) participated in flights 1 and 2. They were seven male cockpit crew members, and one male and eight female flight attendants. Fourteen different subjects (mean age, 30.5 years)

participated in flight 3. They were all flight attendants (8 males, 6 females). All subjects agreed to refrain from taking hypnotics throughout the study.

*Procedure and Measurements.* For each schedule, data were obtained during 5 baseline days, during the layovers, and during 5 "recovery" days after return to homebase. Motor activity was recorded continuously with a wrist-worn, solid-state ambulatory monitor [1, 2], which counts the numbers of suprathreshold movements within 7.5-min intervals. From these data the following parameters were then computed: (a) mean bedtime activity: mean value of all 7.5-min intervals during bedtime; (b) immobility: percentage of immobility periods (i.e., 7.5-min intervals with activity count = 0). Subjective sleep parameters were obtained from questionnaires and self-rating scales (100-mm analog scales). They included the time of going to bed, the time of arising, the estimated sleep latency, the number and duration of waking periods after sleep onset, self-ratings of sleep quality (superficial versus quiet) and the state in the morning (tired versus rested), and for flight 3 only a subjective five-point jet lag scale (none–slight–moderate–strong–very strong). The data from the layover nights of flights 1 and 2 were not analyzed, because sleep was influenced by factors unrelated to the flights (e.g., safaris).

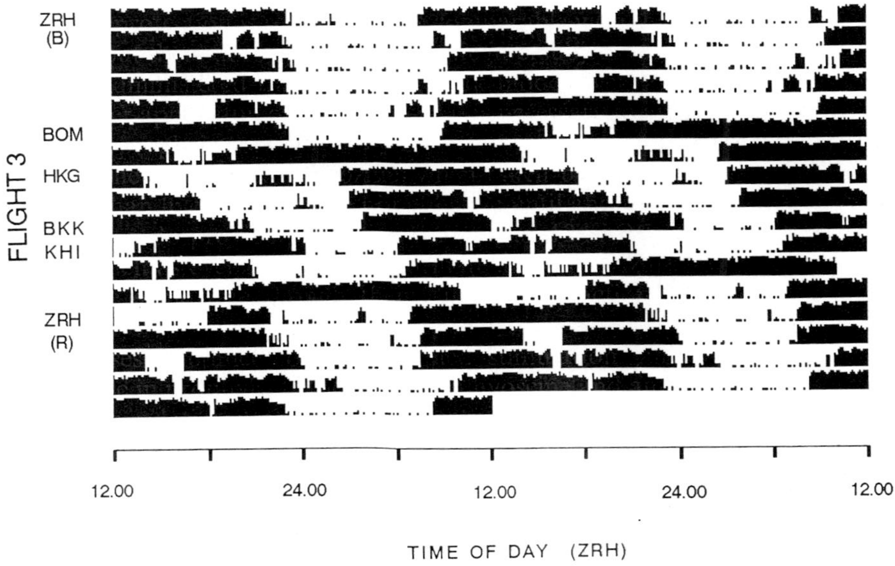


**Fig. 1.** Motor activity of a flight attendant (female, 26 years) participating in flight 3. The records are double plotted on a 48-h time base. Activity counts per 7.5-min periods are plotted for the following 8 bins: 0–5 counts (blank), 6–10, 11–30, 31–75, 76–120, 121–165, 166–210, 211–254. Time of day refers to homebase time. The first night at a new destination is marked *on the left* (ZRH, Zurich; BOM, Bombay; HKG, Hongkong; BKK, Bangkok; KHI, Karachi)

## Results

Figure 1 shows the original motor activity record of one subject for flight 3. The plot shows a clear demarcation of the low activity level during bedtime. Note that the phase of bedtime is advanced from ZRH to HKG.

*Objective and Subjective Parameters During Recovery.* A deterioration of sleep was observed only for flight 2. The mean bedtime activity level (Fig. 2) was increased and the percentage of immobility periods reduced. The subjective sleep parameters showed comparable changes. Both the number and duration of waking periods after sleep onset were elevated in one of the first two recovery nights of flight 2. Sleep was rated less quiet than during baseline, and subjects

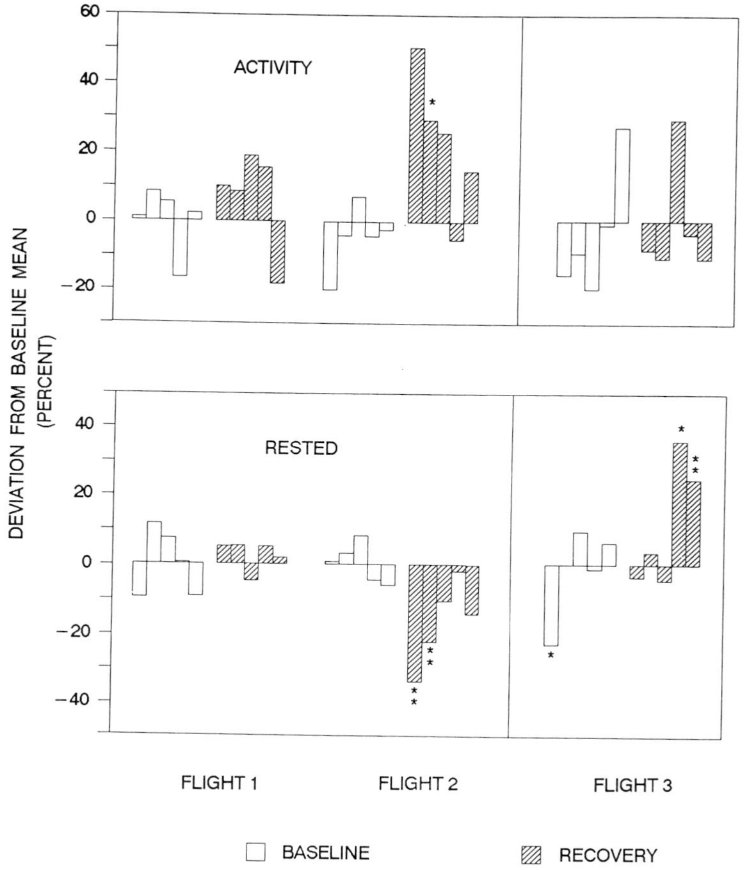


**Fig. 2.** Mean bedtime activity and restedness in the morning during 5 baseline days (*open bars*) and 5 recovery days (*hatched bars*) of the three flights. The values are expressed as percentage deviation from the corresponding baseline mean. Significant differences from baseline mean: * $P<0.05$; ** $P<0.01$ (Wilcoxon matched pairs, signed ranks test, two-tailed)

felt less rested in the morning (Fig. 2). The gradual reversal to baseline during the recovery period of flight 2 was reflected by the trend of mean activity, immobility, quietness of sleep and restedness in the morning. Although sleep was not impaired during the recovery period of flight 1 and 3, the jet lag score was elevated.

*Layover During Flight 3.* Despite time zone shifts of +7 h (HKG), most objective and subjective sleep parameters showed no significant deviation from baseline. The jet lag score increased to a maximum in HKG and then decreased gradually.

## Discussion

A deterioration of sleep was observed after the crew members had returned from NRT via ANC to homebase. The changes reverted to baseline during the first 4 days. Since this flight involved the crossing of 17 time zones with extended layovers, it is likely that the subjects underwent phase shifts in their circadian rhythms. Circadian factors are known to play an important role in sleep regulation. The disturbed sleep after flight 2 and its gradual reversal to baseline may therefore reflect the progressive resynchronization of the circadian pacemaker to the local 24-h cycle. This interpretation is supported by the finding that sleep was not disturbed after flight 1 (only one time zone crossing). It is interesting to note that sleep was little disturbed during and after flight 3. The fact that the subjects had an elevated jet lag score indicates that the jet lag syndrome not necessarily associates with disturbed sleep.

From an operational point of view it is reassuring that after both transmeridian flights sleep disturbances and subjective jet lag symptoms reverted toward baseline within the first 4 days after return to homebase. However, there was a considerable degree of interpersonal variation.

*Acknowledgments.* The study was supported by the Swiss National Science Foundation, grant 3.234-0.85 and by Swissair.

## References

1. Borbély AA (1986) New techniques for the analysis of the human sleep-wake cycle. Brain Dev 8:482–488
2. Borbély AA, Neuhaus HU, Mattmann P, Waser PG (1981) Langzeitregistrierung der Bewegungsaktivität: Anwendung in Forschung und Klinik. Schweiz Med Wochenschr 111:730–735
3. Dement WC, Seidel WF, Cohen SA, Bliwise NG, Carskadon MA (1986) Sleep and wakefulness in aircrew before and after transoceanic flights. Aviat Space Environ Med [Suppl 12]57:B14–B28
4. Graeber RC, Dement WC, Nicholson AN, Sasaki M, Wegmann HM (1986) International cooperative study of aircrew layover sleep: operational summary. Aviat Space Environ Med [Suppl 12]57:B10–B13
5. Graber RC, Lauber JK, Connell LJ, Gander PH (1986) International aircrew sleep and wakefulness after multiple time zone flights: a cooperative study. Aviat Space Environ Med [Suppl 12]57:B3–B9

6. Nicholson AN, Pascoe PA, Spencer MB, Stone BM, Green RL (1986) Nocturnal sleep and daytime alertness of aircrew after transmeridian flights. Aviat Space Environ Med [Suppl 12]57:B42–B52
7. Sasaki M, Kurosaki Y, Mori A, Endo S (1986) Patterns of sleep-wakefulness before and after transmeridian flights in commercial airline pilots. Aviat Space Environ Med [Suppl 12]57:B29–B42
8. Wegmann HM, Gundel A, Naumann M, Samel A, Schwartz E, Vejvoda M (1986) Sleep, sleepiness and circadian rhythmicity in aircrews operating on transatlantic routes. Aviat Space Environ Med [Suppl 12]57:B53–B64

# Motion Sickness and Jet Lag: Their Nature and Treatment

A. J. Benson and A. N. Nicholson

## Motion Sickness

### Introduction

Motion sickness is a condition characterized primarily by nausea, vomiting, pallor and cold sweating, and occurs when humans are exposed to real or apparent motion stimuli with which they are unfamiliar. It is a generic term which embraces sea sickness, air sickness, car sickness, swing sickness, simulator sickness and space sickness. However, despite the diversity of the causal environment, the essential characteristics of the provocative stimulus and the response of the afflicted individual are common.

Nevertheless, "motion sickness" is a misnomer, as symptoms can be evoked as much by the absence of expected motion as by the presence of unexpected motion. "Simulator sickness" and "Cinerama sickness" are examples. Further, motion sickness is a quite normal response of a healthy individual when exposed for a sufficient length of time to unfamiliar motion of sufficient severity. Indeed, after severe stimulus conditions, it is the absence, rather than the presence, of symptoms that is indicative of true pathology, for only those individuals who lack a functional vestibular system are truly immune. It would be better to label the condition as the "motion maladaption syndrome".

Typically the development of motion sickness follows an orderly sequence, the time scale being determined primarily by the intensity of the stimulus and the susceptibility of the individual. The earliest symptom is the unfamiliar sensation of epigastric discomfort. Should the provocative motion continue, wellbeing usually deteriorates quite quickly with the appearance of nausea of increasing severity. Concomitantly, circumoral or facial pallor may be observed, and the individual begins to sweat on those areas of skin where thermal sweating rather than emotive sweating occur. With the rapid exacerbation of symptoms, the so-called "avalanche phenomenon", there may be increased salivation, feelings of bodily warmth, a lightness of the head and, not infrequently, depression and apathy. By this stage, vomiting is not long delayed, though there are some individuals who remain severely nauseated for long periods and do not obtain the relief, albeit transitory, that many report following emesis.

Apart from the characteristic features of motion sickness – pallor, sweating, nausea and vomiting – other signs and symptoms are frequently, though more variably, reported. In the early stages, increased salivation, belching and flatulence are commonly associated with the development of nausea. Hyperventilation is occasionally observed, while an alteration of respiratory rhythm by sighing and yawning not infrequently precedes the "avalanche phenomenon". Headache is another variable prodromal symptom, usually frontal in distribution, though complaints of tightness around the forehead or of a "buzzing in the head" are not uncommon.

Drowsiness is an important, yet often ignored, symptom commonly associated with exposure to unfamiliar motion, even if not necessarily an integral part of the motion sickness syndrome. Typically, feelings of lethargy and somnolence persist for many hours after withdrawal of the provocative motion stimulus and nausea has abated. However, in certain circumstances a desire to sleep may be the only symptom evoked by exposure to motion, especially when the intensity of the stimulus is such that adaptation occurs without significant malaise. The soporific effect of a repetitive motion stimulus on infants has long been recognized. It may be that the drowsiness observed in the adult when exposed to appropriate motion is a manifestation of the same mechanism, though it must be acknowledged that the somnolence in an individual who has suffered overt motion sickness is frequently of abnormal intensity and persistence.

## Incidence

The incidence of sickness in a particular motion environment is influenced by several factors. They are the physical characteristics of the stimulus (frequency, intensity, duration and direction), the intrinsic susceptibility of the individual, the nature of the task performed, and other environmental factors such as odour. It ranges from a fraction of 1% in large civil transport aircraft to 100% during "hurricane penetration flights" in those who had no previous experience of such severe turbulence, but 90% of those who have flown in such conditions before may experience the problem again.

The considerable variability between subjects in their response to provocative motion is an important feature of motion sickness. However, and adult's susceptibility to motion sickness appears to be a relatively stable and enduring characteristic for there is evidence that those who are sensitive to one type of provocative motion are likely to succumb when exposed to another. Motion sickness is rare below the age of 2 years, but increases rapidly to reach a peak between the ages of 3 and 12 years. Over the next decade there is a progressive increase in tolerance which continues, albeit more slowly, with increasing age. This reduction in susceptibility with age has been recorded for both sea sickness and air sickness, but the elderly are not immune. About a fifth of those suffering from sea sickness on a Channel Island ferry were 60 years old or more.

Females are more susceptible to motion sickness than males of the same age, and a higher incidence of vomiting and malaise is reported by female than by male passengers on Channel Island ferries. The difference in susceptibility between men and women is in the ratio of about 1 to 1.7. The reason for this sex difference, which applies both to children and to adults, is not known. It may be that females are more ready to admit to having symptoms. Hormonal factors may play a part as susceptibility is highest during menstruation and is increased in pregnancy.

## Prevention

Passengers in an aircraft can minimize the problem conflict by restriction of head movement, for example, by pressing the head firmly against the seat or other available support, preferably in a reclined position. If space permits, they should lie down on their backs, as this posture has been shown to reduce the incidence by approximately a fifth. Symptoms are decreased by closing the eyes, unless the passenger has a clear view of the horizon or other stable reference outside the aircraft. Attempting to read a book, while a desirable means of occupying the mind and diverting attention from a lack of wellbeing, more commonly accentuates discordant visual cues.

The most useful treatment, at least in the long-term, is to adapt to the provocative motion. This is "nature's own cure" and is the preferred method of preventing sickness, particularly for aircrew who should not fly under the influence of any antimotion sickness drug. The basic philosophy is to be gradually introduced to the provocative motions of the flight environment, and that adaptation, once achieved, is maintained by regular and repeated exposure to the stimuli.

Over the years many medicinal remedies have been proposed for the prevention of motion sickness, but relatively few are effective (Table 1) and none completely prevents the development of signs and symptoms in everyone in all provocative environments. When the motion is relatively mild and only one in ten suffers then *l*-hyoscine is very useful. But when the motion is of such severity and duration that 50% are likely to be sick even a large dose of hyoscine (1.0 mg) may still leave one in ten of the population unprotected. In life rafts, sickness rates approaching 100% have been reported, so it is not sur-

**Table 1.** Adult dose regimen for antimotion sickness drugs

| Drug | Dose (mg) | Time of onset (h) (approx.) | Duration of action (h) (approx.) |
|---|---|---|---|
| Hyoscine hydrobromide | 0.3–0.6 | 0.5–1.0 | 4–6 |
| Cyclizine hydrochloride | 50 | 1–2 | 4–6 |
| Dimenhydrinate | 50–100 | 1–2 | 6–8 |
| Cinnarizine | 30 | 1.5–2.0 | 6–8 |
| Promethazine hydrochloride | 25 | 1.5–2.0 | 24–30 |
| Promethazine theoclate | | | |

prising that a significant proportion of the occupants will still suffer from sea sickness even when the dose of drug given is sufficient to cause side effects.

None of the drugs of proven efficacy in the prophylaxis of motion sickness is entirely specific and all have side effects. Some antihistaminics, such as promethazine and dimenhydrinate, and the anticholinergic, hyoscine, are depressants and can cause impairment of performance. Hyoscine causes decrement on tasks requiring continuous attention and memory storage for new information, and at doses greater than 0.8 mg interferes with motor skills. Promethazine (25 mg) also impairs psychomotor performance. Hyoscine may also lead to blurred vision, sedation, dizziness and dry mouth.

## Prophylaxis

The choice of a prophylactic drug is, in part, dependent upon the foreseen duration of exposure and suceptibility of the individual. In practice, if one drug is not effective or not well tolerated, then another drug or combination of drugs may be indicated. Where the objective is to provide short-term protection, oral *l*-hyoscine hydrobromide (0.3–0.6 mg) is the drug of choice. This acts within 0.5 h and provides protection for about 4 h. However, side effects can be troublesome particularly with repeated administration (at 4–6 h intervals). With the development of transdermal drug-transport techniques it is now possible to provide a loading dose of 200 μg hyoscine with a controlled release at 10 μg/h for up to 60 h. The protection is reported to be comparable with that achieved by oral hyoscine, but there does appear to be some intersubject variability. When hyoscine is administered transdermally, peak blood levels are not reached until 8–12 h after applicaton of the patch, so it is necessary to anticipate the requirement for prophylaxis.

The antihistamines promethazine and meclozine, when taken by mouth, are absorbed more slowly than hyoscine and are not effective until about 2 h after administration, but they do provide protection for at least 12 h. Other drugs in the same group, such as cyclizine, demenhydrinate and cinnarizine, are absorbed at about the same rate though their duration of action is shorter – about 6 h.

D-Amphetamine increases tolerance to cross-coupled stimulation, and there is a synergistic increase in prophylactic potency with hyoscine and antihistamines and a decrease in sedation. Ephedrine is almost as effective as amphetamine in enhancing the efficacy of the antimotion sickness drugs and should be used in preference to amphetamine. Essentially, the combination of *l*-hyoscine hydrobromide (0.3 mg) with ephedrine sulphate (25 mg) is most effective for short-term (4 h) protection, but for sustained prophylaxis promethazine hydrochloride (25 mg) with either ephedrine sulphate (25 mg) or *d*-amphetamine sulphate (5 mg) is recommended.

# Jet Lag

## Introduction

Present-day aircraft operating round northern and southern latitudes cross time zones almost at the same rate as the earth rotates. Journeys between Europe and North America can be completed within a few hours, and a shift of the day or night is experienced. After a westward flight it would have been 8 o'clock in the evening in London, but it is only 3 o'clock in the afternoon in New York, and the day will appear to have been lengthened. On the other hand after eastward flights, which occur mostly overnight, it is 3 o'clock in the morning in New york, but it is 8 o'clock in the morning in London. The night will appear to have been shortened, and several hours rest will have been lost. Clearly, it is in the interest of the intercontinental traveller to avoid or minimize disturbance of sleep during the journey, and the most useful approach, if airline schedules permit, is to travel during the day and arrive in time for bed. However, nearly all flights to Europe from North America are overnight, and so some sleep loss is inevitable.

Even if sleep loss is avoided during the journey there is still the adaptation to the new time zone. After transmeridian flights the individual may have difficulty in falling asleep when it is local time for rest, and there may be spontaneous awakenings during the night as well as early awakening in the morning. Adjustment needs time. There may also be some impairment of alertness or wellbeing during the day either due to poor sleep overnight or to the displacement of the sleep-wakefulness rhythm from the pattern of rest and activity of the new time zone.

Indeed, a period of rest is appropriate before making decisions again. Some journeys from north to south are without a time zone change, and only require a period of rest if the flight occurs during the normal sleep period, but recovery after a transmeridian flight is often delayed and the delay depends on many factors including the duration of the flight, number of time zones crossed, direction and time of departure. In this paper we will be looking at the effects of transmeridian flights on man, in particular on the circadian rhythmicity and sleep-wakefulness pattern, and discussing the usefulness of hypnotics in alleviating the adverse effects on sleep.

## Circadian Rhythms

The reason why there may be difficulty with sleep and, possibly, impaired alertness for several days after a transmeridian flight is that the functions of man vary with time in a periodic and regular manner, and are normally synchronized with the solar day. Conflict of circadian rhythmicity with that of the environment arises when the environmental synchronizers are weak or disappear completely or change their period length, though in man the clock hour and day-related social activities remain important influences.

Transmeridian flights produce rapid and often large time zone changes, and the sudden shift disengages the environmental and biological rhythms.

Subjectively, most people complain of tiredness, impaired appetite and a general loss of wellbeing, while sleepiness is experienced at inconvenient times of the day. Performance may be impaired in the late afternoon and evening of at least the 1st day after a flight in a westwardly direction, and in the morning and early afternoon after travelling eastwards.

Re-entrainment of rhythms to a new time zone occurs gradually. In man social cues and timing of meals are important and, indeed, adopting local times for meals accelerates the phase shift. Nevertheless, individuals differ in the ease and speed of their adaptation. Resynchronization usually takes between 2 and 6 days after westward flights and between 3 and 11 days after eastbound flights, though in some subjects eastbound travel may require even longer for complete adjustment to be attained.

The question arises whether the circadian rhythmicity of man originates from within or is the result on an exogenous influence, and to decide whether a rhythm is endogenous the individual must be studied in an environment free of all time cues. This is difficult because man is not only influenced by the alternation of light and darkness with its almost constant cycle length, but has also developed a pattern of rest and activity with regular meals. Nevertheless, it has been established that under constant conditions such as in caves many physiological and psychological rhythms continue to oscillate, though with a period length somewhat longer than 24 h. Circadian rhythms are endogenous, and are entrained to 24 h by variation in the environment.

## Disturbed Sleep

There would appear to be persistent effects on sleep after flying eastward. Sleep onset is delayed for many days as individuals are attempting to fall asleep earlier than usual, though if the individual does not sleep on the aircraft and works the next day the delay to sleep will overcome any difficulty with falling asleep during the first night. As far as westward flights are concerned there is the possibility that sleep onset is shortened as subjects are falling asleep later than usual, though a definite shortening of sleep onset is seen during the first night due to the additional effect of the delay to the rest period.

There are also subtle changes in rapid eye movement (REM) sleep and slow-wave sleep. Reduction in REM sleep occurs after eastward flights, and this is presumably due to the displacement of sleep to earlier in the natural rhythm of sleep and wakefulness. On the other hand with westward flights there is an increase in the amount of REM sleep, and the normal temporal pattern is established within a day or two. Slow-wave sleep may also be reduced for several days after an eastward flight, but with a westward flight the only change appears to be an increase of slow-wave sleep during the first night due to the delay to sleep.

Wakefulness during sleep is clearly increased during the adaptation to a new time zone. This is seen during the first night after a westward flight, but after an eastward flight increases in wakefulness and number of wakenings are seen for several days and sleep efficiency declines. It would appear that eastward flights involving a 5-h time zone change lead to persistent impairment of sleep, whereas the alterations after a similar westward flight are far less marked, and probably do not persist for more than a day or two. The more pronounced changes in sleep after the eastward flight tend to reflect the relatively slow adaptation of circadian rhythmicity to the new time zone.

## Hypnotics

The question of hypnotics does, of course, arise for the frequent intercontinental traveller. Hypnotics are likely to be of help during long flights, and also during adaptation. Hypnotics are most useful during a flight when there are suitable seats or a sleeperette. However, it must be realized that even transatlantic journeys are unlikely to provide a rest period of more than 5 h, and so the dose should reflect the duration of the journey. The low dose of the normal therapeutic range should be used if the flight is unlikely to provide rest of more than 5 h, but with longer flights a higher one may be appropriate. If a hypnotic is to be used during the flight, it should be tried beforehand to ensure the most appropriate response. In this context temazepam, 10–20 mg (Normison-Wyeth), and brotizolam, 0.125–0.25 mg (Lendormin, Boehringer Ingelheim), are the most useful sedatives.

However, the most relevant issue for the intercontinental traveller is adapting to the new time zone with the drive for sleep and wakefulness only coinciding slowly with the local pattern of rest and activity. The most disturbing effect may be the inability to stay asleep, and so there is need to sustain sleep during the night. In this respect a hypnotic may be useful for the first night or so after flying westward, whereas it may be useful for several nights after an eastward flight. A hypnotic which is likely to sustain sleep without residual sequelae, and which is free of accumulation on daily ingestion, is needed. In this context brotizolam (0.25 mg) is ideal, and zopiclone, 3.75–7.5 mg (Imovane, Rhone-Poulenc and May & Baker), is likely to be equally useful.

Recent studies support the potential of such drugs as brotizolam to sustain sleep, though at the same time, in appropriate doses, they are free of residual effects on performance and of accumulation on daily ingestion. Certainly, studies on the sleep of individuals flying between the United Kingdom and North America have shown that brotizolam reduces wakefulness during the first night after a westward flight, and alleviates the persistent sleep disturbance after an eastward flight. The use of drugs would be very helpful after intercontinental flights, though there is no evidence that hypnotics quicken the alignment of sleep and wakefulness with the rest and activity pattern of the new time zone.

## References

1. Anonymous (1986) Jet lag and its pharmacology. Lancet II:493–494
2. Benson AJ (1984) Motion sickness. In: Dix MR, Hood JD (eds) Vertigo. Wiley, Chichester, pp 391–426

3. Brand JJ, Perry WLM (1966) Drugs used in motion sickness. Pharmacol Rev 18:895–924
4. Money KE (1972) Motion sickness. Physiol Rev 50:1–38
5. Nicholson AN (1986) Hypnotics: their place in therapeutics. Drugs 31:164–176
6. Nicholson AN, Pascoe PA, Spencer MB, Stone BM, Roehrs T, Roth T Sleep after transmeridian flights. Lancet II:1205–1208
7. Reason JT, Brand JJ (1975) Motion sickness. Academic Press, London

# Selected Risk Groups

# Special Aspects for Patients with Preexisting Illness Planning to Stay in Tropical Countries

R. Jansen-Rosseck and R. Steffen

Due to the fact that only few studies illustrate the effect of tropical conditions on prexisting illnesses, fitness for the tropics is not well defined. Of course exposure to health risks varies in healthy persons as much as in ill persons. Therefore it is difficult to define strict rules for people intending to go to tropical countries who have some preexisting illness. Should these people be discouraged from travelling, or should they take additional precautions?

## Available Data

Between 1969 and 1971, 1987 Europeans had to be evacuated from sub-Saharan Africa back to France [1]. Despite the fact that the hygienic conditions were poor, only three (1.6%) cases were due to tropical diseaes, one each to malaria, amebiasis and trypanosomiasis. In contrast, 17% were due to psychiatric and 12% to cardiovascular problems, a large proportion of which could have been noted prior to departure. Ten percent each were due to hepatitis or neurologic affections. Bertrand, the original author of this report, concluded that, above all, persons with mental desequilibration, including alcoholism and drug abuse, need a particularly restrictive selection process. Fatalities were not reported.

Similarly, Joo [2] analyzed 128 evacuations of German foreign aid volunteers in 1972–1977. The leading causes were hepatitis ($n=25$), accidents ($n=24$), psychological or psychiatric disorders ($n=29$), various infections ($n=19$), and low back pain ($n=6$). Again, fatalities were not reported.

On the other hand, Florian [3] described the reasons Siemens workers had to consult doctors in Africa, Asia and Latin America. Out of 3635 medical reports, observed from 1964 to 1980, dental problems predominated ($n=688$), followed by common cold ($n=633$), gastrointestinal disorders ($n=456$), skin diseases ($n=340$) and accidents ($n=268$). Accidents were particularly frequent in Africa. Except for dental problems, preexisting diseases only played a minor role in this workforce of about 450 persons staying abroad, who had a mean age of 32 years.

In one of our earlier studies [4], we interviewed European air passengers, asking whether the status of any preexisting illness had changed, resulting from their holiday in the tropics ($n=10\,929$) or North America (United States or Canada, $n=1379$). Of all travelers coming from tropical destinations, 1.6% reported improvement of their disease, compared with only 0.5% of travelers

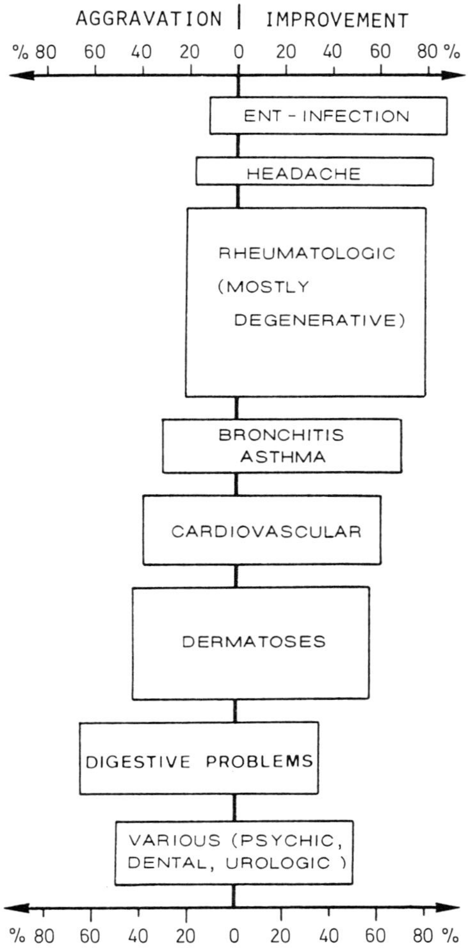


**Fig. 1.** Influence on various groups of preexisting diseases, due to a stay in the tropics, seen in 10929 travelers

visiting North America ($P=0.002$). This was mainly due to a favorable influence on chronic upper respiratory tract infections and chronic rheumatologic impairment (Fig. 1). Aggravation of preexisting disease occurred in 0.9 and 0.7% (NS) in the two groups of travelers respectively and was rarely severe: only three patients had to be admitted to a local hospital, two of them with gastrointestinal complications. Patients suffering from digestive problems in the tropics were adversely affected most frequently. No effect on their preexisting illness was reported by 4.3% of the respondents; this included all diabetics, the majority of people having neurologic disorders or malignancies. Only a minority had diseases influenced by the conditions of a tropical climate.

Other studies are more or less anecdotal, because the authors do not provide exact data showing what influence a stay in developing countries may have on preexisting illness.

This article does not review in-flight incidents, which have been described recently [5], nor does the article review precautions to avoid them [6–8].

## Fitness for a Stay in Tropical Countries

In order to classify the patient's fitness for a stay in the tropics, one can follow Diesfeld's classification, which has four categories [9]:

1. Fit for various tasks under adverse climatic conditions in remote areas (foreign aid volunteers, missionaries, etc.)
2. Fit for various tasks under adverse climatic conditions with either reliable travel facilities to adequate medical care or own medical infrastructure (workforce in large plants, advisors of various organizations)
3. Fit for tasks under good environmental conditions with adequate hygienic infrastructure which alleviate life even under adverse climatic conditions (diplomats, business persons)
4. Fit for short stays in tropical regions under comfortable conditions, characterized by rapid climatic changes (tourists, business persons, government officials)

In practice, only few people who want to travel are not at all fit for any category. Acclimatization is mostly possible within 7–14 days [10]. It can be prolonged in obese, exhausted or elderly persons and in patients with circulatory impairment.

The few people not suitable for any of the categories are those with:

- Severe or unstable cardiovascular illness, e.g., uncontrolled angina, myocardial infarction or stroke within the previous 6 months, persistent congestive heart failure, uncontrolled severe hypertension
- Relevant gastrointestinal illness, e.g. ulcerative colitis
- Immunodeficiency
- Any other severe and unstable illness

Pregnant women are recommended not to visit areas with high transmission of chloroquine-resistant *P. falciparum* malaria.

Additionally not fit for any prolonged stay (categories 1–3) are usually persons with:

- Emotional instability (who often want to escape from their problems)
- Unstable endocrinological diseases
- Chronic or recurrent gastrointestinal illness
- Any other relevant illness or condition, particularly those possibly progressing or leading to complications and those necessitating medical tests not reliably performed in the host country or preferably in the city the patient resides in

Additionally unfit for category 1 and possibly category 2 are usually persons with:

- Chronic or recurrent illness of the eyes or ears
- History of urolithiasis
- History of frequent consultations with doctors at home

Each case has to be judged under consideration of the previous history, health condition, personality, behavior, travel style and epidemiological and environmental situation [11, 12].

## Precautions in Patients with Preexisting Illness

First of all, such patients need detailed counseling. For example, the HIV seropositive person who insists on visiting developing countries needs to know how to avoid an infection. A person with a past history of myocardial infarction, who insists to visit Cuzco, Titicaca Lake and La Paz should restrain from rushing around or from eating opulent meals at altitudes often exceeding 3500 m (10000 ft).

Most contraindications to immunization (Schultz, p. 182) and to malaria chemoprophylaxis (Keystone, p. 102) are listed in this volume. In general, all pre-travel consultations should include the following routine questions:

- Have you had fever (38 °C or more) within the last few days? If so, it is preferable to postpone the vaccination.
- Are you taking any medication?
  Those taking corticosteroids at a dosage exceeding the equivalent of 5–10 mg prednisolone daily for at least 2 weeks [13] or taking immunosuppressants should not receive live vaccines. Patients taking anticoagulants should not receive intramuscular injections. When prescribing malaria chemoprophylaxis, one should consider potential interactions of *d*-penicillamine with chloroquine, of sulfonylureas, anticoagulants, diphenylhydantoin, barbiturates with Fansidar, and of cardioactive substances such as $\beta$-blocking agents with mefloquine. Women taking oral contraceptives should be informed about gastroenteritis possibly causing a prophylactic failure and they should be instructed on action to be taken if this happens [14].
- Do you suffer from allergies?
  Persons hypersensitive to any component of a vaccine (antibiotics, chicken proteins, formaldehyde, phenol, etc.) should not be immunized with these particular vaccines. In the case of possible allergy, 0.1 ml vaccine, diluted 1 : 20 in normal saline and 0.1 ml normal saline as control, should be administered i.c. Persons allergic to particular substances of malaria chemoprophylaxis should take an alternative drug.
- Do you suffer from any acute or chronic illness?
  See above.
- Are you HIV-seropositive?
  Besides the fact that such persons should not be exposed to increased risk of infection, they preferably should not been given live vaccines, even if no increased risk has been documented and WHO for its expanded program on immunization (EPI) considers this restriction unnecessary in EPI-target countries [15] (cf. Lange, this volume, p. 369).

Preexisting illness may present some problems in pre-travel counseling, but hardly ever one will have to discourage somebody or even let him cancel a planned tour. Above all age per se is not a contraindication for a trip, because older people can be experienced travelers, tending to be less prone to illness than younger travellers [16]. In high-risk cases, it may be wise to recommend an insurance policy covering treatment abroad and aero-medical evacuation.

## References


1. Sankalé M (1980) Le malade chronique peut-il voyager? Union Med Can 109(2):7–9
2. Joó S (1979) Prüfung der gesundheitlichen Eignung für den Entwicklungsdienst. Mater Med Nordmark 31:214–222
3. Florian HJ (1981) Arbeitsmedizinische Gesundheitsvorsorge bei Auslandstätigkeit. Mod Unfallverhütung 25:43–46
4. Steffen R, van der Linde F (1981) Intercontinental travel and its effect on pre-existing illnesses. Aviat Space Environ Med 52(1):57–58
5. Cummins RO, Chapman PJC, Chamberlain DA, Schubach JA, Litwin PE (1988) In-flight death during commercial air travel. JAMA 259(13):1983–1988
6. AMA Commission on Emergency Medical Services (1982) Medical aspects of transportation aboard commercial aircraft. JAMA 247(7):1007–1011
7. Mills FJ, Harding RM (1983) Fitness to travel by air. Br Med J 286:1340–1341
8. Steffen R (1984) Reisemedizin. Springer, Berlin Heidelberg New York, pp 131–135
9. Diesfeld HJ (1971) Tauglichkeit für Reisen in warme Länder unter Berücksichtigung der Klimabelastung. Internist (Berlin) 7:268
10. Eyckmans L (1982) Health in a tropical climate (Abstr). Symposium Gesundheit, Reisen, Tourismus, May, Munich
11. Diesfeld HJ (1980) Importierte Krankheiten und ärztliche Untersuchungen vor und nach Tropenaufenthalt. Lang, Frankfurt (Schriftenreihe Medizin in Entwicklungsländern, vol 6)
12. Diesfeld HJ (1985) Tropentauglichkeit von Ferientouristen und Arbeitnehmern. Ther Umsch 42(1):17–22
13. Immunization Practices Advisory Committee (ACIP) (1983) Yellow fever vaccine. MMWR 32:52–58; Weekly Epidemiol Rec (1984) 59:96
14. John AH, Jones AJ (1975) Gastroenteritis causing failure of oral contraception. Br Med J 3:207–208
15. WHO (1987) Expanded programme on immunization. Joint WHO/UNICEF statement on immunization and AIDS. Weekly Epidemiol Rec 62:53–54
16. Steffen R (1985) Epidemiology of health impairments during intercontinental travel. Travel Med Int 3:76–79

# Special Aspects for a Stay in the Tropics: Pregnant and Nursing Mothers

M. S. Wolfe

## Summary

There is considerable confusion and difference of opinion concerning the safety of necessary immunizations and prophylactic and therapeutic drugs for malaria and other diseases in the pregnant and nursing female traveler. The medical literature and travel health guides contain numerous contradictory recommendations and very few of these controversial subjects have been adequately studied. Questions are frequently asked for which there are no definite answers, and decisions must be made on a benefit versus risk basis. Particular important examples will be discussed, including immunizations; malaria prophylactic and therapeutic drugs; antidiarrheals; and treatment of parasitic and other infectious diseases. Longer-term female travelers to and residents in the developing world require advice on adequate nutrition and hygiene for particular situations, which will also be discussed. In all these areas, it is not uncommon for the advice of the travel medicine specialist to differ totally or vary in detail from the very conservative, yet often relatively uninformed, advice given by her obstetrician, leaving her in a most difficult situation.

## Introduction

The pregnant or nursing woman traveling to or living in a tropical developing area presents a number of challenging problems to travel medicine personnel advising her. Major areas of concern include: safety of needed immunizations; adjustment to adverse travel and living conditions; prophylactic drugs for malaria and traveler's diarrhea; acquisition of, diagnosis of, and safety of drugs required, for treatment of tropical (particularly parasitic) diseases; and concerns about adequate prenatal, delivery, and postpartum care [4, 7].

The main problems for the nursing mother involve the safety of necessary immunizations and drugs on the nursing (particularly neonatal) infant. Prior to consulting the travel medicine clinic or specialist, the pregnant traveler usually has received advice on the above problem areas from her obstetrician, personal physician, or nonmedical friends and contacts. Frequently, the advice received either evokes more worry and concern, or extremely conservative, nihilistic or unfounded recommendations are made. Obstetricians in particular are extremely reluctant to recommend any immunization or prophylactic or therapeutic drug during pregnancy, especially in the first trimester. Thus, the prospective pregnant traveler may be advised not go to a developing area until after delivery; or to go but to not take any immunization or prophylactic drugs while pregnant or breast-feeding. She then contacts the travel medicine specialist, whose recommendations usually based on incomplete or nonexistent data, determine whether or not she travels, or, if she does travel, what protective measures she is willing to take.

Certain basic principles must guide the travel medicine specialist in deciding what advice to give. Firstly, in the United States, approximately 2% of births have some congenital abnormality, irrespective of whether or not there has been any use of drug or immunization or a recognized infection. This is the so-called "background noise" against which any meaningful risk of these exogenous factors must be compared. There is also the question of relative disease risk in different parts of the same country. A pregnant woman going to live in Bangkok, where there is virtually no risk of contracting malaria, and who will not venture to any recognized malarious area during her pregnancy, will not require antimalaria prophylactic drugs. However, a woman going to live in West Africa, for example, where malaria risk occurs in both cities and rural areas, requires continuous antimalarial drug prophylaxis. Similar relative risks within a country or region also apply to the need for certain immunizations. Unfortunately, there are minimal data available on the safety (or real danger) of immunizations or drugs during pregnancy. The scanty literature on the subject is based on these inadequate data; it may well be influenced by only anecdotal evidence or personal bias or conservatism, or sometimes by expert consensus. It therefore devolves upon the travel medicine advisor to make the final decision which should be determined case-by-case on a benefit versus risk basis. In the words of President Harry S. Truman, "The buck stops here," i.e., the ultimate decision and responsibility was his.

## Immunizations

### Live-Virus Vaccines

Since a woman may not be aware that she is pregnant until several weeks have elapsed, the travel medicine advisor must first ask her whether pregnancy is possible or have a pregnancy test performed. Should she be pregnant, then there must be particular concern about the use of live-virus vaccines, since many live viruses and live-virus vaccines are able to cross the placental barrier and could possibly infect the fetus. It is therefore, prudent to avoid all routine immunizations with live-virus vaccines during pregnancy unless absolutely required for protection against a mayor threat of infection.

*Yellow Fever*. This is one of two vaccines (the other being cholera) which currently can be required of all entrants to certain countries. In most cases, there is no yellow fever present in the destination country and the requirement is based on the traveler having passed through a yellow fever infected country or zone on the way. In this situation, since the vaccine is not necessary for protection, the pregnant traveler should be given a Letter of Contraindication on a physician's letterhead and signed by him. This is almost invariably accepted in lieu of proof of vaccination. If the pregnant woman is traveling to a country in tropical Africa or South America in which yellow fever risk occurs in specific, usually remote areas, and is willing to restrict herself to cities or other uninfected areas, she should also be given a Letter of Contraindication along with strong admonishment absolutely to avoid traveling to an area with known yellow fever infection.

If it is locally available, she could then receive yellow fever vaccine after delivery. Only if a pregnant woman must for some reason go to a known infected area, or possibly be in a newly occurring epidemic situation, should yellow fever vaccine be indicated. The real risk of yellow fever vaccine to the fetus is unknown, and the prohibition of its use, as with many other vaccines and drugs, is more theoretical. When used during pregnancy, either inadvertently or because of need for protection, it has not shown any detrimental effect on the fetus to my knowledge. Also, extensive inquiries by the World Health Organization failed to show any recognized ill effects in pregnancy [14].

*Poliomyelitis (Live Oral or OPV).* There is definite risk of poliomyelitis infection for an unprotected traveler to the developing world. There is no convincing evidence of adverse effects of either oral or killed? (IPV) polio vaccine in pregnant women or developing fetuses. If protection is needed during pregnancy, due to previous inadequate basic series or booster immunization, authorities agree that oral polio vaccine can be given without any greater risk to the mother or her unborn child than to other persons.

*Measles, Mumps, Rubella.* There is a theorectical risk to the fetus from these live virus vaccines and they are generally not given to pregnant women or those likely to become pregnant within 3 months. They should best be given in the immediate postpartum period. Since measles acquired during pregnancy increases fetal risk, a susceptible pregnant woman exposed to measles should be given immune serum globulin (ISG) in a dose of 0.25 ml/kg (max. dose 15 ml). ISG has not been shown to be effective for post-exposure prophylaxis of mumps, and it is not recommended for this purpose.

Although mumps virus can infect the placenta and fetus, there is no evidence that this virus causes fetal malformations. Mumps vaccine can also infect the placenta, but the virus has not been isolated from fetal tissues from susceptible women who were vaccinated and underwent abortions.

Rubella vaccine should be avoided for theoretical reasons during pregnancy. However, in women inadvertently given rubella vaccine within 3 months of or during pregnancy, evidence to date indicates that the risk of vaccine-associated malformations or congenital rubella syndrome is negligible.

## Inactivated Virus and Bacterial Vaccines, Toxoids, and Immune Globulin

The risk to the pregnant woman of other non-live vaccines, toxoids, and immune globulins is unknown for certain from lack of data, but there is also no confirmed evidence of risk. Thus, a pregnant woman requiring one of these products because of infection exposure should best be given it. Where possible, it is considered prudent to wait until the second or third trimester, on theoretical grounds only; but there need be no prohibition against indicated vaccines if required for protection in the first trimester.

## Traveling

Most airlines and shipping companies refuse to carry passengers in the last 6 weeks or so of pregnancy, even with a permission slip from her doctor. A pregnant woman with a complication of pregnancy (placenta previa, hypertension, diabetes) must carefully consider the increased risk of these conditions to her and the fetus. While on a jet airplane or sitting in a vehicle for long periods, it is important to walk about frequently to maintain circulatory tone. Similar to other travelers, the pregnant traveler must also exert efforts to effect safe water and food intake and to acclimatize to the new environment.

## Malaria Chemoprophylaxis

Malaria infection poses a serious threat to all nonimmune people in malarious areas, particularly pregnant women and their fetuses. Malaria may cause abortion, premature labor, maternal anemia, and congenital infection [3, 10]. A pregnant woman with acute malaria requires treatment with higher doses of chloroquine or other antimalarial drugs than are needed for prophylaxis. Under no circumstance should a pregnant woman be told to go to a malarious area without taking appropriate malaria chemoprophylaxis. She should in addition use other personal protection measures to reduce contact with mosquitoes between dusk and dawn, including: gauze window screens, mosquito nets, long sleeves and trousers, repellants, and a pyrethrum-containing spray.

The complete itinerary should be reviewed in order to determine whether malaria occurs in the specific areas visited. If malaria is present, it must be determined whether chloroquine-resistant *Plasmodium falciparum* malaria occurs.

For travelers who will only be in urban areas of China, Southeast Asia, and Latin America, or who will have only daytime exposure in rural areas, no malaria preventive drugs are necessary as the risk is minimal at best.

For travel to areas of chloroquine-sensitive falciparum malaria, including Central America, Haiti and the Dominican Republic, and the Middle East, and the antimalarial drug of choice is chloroquine. This is taken in a dose of 500 mg salt (300 mg base) once weekly, regularly and without fail, beginning 1 week before, while in, and for at least 4 weeks after leaving the malarious area.

We have studied the safety of chloroquine during pregnancy and found in a cohort of US Foreign Service women that the proportion of birth defects in those taking chloroquine during pregnancy was not significantly different from that in a nonchloroquine-using control group [13]. This observation must necessarily be considered within the limitations of the study which could detect only a strong teratogenic effect, due to the relatively small number of women studied (169 chloroquine users and 454 controls). To obtain the thousands of subjects and a standardized mechanism of reporting to exclude low-grade teratogenicity of chloroquine as malarial prophylaxis would require efforts beyond our means. This study serves as a typical example of why sufficient data have not been obtained on vaccines and drugs used during pregnancy to be able definitely to assure their full safety.

Further confidence on the safety of chloroquine in the recommended 300 mg base weekly dose is the absence of cases of congenital defects in humans reported in the literature with this dose. In a study in which chloroquine was administered intravenously to pregnant mice, chloroquine crossed the placenta and accumulated in the eyes of the fetus at both early and late stages of development. A high accumulation of chloroquine was also observed in the inner ear during late development [11]. Although these effects have not been reported in humans, they may be theoretically possible. It would be of interest to investigate a cohort of infants, whose mothers have taken chloroquine, for evidence of retinal toxicity. Loss of hearing, possibly attributable to intrauterine effects of chloroquine, could be studied at an older age by audiometry. Pyrimethamine (Daraprim) is considered the least effective of the available antimalarial drugs, but it is currently one of the few drugs marketed in the United States. There has been concern over its safety in pregnancy but the current consensus is that it should be considered safe. In over 25 years of use as an antimalarial and antitoxoplasmosis drug it has been used by many thousands of pregnant women and has proved itself perfectly safe to the developing fetus. There has never been any evidence suggesting that pyrimethamine in the doses normally used for malaria suppression might be responsible for fetal damage. Proguanil (Paludrine) can be recommended as an alternative for those unable to tolerate chloroquine or in whom chloroquine is contraindicated, such as in psoriatics. The accepted safety of proguanil in pregnancy is discussed below.

Chloroquine-resistant *P. falciparium* malaria is present in malarious areas of Asia, Oceania, much of tropical Africa, and the para-Amazon region of South America. Many experts believe that chloroquine weekly should be taken in these areas, in addition to other drugs particularly useful against chloroquine-resistant falciparum malaria. These others include: proguanil (Paludrine), and doxycycline (Vibramycin). A dapsone-pyrimethamine combination (Maloprim), though not recommended by United States experts, is recommended by some European and Australian experts. Mefloquine (Lariam) is a newly available drug.

Because of its association with the Stevens-Johnson syndrome, pyrimethamine-sulfadoxine is currently not recommended. The safety of this drug for pregnant women is controversial because of teratogenic effects in laboratory animals; also the sulfadoxine component administered during the last month of pregnancy theoretically could compete with bilirubin for plasma proteins and exacerbate neonatal jaundice. Most experts believe it should best be avoided in pregnancy.

Many years experience with proguanil indicate that it is a very safe drug in pregnancy. However, in recent years it has been routinely used in a 200-mg daily dose and some have concern over whether this dose can be considered as safe in pregnancy as the long-used 100-mg daily dose. As with most drugs, definitive controlled studies remain to be done. Doxycycline is a long-acting tetracycline and like all tetracyclines is contraindicated during pregnancy as it can cause permanent discoloration of children's teeth. Fetal damage has been observed on administration of high doses of mefloquine in mice and rats during early pregnancy. At this time, mefloquine has not yet been licensed for prophylactic use in pregnant women. Since Maloprim contains pyrimethamine, there remains concern by some over its use in pregnancy. However, the only caveat in the package insert is that if Maloprim is used during pregnancy, a folic acid supplement should be given.

Primaquine, for terminal prophylaxis to eliminate any *P. vivax* or *P. ovale* parasites from the liver, is not recommended during pregnancy. This is a conservative recommendation based not on any confirmed evidence of human fetal damage from this drug; but again, as with many other drugs, because not enough pregnant women taking this drug have been adequatedly folllowed to assure complete safety.

## Traveler's Diarrhea – Prophylaxis and Treatment

Measures recommended by some to attempt to prevent or to treat travelers' diarrhea (particularly that due to toxigenic *Escherichia coli*) include the antibiotics doxycycline; trimethoprim-sulfamethoxazole (Bactrim, Septra); and the new quinolones (ciprofloxacin and norfloxacin). Bismuth subsalicylate tablets (Pepto-bismol) are also recommended for these purposes. As discussed under malaria prophylaxis above, doxycycline is not recommended during pregnancy. Trimethoprim-sulfamethoxazole may interfere with folic acid metabolism and is recommended during pregnancy only if the potential benefit justifies the potential risk to the fetus; this is probably not the case in its use in attempting to prevent or treat traveler's diarrhea. Quinolones cause arthropathy in immature animals and are contraindicated during pregnancy. There is no evidence of human teratogenicity from either the bismuth or subsalicylate moieties of Pepto-bismol; its beneficial use in the pregnant women for either prophylaxis or treatment of traveler's diarrhea must, as always, be weighed against any theoretical risk.

## Antiparasitic Drugs

For a thorough review of the safety of antimicrobial agents during pregnancy, reference can be made to the excellent review article by Chow and Jewesson [6] and to a *Medical Letter* summary article [2]. In this presentation, the emphasis will be placed on the management of the commoner parasitic infections in the pregnant woman.

### Malaria Treatment

Treatment of choroquine-sensitive falciparum malaria and *P. malariae* should be with chloroquine alone, which is recognized as being safe in pregnancy. Treatment of *P. vivax* and *P. ovale* should also be with chloroquine, but primaquine should not be given. One approach to attempting to prevent relapses during the duration of the pregnancy could be to continue the woman on suppressive doses of chloroquine. Severe chloroquine-resistant *P. falciparum* in the pregnant woman should be treated with quinine (intravenously or orally) along with either tetracycline or Fansidar. There should be no undue concern for the staining of fetal teeth by tetracycline in this emergency life-saving situation. Neither should there be overconcern about potential (but very rare) induction of abortion in pregnant women when emergency use of quinine is indicated. Here the known benefit must outweigh any possible risk.

## Intestinal Protozoa

For giardiasis, none of the available drugs is considered assuredly safe in pregnancy. If used at all during pregnancy, they should be administered only when severe symptoms are definitely attributable to giardiasis and benefit is judged to outweigh potential risk. When reluctantly forced to treat pregnant women, the author has used both quinacrine and metronidazole and has not recognized any deleterious effects on the fetus. Paromomycin (Humatin), which is poorly absorbed, deserves possible consideration for use against symptomatic giardiasis in pregnancy [9].

In amebiasis infections, asymptomatic cyst-passers should have any treatment deferred until after delivery. Mildly symptomatic intestinal amebiasis could be treated with paromomycin alone. For moderately severe nondysenteric intestinal amebiasis the poor absorption of paromomycin limits its effectiveness with any tissue invasion. This type of infection, along with invasive dysenteric amebiasis and amebic liver abscess, requires tissue-active drugs such as metronidazole or one of the other imidazoles (tinidazole, ornidazole). A number of recent reviews of metronidazole use during pregnancy consider the risk of mutagenicity to be low, if not negligible [8], and in more severe amebic infections the benefit outweighs any potential risk. Follow-up luminal drug treatment can then be with paromomycin. Less confidence of safety is held for iodoquinol, and diloxanide furoate's (Furamide's) safety is not established and it is not recommended. The safety of emetine and dehydroemetine in pregnancy is unknown and they are generally considered contraindicated.

Symptomatic *Dientamoeba fragilis* in pregnant women can be treated with paromomycin. In a nonimmunosuppressed pregnant woman, *Cryptosporidium* infection should be self-limited and not require antiparasitic drug treatment. The present questionable pathogenic potential of *Blastocystis hominis* should restrict drug therapy for this during pregnancy.

## Anthelminthic Drugs

Many helminthic infections are light and, with rare exceptions, multiplication of adult parasites does not occur. Treatment can therefore often be deferred until after delivery.

The intestinal nematodes *Ascaris lumbricoides* and hookworms, and *Enterobius vermicularis*, if symptomatic and troublesome during pregnancy (particularly if not used until after the potentially more vulnerable first trimester) can be treated with pyrantel pamoate (Antiminth). This drug is absorbed in small amounts, with no known fetal toxicity, and is considered probably safe. Mebendazole (Vermox) is teratogenic and embryotoxic in rats and should be used with caution[1] during pregnancy. *Strongyloides stercoralis* can be a potentially dangerous infection during pregnancy. No well-controlled studies during pregnancy have been carried out on the drugs useful for this infection, thiabendazole and albendazole, and they should be used with caution; however, potential benefit probably outweighs any potential risk. *Trichuris* infections are invariably light and asymptomatic in adults, and the drug of choice, mebendazole, should best be withheld until after delivery.

Intestinal cestodes (tapeworms) are usually asymptomatic, but if treatment is considered indicated, niclosamide (Niclocide) can be given. This drug is not absorbed, has no known fetal toxicity, and is probably safe in pregnancy.

Treatment of symptomatic intestinal or urinary schistosmiasis in the pregnant woman with praziquantel (Biltricide) requires careful consideration of benefit versus risk as this drug has an increased abortion rate in rats and no adequate studies have been done in pregnant women. However, no toxic effects have been recognized in pregnant women and many experts consider it probably safe. The use of praziquantel in cerebral cysticercosis during pregnancy seems justified. Praziquantel is currently the drug of choice for other intestinal, hepatic, and pulmonary lung flukes and its use also appears justified in symptomatic pregnant women.

### Filariasis

Troublesome symptoms from the various human filarial infections seldom occur and treatment with diethylcarbamazine or ivermectin can usually be delayed until after delivery. However, in practice no abortifacial or teratogenic effects have been reported with diethylcarbamazine use in pregnant patients. Women of child-bearing potential are excluded from treatment with ivermectin under the investigational protocol.

### Ectoparasites

Scabies and lice in the pregnant woman can be treated with pyrethrin products as these are poorly absorbed, have caused no known toxicity in the fetus, and are considered to be probably safe. Lindane (Kwell) is absorbed from the skin and has potential CNS toxicity in the fetus and is contraindicated in pregnancy.

## Nursing Mothers

Many experts believe breast-feeding should be preferred over bottle-feeding. One advantage in the tropics is the potential for less transmission of infectious

[1] *Caution*: Use only for strong clinical indication in the absence of a suitable alternative. Potential benefit should justify potential risk to fetus.

organisms than with necessary sterilization of bottles and preparation of liquid feedings. It is important for the nursing mother to maintain a high fluid intake.

It is necessary in malarious areas to start appropriate malaria drug prophylaxis for the infant immediately after birth. Insufficient drug reaches the baby through the breast milk of a mother herself taking antimalarial drugs. Chloroquine, proguanil, and primaquine (if G-6PD is normal) are considered safe for the newborn nursing infant. Fansidar, Maloprim, and mefloquine (at this time) are contraindicated for newborn infants, nursing or not. Mosquito nets, as well as other non-drug protective measures, should be employed to avoid mosquito bites.

The same schedule for immunizations should be followed for breastfed as for bottle-fed infants. Inactivated or killed vaccines do not multiply within the body and pose no special problems for mothers who are breastfeeding or for their infants. Live virus vaccines multiply within the mother's body, but most have not been demonstrated to be excreted in breast milk. In the few circumstances where there could be transmission from breast milk, such as rubella, the virus usually does not infect the infant and if it does the infection is well tolerated. Yellow fever virus is not excreted in breast milk after vaccination and this vaccine is not contradicated for breast-feeding mothers [5].

Most drug package inserts contain a warning statement that "no information is known concerning the concentration present in the breast milk of nursing mothers." This statement is sometimes taken to mean that the drug has been shown to be contraindicated for nursing mothers. Actually, it only reflects lack of evidence one way or the other and should be weighed appropriately. There is also general agreement that most drugs deemed safe for a baby in utero when given to the pregnant mother can be given to the lactating mother with reasonable assurance of safety to her breastfed baby. The drug passes into the baby's system much less directly through the milk, if at all, than through the placenta.

With few exceptions, medications prescribed for a mother during pregnancy can be continued after delivery, if the doctor considers it necessary. The best available information regarding questions of a drug's possible effects on a breastfed baby whose mother is taking it is published by the LaLeche League International Inc [12]. While some drugs are found, usually in small amounts, in human milk, available information indicates that most do not have any demonstrable harmful effects on the baby. The major question to be answered is not which drugs are passed onto the infant through the milk, but do they affect the infant in any recognized way. Another summary of drugs in breast milk has been published in the *Medical Letter on Drugs and Therapeutics* [1].

## References

1. Anonymous (1979) Update: drugs in breast milk. Med Lett Drugs Ther 21:21–24
2. Anonymous (1987) Safety of antimicrobial drugs in pregnancy. Med Lett Drugs Ther 29:61–63

3. Bruce-Chwatt LJ (1983) Malaria and pregnancy. Br Med J 286:1457–1458
4. Carter JP, West ED (1971) Keeping your family healthy overseas. DeLacorte, New York, pp 191–207
5. Centers for Disease Control (1988) Health information for international travel. CDC, Atlanta, p 74 [HHS publ no (CDC) 88-8280]
6. Chow AW, Jewesson PJ (1985) Pharmacokinetics and safety of antimicrobial agents during pregnancy. Rev Infect Dis 7:287–313
7. Dawood R (1988) How to stay healthy abroad. Penguin, New York, pp 353–358
8. Finegold S (1980) Metronidazole. Ann Intern Med 93:585–587
9. Kreitner AK, del Bene VE, Amstey MS (1981) Giardiasis in pregnancy. Am J Obstet Gynecol 8:895–899
10. Lewis R, Lauersen NH, Bernbaum S (1973) Malaria associated with pregnancy. Obstet Gynecol 42:696–700
11. Lindquist NG, Ullberg S (1972) The melanin affinity of chloroquine and chlorpromazine studied by whole body autoradiography. Acta Pharmacol Toxicol [Suppl 2] (Cophenh) 31:1–31
12. White GJ, White M (1984) Breastfeeding and drugs in human milk. Vet Hum Toxicol [Suppl 1]26
13. Wolfe MS, Cordero JF (1985) Safety of chloroquine in chemosuppression of malaria during pregnancy. Br Med J 290:1466–1467
14. World Health Organization (1971) WHO Expert Committee on Yellow Fever. WHO Tech Rep Ser 479:31

# Prophylaxis and Treatment of Acute Mountain Sickness

O. Oelz

## Summary

Acute mountain sickness (AMS) can be avoided in most circumstances by "slow ascent", which includes not increasing the sleeping altitude above 2500 m by more than 300 m per 24 h. Care should also be taken to ensure an adequate fluid intake. Warning signs of AMS, such as headache, lassitude, insomnia, nausea, cough, peripheral and periorbital edemas and dyspnea on exertion should be respected and lead to rest days. Travelers who tend to become sick in spite of these prophylactic measures can take acetazolamide as prophylaxis, usually in a dose of 500 mg once a day. The efficacy of dexamethasone in the prophylaxis of AMS has also been demonstrated. Inefficient or dangerous medications include antacids, iron and vitamin preparations, phenytoin, potassium supplements, furosemide and medroxyprogesterone.

Mild cases of AMS can be treated with rest days and symptomatic medications. Severely affected patients should descend, be evacuated to a lower altitude or, if this is impossible, be treated with oxygen. If this is not available, dexamethasone 8 mg initially followed by 4 mg every 6 h alleviates the severity of AMS. This treatment should be reserved for emergencies to facilitate safe descent and is generally more effective for cerebral symptoms than for the pulmonary manifestations of AMS.

Acute mountain sickness (AMS) is a syndrome initially characterized by peripheral edema, headache, lassitude, insomnia and nausea (Table 1). Although this complex of symptoms is usually self-limited, it may progress to vomiting, ataxia, severe lassitude and breathlessness. Such patients may already have or can rapidly develop frank high-altitude pulmonary edema (HAPE) and high-altitude cerebral edema (HACE) [8, 9, 11]. HAPE and HACE rapidly lead to death unless appropriate measures are taken. AMS occurs in subjects who rapidly ascend to altitudes of 2500 m or more, and takes from a few hours to a

**Table 1.** Altitude-related illness

| |
|---|
| *Symptoms and signs:* Headache, lassitude, dizziness, insomnia, anorexia, nausea, vomiting, dyspnea on exertion/at rest, ataxia |
| *Acute mountain sickness* (AMS): Several of the symptoms/signs |
| *High-altitude pulmonary edema* (HAPE) |
| *High-altitude cerebral edema* (HACE) |
| *Complications:* Thrombosis (venous, arterial), pulmonary embolism, frost bites, retinal hemorrhages |

few days to develop. The actual prevalence varies with rate of ascent and the altitude attained. Studying 460 random climbers at four locations in the Swiss Alps, Maggiorini et al. [18] found that 34% suffered from AMS. The prevalence correlated with the altitude at which the subjects were studied. Approximately 67% of climbers on Mount Rainier (4392 m) suffer at least from a mild form of AMS due to a very rapid ascent [22]. The prevalence of HAPE and HACE in two different studies in Nepal was 2.5% and 4.5% respectively [9, 11]. In the Swiss Alps approximately ten patients have to be rescued annually by air-rescue services due to HAPE. In the highest mountain hut, the Capanna "Regina Margherita" at 4559 m, 1 out of 600 climbers who stay there overnight have to be evacuated [13]. Annually several deaths due to HAPE or HACE occur in the higher regions of the Himalayas and the Andes.

## Prophylaxis

The most effective preventive measure to avoid AMS is gradual acclimatization and slow ascent. Gradual acclimatization should be achieved at an altitude between 1500 and 2500 m for 2–4 days before ascending to a higher elevation [10, 20]. Once ascending above 3000 m particular care should be taken not to increase the sleeping altitude by more than 300 m/24 h. In general a climber is safe if he sticks to these simple rules even if he does higher ascents during the day.

However, some people habitually develop AMS and even HAPE, although they observe these precautions. The main pathogenetic factor for the development of AMS in these individuals seems to be a blunted hypoxic ventilatory response and periodic breathing during sleep, resulting in further oxygen desaturation. Therefore there have been a number of well-controlled studies assessing the efficacy of the respiratory stimulant acetazolamide in the prevention of AMS [2, 3, 6, 7, 17]. In general most studies found that ventilation and partial arterial oxygen pressure were increased during altitude exposure in humans pretreated with the drug and also fewer symptoms of AMS were observed. Sutton et al. [25] found on Mt. Logan that acetazolamide reduced periodic breathing during sleep, improved arterial oxygenation at high altitude and increased ventilation at any percentage of oxygenation at sea level. Further double-blind crossover studies also demonstrated that subjects on acetazolamide were able to reach a higher altitude while ascending peaks like Kilimanjaro and trekking peaks in Nepal. During a prolonged journey in Nepal, Bradwell et al. [2] observed that subjects on acetazolamide had less weight loss, better exercise performance and less loss of muscle mass than controls. Once again the acetazolamide group had fewer symptoms of AMS. Anecdotal reports from extreme altitude climbers suggest that even while attempting 8000-m peaks acetazolamide may improve performance and reduce the discomfort associated with severe hypoxia.

There is some discussion about the most appropriate dose of acetazolamide. Studies have been performed with 500, 750 and 1000 mg. The higher doses are frequently associated with side effects like paresthesias, unpleasant taste and more serious dehydration. Most mountaineering doctors now agree that a single dose of 500 mg acetazolamide slow-release preparation in the morning is the best prophylactic dose against AMS.

Other respiratory stimulants such as methazolamide and almitrine have been tested but not found to be superior to acetazolamide [12, 27]. Since many of the symptoms of AMS are probably due to some degree of cerebral edema, and since dexamethasone (DXM) is used for treating some forms of cerebral edema, Johnson et al. [14] investigated its efficacy in preventing AMS in a hypobaric chamber. DXM in a dose of 4 mg every 6 h significantly reduced the symptoms of acute mountain sickness as assessed by questionnaire and by an interviewing physician. The cerebral symptoms score was decreased by a factor of four in subjects receiving DXM. These investigators also observed a reduction in the width of the retinal arteries under DXM, suggesting an effect on cerebral edema. These chamber studies were subsequently confirmed by the same workers during actual altitude exposure up to an altitude of 4300 m [23]. During rapid ascent DXM treatment reduced the incidence of AMS from 60% in subjects on a placebo to 30% in subjects receiving DXM. It has to be emphasized that after cessation of DXM treatment mountaineers experienced a progressive development of symptoms of AMS which lasted throughout the altitude stay, indicating that DXM does not provide rapid acclimatization and that AMS can occur if the drug is suddenly stopped.

When comparing the prophylactic efficacy of DXM and acetazolamide, Ellsworth et al. [4] found comparable effects. However, subjects on acetazolamide experienced more unpleasant side effects of the treatment and missed the euphoric effects of DXM. This study was performed with 750 mg acetazolamide/day and different results might have been obtained with a more appropriate dose of 500 mg

Several drugs have been tried or recommended in the past which should at the present time no longer be used for the prophylaxis of AMS, since they are either inefficient or dangerous. Among these drugs are antacids, phenytoin, iron preparations, potassium supplements, furosemide and medroxyprogesterone [15, 20, 22, 26].

## Therapy

The most important treatment modality is knowledge about the symptoms and signs of AMS, which leads to appropriate therapy when the first symptoms occur. Most cases of mild AMS will improve and become asymptomatic upon simple modalities like rest days, leisure and eventually a descent of a few hundred meters. Mild symptoms like headache can also be treated with aspirin or acetaminophen. Insomnia should not be treated with sleeping pills, since they tend to aggravate oxygen desaturation during sleep. Mild cases of AMS can also be treated with acetazolamide although there are no controlled studies available proving its value in established AMS.

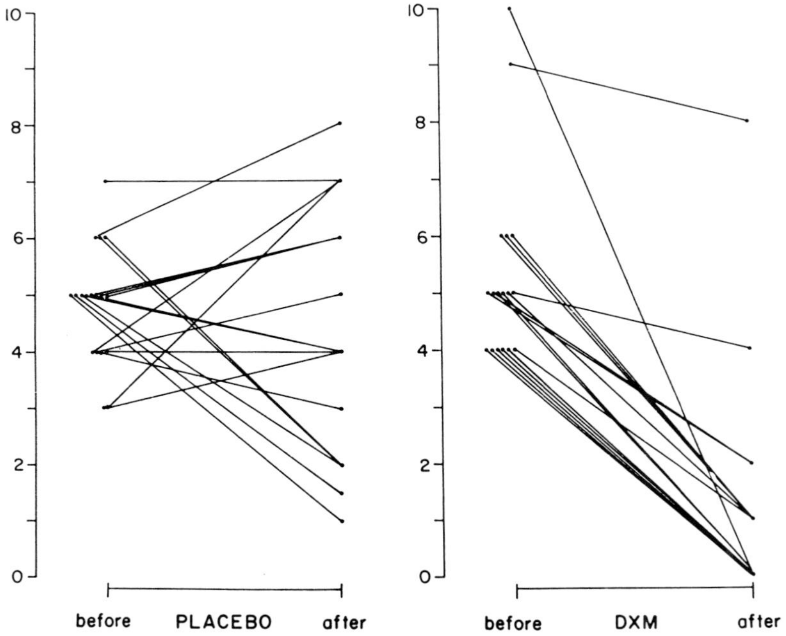


**Fig. 1.** Acute mountain sickness score of mountaineers before and after 12–16 h of treatment with placebo or DXM

The most effective and immediate measure in patients with severe AMS, HAPE or HACE is descent or evacuation to a lower altitude. This should be insisted upon by all means available and with no loss of time. Frequently a descent of 500–1000 m is sufficient to improve the condition of the patient remarkably. The following warning signs of cerebral edema should indicate an immediate descent: severe headache not relieved by aspirin, ataxia, repeated vomiting and impaired consciousness. The same is true for signs of pulmonary edema like dyspnea at rest, cyanosis and physical signs of pulmonary edema. Even patients without evident pulmonary rales can already be suffering from serious interstitial edema, with marked impairment of oxygen diffusion and blood shunting [1].

If descent or evacuation is impossible, oxygen should be given at a flow rate of 2–3 liters/min. Occasionally descent or evacuation may be prevented by weather or avalanche conditions and oxygen equipment is not available. In such circumstances a simple drug regimen with dexamethasone (8 mg initially followed by 4 mg every 6 h can be used [5]. In a double-blind placebo-controlled trial of patients with established severe AMS, this treatment significantly reduced the score of symptoms and signs of AMS in all patients studied (Fig. 1). The mean score decreased significantly from 5.4 to 1.8, and 8 of 17 patients became totally asymptomatic. There was also a rise in arterial oxygen saturation and a small increase in standard spirometric measurements in climbers treated with DXM, whereas none of these parameters changed significantly in climbers on a placebo. Comparable results have independently been obtained by Hackett and Roach [10] in a study of sick climbers on Mt. McKinley. DXM seems to be more effective for cerebral than for pulmonary symptoms of AMS.

Since breathing against positive end expiratory pressure has been used to improve gas exchange in many forms of pulmonary edema, positive end expiratory pressure has been evaluated in studies involving climbers with HAPE at 4400 m on Mt. McKinley. Short-term treatment increased oxygen saturation and improved exercise tolerance probably due to opening of microatelectatic alveoli [16, 24]. This treatment should not be used for prolonged periods since the development of HACE after the improvement of HAPE has been reported under these circumstances [19].

A recent anecdotal report suggests that the calcium channel blocker nifedipine improved the symptoms of a patient with HAPE at 7000 m [21]. It was postulated that this effect was due to a reduction of pulmonary hypertension associated with HAPE. Controlled studies are necessary to evaluate the role of nifedipine in the treatment of HAPE.

Furosemide has been frequently used in the past to treat HAPE, particularly in patients who were evacuated by helicopter at the same time. There is no convincing evidence that this treatment improves the permeability edema of HAPE. On the contrary it might favor the development of peripheral and cerebral thrombosis due to hemoconcentration. Other dangerous drugs for the treatment of HAPE include morphine and other respiratory suppressants.

## Conclusion

High altitude can be uncomfortable for many people and dangerous for some. The headache, nausea and other symptoms of AMS, which usually subside in a few days, can be avoided by proper acclimatization and if necessary by taking acetazolamide or dexamethasone. HAPE or HACE, which occur in a small percentage of people who ascend quickly to altitudes above 2500 m, can be rapidly fatal in previously healthy young people. Again gradual ascent and sleeping at altitudes below 2500 m can decrease the incidence of this catastrophic event. Serious cases of AMS and patients with HAPE or HACE should descend or be evacuated to lower altitudes immediately. There is no substitute for this simple regimen.

## References


1. Bärtsch P, Waber U, Haeberli A, Maggiorini M, Kriemler S, Oelz P, Straub WP (1987) Enhanced fibrin formation in high altitude pulmonary edema. J Appl Physiol 63:752–757
2. Bradwell AR, Coote JH, Milles JJ, Dykes PW, Forster PJE, Chesner I, Richardson NV (1986) Effect of acetazolamide on exercise performance and muscle mass at high altitude. Lancet I:1001–1005
3. Cain SM, Dunn JE II (1966) Low doses of acetazolamide to aid accommodation of men to altitude. J Appl Physiol 21:1195–1200
4. Ellsworth AJ, Larson EB, Strickland D (1987) A randomized trial of dexamethasone and acetazolamide for acute mountain sickness prophylaxis. Am J Med 83:1024–1030
5. Ferrazzini G, Maggiorini M, Kriemler S, Bärtsch P, Oelz O (1987) Successful treatment of acute mountain sickness with dexamethasone. Br Med J 294:1380–1382
6. Forwand SA, Landowne M, Follansbee JN, Hansen JE (1968) Effect of acetazolamide on acute mountain sickness. N Engl J Med 279:839–845
7. Greene MK, Kerr AM, McIntosh IB, Prescott RJ (1981) Acetazolamide in prevention of acute mountain sickness: a double-blind controlled cross-over study. Br Med J 283:811–813
8. Hackett PH (1980) Mountain sickness. Prevention, recognition and treatment. Am Alpine Club
9. Hackett PH, Rennie D (1979) Rales, peripheral edema, retinal hemorrhage and acute mountain sickness. Am J Med 67:214–218
10. Hackett PH, Roach RC (1987) Medical therapy of altitude illness. Ann Emerg Med 16:980–986
11. Hackett PH, Rennie D, Levine HD (1976) The incidence, importance, and prophylaxis of acute mountain sickness. Lancet II:1149–1154
12. Hackett PH, Roach RC, Harrison GL, Schoene RB, Mills WJ Jr (1987) Respiratory stimulants and sleep periodic breathing at high altitude. Almitrine versus acetazolamide. Am Rev Respir Dis 135:896–898
13. Hochstrasser J, Nanzer A, Oelz O (1986) Das Höhenödem in den Schweizer Alpen. Beobachtungen über Inzidenz, Klinik und Verlauf bei 50 Patienten der Jahre 1980–1984. Schweiz Med Wochenschr 116:866–873
14. Johnson TS, Rock PB, Fulco CS, Trad LA, Spark RF, Maher JT (1984) Prevention of acute mountain sickness by dexamethasone. N Engl J Med 310:683–686
15. Kryger M, Glas R, Jackson D, McCullough RE, Scoggin C, Grover RF, Weil JV (1978) Impaired oxygenation during sleep in excessive polycythemia of high altitude: improvement with respiratory stimulation. Sleep 1:3–17
16. Larson EB (1985) Positive airway pressure for high-altitude pulmonary oedema. Lancet I:371–373
17. Larson EB, Roach RC, Schoene RB, Hornbein TF (1982) Acute mountain sickness and acetazolamide. Clinical efficacy and effect on ventilation. JAMA 248:328–332
18. Maggiorini M, Bühler B, Walter M, Oelz O (1986) Inzidenz und Erscheinungsformen der akuten Bergkrankheit in den Schweizer Hochalpen. Schweiz Med Wochenschr [Suppl 20]116:24
19. Oelz O (1983) High altitude cerebral oedema after positive airway pressure breathing at high altitude. Lancet II:1148
20. Oelz O (1985) Prophylaxe und Therapie der akuten Bergkrankheit. Ther Umsch 42:52–57
21. Oelz O (1987) A case of high-altitude pulmonary edema treated with nifedipine. JAMA 257:780
22. Roach RC, Larson EB, Hornbein TF, Houston CS, Bartlett S, Hardesty J, Johnson D, Perkins M (1983) Acute mountain sickness, antacids, and ventilation during rapid, active ascent of Mount Rainier. Aviat Space Environ Med 54:397–401

23. Rock PB, Johson TS, Cymerman A, Burse RL, Falk LJ, Fulco CS (1987) Effect of dexamethasone on symptoms of acute mountain sickness at Pikes peak, Colorado (4300 m). Aviat Space Environ Med 58:668–672
24. Schoene RB, Roach RC, Hackett PH, Harrison G, Mills WJ Jr (1985) High altitude pulmonary edema and exercise at 4400 m on Mount McKinley. Effect of expiratory positive airway pressure. Chest 87:330–333
25. Sutton JR, Houston CS, Mansell AL, McFadden MD, Hackett PM, Rigg JRA, Powles ACP (1979) Effect of acetazolamide on hypoxemia during sleep at high altitude. N Engl J Med 301:1329–1331
26. Wohns RNW, Colpitts M, Clement T, Karuza A, Blackett WB, Foutch R, Larson E (1986) Phenytoin and acute mountain sickness on Mount Everest. Am J Med 80:32–36
27. Wright AD, Bradwell AR, Fletcher RF (1983) Methazolamide and acetazolamide in acute mountain sickness. Aviat Space Environ Med 54:619–621

# Helicopter Rescues and Deaths Among Trekkers in Nepal

D. R. Shlim, R. Houston, and M. Motamedi

Trekking in Nepal has become an increasingly popular vacation activity. The number of foreigners taking out trekking permits in this Himalayan kingdom has increased from 14 000 in 1976 to almost 50 000 in 1986 [1]. A trek in Nepal involves hiking for a number of days over hilly terrain that can vary in altitude from 200 m to over 5500 m.

Our study is the first attempt to establish the reasons for helicopter evacuation and death in trekkers in the Nepal Himalaya. Data on age, sex, location, altitude, and types of accident or illness provide the first guidelines for physicians and others who are asked to advise prospective adventure travelers.

## Methods

All helicopter evacuations and deaths among trekkers in Nepal which occurred between 1 January 1984 and 30 June 1987 were reviewed retrospectively through records obtained from trekking agencies, embassies, the Royal Nepalese Army Rotary Wing Command, the Himalayan Rescue Association, and local hospitals and clinics. The number of trekkers in Nepal each year was obtained through the Ministry of Tourism in Nepal.

For the purposes of this paper, a trekking death is defined as anyone who died while on trek in Nepal. An evacuation is defined as anyone who was ill or injured and obtained a helicopter to fly them to Kathmandu. Hundreds of other people are known to become ill or injured in Nepal, but if they do not fly out by helicopter there is no way to record these events. We excluded anyone who was working in Nepal, unless they were on vacation, and we excluded all mountaineering accidents, and evacuations from mountaineering base camps. We did not include trek-related evacuations and deaths among Nepalese citizens.

## Results

Approximately 148 000 people took out trekking permits during the time span of the study. Twenty-three people died. One hundred and eleven were rescued by helicopter. Only one person who was rescued by helicopter subsequently died (cerebral hemorrhage). The trekkers who required rescue ranged in age from 15 to 73 years, and came from 19 countries. The risk of dying while trek-

**Table 1.** Causes of rescue and death while trekking in Nepal, January 1984 to June 1987

| Cause | Rescue ($n=111$) | Death ($n=23$) |
|---|---|---|
| Acute mountain sickness | 38 | 3 [a] |
| Trauma | 29 [b] | 11 |
| Fall | 16 | 6 |
| Rockfall, avalanches | 2 | 4 |
| Assault | 2 [c] | 1 |
| Airplane | 1 [d] | – |
| Rhinocerous | 1 [e] | – |
| Frostbite | 1 | – |
| Rafting | 1 | – |
| Unknown | 5 | – |
| Illness | 29 | 8 |
| Respiratory | 6 | – |
| Cardiac | 6 | – |
| Diarrhea | 5 | – |
| Exhaustion | 4 | – |
| Asphyxiation in tent | – | 2 |
| Meningococcal meningitis | 2 | 2 |
| Cerebral hemorrhage | – | 2 |
| Appendicitis | 1 | – |
| Skin infection | 1 | – |
| Psychiatric | 1 | – |
| Vertigo | 1 | – |
| Hepatitis | 1 | – |
| Orthopedic (nontraumatic) | 11 | – |
| Back pain | 5 | – |
| Knee pain | 5 | – |
| Ankle pain | 1 | – |
| Unknown | 5 | 2 |

[a] Two cerebral edema, one pulmonary edema
[b] Eleven with fractures
[c] Attacked by Nepalese
[d] Motorized hangglider crash at 4900 m
[e] Attacked by rhinocerous in jungle area of Nepal

king was 15/100000. The risk of being evacuated by helicopter was 75/100000. In contrast, the risk of dying among foreigners who attempted to climb Himalayan peaks during the same study period was 2900/100000 (2.9%) (Hawley 1987, personal communication).

Surprisingly, there was no correlation between the number of deaths and altitude, through a range of over 5000 m. The causes of rescue are shown in Table 1.

Table 2 shows the age of the trekker in relation to number of deaths and number of rescues. Among persons 20–29 years old, there were two rescues for every death. Among persons age 50–59, there were 17 rescues for every death. Twenty-eight percent of people rescued for acute mountain sickness (AMS)

**Table 2.** Age (where available) of persons who died, were rescued, and the total

| Age | Died ($n=19$) | Rescued ($n=101$) | All ($n=120$) |
|---|---|---|---|
| 0– 9 | 0 | 0 | 0 |
| 10–19 | 1 (5)[a] | 3 (3) | 4 (3) |
| 20–29 | 8 (42) | 16 (16) | 24 (20) |
| 30–39 | 5 (26) | 36 (36) | 41 (34) |
| 40–49 | 3 (16) | 16 (16) | 19 (16) |
| 50–59 | 1 (5) | 17 (17) | 18 (15) |
| 60–69 | 0 | 9 (9) | 9 (8) |
| 70–79 | 1 (5) | 4 (4) | 5 (4) |

[a] Percentages in parenthesis

were over age 50, while 78% of people rescued for trauma were under age 50. Even though less than 16% of all visitors to Nepal are over age 50 [1], 45% of people rescued for illness were over that age.

Ninety-six percent of trekking permits were taken out for the three main trekking regions in Nepal: Everest (30921), Annapurna (94812), and Langtang (17277). Only 5286 people trekked in other parts of Nepal, but their risk of dying was four to ten times greater than in the usual trekking areas.

## Discussion

Less than seven people die each year while trekking in Nepal, out of an average of 42000 trekkers/year. Although AMS is the most publicized risk of trekking in Nepal [2, 3], the number of deaths from trauma is three times greater than the number of deaths from AMS. In fact, the number of deaths from AMS has averaged about one/year for the last 10 years despite the fourfold increase in tourism (Himalayan Rescue Association data 1987). The three AMS deaths in the study were completely preventable if early symptoms had been heeded. The frequent evacuations for AMS and the low death rate suggest that efforts to educate trekkers about this hazard are succeeding.

The issue of whether altitude provokes previously undiagnosed heart disease is unresolved. Our data show that there was only one unknown death and no proven cardiac deaths. Among the cardiac evacuations were two men in their late fifties with known severe cardiac disease who had been advised not to trek. A third cardiac evacuation was a 27-year-old man with frequent ectopic beats, which persisted after descent. Three other men (ages 39, 41, and 55) were evacuated for "chest pain," but no follow-up was available. High-altitude pulmonary edema can cause substernal chest pain and dyspnea, and can be difficult to distinguish from angina at altitude. People with known cardiac disease should not trek in Nepal due to the difficult terrain and the lack of medical facilities, but our study does not demonstrate an increased risk for people with no history of heart disease.

Meningococcal meningitis has been an increased risk in Nepal since 1983, and the Centers for Disease Control in the United States advised meningococcal meningitis vaccine for all travelers to Nepal in March 1985 [4]. The two deaths from apparent meningococcal septicemia occurred in people ages 24 and 28. Both deaths occurred before the advisory about meningococcal vaccine was issued.

There seemed to be an increased incidence of rescue among older trekkers, but not an increased risk of death. These data would suggest that younger trekkers are able to keep going until they are very seriously ill, or are involved in serious trauma. Older trekkers (over age 50) may not be as resilient when affected by illness (requiring evacuation more often), but may be more cautious in their travels, thus avoiding frequent death from trauma. There seems to be no reason to discourage older people from trekking if they are fit and have experience in the mountains.

In summary, the major risks of trekking in Nepal over the past 3½ years are now known. A decision to embark on a trek in Nepal should be individualized, understanding the problems related to remoteness, altitude, and illness in the absence of medical facilities.

## References


1. His Majesty's Government of Nepal (1986) Nepal Tourism Statistics 1986. Asian Printing Press, Kathmandu
2. Hackett PH, Rennie D (1976) The incidence, importance, and prophylaxis of acute mountain sickness. Lancet II:27
3. Hackett PH et al. (1979) Rales, peripheral edema, retinal hemorrhage and acute mountain sickness. Am J Med 67:217–218
4. Centers for Disease Control (1985) Epidemic meningococcal disease: recommendations for travelers to Nepal. MMWR 34:9–119

# Drug Therapy of Patients with Coronary Heart Disease During Exposure to Moderate Altitude

H. J. Deuber

Increased travel of older patients has posed the question of whether preexisting diseases, especially coronary heart disease, require restrictions in these patients in respect of traveling by air or tolerating mountaineering at moderate altitudes of up to 10000 ft. As there is little experience with this problem [1, 3, 6], this study was initiated to investigate the influence of altitude-related hypoxia on patients with coronary heart disease using different therapies.

## Methods

Thirty-four patients, aged 41–69 years, having angiographically proven coronary heart disease, were investigated. They had to perform bicycle ergometry in a sitting position in a hypobaric chamber at normal environmental conditions (i.e., 1000 ft) and at an altitude of 10000 ft. Fourteen patients were randomly chosen to investigate the effects of treatment with nifedipine (Adalat SL, Bayer AG, FRG) or isosorbide dinitrate (Isoket Ret, 120 mg, Schwarz-Pharma GmbH, FRG) on myocardiac ischemia and therefore working capacity. These patients had to perform ergometry 90 min after drug intake. All ergometry was performed at the same time on different days. It was started with 50 W and every second minute 25 W was added until one of the usual criteria for discontinuation of ergometry were fulfilled. During ergometry there was a continuous recording of a 12-lead ECG and every 2 min heart rate and blood pressure were measured. Evaluations were made of the maximum working capacities, the ST-segment depressions, heart rate and blood pressure as well as patients' complaints.

## Results

Cardiac arrhythmias did not occur. Heart rate remained comparable with and without therapy whereas systolic blood pressure was lowered significantly ($P<0.05$) from $138\pm15$ mmHg to $134\pm11$ mmHg (rest, isosorbide dinitrate), from $185\pm20$ mmHg to $170\pm25$ mmHg (work, isosorbide dinitrate), from $136\pm14$ mmHg to $131\pm14$ mmHg (rest, nifedipine) and from $181\pm22$ mmHg to $164\pm22$ mmHg (work, nifedipine). Blood pressure was compared at the mean work of $475\pm278$ Wmin, a stage that was tolerated by all patients at each examination.

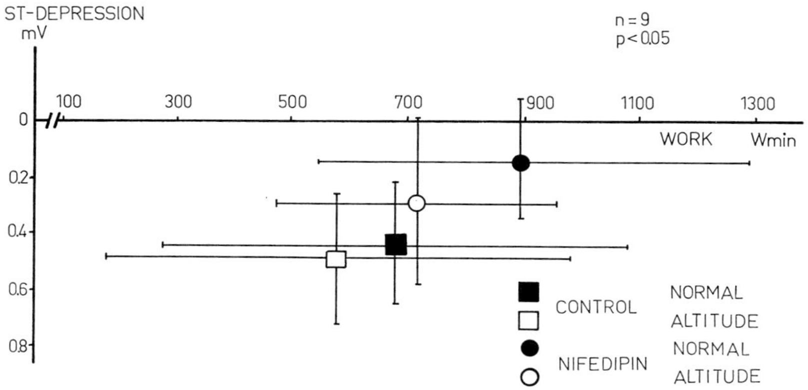


**Fig. 1.** Working capacity and ST depression after nifedipine treatment compared with therapy-free working capacity and ST depression of patients with coronary heart disease

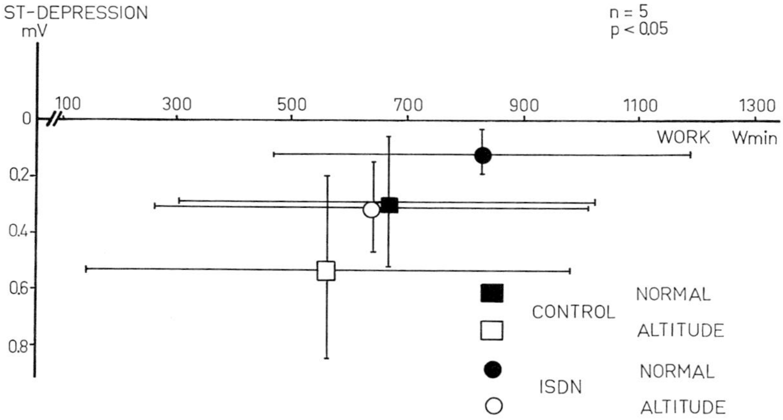


**Fig. 2.** Working capacity and ST depression after isosorbide dinitrate treatment compared with therapy-free working capacity and ST depression of patients with coronary heart disease

At altitude working capacities were significantly ($P < 0.05$) reduced (Figs. 1, 2). Due to significantly ($P < 0.05$) reduced ST depressions as a sign of reduced myocardiac ischemia, both nifedipine (Fig. 1) and isosorbide dinitrate (Fig. 2) were able to improve working capacities of patients with coronary heart disease significantly ($P < 0.05$) both at normal environmental conditions of 1000 ft and at a moderate altitude of 10 000 ft.

## Discussion

Both isosorbide dinitrate [4] and nifedipine [2, 5] are effective in reducing myocardiac ischemia. Therefore these drugs are generally used in the therapy of coronary heart disease. Both have the concomitant effect of lowering blood pressure, which was also demonstrated in this study.

The study shows that at altitude working capacities of patients with coronary heart disease are reduced regardless of therapy, probably because of reduced oxygen pressure. Treatment with either nifedipine or isosorbide dinitrate improves physical performance by reducing myocardiac ischemia. The results of the limited number of patients investigated suggest that antiischemic therapy enables patients to perform approximately the same work at 10000 ft as at 1000 ft without therapy.

According to general medical opinion, patients with coronary heart disease should avoid staying and working at altitude. Therefore patients are often advised not to travel by air or go mountaineering. The results of this study strongly suggest that there is no major impairment in patients with coronary heart disease who stay and even work at moderate altitudes of up to 10000 ft, an altitude that corresponds with the cabin pressure of commercial aircraft, if these patients are properly treated with antiischemic drugs and show physical reserves during labor at environmental conditions. Similar advise is given by Lomazzi and Gurtner [6].

## References

1. Deuber HJ, Wortmann A, Bachmann K (1985) Exercise-induced myocardial ischemia at high altitude simulated in a negative pressure chamber. 2nd International Conference on Space Physiology, 20–22 Nov, European Space Agency
2. Hausmann A et al. (1981) Mod Med 10:732–740
3. Inama K, Halhuber MJ (1975) Der Herz-Kreislaufkranke im Hochgebirgsklima. Deutsche Zentrale für Volksgesundheitspflege, Frankfurt
4. Kukovetz WR, Holzmann S (1983) Mechanism of nitrate-induced vasodilation and tolerance. Z Kardiol [Suppl 3]72:14–19
5. Lehmann HU, Hochrein H (1985) Differentialtherapie mit Calciumantagonisten. Dtsch Med Wochenschr 17:674–680
6. Lomazzi F, Gurtner HP (1981) Höhenaufenthalt und Flugreisen bei Herzkranken. Schweiz Med Wochenschr 111(18):618–624

# Practice of Medicine on a Sailing Ship from England to Australia

D. M. K. Keefe

The STS "Young Endeavour" was Britain's bicentennial gift to Australia. The ship's company for her delivery consisted of three different groups. Firstly, the "voyage crew" (or trainees) were 12 young Australian and 12 young British men and women, selected by special committees in Australia and the United Kingdom. Secondly, there were 11 "staff crew," selected from the British and Australian Navies, and civilian sailing fraternities. Finally, 3 film crew brought the total to 38. All voyage crew were between the ages of 18 and 24 years, with all staff being under 42 years.

A vigorous selection procedure, including special weekends where people were observed in a variety of situations, especially with respect to their reaction to living in a group, was carried out for all except the film crew, who were seconded from the Australian Broadcasting Corporation. In addition to my role as Medical Officer, I was also one of three "Watch Officers," responsible for sailing the ship for 8 h each day.

The route taken was from Cowes, Isle of Wight, via Tenerife, Rio de Janeiro, Tristan da Cunha, Cape Town (as an emergency only) to Fremantle, and thence 12 Australian ports before handover in Sydney on Australia Day 1988.

## Planning

Planning began 6 months before departure, the Medical Officer being responsible for medical stores. Advice was sought from senior colleagues, one in each relevant field. They all agreed that:

1. One should only take equipment one was happy (and able) to use oneself.
2. General rather than specific drugs and equipment were best, for example broad-spectrum antibiotics.
3. Operations are very dangerous at sea. One must be prepared to perform an appendectomy but almost never do so. The order of action is conservative treatment, followed by a request for outside help. Only if both these fail should operation be considered.

To ensure crew fitness before the trip, the ship's company were obliged to have medical and dental examinations 3 months before joining, and to ensure any necessary treatment was completed before departure. Immunizations required included yellow fever, cholera, typhoid and hepatitis A.

The expected problems, in order of frequency, were psychological, traumatic, infective and other.

The Stores were a combination of a surgical kit carried by Royal Australian Naval destroyers; the merchant shipping requirement for the United Kingdom; and a list compiled with the help of the advisors. The first two only catered for ships without a doctor, so the latter was more relevant to our case. Dental instruments were carried in addition, as tooth extraction was likely to be necessary. Psychosis would be very serious if occurring at sea, so major tranquillizers were carried. Minor tranquillizers would be used to ensure rest during illness, as isolation would not be possible. Modern, big sailing ships do not regularly provide much exercise. There can be many days when no sail-handling is required. A keep-fit programme was therefore set up incorporating a readily available foredeck "gym".

## Reality of the Trip

On board ship, access to all drugs except aspirin and cinnarizine was solely through the Medical Offier – leading to more consultations than on land; and crew members had to have the Medical Officer's permission to miss duty. There were 236 new consultations from August 1987 to January 1988; the majority occurring during the longer passages, and mostly for minor problems. Interestingly, there were more consultations on Mondays than any other day. The voyage crew averaged six consultations to the staff's four – mainly due to differences in age and experience of the sea. In both the staff crew and the voyage crew, the females averaged twice as many consultations as the males; the difference not being accountable to "female problems". However, with only two females on the staff, that figure is less significant.

The breakdown of cases differed from the expected one of psychological followed by traumatic and infective (Table 1). Infections were commonly skin abscesses and upper respiratory tract infections. Trauma was most often to the hand, with fingers being caught in blocks or ropes. The allergies were mostly to the strong galley detergents, and most of the foreign bodies were metal filings or glass. Most women on board had stopped taking the oral contraceptive pill prior to the trip. Seven restarted during it. Only one male sought contraceptive advice. My perception of the work was also that there had been more psychological problems than any other. This was because these tended

**Table 1.** Nature of consultations

| | |
|---|---|
| 1. Infection | 90 cases = 38% |
| 2. Trauma | 60 cases = 25 ½% |
| 3. Psychology | 18 cases = 7 ½% |
| 4. Allergy | 13 cases = 5 ½% |
| 5. Foreign body | 11 cases = 4 ½% |
| 6. Contraception | 9 cases = 4% |
| 7. Other | 35 cases = 15% |

to endure – requiring several follow-up consultations each; whereas minor infections and minor traumas were easily dealt with. Seasickness was never a large problem – everyone adapted to the ship's motion very quickly and never had enough time to lose their sea legs. Although successful during the warm weather, the keep-fit programme faltered in the cold southern ocean. Once in Australia, the crew began to participate in sports ashore and the programme restarted. Many of the males lost weight (apparently muscle) while the girls tended to gain it.

## Major Medical Problems

1. When one of the film crew presented with anxiety-depression and auditory hallucinations, we were one day from Tristan da Cunha but unable to land due to inclement weather. A major detour to Cape Town was necessary, the patient being nursed for the 10 days in a cabin shared with five others. The medical history taken prior to the trip had not been probing enough psychologically – and the film crew selection had not been strict enough.
2. Another crew member suffered from a series of infections, including several skin abscesses and rashes, dacryocystitis and an infective phymosis. Each was treated individually. His blood sugar was normal but no other investigations were possible.
3. Several crew members sustained back injuries – and all were treated with bedrest and analgesia. A pitching, rolling ship is not the ideal environment especially for people in upper bunks.
4. One of the crew found changes in routine hard to accept; becoming angry and frustrated and inflicting physical pain on himself as a relief. He was sedated for 18 h, giving him an escape and gradually recovered from his anxiety.
5. Two of the crew developed a stormy heterosexual relationship in which physical violence was not unknown. This led to isolation from the rest of the ship's company. Both had frequent consultations for very minor physical problems – leading on to discussion about their relationship. Counselling here was not successful. They stayed violently together and remained isolated.
6. One of the girls developed abdominal pain which was diagnosed as cholecystitis. As we were only 2 days from land, she was referred to a surgeon on arrival. She rejoined the ship 10 days after a cholecystectomy and convalesced on board.

In summary, the major problems were, naturally, due to the isolation, both with respect to distance and to weather. The lack of sterile environment was countered by the use of antibiotic cover for procedures such as suturing. Indeed, antibiotics were generally prescribed earlier than on land. The selection procedure was, in retrospect, not perfect. If a more detailed questionnaire had been included in the medical examination, one unsuitable person at least would not have been selected.

## Conclusion

The lessons learned, or rather reinforced, were as follows:

Firstly, some of the equipment – namely surgical instruments – could safely have been left behind but this is more easily said with hindsight. Secondly, more of the Medical Officer's time was spent dealing with psychological problems than with any other. Thirdly, the threshold for antibiotic treatment of infection is lowered when in an isolated, crowded environment because infections spread very quickly here and are harder to treat later. The major lesson, however, was that the group behaved like a mini-society. At sea and out of contact with the rest of the world, the ship and ship's company became all-important. The group had its hero (the Captain) and its outcasts (various people at different times during the voyage). As Medical Officer, one was a sounding-board for many of the crew, as well as the provider of health care.

# Passenger Travel on Freighters

C. J. Urner

Up to 12 passengers enjoy traveling on Lykes' cargo liners to ports all over the world on voyages which may last up to 90 days. There are no physicians on board these vessels. As in the past, medical care is provided by the ship's Captain or First Mate. These officers main duty is to handle the affairs of the ship and cargo, with medical care to crew and passengers being only a small aspect of their overall responsibilities. This is further complicated by the fact that usually little or no medical information on their charges is available to them. The crew is provided with sign-on medical examinations, a copy of which they bring on board. A similar form was developed for our passengers to provide better service. Most of our Masters and First Officers have obtained training in shipboard medical care [1] and are nationally certified Emergency Medical Technicians with knowledge on how to use this information in an isolated environment. On board ship they have access to our standardized medicine chest [2], which is stocked according to the recommendations of the United States Public Health Service (USPHS) [3], the USPHS book *The Ship's Medicine Chest and Medical Aid at Sea* [3], and medical advice by radio [4].

## Health Status of the Passengers

A passenger applying for travel aboard one of Lykes' ships is furnished a packet with various information including a health form, in which the passenger completes the history part, and the physician the physical examination results, and gives recommendations. This form is reviewed by the Medical Department prior to accepting the passenger, and is available on board ship in case of need. In addition passengers are urged to provide a copy of a recent EKG tracing, and a report on a recent chest X-ray. This is the only medical information available during the voyage and has proven generally helpful in treatment both on board as well as ashore. Restrictions from freighter travel include the need for canes, crutches, prosthetic limbs, and certain medications (e.g., coumadin, long-term steroids), as well as difficulty with balance or grasp, serious medical problems, or age over 80. Should serious questions arise, the prospective passenger's physician is consulted before final acceptance of travel is offered. In most cases such questions are answered satisfactorily. The actual rejection rate has been only six in 5 years, probably because of self-selection and recommendations offered by the passenger's own physician.

**Table 1.** History and physical findings: passenger please complete

| | Yes | % | | Yes | % |
|---|---|---|---|---|---|
| Have you ever had or do you now have: | | | | | |
| Anemia/blood disorders | 84 | 3% | High/low blood pressure | 524 | 17% |
| Angina (heart pain) | 110 | 4% | Kidney/urinary trouble | 144 | 5% |
| Arthritis/joint trouble | 497 | 16% | Malaria/tropical fever | 56 | 2% |
| Asthma/lung problems | 112 | 4% | Nervous trouble | 21 | 1% |
| Back trouble | 251 | 8% | Pneumonia/pleurisy | 200 | 7% |
| Cancer/tumor | 233 | 8% | Rheumatic fever | 19 | 1% |
| Depression (frequent fears) | 16 | 1% | Skin trouble | 95 | 3% |
| Diabetes | 81 | 3% | Tuberculosis | 22 | 1% |
| Epilepsy or fits | 5 | | Ulcer/stomach trouble | 136 | 5% |
| Eye, ear, nose, throat trouble (loss of hearing) | 239 | 8% | Varicose veins | 149 | 5% |
| | | | Veneral disease | 1 | |
| Eye glasses/contact lenses (loss of vision) | 2049 | 68% | Yellow jaundice | 59 | 2% |
| | | | To what extent do you use: | | |
| Fainting or dizzy spell | 33 | 1% | Alcohol moderate | 998 | 33% |
| Heart trouble | 147 | 5% | Tobacco | 393 | 13% |
| Hernia (rupture) | 204 | 7% | Drugs | | |
| | | | Passengers | 3021 = 100% | |

Physical examination

| NOR | ABN | NOR | ABN |
|---|---|---|---|
| Nose | 20 | Genitalia | 20 |
| Mouth | 51 | Hernia | 36 |
| Teeth | 66 | Venereal | |
| Tonsils | 25 | Hemorrhoids | 58 |
| Throat | 1 | Spine | 52 |
| Neck/thyroid | 36 | Extremities | 14 |
| Chest/lungs | 56 | Varicosities | 46 |
| Heart | 129 | Tremor | 25 |
| Abdomen | 29 | Neurology | |
| Psychiatric (severe anxiety, depression, alcoholism, etc.) | | | |

The health records of 3021 passengers who traveled between 1983 and 1987 were reviewed for self-indicated problems and physician findings (Table 1). In addition to the check-off items passengers wrote in comments indicating present or previous treatment for a variety of conditions. The biggest number of these were cancer of the breast (22) and colon (10). Of the 326 surgical procedures listed the majority were for cancer. But also included were 15 cardiac bypasses, 8 pacemakers and 3 cardiac valve surgeries. Also there were 5 colostomies, 18 back surgeries and 7 hip replacements. Some provided full workups. EKGs were brought by only 105 passengers.

## Illness and Injuries During the Journey

Analysis of our passenger population by age (Table 2) shows that the majority of our passengers fall between the ages of 60 and 79 (83% of passengers). Similarly this group shows the highest incidence of illnesses/injuries. The 80-year-old passengers usually reached that age during the voyage, and this group never had any problems.

The 5% total of illnesses/injuries in all passengers was further checked for systems affected (Table 3). There were some particularly difficult instances and one death. In 19 of all cases (12%) medical advice by radio had to be obtained. There were two health-related ship diversions. For the same reason 16 passengers had to interrupt their voyage and were sent home. Repatriations are tabulated in Table 4, with the reason for obtaining medical advice by radio indicated. However, such advice was also obtained for ulcers, dental, asthma, sprains, herpes zoster (chest pain) and other instances where passengers were able to continue their voyage. In all instances the prompt and effective advice received was of material benefit to the treatment of the patient. Medical advice by radio was not obtained when the problem could be adequately dealt with on board or through a port physician. Among the major illnesses were painless jaundice (cancer of the pancreas), vaginal bleeding (cancer of the uterus), urinary tract obstruction, and chest pain. Several fractures happened while going ashore or sight-seeing, or during the roll of the ship. One passenger had urinary incontinence to the point of debility. One passenger died of an apparently acute cardiac event.

**Table 2.** Age distribution

| Age (years) | Number | % | Illness/injury | % | % of passengers |
|---|---|---|---|---|---|
| 0– 9 | 4 | 0.1 | | | |
| 10–19 | 11 | 0.4 | | | |
| 20–29 | 18 | 0.6 | | | |
| 30–39 | 63 | 2.0 | | | |
| 40–49 | 67 | 2.2 | 1 | 0.6 | 1.5 |
| 50–59 | 271 | 9.0 | 4 | 2.5 | 1.5 |
| 60–69 | 1314 | 44.0 | 34 | 21.6 | 2.6 |
| 70–79 | 1180 | 39.0 | 75 | 47.7 | 6.4 |
| 80 | 24 | 1.0 | | | |
| Age unknown | 69 | 2.0 | 43 | 27.4 | |
| No history | 9 | 0.3 | | 100 | |
| Total passengers | 3021 | 100 | 157 | | 5.2 |
| Total passengers traveled | 3171 | | | | |
| No data | 41 | | | | |
| Medical advice by radio (none in 1986) | | | 19 | 12% of illness/injury | |

**Table 3.** Illness/injury passengers 1983–1987

| Classification | Number | Distribution (%) |
|---|---|---|
| Infectious disease | 9 | 6 |
| Endocrine (diabetes) | 1 | |
| Mental | 1 | |
| Nervous system/sense organs | 4 | 3 |
| Circulatory | 9 | 6 |
| Respiratory | 34 | 22 |
| Digestive | 19 | 12 |
| Genitourinary | 5 | 3 |
| Skin | 14 | 9 |
| Musculoskeletal | 11 | 7 |
| Ill-defined symptoms | 19 | 12 |
| Injuries | 28 | 18 |
| Total | 157 | 100 |
| Medical advice by radio | 19 | 12 |
| Inoculations | 20 | 13 |
| Medication refills | 2 | 1 |
| Total illness/injury for 3021 passengers | 157 | 5 |

**Table 4.** Repatriation cases by age and reason

| Age (years) | Sex | |
|---|---|---|
| 72 | F[a] | Vaginal bleeding – carcinoma, uterus |
| 76 | M[a] | Mild stroke affecting right side |
| 73 | M[a] | Fracture right hip |
| | M[a] | Rash secondary to medication |
| 76 | M | Fractured clavicle |
| 79 | F[a/b] | Digitalis toxicity |
| 65 | M[a] | Bladder obstruction |
| 76 | M[a/b] | Melena, on cimetidine; alcohol abuse suspected |
| | M[a] | Delirium tremens |
| | M[a] | Acute bladder obstruction |
| | F | Alcohol abuse, foul language |
| 76 | M | Appendicitis |
| 76 | F | Severe radicular sciatica |
| | M | "Medical reasons" |
| 72 | M | Jaundice – carcinoma pancreas |
| 61 | F | Heart attack – death |

[a] Radio advice obtained
[b] Ship diversion necessary

## Comments

In all cases reviewed the properly completed initial health form was helpful in providing data for potential treatment aboard ship, for radio advice to ships at sea, and for treatment in foreign ports. They were also helpful for finding potential passengers with obvious limiting health problems, passengers who then were not accepted. Some of the forms submitted were only cursorily filled out, necessitating follow-up before accepting the passenger. On the other hand, difficulties mentioned often allowed fruitful consultation with the personal physician. In some cases the forms obviously did not represent the actual health status of the passenger, which was discovered only after embarkation. This was a disservice to the passenger and to the shipping company. In the cases of shipboard illnesses/injuries observed the health forms proved not to be predicitive of the actually occurring medical problems.

Age per se certainly is not a limiting factor. Although most of our passengers are above the age of 60, the overwhelming majority never experienced problems during freighter travel which could have been predicted and which would force them to interrupt travel. Severe instances totaled 16 (10.2% of all occurrences on board), or 0.5% of all passengers traveling during these 5 years. Those that chose this mode of travel like it and many make more than one voyage. Increased stress and education on safety aboard ship for passengers could help. Passengers must be consciously aware of the hazards with slips, trips and falls, useage of chairs and doors, and just walking and climbing when traveling aboard freighters.

## Conclusions

The great majority of passengers of all ages including those of 60–80 years can travel on freighters without difficulties. Even though the health history form does not provide predictive data except in very obvious circumstances, it will eliminate severe risks for travel on freighters when conscientiously completed. It is, however, primarily useful for assuring that health data are available on board when needed for treatment on the ship or in a port, or for medical advice by radio. The use of a health history and physical examination form, and EKG and a chest X-ray report, and attention to details of safety taken for granted by shipboard personnel should reduce the incidence of passenger medical problems on freighters. The availability of specialized 1-month shipboard medical care training for Masters and Mates,[1] a properly stocked medicine chest according to USPHS recommendations, and adequate radio advice to ships at sea benefit passengers and crew alike.

[1] Training in shipboard medicine is being provided by the Maritime Institute of Training and Graduate Studies, Linthicum Heights, MD. Medical advice to ships at sea is provided through Marine Advisory Systems, Inc., Owens MD.

## References

1. Merkle DL, Urner CJ (1980) Emergency maritime service training for distress at sea. Emergency 12:91–96
2. Urner CJ, Staton AB (1983) The ship's medicine chest. Natl Safety News 128:36–44
3. DHEW (1978/1984) The ship's medicine chest and medical aid at sea. DHEW, Washington [Publication (HSA) 84-2024]
4. Hall TM, Herring SA, Jozwiak TJ (1984) Basic elements of maritime health care. J Occup Med 26:202–209

# Health Problems of Seafarers – "Professional Travelers"

S. Tomaszunas

From the point of view of travel medicine, seafarers may be considered as a special risk group of travelers. Their occupation and the type of their work exposes them to a number of health risks, some of which are the same or similiar to those which are typical for other groups of travelers, such as tourists and businessmen.

For nonimmune seamen malaria is a serious risk, when their ships call to ports in East and West Africa, and in Southeast Asia. In 1983, there were 12 cases of malaria with 2 fatalities reported in crews of 25 ships of the African lines of a national shipping company in Poland. The estimated total number of crews of those 25 ships was about 1000 men. Although antimalarials were available on all ships and seamen were advised to take them, malaria prophylaxis was not satisfactory [1]. Many malaria infections in seafarers have been treated in hospitals in Rotterdam [2], in Hamburg and in other ports.

There are many health risks connected with specific working environment and with living conditions on board ship, which is a place of work and at the same time a home for seamen. They are exposed to most of these risks on and off duty, for long periods. During intercontinental voyages, crews are exposed to frequent time zone and climatic changes. Combined with the traditional pattern of shift work including night work, and with limited recreational opportunities, these changes create stress, interfere with the working of biological mechanisms of the body, and contribute to increased morbidity. Another factor is a very high temperature in engine rooms of ships. The high level of noise and vibration in engine rooms, and also in living quarters of some ships, adversely affects the health of crew members. Many ships carry dangerous cargo such as chemicals, gases, petroleum products, and raw hides. Their crews are exposed to additional health risks.

Health services for seafarers are available in ports and on board ships. Medical officers are usually employed only on passenger ships. In some countries, however, the they also work on cargo ships and on large fishing trawlers-factory ships [3], with crews numbering 60–100 men.

On most cargo ships, first aid and primary health care is provided by one of the (nonprofessional) crew members, trained for this additional responsibility. To facilitate his task, he usually has a copy of a medical guide for ships; he can also request and obtain radio-medical advice from shore.

Since qualified medical assistance is not available on the great majority of ships, the prevention of diseases is essential in seamen: through pre-employment and periodic medical examinations, vaccinations, health education, malaria prevention, accident prevention, fresh water supply for ships, food hygiene, etc.

Modern ships are highly automated, the loading cargo in ports takes less time than before, and hence there is not much time available for seamen to visit doctors in ports.

The number of crew of a cargo ship has decreased during the past 20 years, from about 40 men previously to 16–24 at present; and this number may be reduced even more in the near future. With the decreasing number of men on board a modern ship, it becomes more important to maintain the high level of health of all people employed at sea. A sudden illness of several crew members at the same time, during a voyage, may seriously affect the operation of the ship.

The international collaboration in the study of health problems of seafarers has been well established, and has been supported by governments, and by international organizations: WHO, ILO, and IMO.

## References

1. Tomaszunas S (1984) Malaria in Polish seafarers in 1983. Bull Inst Marit Trop Med Gdynia 35:41–46
2. Stuiver PO (1983) Problems with malaria. 4th European Maritime Medical Officers Meeting, 19–22 Sept, Rotterdam
3. Tomaszunas S, Filikowski J, Jankowski A (1975) The organization of health services for seafarers in Poland. Bull Inst Marit Trop Med Gdynia 24:265–274

# Uprooting – The Psychosocial Problems of the International Student

A. D. G. Gunn

International students enroll in the universities and colleges of the world in ever-increasing numbers and it is here in Europe that the history of care for these specially "uprooted" individuals – migrants in the cause of higher education – was actually started. In the thirteenth century a special college was founded for students from the diocese of Avignon who wanted to study in Bologna and in the fourteenth century 24 Spanish students had two special chaplains appointed for their care because of the difficulties these expatriates were experiencing. Thus, historically "international student care" started in Europe 700 years ago. Since then the pattern of migration and the need for special care has escalated until today there are, for example, over 150 000 international students in the United Kingdom, 350 000 in the United States and in western Europe over a million students enrolled for higher education whose homes are originally "abroad" [1].

Governments encourage this migration at one level for diplomatic reasons, and there are now quotas being developed, in the United Kingdom and western Europe, to accept students, directly apportioned according to the amount of economic aid that that country receives. Countries around the world also accept international students for economic reasons that are of benefit to the whole community. For example, in the United Kingdom at the present time the "international" student is a one billion pound a year industry, in terms of the fees and funds they "import". (The United Kingdom receives from tourism 6 billion pounds a year). Similarly, there is a growing feeling in the western and developed world that we "owe it" to the less-developed worlds to give them aid and what we have got to offer is higher education, so there are an increasing number of "student packages" as agreements between different countries that are part of a formal aid pattern.

## The Price and The Consequences

The picture of consequent psychosocial distress with regard to migration in higher education and further advancement in careers in universities and colleges is mirrored in commerce worldwide. In banks, in oil firms, in airlines, in the diplomatic corps, and in organizations associated with exploration in civil engineering development in the third world, "expatriate stress" is now becoming a very frequently used term [2]. There is a similarity here to the problems which we (i.e. student health physicians) are seeing in the health care of overseas students. We, the doctors, who care for the "uprooted", are all finding similar casualty and mental breakdown rates.

Commercial organizations try to select the flexible and patient individual as being the one that might cope better with differences in the environment and employment demands when they are away. The person who is willing to learn, the person who is non-political, the person who is sociable and the person who copes with stress are all high in priority on the selection list.

The military, from long experience, look after families who are sent abroad, and their authorities now initiate a rigorous selection technique because historically 25% of the wives and families sent abroad to be present with their husbands on overseas postings have to be brought back within 1 year, and that is expensive as well as disruptive for the husband, who often has to be repatriated too [3]. Learning from experience, the US Navy, for example, now will *not* send out a Naval wife who has recently married; there is a minimum of 2 years before she is allowed to accompany her husband to an overseas posting. Experience has shown that a new marriage will not stand up to the extra stress of a totally foreign environment. Similarly, they will not send anybody where there is any evidence of a crumbling mariage. They will not send anybody within 1 year of their first pregnancy, and they will not send anybody within 6 months of a recent close family bereavement [3]. For students, however, we cannot impose any such personal requirements – their selection is often based on academic ability alone.

## When and Why "Disturbance" Occurs

From the point of view of selection, we can quite quickly dismiss the idea that international students arrive "ill". Many of our international students arrive in our countries fitter and possibly even healthier than many of our own students. They are an "elite". Nevertheless, within the short period of arrival, there are indications of disturbance. Dr Donald Char of the University of Hawaii (who is probably one of the most experienced physicians in coping with "international" students), states that most international students tend to have a 2–3 months "honeymoon" period in their new host country which they enjoy [4]. This has also been confirmed by colleagues in Israel, who say that both the new Israeli immigrant and the international student thoroughly enjoys being there, for 2–3 months before any psychosocial problems develop [5]. Employers of expatriate staff say they notice a "mid-term slump", again after 2–3 months, and in the United Kingdom we in student health have noticed remarkably over the years a peak in the presentation of depressive symptoms and the depressive psychotic reactions that occur 3 months after the students' arrival [6].

Migration is, for many, something that they yearn for and the uprooting experience in itself need not necessarily be harmful but there are, in association with this, certain phenomena that are inevitable, and which any student or any immigrant will encounter. They are as follows:

## Inevitable Problems

| | |
|---|---|
| Local peculiarities | Sexual problems |
| Racial discriminations | Career choice restrictions |
| Accommodation difficulties | Study method discrepancies |
| Separation reactions | Dietary difficulties |
| Age-determined problems | Personality problems |
| Language and adjustment | Local climate |

Anybody in the world can meet racial discrimination. It exists everywhere and it is expressed in one way or another, either overtly or subtly.

Another inevitable problem is that of accomodation difficulties. There will be separation reactions from mother, loved ones, relatives, wives, children or friends.

There will be language and consequent adjustment difficulties. Until everybody speaks the same international language, there always will be language adjustment difficulties. There are sexual problems, and these are enhanced when you are abroad. Inevitable problems for any international student are career choice restrictions and difficulties after qualification.

Study difficulties are also a major problem for most international students, for there are special problems when students come from the developing world where there are different accepted patterns of behaviour in learning, tuition and examining.

Dietary difficulties and problems are another inevitability of migration. Similarly with climate, there is quite severe adjustment to be made for people who come from a country which is tropical to a cold northern clime. These therefore are just a few of the major, but inescapable, consequences of "uprooting".

## Avoidable Problems?

What about problems that might be avoided, and about which we really ought to try and do more, in order to smooth the transition? We cannot, however, change the weather. We cannot change the life-style of the host population.

These are the avoidable problems:

| | |
|---|---|
| Financial stress | Over-identification |
| Misunderstanding and mistrust | Academic inadequacy |
| Teacher-student difficulties | Ethnocentricism |
| Vocational guidance | Disillusionment |
| Loneliness | Employment difficulties |
| Married student difficulties | Inadequate embassy support |

Financial stress is an avoidable problem. The "western" degree is, in my opinion, somewhat over-evaluated. It is a "status" degree. In theory, back home in Egypt, for example, a "western" degree is better than the one that you got at Cairo University and therefore this is why you struggle to achieve one. Inevitably in this "value order" this leads to a degree of financial stress on students seeking to achieve something which they perceive as being so important to them. Thus often desperate financial struggles develop for parents and families to send their children abroad to study so that they may come back with the extra "cachet". Thus you may have your Chinese student who is well aware that the rest of the family's future seemingly depends on his graduation in law from the University of Vancouver, for example, before he returns to Hong Kong. The extra stress is thus not personal satisfaction but it is striving for the satisfaction of parental ambition and the reward for their financial deprivation that motivates. Thus you are not studying to enjoy yourself and integrate into the host society, you are doing it for the family back home.

The recognition, therefore, not just of any illness in the international student who is socially dislocated or uprooted, but the earlier recognition of the one who is doing less well academically is crucial.

Loneliness is another major problem that tends to be reported in nearly all surveys of international student risk [6] that one pursues. We should constantly be asking "What can we do to mitigate this common experience of loneliness?"

Academic inadequacy is also frequently reported [6]. This, in itself, is avoidable. There is a need for the rigorous imposition of minimum educational standards.

Among the avoidable problems is what may be called "inadequate embassy support". Without adequate support we have nobody to turn to who might be much more in tune with the ethical, social, and language needs of a particular student in distress.

We must also always remember the impact of the current role of the female in our western society. This in itself for Middle Eastern female students can prove to provide a shock reaction if they come from a fundamentalist protective society. Western women's life-style is a stark contrast to what they are used to. There are those who grew up in the protective society of their homeland who find ours a total, but perhaps unwelcome or uncomfortable, "liberation". This in itself can disrupt their attitudes and change their personality for their return. It may, in consequence, make them want to return earlier because they find the role of the western female too uncomfortable and difficult to assume.

## Recommendations for Prevention of a Severe Uprooting Experience

1. Firstly, we should all attempt to overcome the barriers in delivery of health care, to people familiar only with their own system.
2. There should be better written information about how to obtain health care in the language of the "guest" student.
3. More "peer" helpers are needed to deal with emotional stress, as is better advice on exercise, nutrition, and stress reduction counselling.
4. Earlier recognition of study and psychosocial difficulties in the international student is necessary with better communication between the academic/medical/counselling services.

5. Special skill training is necessary in dealing with pathological "uprooting" reactions.
6. "Casualty evacuation" services are necessary to ensure swift, easy and dignified repatriation where academic failure is inevitable and life's survival (i.e. suicide threat) is prejudiced.
7. Preparation for return home is as necessary as preparation for arrival.
8. Follow-up research must be increased in order to reduce the current casualty rate.

## Conclusion

Psychosocial change as a result of migrating to study is inevitable, but damage and disruption to the personality is not. Travel broadens the mind. It is not supposed to disrupt it.

## References

1. Bull Int Bur Educ (1985) 9:236–237
2. Expatriate stress and breakdown. Symposia held at Roy Coll Phys London 1983, 1984 and 1985
3. Fowler SM (1985) Prevention and assistance. In: Symposium on Expatriate Stress and Breakdown. Royal College of Physicians, London
4. Ebbin AJ (1986) International versus domestic students. Am J Coll Health 34:177–182
5. Kaplan B (1985) Immigration to Israel. Summer Conference on International Student Care, Hebrew University, Jerusalem
6. Zwingmann C, Gunn ADG (1983) Uprooting and health: psychosocial problems of students from abroad. WHO, Geneva

# Sojourners and Health – Providing Health Care for International Students

D. F. B. Char

Annually, over one million students travel abroad and overseas in pursuit of higher educational opportunities. As seen in Table 1, these students generally go from the developing third world regions to the developed countries for this higher education.

Although the vast majority of these students are successful in attaining their education, they nonetheless often undergo varying degrees of stress and hardship in coping with life as an alien student in a foreign society and culture.

Compounding their dilemma of having to negotiate with interpersonal, social needs of achieving adulthood in a foreign culture and needing to be accepted by peer groups that may have very different, life-styles, habits, interpersonal values and beliefs, many of these students encounter real difficulties in adapting. In addition, the questions of migration into a country with higher standards of living (or having to return to one with lower living standards), the questions of love and marriage, the gaining of an enhanced role by achieving the higher degree in education and many other problems confront these foreign students.

Much has been written about "culture shock" and the "brain drain," but most of the accounts are based upon anecdotes and personal experiences and little scholarly work has been done to evaluate this important subject. The world is finally beginning to realize that international education must be more carefully considered and evaluated, and some scholarly organizations are beginning to address these questions. With these vast numbers of students involved in higher education abroad, it behooves the health care providers to become more fully informed and knowledgeable about the health needs of international students.

In addition to realizing they may have difficulties with poor language, financial and housing conditions, lacking normal supportive social networks and having a tendency to accept unquestioned authority, it must also be recognized that these foreign students generally lack comprehension and understanding of the host country's medical care system and complex medical economic framework.

Hopefully, physicians, nurses and other health professionals knowledgeable about these special care problems can better assist these transients or sojourners in our colleges and universities to achieve their higher educational objectives with the minimum amount of discordance and illness.

**Table 1.** UNESCO world region of origin of foreign students within host country

| Host country | World region of origin | | | | | | | | Total Enroll-ment |
|---|---|---|---|---|---|---|---|---|---|
| | Africa | Europe | Middle East | North America | Oceania | Latin America | South and East Asia | USSR | |
| United States (84) | 12 | 10 | 14 | 5 | 1 | 16 | 42 | 0.1 | 342110 |
| France (83) | 58 | 17 | 9 | – | 0.1 | – | 0.7 | 15 | 128350 |
| Germany, Federal Republic (83) | 6 | 40 | 14 | 6 | 0.2 | 4 | 27 | 3 | 74267 |
| USSR (78) | | | | | | | | | 62942 |
| United Kingdom (83) | 24 | 8 | 16 | 8 | 2 | 4 | 37 | 2 | 43267 |
| Canada (83) | 13 | 13 | 4 | 9 | 1 | 8 | 50 | 1 | 35365 |
| Lebanon (82) | 25 | – | 43 | – | – | – | – | 33 | 29480 |
| Italy (83) | 7 | 57 | 28 | 4 | 0.1 | 3 | 0.5 | 0.7 | 28068 |
| Belgium (83) | 35 | 48 | 6 | 2 | – | 4 | 4 | 2 | 21188 |
| Egypt (82) | 52 | 1 | 23 | 0.1 | – | 0.1 | 1 | 24 | 17062 |
| Switzerland (80) | 6 | 77 | 5 | 4 | 0.2 | 4 | 3 | 1 | 16830 |
| Saudi Arabia (83) | – | 0.1 | 40 | 0.3 | – | – | 14 | 46 | 16529 |
| Austria (84) | 4 | 65 | 17 | 3 | 0.2 | 2 | 6 | 3 | 14858 |
| India (79) | – | 2 | 28 | 1 | 1 | 0.2 | 29 | 39 | 14710 |
| Australia (80) | 2 | 3 | 0.2 | 2 | 9 | 0.2 | 81 | 3 | 12078 |
| Japan (84) | 2 | 4 | 1 | 8 | 1 | 4 | 80 | 0.2 | 10697 |

## References

1. Glaser W (1978) The brain drain. Emigration and return. Pergamon, Oxford
2. Goodwin CD, Nacht M (1983) Absence of decision. Foreign students in American colleges and universities. Institute of International Education, New York
3. Kleinman A (1980) Patients and healers in the context of culture. University of California Press, Berkely
4. Kleinman A, Kundstadter P, Alexander ER, Gate JC (1978) Culture and healing in Asian societies. Scheukman, Cambridge, MA
5. Reed B, Hutton J, Bazalgette J (1978) Freedom to study. Requirements of overseas students in the U.K. Overseas Student Trust, London
6. Zwingmann CAA, Gunn ADG (1983) Uprooting and health. Psychosocial problems of students from abroad. WHO, Geneva

# Health Risks of Children and Adolescents in Short-Term Travel or Temporary Residence in Developing Countries

F. Sabate

In increasing cooperation between developed and developing countries, as well as the facilities for intercontinental travel, and the attraction for young people of adventure, result in expatriate children and adolescents going more frequently to developing countries and they should be considered as a selected risk group regarding health aspects. The aim of this study was to assess the prevalence of major pathological conditions in expatriate children and adolescents, as seen in our field day clinic.

Arusha, the third largest city in Tanzania, at the foot of Mt. Kilimanjaro, and near the world's famous Serengeti National Park, is a very active tourist center. There, we had the opportunity to see 493 expatriate children and adolescents, between 0 and 19 years old, over the period January 1984 to December 1985.

## Results

The group of 335 children, between 0 and 14 years old, were mainly temporary residents though some of them (25%) were born locally. The major health problems that motivated consultation, by order of frequency were:

| | |
|---|---|
| Parasitic diseases | 75 patients |
| Health advice and preventive medicine | 73 patients |
| Digestive system including acute infective gastroenteritis (27), diarrhea (19), and hepatitis (12) | 56 patients |
| Respiratory infections | 54 patients |
| Neonatology | 12 patients |
| Allergy | 11 patients |
| Psychosocial or behavioral disorders | 9 patients |
| Others | 45 patients |

The group of 158 adolescents, between 15 and 19 years old, were mainly short-term travelers. The health problems they faced were:

| | |
|---|---|
| Digestive problems including acute diarrhea (19), traveler's diarrhea (7), and food poisoning (9) | 52 patients |
| Parasitic diseases | 35 patients |
| Sexually transmitted diseases | 12 patients |
| Accidents/traumas | 12 patients |

| | |
|---|---|
| Health advice/vaccinations | 11 patients |
| Skin diseases | 9 patients |
| Dental, eye and ENT complaints | 10 patients |
| Miscellaneous | 17 patients |

The group of adolescents showed a different pattern of health risk.

First came the digestive problems, with the main symptom diarrhea. The source is almost always food or water which is contaminated with pathogens. Also the different ionic composition of food and water abroad can change the osmotic balance in the gut and facilitate the proliferation and penetration of enteropathogens.

Parasitic diseases were second in importance by number of cases. Malaria was the most frequent (31), due to lack of chemoprophylaxis (10), chloroquine-resistant strains of the *Plasmodium falciparum* (9), and inappropriate use or dose of antimalarial drugs (12). Others included: schistosomiasis (1), amebiasis (1), and worms (2).

Sexually transmitted diseases (12) were mainly acute conditions such as: urethritis in males (2) or urinary tract infection (2) and genital herpes (1); while in females diseases seen were pelvic inflammatory disease (1), genital herpes (1), vulvovaginitis (1), molluscum contagiosum (1), syphilis (1) and urinary tract infection (2).

Parasitic diseases are the most relevant for expatriate children, since the majority of affected children (40) had not taken malaria chemoprophylaxis. Roundworms of the digestive tract were most frequently found in those with close contact with native children. Schistosomiasis was seen in five children living near dams.

Health advice (75) was requested mainly by the parents of children recently arrived from overseas and for the newborns. The main concern was related with nutrition and other environmental problems (waters, climate, immunizations).

Acute gastroenteritis was related mainly to rotavirus infections. Mild dehydration was seen in cases of severe diarrhea. Malabsortion was related to chronic diarrhea. Isolated cases of mild malnutrition or vitamin deficiency (ascorbic acid) could be seen in expatriate children whose parents were living in critical areas. Hepatitis is a significant problem for expatriates in developing countries, and we suggest the convenience of vaccination for children living in endemic areas.

The morbidity of expatriate children abroad is no higher than "at home." The source of the majority of problems is neglect of preventive rules and close contact with contaminated environments. The morbidity of expatriate adolescents abroad is a little higher than "at home," reasons being promiscuity, weakness of personal hygiene, lack of preventive measures and more aggressive behavior. To avoid or minimize the health risks of expatriate children and adolescents abroad, it is necessary to strengthen their health education and preventive measures. It is necessary for pediatricians and public health workers to be acquainted with the health risks of children and adolescents living or traveling abroad in order to treat or prevent such problems, in developing or developed countries.

# Mental Health Care of Expatriates

M. Foyle

These observations are based on a group of mainly self-referred long-term expatriates examined in Southeast Asia and in their home countries (United States, Canada, Europe).

## Data Collection Period 1981–1987

The age range of the patients was 4–75 years and the male: female ratio was 69:153. They came from 12 different countries. The patients were categorized into four groups:

1. Patients with age-related illnesses such as presenile dementia, whose onset was not related to expatriate service (14 patients).
2. Patients with stress-induced illnesses, i.e. those who had coped adequately with stress in their own countries but had been unable to cope with the various stresses of expatriate life (52 patients).
3. Patients who required only simple counselling. These cases usually had only one major problem, which was amenable to counselling (45 patients).
4. Patients with selection problems. These patients had experienced problems before their selection for expatriate service, and had often received little or no professional help. The problems experienced were exacerbated by expatriate service (120 patients).

## Frequent Causes of Stress in Expatriates

The stress may be job related: the work is different from expectations, the training received was not suitable for local conditions, or there were conflicting priorities between the home and family versus the job. Stress may be caused by difficulties in interpersonal relationships such as problems between nationals and expatriates due to different working patterns, language and cultural misunderstanding; or problems between different national expatriate groups due to language and cultural misunderstandings, different training patterns and life-styles; or marital problems and parent/child conflicts. Often cultural problems contribute to the stress and may be aggravated by loss of home support systems, leading to loneliness and insecurity.

## Methods of Preventing and Reducing Stress

Use of better selection procedures prior to departure are important. Certain factors may increase mental health risks for expatriates such as current or previous mental illness, heavy genetic loading, marital instability, personality problems severe enough to have created problems at home and drug and alcohol abuse. "In the ambiguity and stress of another culture, past experience and events tend to shape how the individual will respond" [1]. Adequate psychological screening (interviews and tests) should be included, in addition to physical and professional screening. Good preparation for the assignment abroad should include briefing, orientation, a preliminary "looksee" visit if in doubt, suitable professional experience, and advice on special needs such as children's education, working roles and housing. Development of good relationships with the sending agency is also of importance.

During overseas service adequate support should be provided. This includes giving of local assistance (twinning with established workers), making personnel available as troubleshooters, establishing pre-planned emergency procedures, outlining clear lines of communication with the administration, preparing clear contracts and terms of service, and providing end of contract planning and help.

After return home, either permanently or between contracts, some support needs to be given. This includes debriefing of both husband and wife, providing practical advice especially after long-term service, and adequate health care on arrival and before a new contract.

## Reference

1. Britt G (1983) Pretraining variables in prediction of success overseas. J Psychol Theol 11(3):203–212

# Parasites and Pregnancy

R. V. Lee

Acquisition of parasites is a medical complication of travel for pregnant women. Two features of parasitic infection can classify risk to pregnancy: (1) residence – whether the organism is a surface dweller only or is capable of invasion or prolonged residence in tissues or in cells – and (2) reproduction – whether the organism is capable of completing its life cycle within the human host. Invasive parasites (plasmodia, *toxoplasma*) that multiply pose the greatest threat by producing severe maternal disease and placental or transplacental infection. Tissue-dwelling helminths (filarial nematodes, schistosomes) produce vast numbers of eggs which amplify the impact upon the mother. Circulating or migrating eggs or larvae may interfere with placental function or traverse the placenta. Surface-dwelling intestinal parasites (*Diphyllobothrium latum, Giardia*) may interfere with maternal nutrition.

The effect of transplacental infections on the fetus is determined by the time during pregnancy when the mother acquires the infection. Early in gestation infection of the fetus is uncommon, but when it does occur the results are grave: fetal demise and teratogenesis. Late in gestation infection of the fetus is less likely to cause teratogenesis or intrauterine fetal death but more likely to cause debilitating infection of the neonate with chronic disease or demise.

Parasites that never penetrate the surfaces of the patient, the skin or the gastrointestinal tract are not likely to cause transplacental infection. *Trichomonas vaginalis* despite its noninvasive mode of existence is capable of altering the ecology of the cervix and has been associated with increased risks of premature labor and premature rupture of the membranes.

Surface-dwelling parasites like the hookworms have a larval migration during which placental and transplacental infection can occur. While the larval form can produce serious placental or fetal disease its life is short unless it can regain the gastrointestinal lumen.

Tissue-dwelling or -persisting organisms like *Trichinella* and the filarial nematodes may be able to establish infection of the fetus. The protozoan *Toxoplasma gondii* can produce devasting acute and chronic infection of the fetus when the mother is infected for the first time during pregnancy.

Maternal health is injured most by organisms completing their life cycle within the host. Enormous increases in parasite burden can occur, as with *Strongyloides stercoralis* hyperinfection syndrome. Extension of the infection may be local, as with *Giardia lamblia*, or metastatic, as with *Entamoeba histolytica*.

**Table 1.** Some parasites of importance during pregnancy

| Life cycle in or on human host | Residence of parasites | |
|---|---|---|
| | Surface dwellers | Invasive tissue dwellers |
| No maturation and no increase in parasite population | Ticks<br>Maggots | *Larva migrans: Toxocara* spp.<br>*Gnathostoma spinigerum,*<br>*Dirofilaria immitis,*<br>*Trichobilharzia* spp. |
| Maturation but no increase in parasite population | *Enterobius vermicularis*<br>*Trichuris trichiuria*<br>*Taenia* spp.<br>*Diphyllobothrium lata*<br>*Fasciolopsis buski* | Hookworm spp.<br>*Ascaris lumbricoides*<br>*Anisakis* spp.<br>*Dracunculus medinensis*<br>*Fasciola hepatica*<br>*Cysticercus cellulosae (T. solium)* |
| Maturation and increase in quantity of larvae or eggs but no increase of infective stage | *Tunga penetrans*<br>Chiggers (Trombiculid mites) | *Angiostongylus cantonensis*<br>*Trichinella spiralis*<br>Filarial nematodes:<br>*Wuchereria bancrofti,*<br>*Brugia malayi,*<br>*Onchocherca volvulus,*<br>*Loa loa*<br>*Schistosoma* spp.<br>*Clonorchis sinensis*<br>*Opisthorchis viverrini*<br>*Paragonimus westermani*<br>*Echinococcus granulosus* |
| Maturation and reproduction with increase in quantity of infective stage, eggs, larvae, and adults | *Pediculus* spp.<br>*Sarcoptes scabiei*<br>*Giardia lamblia*<br>*Trichomonas vaginalis* | *Entamoeba histolytica*<br>*Toxoplasma gondii*<br>*Plasmodium* spp.<br>*Babesia* spp.<br>*Trypansoma* spp.<br>*Leishmania* spp.<br>*Capillaria philippinensis*<br>*Strongyloides stercoralis*<br>*Hymenolepsis nana*<br>*Echinococcus multilocularis* |

At the other extreme are organisms that cannot increase their parasite burden because the life cycle requires steps outside the host. The quantity of hookworms (*Ancylostoma* and *Necator*) in the pregnant patient's gut will not increase unless she acquires a new inoculum of rhabditiform larvae from the soil.

In the middle are parasites like the schistosomes which increase the parasite burden by producing enormous quantities of eggs, but which are unable to increase the number of egg-laying adults whithout a new inoculum of miracidia. Parasite burden may not be measurable by the number of adult or immature forms present; for example, parasites like *Diphyllobothrium latum* can compete with the host for essential nutrients and impose a severe biologic burden upon the mother without an increase in the quantity of the parasite.

## Reference

1. D'Alauro F, Lee RV, Pao-In K, Khairallah M (1985) Intestinal parasites during pregnancy. Obstet Gynecol 66:639–643

# The Pregnant Traveler

R. V. Lee

Giving good health advice to the pregnant traveler requires attention to factors that are intrinsic and extrinsic to the pregnant patient. Intrinsic factors include (1) maternal health (medical and immune status, physical conditioning and acclimatization, etc.), (2) physiologic and anatomic changes of pregnancy, and (3) obstetrical risk factors. Extrinsic factors include (1) method and duration of travel, (2) destination and duration of stay, (3) objectives of travel or residence, and (4) accidents and trauma. The major health hazards of travel during pregnancy are trauma, infections acquired during travel, premature labor or rupture of membranes, and problems associated with the mechanical effects of the gravid uterus. Multiple pregnancy, uterine abnormalities, prior premature delivery or rupture of membranes, prior poor pregnancy outcome, history of sexually transmitted disease including cervicitis and vaginitis, medical complications of pregnancy, and prolonged sitting posture are factors that are commonly present in travelers admitted to our hospital with pregnancy com-

**Table 1.** Factors intrinsic to the pregnant patient

I. Maternal health
   - A. The alteration in clinical course of maternal conditions such as diabetes mellitus produced by pregnancy requires increased vigilance and should restrict any but the most essential travel
   - B. Nonimmune mothers ought not to travel to areas with endemic infection (vide infra)
   - C. Pregnancy increases blood volume, cardiac output, and glomerular filtration rate. Pregnant women with stenotic valvular lesions and hypertension may not tolerate the additional stress of travel. Women with congenital cyanotic heart disease should not travel even in pressurized aircraft. Altered pharmacodynamics requires careful monitoring of drug levels and alteration in dosing regimens

II. Physiologic and anatomic changes of pregnancy
   - A. Mechanical effects of the gravid uterus
   - B. Systemic effects of pregnancy
   - C. The pregnant patient tends to collect edema because of diminished colloid oncotic pressure and increased hydrostatic pressure. Pregnant women tend to develop hyperventilation symptoms (paresthesias, muscle cramps, lightheadedness, dyspnea) with minimal changes in respiratory rate or depth

III. Obstetrical risk factors: see text

**Table 2.** Factors extrinsic to the pregnant patient

I. Method and duration of travel

A. Travel requiring prolonged sitting or restricted access to recumbent posture is a special problem for pregnant women; a problem that increases as the uterus expands in volume. Pregnant patients should be advised to wear support, waist or chest high, stockings and to interrupt the sitting position every ½ to 1 h

B. Air travel in pressurized jet planes does not pose a hypoxic risk to the healthy pregnant mother or her fetus. However, women with conditions jeopardizing placental function (lupus, hypertensive state, placental separation, etc.) may be at risk; the above 2000 m reduction in ambient partial pressure of gases may be sufficient to produce further placental or fetal deterioration

II. Destination and duration of stay

A. Prolonged absence from home and interruption of established medical care is a hazard during pregnancy. Patients should seek prenatal care upon arriving at their destination

B. Visits or residence in areas of endemic infection by organisms capable of transplacental infection or by organisms capable of capitalizing upon altered maternal immune status are hazardous. For example, the risk of infection by multiple drug resistant *Plasmodium falciparum* is sufficient to actively discourage travel by a pregnant woman to an area with known *P. falciparum* malaria. Live virus immunizations (yellow fever, polio, rubella, smallpox, etc.) are required for some travelers and for travel to certain areas. In general, live virus vaccines are relatively contraindicated during pregnancy

C. Pregnant patients may not tolerate climatic extremes as well as nonpregnant women although there is no special risk from extremes of temperature and humidity if the patient dresses properly

III. Objectives of travel

A. Pregnant patients traveling with their spouse for pleasure may have an increase in sexual activity which may have increased risks for the pregnancy

B. Adventure travel to areas of physiologic (high-altitude, hiking or climbing, scuba diving, etc.) or infection risk may be particularly dangerous for pregnant patients

IV. Accidents and trauma

A. Vehicular injuries are still the most common cause of serious illness. Pregnant women need to be reassured that lap and shoulder seat restraints are effective and safe and should be used

B. The gait and posture changes of pregnancy enhance the risk of musculoskeletal injury in pregnant women not accustomed to physical exertion

---

plications. For travelers outside the United States the risk of acquiring serious infection is proportional to the duration of the travel or residence in endemic areas and the intensity of exposure to vectors or sources of infection. The immune changes of pregnancy may contribute to grave clinical illness from pathogens cleared or neutralized by cell-mediated immunity.

*Obstetrical Risk Factors.* During 1985 and 1986, 20 pregnant travelers were admitted to Children's Hospital of Buffalo. Only patients living beyond the usual limits of referral to our high-risk pregnancy service and identified as travelers or maintaining prenatal care at facilities close to their home were included. Three-quarters of the patients required admission because of premature labor, premature rupture of the membranes, vaginal bleeding, or a combination of these problems. The majority of these 15 patients had readily identifiable obstetrical risk factors. Eight (53%) had had one or more operative cervical procedures (dilatation and curettage or elective termination of pregnancy). Six (40%) had experienced premature labor, premature rupture of the membranes, stillbirth, or ectopic pregnancy during previous pregnancies. Only five (33%) had no previous reproductive complications or were primigravidae. Ten (66%) of the patients with problems related to the uterus or its contents were delivered on the same admission, only a minority by cesarean section. All infants beyond 29 weeks gestation survived. Only one of the three neonates less than 29 weeks gestational age survived.

Of the five remaining patients, two were admitted because of suspected deep vein thrombophlebitis of the calf following prolonged sitting during international air travel. Both of these women had a history of intense nocturnal calf muscle cramps during the pregnancy; neither had evidence of obstructive venous disease by Doppler plethysmography or clinical course.

This and another small series from Hawaii [1] indicate that travel is a potentially greater risk to women who have had previous adverse pregnancy outcomes or operative procedures involving cervical dilatation. We routinely inquire about such events when pregnant women or their obstetricians ask about travel; and we are routinely cautious about allowing travel for patients with a positive past history.

## Reference

1. Easa D, Ash K, Boychuk R et al. (1985) Preterm delivery in tourists: the Hawaii experience. Hawaii Med J 44:173–178

# Counseling the HIV Antibody Positive Traveler Relative to Immunization Protection and Malaria Prophylaxis

W. R. Lange, S. D. Kreider, and E. M. Dax

The principal concern relating to international travel by those infected with the human immunodeficiency virus (HIV) is the impact that such activities might have on their health, not the threat such travel could theoretically impose on others. Since there continues to be no evidence of nonspecific transmission of HIV through casual contact, insect bites, or foodborne, waterborne, or other environmental mechanisms [1], travel on public conveyances by infected individuals as well as their eating in restaurants and residing in hotels does not create a risk for others. The risks of travel depend on the severity of clinical illness, and would be directly proportional to the progression of symptoms and inversely related to the number of circulating CD-4 cells. Regardless, all HIV-infected travelers are exposed to a variety of real and theoretical risks, and many of these can be reduced by both vaccine administration and prophylactic medication.

In deciding on immunization strategies for persons at risk of HIV infection or disease, the risks and benefits of the particular vaccines must be weighed against the risks posed by the respective diseases. Even though, in general, the effectiveness of vaccines may be reduced in the presence of HIV, the risk of vaccine-preventable disease is often substantial. To date, adverse reactions attributable to vaccines appear to be minimal. In structuring an immunization program for the HIV-infected international traveler, a reasonable approach would be to first consider baseline immunizations appropriate for the patient's age, next to reflect on vaccine protection indicated as a consequence of immunocompromise, and finally to contemplate vaccines specific for the travel itinerary.

## Childhood Immunization and HIV Infection

Baseline pediatric immunization schedules will not be discussed in this review, and excellent monographs have recently been published which outline experience with and recommendations for various vaccines in the face of HIV infection [2, 3]. The consensus appears to be that immunization against diphtheria, pertussis, tetanus, *Haemophilus influenzae B*, and measles is indicated, as would be protection against poliomyelitis.

In regions of the world where the risk of polio is enhanced, live oral polio vaccine may be used, whereas, in areas of lower risk, inactivated polio vaccine would be appropriate. Mumps and rubella vaccines would not be contraindicated, but, as will be discussed, BCG may have associated with it an increased element of risk.

Of theoretical concern is the potential for an iatrogenic infection following the administration of live virus vaccines to individuals with leukopenia or a depressed CD-4 cell count. Nevertheless, immunocompromised children may actually be at greater risk if they are not immunized. Measles infection, for example, among patients with immune deficiency may be severe, protracted, and fatal [4]. Similarly, concern that immunization might somehow activate T-helper cells, stimulate viral replication, and accelerate the course of HIV infection do not appear to be substantiated by clinical experience.

## Adult Immunization

Baseline adult immunization recommendations are age specific [5, 6]. All adults, including those with immune deficiency as well as those traveling abroad, should have adequate immunity against tetanus and diphtheria and should receive a Td booster every 10 years, such as in conjunction with the mid-decade birthday. All young adults should manifest evidence of immunity against measles, mumps, and rubella, or else they should be immunized unless there is a clear contraindication such as clinical evidence of immune deficiency. All elderly individuals should avail themselves of an annual influenza inoculation and be protected against pneumococcal disease.

Adults who are immunocompromised would be candidates for selected vaccine protection. Both influenza and pneumococcal pneumonia vaccines have been recommended for immunodeficient patients [7], and this would include those with AIDS and ARC, whether traveling or not. There is less agreement as to whether this protection should also be afforded to asymptomatic carriers whose only manifestation of infection is a positive assay for HIV antibodies.

Many adults at risk of HIV infection are also at risk of hepatitis B virus infection, and susceptible high-risk individuals should be protected with hepatitis B vaccine whether traveling or not. The evidence to date is mixed as to whether the plasma-derived vaccine or the recombinant product is more immunogenic in this population. There does not appear to be any risk associated with the administration of inactivated virus or viral-particle vaccines [8], although the efficacy of immunization may be decreased [9].

There is less clinical experience with live virus vaccines in HIV-infected adults than with pediatric-age patients. This is particularly true for patients with clinical illness. Data relative to the safety and efficacy of yellow fever vaccine in HIV-infected individuals are unavailable. It has been recommended that this vaccine not be administered to persons who are immunocompromised as a result of immune deficiency diseases [5, 6]; however, the situation with asymptomatic HIV infection is less clear. The US military appears to have immunized several hundred HIV-positive recruits with multiple vaccines without ill effect before routine screening and exclusion of seropositives became standard operating procedure [10, 11]. Disseminated vaccinia has been reported in a military recruit who was vaccinated against smallpox [12], but no adverse sequelae to yellow fever vaccine were identified. Nevertheless, many believe that, in conjunction with international travel, it is prudent for symptomatic and immunologically compromised seropositive adults to avoid live virus vaccines, and at the same time to avoid traveling to less-developed areas of the world where these agents are either required or recommended.

## Tuberculosis

Disseminated *Mycobacterium bovis* infection has been reported in an AIDS patient following the receipt of BCG vaccine [13]. There appears to be a special liaison between HIV and mycobacterial infection, including both atypical strains, notably *Mycobacterium avium intracellulare* [14], as well as disease caused by *M. tuberculosis* [15].

Even though many of the atypical strains are ubiquitous in the environment worldwide, disease caused by *M. tuberculosis* is often more prevalent in regions frequented by world travelers, with the subsequent greater risk of exposure [16]. Even though BCG is not indicated as an immunoprophylactic agent for international travelers, pre-departure and follow-up skin testing with PPD is indicated in selected circumstances. Even though it is arguable that HIV infection might adversely impact upon the capability of responding to a tuberculin skin test challenge, it has been reported that 55% of AIDS patients with disseminated tuberculosis have tested positive with purified protein derivative (PPD) challenge [17].

## Malaria

Malaria is an infection worthy of specific comment since this is a disease about which all travelers should be cognizant and appropriately prepared. Chloroquine, the standard antimalarial chemoprophylactic agent, is not contraindicated in persons infected with HIV. The drug can produce a dose-related retinopathy, and AIDS patients with cytomegalovirus retinitis are neither candidates for chloroquine nor international travel to malarious areas. Sulfadoxine and pyrimethamine (Fansidar) is an agent often employed in situations when chloroquine resistance is encountered. This product, which can also protect against toxoplasmosis [17], is of concern because of its capacity to induce blood dyscrasias and Stevens-Johnson syndrome.

The use of Fansidar in patients with HIV infection is controversial. The drug has successfully been used for periods up to 12 months in AIDS patients as an effective prophylaxis against *Pneumocystis carinii* [18]. However, side effects, including the Stevens-Johnson syndrome, appear to be more common and more severe in this population, and, as a result, many believe the drug to be contraindicated in situations of advanced HIV-associated disease [19]. Symptomatic patients with HIV as well as asymptomatic carriers with abnormal hematologies should avoid both Fansidar as well as travel to chloroquine-resistant areas. Because of the vital, yet incompletely understood, role of the T cell in defending the host against plasmodial infection [20], the best advice for all HIV-infected travelers might be to avoid malarial regions altogether unless their hematologic profile is completeley within the limits of normal.

## Travelers' Diarrhea

To date, there is not a licensed vaccine available to protect against any of the common pathogens responsible for travelers' diarrhea. However, since chemoprophylaxis against malaria in HIV-infected travelers has been reviewed, the issue of the potential role, if any, of antibiotic prophylaxis for travelers' diarrhea in this population will be raised. Whether HIV disease or infection constitutes an appropriate indication for such therapy is controversial. However, in selected circumstances, prophylaxis with trimethoprim-sulfamethoxazole appears to be justified. Not only would such intervention afford some short-term protection against many strains of enteric pathogens, but is would also provide an element of protection against *Pneumocystis carinii*, an agent which may well pose an equal or greater threat in the international traveler infected with HIV. In addition, prophylaxis with doxycycline would protect against sensitive enteric pathogens as well as plasmodial infection.

## References

1. WHO (1987) International travel and HIV infection. Bull WHO 65:739–740
2. Immunization Practices Advisory Committee (1986) Immunization of children infected with human T-lymphotropic virus type III/lymphadenopathy-associated virus. MMWR 35:595–606
3. Von Reyn CF, Clements CJ, Mann JM (1987) Human immunodeficiency virus infection and routine childhood immunisation. Lancet II:669–672
4. Cherry JD (1981) Measles. In: Fergin RD, Cherry JD (eds) Textbook of pediatric infectious diseases. Saunders, Philadelphia, pp 1210–1231
5. American College of Physicians (1985) Guide for adult immunization. ACP, Philadelphia
6. Immunization Practices Advisory Committee (1984) Adult Immunization. CDC, Atlanta [HHS publ no (CDC) 84-8017]
7. Drotman DP (1986) Vaccination for AIDS patients. JAMA 256:1051–1052
8. Zagury D, Bernard J, Leonard R et al. (1986) Long-term cultures of HTLV-III-infected T-cells: a model of cytopathology of T-cell depletion in AIDS. Science 231:850–853
9. Simberkoff MS, El Sadr W, Schiffman G, Rahal JJ (1984) *Streptococcus pneumoniae* infections and bacteremia in patients with acquired immune deficiency syndrome, with report of a pneumococcal vaccine failure. Am Rev Respir Dis 130:1174–1176
10. Halsey NA, Henderson DA (1987) HIV infection and immunization against other agents. N Engl J Med 316:683–685
11. CDC (1986) Human T-lymphotropic virus type III/lymphadenopathy-associated virus antibody prevalence in U.S. military recruit applicants. MMWR 35:421–424
12. Redfield RR, Wright DC, James WD, Jones TS, Brown C, Burke DS (1987) Disseminated vaccinia in a military recruit with human immunodeficiency virus (HIV) disease. N Engl J Med 316:673–676

13. CDC (1986) Disseminated *Mycobacterium bovis* infection from BCG vaccination of a patient with acquired immunodeficiency syndrome. MMWR 34:227–228
14. Macher AM, Kovacs JA, Gill V et al. (1983) Bacteremia due to *Mycobacterium avium-intracellulare* in the acquired immunodeficiency syndrome. Ann Intern Med 99:782–785
15. Maayan S, Wormser GP, Hewlett D et al. (1985) Acquired immunodeficiency syndrome (AIDS) in an economically disadvantaged population. Arch Intern Med 145:1607–1612
16. Nolan CM (1987) Tuberculosis in travelers and immigrants. In: Jong EC (ed) The travel and tropical medicine manual. Saunders, Philadelphia, p 106
17. Volberding PA, Kaplan LD (1988) AIDS controversies. Annual Session, American College of Physicians, New York
18. Gottlieb M, Knight S, Mitsuyasu R, Weisman J, Roth M, Young LS (1984) Prophylaxis of *Pneumocystis carinii* infection in AIDS with pyrimethamine-sulfadoxine. Lancet II:398–399
19. Navin TR, Miller KD, Satriale RF, Lobel HO (1985) Adverse reactions associated with pyrimethamine-sulfadoxine prophylaxis for *Pneumocystis carinii* infection in AIDS. Lancet I:1332
20. Plorde JJ (1983) Malaria. In: Petersdorf RG; Adams RD, Braunwald E, Isselbacher KJ, Martin JB, Wilson JD (eds) Harrison's principles of internal medicine, 10th edn. McGraw-Hill, New York, p 1189

# Health Advice

# Health Advice to Travelers

P. Grimes


## Summary

Health risks are increasing for travelers to developing countries. They can easily be overcome, however, through the dissemination of accurate information.

In an insatiable quest to see new places and have new types of experiences, Europeans and Americans, using increasingly sophisticated means of travel, are adventuring into primitive and disease-ridden areas, many of which were inaccessible a decade ago. Meanwhile, malaria and other disease have spread, gastrointestinal disorders are rampant and AIDS has produced widespread fear.

Public health organizations have excelled in gathering information on the extent of disease and on prevention and treatment. They have readily made such knowledge available to hospitals, physicians and the travel industry. The problem is that the industry frequently ignores or undervalues it. In organizing and marketing travel to the developing world, the profit motive is dominant. Customers are often accepted, indeed welcomed, for travel that is far beyond their physical ability. Health warnings are often not passed on to travel agents, or by agents to their clients. Conversely, private physicians, acting on misinformation about health conditions beyond what they encounter in everyday practice, have sometimes cautioned patients against travel that the patients could handle very well.

This situation can and must be overcome. The news media can play a leading role. And they can do so in ways to enhance the enjoyment of travel to the developing world, not to frighten people away.


Twenty-seven years ago I had the great challenge and privilege to live in a choice suburb of New Delhi, India. My wife and I lived well there. We had a large modern home in which each of the four spacious bedrooms had its own private bath. We had eight servants to pamper us and our three small children. They kept the premises immaculate and our Bengali cook took all the usual health precautions of the day: for example, he served no unpeeled fruits and no lettuce that had not been thoroughly soaked in potassium permangenate.

Because I was then the chief correspondent of The New York Times for South Asia, we entertained frequently. We were eagerly sought out by American visitors bearing letters of introduction, often from people whom I knew ony slightly, if at all.

Ruth Selden, however, was different. That's not her real name – I don't want to embarrass her, even 27 years later – but I remember her visit vividly. She wanted to meet me very badly, she said, so couldn't my wife and I have tea with her at the Ashoka Hotel? I had a better idea – at least I thought I did. Why not come to our home for dinner? "Oh no," she replied, "I couldn't possibly do that. My doctor in New York told me not to eat anywhere in India except in five-star hotels."

Unfortunately, such inhibitions were not unusual in those days, and I fear that they are not particularly unusual even today. They make me wonder why some people – and even some physicians – bother to travel, or even to think about travel, at all. somewhere, somehow, abstinence has been confused with precaution. Untold numbers of people are being deprived of the physical and intellectual excitement in travel because of needless fear. They don't understand that whatever health dangers there are, no matter how formidable, they can usually be overcome easily by realistic guidance, prophylaxis and common sense.

Now there's no question that India, like many developing countries, is ridden with disease. But it's also true that much of this disease is being avoided. If that was not the case, I hardly think there would be twice as many Indians today as there were when I first went there in 1950.

I haven't come out completely unscathed. While living in India, I had amebic dysentery and bacillary dysentery and hepatitis and pneumonia and worms – not all at once, thankfully, but one by one over a period of 13 years. I probably would have suffered more if not for what they called "Molotov cocktails": syringes full of vaccine against cholera and typhoid and tetanus that were periodically emptied into my arm. I was also immunized against yellow fever and typhus and the plague: why, I'm not so sure, since the threat of those diseases in South Asia was minimal to nonexistent.

While traveling about the five countries in my area, I was careful about where and what I ate and drank. In rural areas, I slept under mosquito netting, although in that period, thanks largely to DDT, as I recall, malaria had been virtually eliminated, though only to return a generation later. But most important of all, I had fun. I rode river boats through the jungles of Kerala, trekked high into the Himalayas between Sikkim and Nepal, bounced 6 days on muleback into the heart of Bhutan, rode with my wife in the back of an apple truck through northern Afghanistan. My wife joined me in India with our two infant sons – her New York pediatrician advised against it – and our third son was conceived on a houseboat in Kashmir and born in Okhla in the southern extremities of New Delhi. We explored, we absorbed the local scene and culture where ever we went and, in general, our lives were a grand adventure. And as you can see by our presence here today – my wife is out there among you – we lived to tell about it.

Although I was doing an enormous amount of traveling in those days, I wasn't writing much about travel. For the New York Times, much of my focus was on politics and international affairs. Only relatively lately, just a little more than a decade ago, did I become primarily a travel writer and editor.

Much of my attention in the last 10 years has been on travel and health. Obviously, I know first-hand how important it is, when traveling, to be healthy. Everybody knows that. But I have seen instance after instance where knowledge has been overriden by foolhardiness, misinformation or no information at all when it is badly needed.

Now, I am not an epidemiologist. I have little talent in the sciences. In fact, as a university undergraduate, the only science course that I took, Zoology 101 at Cornell, was the only course that I failed. But I am a communicator. I know enough about epidemiology to know how important it is and, having seen what I have seen about health in the developing world, I know how important it is to communicate the vital truths about health and travel in ways that the public cannot ignore them.

Here are a few realities, some of which are figuring prominently and urgently in this international conference. One is that no part of the world is really remote any more. I was in India when the summit of Mount Everest was scaled for the first time. Today climbs up its slopes, though perhaps not to the very top, are commonplace. In fact, I heard recently that several discotheques have opened in Namche Bazar, the town near Everest's base on the Nepalese side.

In short, Europeans and Americans and Australians and Japanese – almost everyone who can get a passport and enough money – are going everywhere. They are using every conceivable means of transportation – from pickaxes and ropes for mountain climbing to bicycles to white-water rafts to camel back to helicopters to jumbo jetliners – even to hot-air balloons – to adventure into areas that until recently were firmly sealed to outsiders.

Unfortunately, living conditions in many of these areas are primitive indeed. Shelter often means what your ingenuity and the supplies that you carry on your back enable you to erect on the spot. Often such areas are ridden with disease. Prophylaxis is important and appropriate means of treatment and emergency evacuation are essential.

Travelers are being exposed to diseases today that rarely threatened them before. Schistosomiasis, brucellosis, Chagas' disease and other maladies are ready to strike adventurers who, for example, can be found swimming in the inviting still waters of African oases, places that few would have gone near a few years ago. Meanwhile, chloroquine-resistant malaria has spread through many parts of the world that, until recently, were believed to be malaria-free. There are recurrent reports of the disease afflicting travelers who were in a malaria zone only long enough to change planes at an airport at dusk.

Gastrointestinal disorders are rampant today and are a major topic for discussion this week. All of us know how discomforting and how disruptive of travel they can be. And then there is the threat of AIDS. It's easy to say beware of the tainted needle – although perhaps not so easy to heed if you need emergency assistance in areas less fastidious about health. Realistically speaking, however, it is not easy at all to convince travelers not to have sex.

Having said all this, I must commend public health organizations for gathering information on the extent of disease and on prevention and treatment. They have readily and exhaustively made such knowledge available to hospitals, physicians and the travel industry. The problem is that the travel industry frequently ignores or undervalues it. For example, in the United States the Centers for Disease Control offer travel agents and tour operators free information on disease and sanitation. All agents have to do is ask for it. According to statistics from CDC headquarters in Atlanta, relatively few of them do.

In organizing and marketing travel to the developing world, the profit motive tends to be dominant. Passengers are often accepted, indeed welcomed, for tours that are far beyond their physical ability. Health warnings are often not passed on by tour operators to travel agents, or by agents to their retail clients.

Conversely, private physicians, acting on noninformation or misinformation about health conditions beyond what they encounter in everyday practice, sometimes caution patients about travel that the patients could handle very well.

The next time you are in a travel agency, pick up a brochure about a wildlife safari in East Africa. Does it contain a warning, in reasonably prominent type, about the need for antimalaria prophylaxis? If it does, that is a sign of the tour operator's responsibility. If it does not, I would certainly not go on that operator's tour. In these adventurous days, advising somebody to take a pill against malaria will hardly scare him or her away from a tour. It's as easy as taking a multivitamin in the morning. It will not scare clients away, but rather, I believe, reassure them that adventure travel can be easy on the body as well as stimulating to the spirit.

Of course, a major part of the responsibility for maintaining good health lies with the individual traveler. Before going abroad – anywhere abroad, or for that matter even to many parts of one's own country – it is important to ask about health conditions, particularly if you have a chronic ailment or debility. If information is not volunteered, ask your travel agent, ask the operator of whatever tour you may be going on, ask your physician. If none of these sources seems adequate, go to your local public health authorities; if they don't have literature, they at least should be able to put you in touch with appropriate sources of information.

Above all, know yourself. Don't take on more than you are sure you can handle. In adventure travel, a good tour operator will require that you submit a medical report before you are accepted. Of course you can lie, and in this crazy world, some unethical physicians will lie for you. But in the end, who suffers when you have a heart attack at 15,000 feet?

Responsibility also lies with the practicing medical community. Increasingly, physicians specialize; even generalists cannot be expected to have more than a general smattering of across-the-board information. But they should know where to get more and, when the care of a patient demands it, they should go out and get it or at least refer the patient to an appropriate specialist or information source.

At many hospitals in America, it has become a vogue these days to sponsor clinics for travelers. For a fee – sometimes a rather steep one – you can get all sorts of immunizations, prophylactic medicines and advice. While I cannot really fault such clinics, I sense a profit motive lurking behind the scenes and wonder whether information offered free from the WHO or the Centers for Disease control to your personal physician cannot be just as effective.

And, finally, responsibility lies with the news media. We, too, have access to the some of the best-possible information on travel and health. We have ready access to authoritative reports on the spread of disease, on sanitation on land and at sea, on medical research, on emergency services in the field. We have the publishing and broadcasting ability – and responsibility – to disseminate this information widely. Not all of it is rosy, but the most important factor is truth. Ultimately, constructive truth will promote travel, not drive people away.

# Various Approaches to Providing Health Information for Travelers

P. D. Clarke

## Introduction

Travelers require information to reduce the risks to their health while abroad. The information is both factual and advisory. Much of the information is stable and can be provided in printed form well in advance. Other information changes frequently and the latest situation must be communicated prior to each journey. The delivery of this current health information is the main subject of this paper.

## Route of Delivery

Because of the relatively low incidence of disease in travelers, current health information must reach a high proportion of the very large number of travelers if it is significantly to reduce this incidence. The main practical problem is to decide the route by which travelers are best reached.

*Health Care Professionals.* Most travelers look to their doctors for advice on issues such as immunization and malaria tablets. Many of these doctors are in a poor information state for supplying accurate up-to-date advice, as they have no single credible source. If a central database was easy to access and doctors were able to do so without much cost to themselves, then this route would probably be the best route to follow. In practice the costs and the relative naivety of most practitioners in using electronic databases makes the route poorly used when it has been provided in the past. As to cost, many doctors, particularly in the United Kindom, are quite unused to charging for services and have no real mechanism for doing so. Thus unless it is provided without charge by Central Goverment it is difficult to see how it will gain sufficient support amongst GPs. In the United States the possibility is greater as the whole health care system is orientated to a fee-based service. One major problem faced by health care professionals is that the call for an information service is relatively small and sporadic in any one practice. As speedy computer use requires regular practice, access routines have to be extremely simple and quick if they are to be used on an ad hoc basis. In this respect it is important that health care professionals are educated to make such routine enquiries. In order to overcome this it would be better to set up busier travel clinics in each locality to ensure that there is sufficient turnover.

*Travel Agent.* At first glance, this might seem a particularly useful route for providing health information. In practice travel agencies do not take a major interest in health risks for two main reasons. Firstly, it is seen as potentially detracting from the prime objective of selling tickets and, secondly, most travel agents do not wish to be seen to be taking responsibility for an area which they essentially believe is outside their knowledge base. Most travel agents regard health advice as a specialized matter for the medical profession and can see little to be gained by accepting responsibility for it. Such an attitude is not unreasonable and is indeed promoted by the profession in many countries. To deliver information through travel agents, a completely automated system is required which will deliver information through existing computer networks but without any requirement for interpretation on their part. With it must come a clear indication that responsibility for application and implementation of the advice to any given individual lies firmly and solely with his/her own doctor. This implies that the doctor will be well enough educated in the specific problems of applying such information and be able to implement it. Where, for example, a more unusual vaccine may be recommended the doctor may not have means to implement the advice and credibility is lost.

*Airlines.* Airlines have a greater interest than their travel agents in promoting the good health and wellbeing of their passengers. This comes in part from their international responsibility as carriers and the fact that many are involved in repatriation of sick people. Many airlines, too, are promoting a much more caring image which is perceived as a prerequisite for being a player in this lucrative commercial field. However, the same limitations as for travel agents apply if delivery of information is purely electronic. It is likely therefore that airlines would look to form a liason with clinical groups to develop travel centres where clinical interpretation as well as post travel care can be undertaken.

*Direct to the Traveler.* The traveler is usually the prime mover in seeking information, although too many still remain unaware of the need to do so. Direct advice to the traveler has the advantage that if personal details can be elicited then a much more comprehensive "briefing" can be achieved. Such "health briefs" can be sent by mail and include both stable and current information. The main limitation is to achieve sufficient penetration into the large traveler population in order significantly to affect the incidence of disease. It is also extremely important that such a system must take into account the different groups that make up the traveling population. These different groups include regular travelers, expatriates, businessmen, and holidaymakers, and all have different requirements. A regular traveler, for example, needs a system of simple updating of current information for any given trip while having a basic manual of stable information for reference. Dealing direct with the traveler has the same limitation as via the travel agent, namely that there is still the requirement to visit the health care professional for implementation of immunization schedules, prescriptions for tablets and interpretation of information for the individual.

## Verbal Versus Printed Advice

An increasing number of recent publications emphasize that advice is most effective if in a written format. Ideally such advice should be seen to emanate from a credible authority, be concise and relatively dogmatic with its clarity enhanced by the removal of information "clutter".

### Verbal

*Telephone.* Most travelers would choose a telephone advisory service as their preferred option. It has the personal touch which is important in clinical medicine and allows interaction between enquirer and provider with selection of particular topics of interest. For the traveler it is a cost-effective way of making a specific enquiry but for the provider it is extremely expensive. Manning sufficient telephone lines to cope with the volume of enquiries that would result if all travelers called for advice almost excludes it as a realistic option on a national scale unless it is very heavily subsidised. An alternative is to try to find a way to charge callers but this has so far eluded most who have tried.

It is a much more practical proposition to provide a telephone advisory service for health care professionals who wish to discuss specific matters. Even these, however, can become extremely busy and require a major commitment by staff in the national centre of expertise. One of the major concerns about telephone advice is the maintenance of the quality and continuity of that advice.

*Personal Consultation.* Although this is the time-honoured standard by which all others are judged, it does have serious limitations in the field of mass advice. Only a very limited number of travelers can be advised in this way, and it is extremely expensive to provide even this. On the other hand, charging mechanisms can be applied which mean that it does not have to be subsidised to the same extent as a telephone consultancy service. Many companies already have occupational health departments that undertake this work and combined with a current computer advisory service they represent one of the ideal means of complete patient care. Such "travel clinics" should be the eventual aim of any national system.

The use of pre-recorded telephone tapes to give out information on health matters is a new development that overcomes some of the limitations of a person to person call. It has the enormous advantage of being able to deal with a very large number of callers, most of whom will get the simple information that they require and the quality of that information is consistent. The tapes can be readily updated and out-of-date information is not therefore perpetuated. The Ross Institute in the United Kingdom currently have such a system for malaria advice which is widely used. The limitation as mentioned earlier is the relative weakness of verbal over written advice in inducing compliance in the traveler.

## Printed

This is the traditional means of information dissemination and many avenues of delivery have been exploited in the past.

### Travel Agent/Traveler

*Books*. There are many travel books which offer health advice and these are quite good for stable advice although they usually suffer from information "clutter" as the author tries to appeal to as wide a readership as possible. They have the great advantage of all written material, namely that it can be referred to at a later date. The main disadvantage is that outdated books may be used for a long time.

*Annual Publications*. These vary from Government pamphlets to travel agents and airline guides. The main problem is that most try to summarize current information but because of the preparation time and relative infrequency of publications are often much out of date. Many take a whole year to prepare and then are in use for the whole of the following year if not longer. This is much too insensitive a system for disseminating anything but the most basic stable information. In order to overcome information "clutter" it is commonplace for authors to oversimplify and trivialize information in an attempt to clarify and become more dogmatic. The subject has long suffered these "half-truths", which eventually lead to a breakdown in credibility of all sources. A number of pharmaceutical companies produce publications as well but there is always the added concern over vested interest in these circumstances.

*Monthly Publications*. These are a much more effective tool for disseminating current advice provided they are actively maintained. This major task is often poorly carried out particularly in those publications which are primarily designed to help travel agents plan itineraries and sell tickets rather than reduce ill health abroad. Such publications do little to add credibility to efforts to maintain a national standard as they often lead to confusion. The discerning individual can readily identify conflicting statements which often result from poor maintenance.

*Newspaper and Travel Magazines*. It is a sad reflection that these are amongst the most influential of means for publicizing travel health problems. This is because of their enormous readership and penetration into the traveling population. All too often, however, the thirst for sensationalism distorts the message putting perceived risk into a higher profile than actual risk. No clearer example of this can be found than in the press coverage of the current AIDS epidemic contrasted with the extreme difficulty in promoting an interest in the figures for imported malaria cases into the United Kingdom.

### Health Care Professionals

*Books*. There are many manuals of travel health which are excellent sources of advice on the more stable aspects of diseases that can affect travelers as well as pre-travel advice. Nearly all suffer from the problem of currency and are very dependent upon regular editions being produced.

*Annuals*. Publications such as the *WHO Yellow Book* and the equivalents produced by several individual national goverments can put across a policy with considerable credibility. The major problem is ensuring that health care-professionals retain and use these documents properly. It may well be that more attention should be paid to this in medical education. There are very real problems in addition, where the decision-making process requires additional current information. Thus a busy general doctor may be required to keep abreast of the progress of chloroquine-resistant malaria in order to make decisions on antimalarial tablets, but in practice is unlikely to do so. There are also the limitations set by the politics of producing government publications; thus the practical requirements to have a cholera certificate to enter Tanzania are well known by those that go there despite assurances that they are not officially required.

*Monthly's and Weekly's*. These publications vary enormously in their purpose and authority. Those from government sources such as, Weekly Epidemiological Records, Communicable Diseases Reports and Morbidity Mortality Weekly Reports often contain much useful information but they are rarely read by the primary care physician who is only advising a few travelers and they are not priority reading. He is much more likely to read the "free" doctors' newspapers that commonly provide "charts" of standardized recommendations. Unfortunately, such charts have severe limitations which are quite often mentioned in the small print but are rarely read by the busy physician. They are inappropriate for advising people undertaking journeys "off the beaten track" or involving several countries because they have been so simplified for ease of reference that they cannot take into account the complexities of such journeys. This trivialization of the overall problem of advising travelers leads in the long run to loss of credibility when such sources become the quoted authority. Unless they are very actively maintained they can often lead to the perpetuation of myths and perhaps the best example of this is the continuing difficulty WHO is having in stamping out the excessive use of cholera vaccine.

*Personal Electronic Printing*. This is much the most exciting area of development at the present moment as it allows the selection of information from a textural and logical database for any individual for a given journey. This greatly reduces information "clutter" yet ensures sufficient depth, accuracy and currency to allow a true appreciation of the appropriate preventive action that should be taken. Examples of this are now to be found in Canada (CATIS), United States (Immunization Alert), Federal Republic of Germany (MEDIDAR) and the United Kingdom (MASTA).

## Electronic Communication

The growth of information technology has led to the development of several systems of health advice to travelers which use electronic communication.

These can be broadly divided into two groups dependent on the method of distributing the information.

*Discs.* Distribution of a database using discs is a cheap method of allowing many centres to use the information at the same time, but it has drawbacks also. Computer compatability still presents problems, most particularly if any processing is to be done. Industry standards are slowly being sorted out in this area and intercompatability is improving. Discs are also prone to damage and corruption and out-of-date discs can continue to be used in the same way as out-of-date annual publications. The major problem therefore is to maintain control over the information. Errors can never be reliably corrected and response times to alterations are not known.

*Online.* The growth of rapid data transmission has revolutionized distribution from centrally maintained databases. The networks required to distribute the data are the subject of intense competition and are now relatively cheap for the customer. The development of "gateways" between the standard telephone network and such fast packet switching networks means that rapid, cheap, data access is now available to almost everyone, worldwide. One major area of difficulty in on-line systems remains the format of information. There are two principle systems. The first is *Video text*, in which information appears screen by screen. This quite severely limits the freedom of interreaction between users and host, although better systems are being developed to overcome this. Line-lengths are currently limited to 40 characters, which is a major restriction on presentation. Many travel agents use the videotext system, but some believe that its future is limited. The second format is *Continuous text* – which has the advantage of 80 character lines and greater ease of interreaction. This system is usually transmitted using the standard ASCII code.

Interactive databases allow the user to input data allowing the host computer to select out all the relevant information, sort it and present it in a usable format. Thus account can be taken of such parameters as the patient's age, pregnancy, allergies, past immunizations, living conditions in each country and sequence of countries being visited in a journey. The final advice is then tailored to the individual's requirements. Such information can be printed directly in the travel clinic or if too lengthy it may be printed "off-line" using fast laser printers and then sent by mail to be used as a reference document during travel.

## Conclusion

The opportunity now exists through computerization for any country to set up an integrated system of information and clinical services in a national network of travel clinics. Such integration will allow a national policy to be developed and promoted from a selected centre of expertise and carried out in a network of designated travel clinics. This will ensure control and credibility that should lead to a reduction in the incidence of illness in travelers.

# Health Information for Spanish Intercontinental Travelers

R. Abós, G. Añanos, P. Navarro, X. Blanche, and M. Corachan

A cohort of 910 Spanish travelers to tropical and subtropical areas were interviewed at Barcelona Airport with a questionnaire designed to evaluate the health information received prior to their trip as well as questions concerning malaria prophylaxis. The objectives of the study were:

- To determine the profile of the travelers including reasons for travel and country of destination
- To investigate the sources of health information
- To assess required and optional vaccines received
- To analyse the adequacy of the malaria prophylaxis (dose by weight and drug by destination)
- To study the occurrence of adverse reactions to antimalarials

The study was carried out during the summer of 1987 by contacting the tour operators located at the airport 3 days a week. Travelers completed their interview forms before embarking. Only 15 persons refused the interview. A total of 894 travelers were contacted by telephone during the first trimester after returning home to assess use of prophylaxis after travel.

## Results

The male : female ratio was 46 : 54. Most travelers (94%) were going abroad as tourists and 55% of these were in the 27–40 year age group. Final destinations were: Indian subcontinent (21.5%), China (4.5%), Southeast Asia (22%), Turkey (1%), Egypt (37.5%), Kenya (10.5%), and Brazil (3%).

The pretravel health information sources for these travelers is shown in Fig. 1. One-third of the respondents had received information from more than one source. Only 23% had not received any information.

*Vaccinations.* No vaccine had been given to 510 (57%) of 889 travelers. No yellow fever vaccine had been received by 73 of 94 (68%) travelers to East Africa and 19 of 30 (63%) to Brazil.

Recommended vaccinations received included cholera by 271 (30%) travelers, typhoid by 110 (12%), tetanus by 86 (10%), poliomyelitis by 11 (1%) and hepatitis by 4 (0.4%) of travelers.

*Malaria Chemoprophylaxis.* Only 33% of the respondents intended taking antimalarial drugs. Of these, 8% discontinued prophylaxis during the travel, 8% discontinued prophylaxis during the 1st week after return, 11% during the

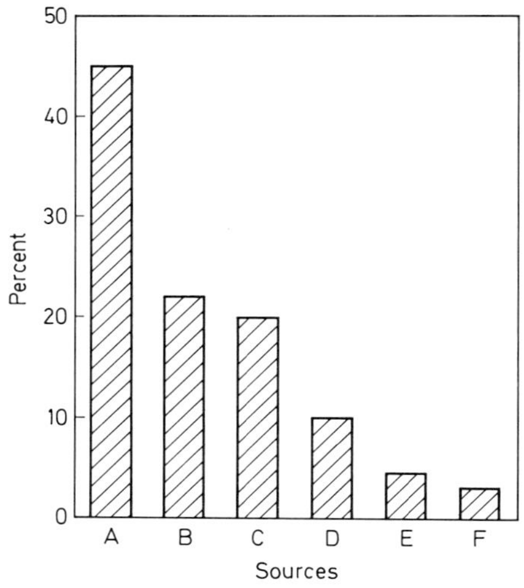


**Fig. 1.** Sources of health information: *A*, travel agencies; *B*, official centre; *C*, practicing physicians; *D*, acquaintances; *E*, pharmacies; *F*, Departments of Tropical Medicine

**Table 1.** Prophylaxis in travelers to areas with chloroquine-resistant *P. falciparum*

| Geographic areas | Indian subcontinent | Southeast Asia | East Africa | Brazil | Total |
|---|---|---|---|---|---|
| Number of travellers | 194 | 196 | 96 | 30 | 519 |
| No prophylaxis | 61 | 148 | 21 | 12 | 242 |
| Chloroquine only | 47 | 27 | 14 | 9 | 97 |
| Chloroquine combined | 86 | 21 | 61 | 9 | 177 |

2nd week, 13% during the 3rd week and 21% during the 4th week. Only 39% of those taking drugs completed their prophylaxis for 4–6 weeks after return as recommended by the World Health Organization. Chloroquine prophylaxis was used by 300 travelers visiting malarious areas. Of these 118 (39%) received a low dose for their weight. This was mainly due to the standardized advice that is given by vaccination centres, travel agencies and general practitioners. Of 516 travelers going to areas where *Plasmodium falciparum* is resistant to chloroquinine, 242 (47%) took no prophylaxis at all and 97 (19%) were advised to take chloroquinine alone. Only 177 (34%) were correctly advised regarding drugs. Overall, 12% of the travelers reported some kind of intolerance to antimalarials, mostly involving the GI tract. One case of blurred vision and two cases with rash were also reported. One rash was due to pyrimethamine-sulphadoxine and the other to chloroquinine (centrifugal annular erythema).

## Conclusions

Tourism to the tropics is a recent development in Spain, because there are relatively few trade and aid relations with African and Asian countries. This is likely to change, however. The low use of vaccinations and chemoprophylaxis as found in this survey may be attributed to the use of non-specialized sources of information. We believe that individualized information on a case-by-case basis is needed, which requires training in tropical medicine and imported diseases. A strengthening of these specialized services is therefore urgently needed within the framework of Spanish Health Care.

# A Survey of Health Risks of North American Mission Personnel Serving Overseas *

W. R. Lange and S. D. Kreider

It has been estimated that there are approximately a quarter of a million Christian missionaries at work in the world today; however, despite their numbers, the health status and medical problems of missionaries are areas about which there is relatively little clinical information. Nevertheless, there is reason to believe that the missionary calling has associated with it increased and unique health risks [1]. A study was undertaken to identify and prioritize medical problems of overseas protestant mission personnel, to differentiate health risks of medical missionaries from those of missionaries as a whole, and to delineate preventive measures that might be pursued to improve health status.

## Methods

The *Mission Handbook: North American Protestant Ministries Overseas* is a descriptive and statistical reference of North American protestant overseas ministries [2], which lists 137 organizations which provide medical, dental and/or public health services. The medical director or overseas coordinator of these boards was asked to describe the nature and scope of their overseas activities, including common and serious health problems affecting missionaries and regions of the world where the health of mission personnel was most in peril.

Since both anecdotal reports and published accounts [3–6] have suggested that viral hepatitis is a significant health problem of missionaries, boards were asked a series of questions specifically on this topic. Additionally, they were asked to render an opinion concerning their recommendation of a number of frequently used preventive measures, and to describe various strategies for improving missionarie's health.

## Results

Of the 61 boards which responded, the median number of overseas personnel was 216 (range 3–3400). Eighty-five percent of the boards had their own medical personnel overseas, and the median number of such staff was 31 (range 1–172). The ten largest boards with a health component to their ministry participated in this survey.

---

* Parts of this paper originally appeared in the *American Journal of Preventive Medicine*

**Table 1.** Health problems of mission personnel

| Ranking | Most frequent | Most serious |
|---|---|---|
| 1 | Malaria | Viral hepatitis |
| 2 | Viral hepatitis | Malaria |
| 3 | Helminths | Neoplasia |
| 4 | Amebiasis/giardiasis | Accidents |
| 5 | GI disorders (not parasitic) | Typhoid fever |
| 6 | Dental problems | Stress/burnout |
| 7 | Worsening of CMC[a] | Depression |
| 8 | Depression | Worsening of CMC |
| 9 | Stress/burnout | Dental problems |
| 10 | Accidents | Chronic diarrhea |

[a] Chronic medical condition

**Table 2.** Use of select preventive medicine measures by mission boards

| Preventive practice | % recommending use |
|---|---|
| Malaria prophylaxis | 72.1 |
| Water purification measures | 70.5 |
| Typhoid immunization | 68.9 |
| Polio vaccine booster | 65.6 |
| Immune globulin inoculations | 57.4 |
| Yellow fever vaccination | 55.7 |
| Cholera immunization | 50.8 |
| Hepatitis B immunization | 31.1 |
| Diarrhea prophylaxis | 18.0 |

Table 1 ranks the most frequent and the most serious health problems of overseas mission personnel for which medical attention was sought. The "frequent" problems tabulated do not include trivial complaints, but rather consist of conditions that caused a staff person to miss 2 or more days from the field, either because of personal illness or illness in a family member also on assigment. A "serious" problem was defined as one producing loss from duty for at least a week and/or medical evacuation from the field. There were no differences in the nature of the health problems befalling medical missionaries and missionaries in general, suggesting that both are subjected to similar risks.

The majority of responses did not designate a particular region of the world where it was felt that the health of missionaries was most in peril. However, of the 41% who felt there was such an area, 50% indicated sub-Saharan Africa and 25% selected the Asian subcontinent.

Table 2 lists various preventive health practices and tabulates the percentage of responding mission boards which recommend their use. Table 3 sum-

**Table 3.** Mission board suggestions for improving missionary health status

| Stage | Recommendations | Percent |
|---|---|---|
| Before departure | Health education: clinical DX and RX | 30 |
| | Health education: public health and sanitation | 25 |
| | More comprehensive initial health assessment | 22 |
| | Increased immunization protection | 12 |
| | Other | 11 |
| | | 100 |
| While abroad | Improved periodic health assessment | 44 |
| | Ongoing health education: public health | 24 |
| | Improved scheduling: more relaxation time | 10 |
| | Ongoing health education: clinical DX and RX | 8 |
| | Greater use of malaria prophylaxis | 6 |
| | Other | 8 |
| | | 100 |
| Upon return | More comprehensive health assessment | 60 |
| | Follow-up stool parasitology | 14 |
| | Time for rest and readjustment | 9 |
| | Specific debriefing | 6 |
| | Other | 11 |
| | | 100 |

marizes board responses as to methods which might be employed to improve the health status of mission personnel.

## Discussion

Of medical problems resulting in time lost from work, malaria was regarded as the most frequent complaint. It was disconcerting that only 72% of the boards recommended malaria prophylaxis, including many who had personnel in high-risk regions. Viral hepatitis was regarded as the most serious health concern as well as the second most common. Earlier studies have documented that hepatitis is a common occupational hazard for missionaries [3–6], and the magnitude of disease has been substantial.

Early investigations have substantiated that immune globulin (IG) can dramatically decrease the incidence of icteric illness in personnel on long-term assignment overseas [7]; nevertheless, of the boards surveyed, only 57% recommended regular IG administration, and only 31% advocated hepatitis B immunization. In the United States, the Immunization Practices Advisory Committee (ACIP) advocates IG use for the prevention of hepatitis A in travelers to developing countries who will be visiting extensively with local persons [8], and this would include most missionaries. The use of hepatitis B vaccine is definitely indicated for all medical missionaries as well as for selected others assigned to certain high-risk regions of the world. The ACIP recommends hepatitis B vaccine for international travelers who will be residing in a high-risk region for more than 6 months [8], and other authorities have specifically advocated hepatitis B vaccine use in missionary personnel [9].

The finding that psychological conditions, including depression, stress, and burnout, are considered among the most common and most serious conditions is important. Even though others have described expatriate psychopathology in missionaries [10], there is often substantial denial that such problems exist in this population. Nevertheless, both individual and family stressors appear to be important problems and appropriate for attention at all phases and stages of a missionary's career.

Accidents were also considered to be among the most common and most serious conditions. Frequent comment was made that motor vehicle accidents account for the majority of the more serious incidents, and that seat belt use was infrequent, often because restraints were not available. Cancer was also regarded as a serious health problem, but the various types of malignancies occurring in missionaries were not tabulated in this survey.

Even though typhoid fever was regarded as a serious health threat, the magnitude of enteric fever among missionaries is unknown. Although typhoid immunization has its limitations, particularly in adults, the living conditions of the majority of missionaries would make them candidates for typhoid vaccine [11], but only 69% of mission boards utilize this preventive measure with their staff.

Concern over AIDS was apparent, but the logistical constraints imposed on many boards precluded the adoption of the standard accepted safeguards. However, modified health care delivery practices and evacuation procedures for staff are being implemented. AIDS education and precautions will warrant increasing attention, and the scope of the pandemic will mandate that the same precautions advocated for other professionals ministering to and caring for AIDS victims be extended to missionary personnel.

The survey responders gave a comprehensive overview of suggestions for improving missionary health status; however, during the predeparture phase, only 12% felt that more attention should be given to increased immunization protection. Many acknowledged the importance of preexposure rabies prophylaxis; however, few appear to be doing this routinely even though the rate of exposure to animal bite is at least ten times higher abroad than it is domestically in the United States [12]. Sixty percent of those offering an opinion as to how to improve missionary health upon returning to North America felt that a more comprehensive medical assessment was in order. Both while abroad and upon return, there is a growing awareness that attention should be given to the mental health and total well-being of the missionary family, including improved scheduling with increased time for relaxation.

In conclusion, strategies for improving missionary health not only include appropriate interventions to reduce infectious disease risks, but also increased attention to mental health issues, accident prevention, health education, and health care provision.

## References

1. Lange WR, Kreider SD, Kaczaniuk MA, Snyder FR (1987) Missionary health: the great omission. Am J Prev Med 3:332–338
2. Wilson S (ed) (1980) Mission handbook: North American protestant ministries overseas, 12th edn. Missions Advanced Research and Communications Center, Monrovia
3. Cline AL, Mosley JW, Scovel FG (1967) Viral hepatitis among American missionaries abroad (a preliminary study). JAMA 199:119–121
4. Frame JD (1968) Hepatitis among missionaries in Ethiopia and Sudan (susceptibles at high risk). JAMA 203:99–106
5. Woodson RD, Cahill KM (1972) Viral hepatitis abroad (incidence in catholic missionaries). JAMA 219:1191–1193
6. Kendrick MA (1974) Viral hepatitis in American missionaries abroad. J Infect Dis 129:227–229
7. Woodson RD, Clinton JJ (1969) Hepatitis prophylaxis abroad. Effectiveness of immune globulin in protecting Peace Corps volunteers. JAMA 209:1053–1058
8. Immunization Practices Advisory Committee (1985) Recommendations for protection against viral hepatitis. MMWR 14:313–335
9. Seeff LB, Koff RS (1984) Passive and active immunoprophylaxis of hepatitis B. Gastroenterology 86:958–981
10. Littlewood R (1985) Jungle madness: some observations on expatriate psychopathology. Int J Soc Psychiatry 31:194–197
11. CDC (1985) Health information for international travel 1985. CDC, Atlanta [DHHS publ no (CDC) 85-8280]
12. Banta JE, Jungblut E (1966) Health problems encountered by the Peace Corps overseas. Am J Public Health 56:2121–2125

# Attitudes Towards Prevention of Communicable Diseases Among French Travelers

O. Obrecht, E. Bouvet, C. Saout, J. Perrin, A. Andremont, and M. Kermorvant

A survey was conducted to investigate pretravel medical advice received by travelers, the use of prophylaxis against malaria and diarrhoea, and their vaccination status. The survey was conducted among French-speaking travelers departing from Paris by air between December 1984 and March 1985.

## Methods

A random sample of 150 flights was selected and an average of 11 questionnaires were collected per flight. The questionnaires were distributed at random to passengers by French Border Health Service agents and were completed by the passengers. A total of 1449 completed questionnaires were collected. For the study four main areas of destination were selected: northern Africa (5 countries), tropical Africa (26 countries), Middle East (12 countries) and Southeast Asia (13 countries).

## Results

The numbers and percentages of travelers to each area are shown in Table 1. The questionnaires sollicited the following information: personal characteristics, details of purpose and length of travel, destination, pretravel health information received, intended prevention measures concerning eating and drinking, malaria prevention, and immunizations received.

**Table 1.** Numbers of percentages of travellers going to each area

| Area | Number | Percentage |
|---|---|---|
| Northern Africa | 387 | 26.8 |
| Tropical Africa | 505 | 34.8 |
| Middle East | 255 | 17.6 |
| Southeast Asia | 283 | 19.5 |
| Other countries | 16 | 1.1 |
| Not stated | 3 | 0.2 |

## Traveler Characteristics

The traveler's characteristics were similar to those of French travelers leaving Paris airports based on French airline statistics. The male: female ratio was 65:35, the average age was 42 years; 53% traveled for less than 15 days and 73% for less than 45 days. Business travel accounted for more than 80% of travelers to the Middle East, less than 40% of travelers to northern Africa and Southeast Asia, and 50% of travelers to tropical Africa.

## Pretravel Health Information

Overall, 87% of travelers had asked for information before leaving. The sources of information included medical doctor (48%), vaccination centre (26%), company (20%), travel agency (17%), the French Border Health Service (17%), and other sources such as a pharmacist or friends accounted for 10%. Often multiple sources provided advice. Receiving advice was not associated with sex, age, length of stay, or destination, but was dependent on social level: workers received less information than other social groups ($P < 0.001$). An information leaflet had been received by travelers. Travel agencies and vaccination centres were the main sources of these leaflets. Medical sources accounted for only 8% of the leaflets received.

## Prophylaxis Against Malaria

One-third of the travelers said they would take prophylaxis against malaria. Significant differences occurred depending on destination (Table 2).

Only 65% of travelers going to malarious areas in tropical Africa took prophylaxis. Chloroquine was used by 90% of travelers who intended to take chemoprophylaxis. Use of prophylaxis was associated with destination, sex (women protect themselves better), and reason for the trip: tourists were more likely than business travelers to use prophylaxis. Prophylaxis use was also associated with receiving a leaflet to vaccinations received for this trip, and not for a previous one.

**Table 2.** Travelers taking prophylaxis for malaria

| Area | Percentage |
|---|---|
| Northern Africa | 5.2 |
| Tropical Africa | 59.3 |
| Middle East | 6.7 |
| Southeast Asia | 43.1 |

## Precautions Regarding Food and Drink, Prophylaxis Against Diarrhoea

Passengers were asked whether they intended to take precautions regarding food and drink: 82% said they would be cautious about food and drink and only 16% said they would not take special precautions. Only 5% of passengers would take daily prophylaxis against diarrhoea and 12.5% carried antidiarrhoea drugs without taking them systematically. The daily use of drugs was associated with sex (more women), age (older travelers used more prophylaxis), length of stay (higher among short-term travelers), tourists, and destination: travelers to northern Africa and Southeast Asia used chemoprophylaxis more than travelers to other destinations.

## Vaccinations

There was a high level of yellow fever vaccination among travelers to tropical Africa (98%). Low coverage was observed for the usual recommended vaccinations such as poliomyelitis and tetanus; 29% of travelers were not vaccinated although one-fourth of the vaccinated travelers had received their vaccinations before departure. Vaccination status was associated with age (young people were better vaccinated), length of stay (long-term travelers were better vaccinated), and professional status (workers were less vaccinated than other social groups). (Table 3).

**Table 3.** Percentages of travellers who said they had been vaccinated

| Vaccination | This trip | Previously | Total |
|---|---|---|---|
| Yellow fever | 20.7 | 41.4 | 62.1 |
| Diphtheria | 7.4 | 29.7 | 37.1 |
| Poliomyelitis | 12.9 | 42.8 | 55.7 |
| Tetanus | 16.9 | 54.3 | 71.2 |

## Conclusions

This survey provided a good methodology to assess the use of preventive measures of travelers. Our sample appeared to be a representative sample of travelers. The major preventive attitudes were associated and related to the information travelers received. This demonstrates the importance of such information: one-half of the travelers received information from private physicians and one-third went to a vaccination centre before departure.

A new survey should provide interesting information regarding chemoprophylaxis among travelers to areas with chloroquinine resistance in Africa. All travelers need to be given accurate advice on existing risks and prevention measures.

# Acquisition of Knowledge by Travelers Receiving Pre-Travel Advice

E. D'Agata, J. S. Keystone, L. Sawyer, and P. Scappatura

As increasing numbers of travelers search for sun, sand and sex in more exotic tropical locations, there is a growing need for up-to-date health information for international travel.

In the summer of 1987 a prospective study was carried out in the Travel and Inoculation Clinic at Toronto General Hospital to ascertain the knowledge base of travelers seeking advice from this travel clinic and to determine whether or not such travelers increased their knowledge by visiting the clinic.

## Method

Travelers over 18 years of age who were traveling to a malarious area and who required two visits to complete their pre-travel immunization were asked to participate in this study. The purpose of the study was explained by an interviewer and a signed consent was obtained. Volunteers who agreed to participate in the study were asked to complete a questionnaire which included 10 questions concerning demographic information and an additional 15 multiple-choice questions on health precautions to ensure safe travel. The majority of questions were concerned with safety aspects of food and water and ways to prevent malaria.

The pre-visit questionnaire was completed by the traveler before he or she received advice from a member of the clinic staff. A post-visit questionnaire, identical to the pre-visit one, was completed by the traveler immediately before the first follow-up clinic visit. To ensure that the pre-test questionnaire itself was not biasing the study, a group of travelers was given a post-visit questionnaire only. The statistical analyses were carried out by means of multivariate analysis and Student's *t*-test.

## Results

Out of 385 travelers who were asked to participate in the study, 10 (3%) refused to enter it. One hundred and ninety travelers completed the study successfully. The remaining 185 did not require a follow-up visit and hence were excluded from the present analysis. One hundred travelers completed both pre- and post-visit questionnaires while 90 completed post-visit questionnaires only.

No difference was detected between the scores on the post-visit questionnaires of those receiving the pre- and post-visit questionnaires compared with the group receiving the post-visit questionnaire only. Our demographic information showed that the average age of our travelers was 33 years and approximately equal numbers of males and females participated. Sixty-one percent of the participants were single and 61% had university education. Forty-three percent of the individuals had traveled previously in the tropics but only 9% had visited our clinic in the past. Ninety-four percent of the travelers cited tourism as their main purpose of their travel. Thirty-one percent of the travelers were considered to have a high risk of illness in that they were planning to travel off the usual tourist routes, in rural areas, or live in a third-class accommodation or lower. The mean duration of the present trip was 3 months (5 days to 3 years), but the median was 1 month. The average time elasped between the first and second clinic visit was 25 (7–58) days.

Out of the 15 questions, the mean pre-visit score of 8.9 (59% correct) was significantly lower than the post-visit test score of 10.2 (68% correct responses) ($P \leqq 0.0001$). The knowledge level of the study participants increased by only 20% following the clinic visit. The pre-visit test showed that a majority of travelers were knowledgeable about food and water precautions (mean score 10%) whereas knowledge about the prevention of malaria was poor (mean score 46%). There was a greater acquisition of knowledge about malaria prevention than about food and water precautions. It was interesting to note that previous travel had no effect on the base-line knowledge of travelers. For example, the average score of those who traveled previously was 68% in the area of food and water precautions whereas those with no previous travel scored an average of 72% on the same six questions.

Acquisition of knowledge did not correlate with age, sex, marital status, education level, risk of travel, duration of the trip or number of previous clinic visits. The only variables which correlated with acquisition of knowledge were the education level of travelers and whether or not they read printed material which was made available. The overall score increased by 10% in those 75 individuals who read the pamphlets compared with 1% in the 18 individuals who did not ($P \leqq 0.05$).

## Conclusions

We concluded that the travelers attending the Travel and Inoculation Clinic at Toronto General Hospital were relatively knowledgeable about food and water precautions but not about malaria prevention. Using present methods, our clinic succeeded only to a limited extent in improving the knowledge of travelers concerning health aspects of travel. We believe that the relatively low acquisition of knowledge might have been related to use of printed material which was too detailed and hence difficult to remember. It is also possible that the multiple-choice questions were too difficult for travelers who were not used to this format of questionnaire.

Acquisition of knowledge was correlated with the travelers' education level and the use of printed material. We believe that travel health advisors should concentrate less on food and water precautions and more on malaria prevention, using concise, printed material which highlights the most important aspects of health precautions.

# Advice on Prophylaxis for Travelers Dispensed by Telephone at the Pasteur Hospital Vaccination Center

C. Goujon

## Introduction

Providing information by telephone represents an increasingly important part of the International Vaccination Center's activity. Data presented are based on a survey at the vaccination center of the Pasteur Institute from November 1987 to January 1988. This center is part of the medical department of the Pasteur Institute. A similar survey was conducted in this center from January to February 1985. Comparison of the results of the two surveys enables the development of this activity to be observed.

## Description

The center is open from 9 a.m. to 5 p.m. from Monday to Friday and from 9 a.m. to noon on Saturday. A switchboard receives phone calls and passes them on to different extensions. There is a doctor permanently available during working hours to answer medical questions. Most phone calls come from the general public, followed by, in decreasing order, medical staff, pharmacists, and travel agencies.

## Results

A total of 2969 calls were recorded, at an average of 54 calls a day. These calls only include questions related to travel overseas. Enquiries were either general (82%) or medical (18%). Analysis indicated that the questions were rather stereotyped and that they could be categorized into a few groups. The general enquiries fall into three main categories:

1. Vaccinations and/or malaria prophylaxis in accordance with the visited country(ies) 89%
2. Immunization schedules and possible vaccine associations 10%
3. Other preventive measures and hygiene rules to use in tropical countries 1%

For the first category, the countries visited were recorded. The parts of the world about which questions were frequently asked included: countries of Southeast Asia, especially Thailand, 23%; countries of West Africa, mainly Senegal, 11%; India and Nepal, 10%; Kenya and Tanzania, 8%; Egypt, 6%; Mexico, 5%; and Brazil, 4%. The questions pertained to almost all countries of tropical and subtropical areas.

The medical questions were categorized as follows:

1. Vaccinations and/or malaria prophylaxis in pregnant women
2. Vaccinations and /or malaria prophylaxis in young children
3. Yellow fever (or other) vaccination of patients with different conditions, such as immunization against yellow fever for HIV-positive patients, patients treated with antibiotics or for allergies, and patients having had surgical treatment and radiotherapy for breast cancer.
4. Malaria prophylaxis for patients with different conditions such as chloroquine prophylaxis for patients with retinopathy or mefloquine prophylaxis for patients with migraine.

## Discussion

When comparing the results with the data from the survey conducted in 1985, we noted that the type of enquiry had not changed appreciably but the number of daily calls had increased considerably from 30 in the 1985 study to 54 in 1987. Our experience indicates that only simple and concise information can be given by phone. Lengthy and complicated explanations are often misunderstood or wrongly recorded by persons without medical knowledge.

This applies especially to malaria prophylaxis for travel in areas of resistance to chloroquine where the recommendations may vary depending on several different criteria. Medical advice from a general practioner is then advised. However, French Gps may be misinformed about tropical diseases.

## Conclusions

Advice by telephone for the general public can be useful but has limitations. For special cases we suggest an appointment so that medical advice can be discussed with the traveler.

*Acknowledgments.* We would like to thank all members of the Pasteur Institute's Vaccination Center for their help in this survey.

# Advisory Services for Travel and Tropical Medicine

A. Fidler and K.-L. Hitze

As a result of increased business travel between the Vorarlberg and tropical countries advisory services for travel and tropical medicine are being developed. The Vorarlberg, in the western part of Austria, has a population of more than 350 000. It is next to Vienna, the most industrialized part of Austria, and 60% of its production is exported. This represents more than 2.5 billion US $ worth of products, primarily textiles and machinery. This high level of industrialization and exports results in many foreign contacts and business trips, and the sending of personnel abroad. In addition, there is more travel to tropical countries for tourism, trekking, expeditions and adventure including the so-called sex tourism. The most popular destinations include Southeast Asia, East Africa and tropical South America. Travelers to such destinations need medical advice for prevention and follow-up care. Travel to distant places may evoke the feeling that certain things are permissible, including sexual contacts, which are not part of usual behavior or life at home. Thus, travel may lead to a sense of liberation from usual cares and responsibilities and may lead to the so-called "cruise romance syndrome." It is especially important that travelers are aware of the basic aspects of transmission of AIDS and that they realize that precautions that should also be taken at home are especially important abroad. If one decides to have sex with an unknown person or casual aquaintance, it is essential to use a condom properly, i.e., each time and from start to finish because appearance cannot indicate whether someone is infected. Therefore, a suitable supply of condoms needs to be carried. AIDS infection may also be acquired by blood transfusion if the blood is not screened for HIV, or by the use of contaminated needles, syringes or other instruments that perforate the skin.

It is essential to reduce the risk of needing a blood transfusion during travel. Seat belts should be worn when driving, and caution and care should prevail: drinking and driving is to be avoided. It is advisable to learn how to say "slow down" or "stop" in the local language. If a blood transfusion is unavoidable, only screened blood should be used. Injections should be avoided unless absolutely necessary. It should then be ensured that syringe and needle are new and come directly from an unopened sterile package. This may be difficult and, it is therefore strongly advisable to carry a small supply of sterile disposable syringes and needles. These can be readily obtained from a pharmacy before departure.

The general practitioner may find little information regarding travel and tropical medicine. Only recently has this subject received attention by universities in Austria. The opportunities for education and training for the general practitioner in this important area have been limited. Two years ago, a post-graduate study progamme of tropical medicine was established between the Universities of Innsbruck, Austria, and Bangkok, Thailand. This effort will increase the knowledge of physicians in training; however, it does not help the practicing physician who is consulted by a traveler for advice.

The role of advisory services for travel and tropical medicine will to educate these physicians and to increase the understanding of the population regarding medical and social problems in developing countries. Another goal is to provide medical information to organizations. The advisory services part of the Association for Preventive and Social Medicine (AKS) comprises 250 practicing physicians.

The urgent need for advisory services is illustrated by three cases, in which lack of information for the traveler resulted in illness, and insufficient knowledge of tropical medicine by the physician resulted in dangerous delays of optimal therapy. A 40-year-old electric company employee was sent to Saudi Arabia without proper prior medical advice. After several months he returned to the Vorarlberg because of refractory bloody diarrhea, which subsequently ceased. He then developed acute upper abdominal symptoms and was hospitalized with a presumed diagnosis of acute cholecystitis. Despite the history of possible exposure to infectious disease, further diagnostic tests were not performed. After clinical deterioration, the patient was transferred to the regional medical center. The attending physician was trained in tropical medicine and diagnosed extraintestinal amebiasis, demonstrating five amebic liver abscesses sonographically. Appropriate therapy was initiated.

The second case was a 2-year-old child of Austrian parents who was admitted with the diagnosis of malaria a few days after returning from Nigeria. Quinine for intravenous administration was not available in the Vorarlberg be and had to be obtained from a neighboring country resulting in loss of time. The physicians were unaware that an equally effective drug would have been readily available by using the antiarrhythmic agent quinidine.

A third case involved a traveler to Borneo, who, due to incorrect advice, took chloroquine for prophylaxis. He aquired falciparum malaria and after return to Austria he was hospitalized with cerebral malaria. In this case, there was uncertainty as to therapy and difficulties to obtain the appropriate antimalarial drug.

Such problems are common in Austria, due to the unavailability of certain antiparasitic drugs, such as quinine, dehydroemetine and praziquantel. In emergencies much time is unnecessarily lost as these drugs have to be obtained from obroad.

The advisory services for travel and troical medicine are organized by specialists in tropical medicine and hygiene who collect, sort and distribute information to the consumers. Because there is no medical school in the Vorarlberg, collaboration with the institutes in Vienna (Austria), Hamburg (Germany), and Basel or Zurich in Switzerland is established. One project is a health advice brochure for travelers. A small edition is printed for each travel destination. Because the production is computerized new information can easily be added or introduced.

# “Health Passports”: Changes and Trends

T. Strasser

Vaccination certificates are the prototype of international travel-related personal health documents. The International Sanitary Convention proposed such a document, the International Certificate of Vaccination against Smallpox, in 1944 [1]. This was extensively amended by the World Health Organization and subsequently developed into a more comprehensive vaccination “passport”, including, among others, vaccination against cholera, typhoid and yellow fever. After WHO’s historic declaration on 8 May 1980 of the eradication of smallpox [2], the smallpox page in the booklet was replaced by the statement that such vaccination is no longer required, and in fact could be harmful. Yellow fever vaccination is now the only one required in international travel, and only to selected countries [3]; nevertheless, space is also provided for certifying cholera and other vaccinations, and WHO’s “yellow booklet” is likely to remain part of international travelers’ personal documents for many years to come.

Mass tourism is a characteristic of modern times. Masses of pets, mainly dogs and cats, became man’s fellow travelers during the late twentieth century travel boom. In consquence, “health passports” for dogs and cats were developed, certifying vaccination against rabies and distemper, and hepatitis and leptospirosis (for dogs) as well as infectious enteritis (panleukopenia) (for cats).

In the travel boom, persons with health problems no longer refrain from long-distance journeys. For individuals with chronic conditions who fly repeatedly, member companies of the International Air Transport Association (IATA) have developed the Frequent Traveler’s Medical Card (FREMEC), containing a description of the passenger’s incapacitation; the aim is to facilitate the travel arrangements and to preserve both the passengers and the companies from taking excessive risks.

Patients suffering from chronic diseases such as coronary heart disease or diabetes mellitus are at high risk of developing acute complications. Although this risk is not necessarily higher when traveling, emergency treatment given in the absence of the physician familiar with the patient may be inappropriate, unless information on the underlying disease is readily available. Emergency health cards have been developed therefore for patients with specific diseases, such as the “Cardiocard” for heart patients (recommended by WHO and issued by International Green Cross), or that for diabetic patients (e.g. by the Swiss Association against Diabetes).

In case of traumatisms, such as traffic accidents, information on the blood group of the victim may be vital; in some countries the identity card issued by the police authorities specifies the individual's blood-group.

An individual may be exposed to accidents *and* suffer from several chronic diseases. In addition to single disease cards, comprehensive "health passports" were developed therefore in the 1970s. More recently, such a comprehensive emergency health card (health passport) has been adopted by the European Communities in May 1986 [4]. This 12-page booklet is valied in all members countries of the European Communities; it is multilingual (written in nine languages) and, therefore, somewhat heavy.

Some personal health documents contain information on chronic diseases risk factors. These may help both patient and physician in managing a condition, such as hypertension or diabetes. In some places, for example in Japan, even comprehensive health records are handed out to patients and healthy people, such as, in Akabana town, a 60-page pocket book. Only one further step leads to the use of such documents for didactic purposes, as done by the American Health Foundation with its "Health Passport", serving exclusively health educational purposes.

The classical passport-type booklet is increasingly being replaced by wallet cards. Some are even sensing business in the production of such cards: in Switzerland, for example, mail-box publicity offers for 25 Swiss francs such a card testifying, among other items, that its carrier does not carry the AIDS virus. On the more serious side, high technology is pervading the field with supersonic speed. Microfiche cards, magnetic stripe cards and microchip cards developed in recent years contain increasing amounts of information, some of them of astonishing detail, and the last hit, the Opitcal Memory Card (LaserCard), holds up to 800 pages of data, retrievable at a computer terminal [5]. Such an "omnicard" may be of value in a specially equipped hospital, but is flimsy and futile on the highway, in a plane or in the midst of a safari.

Medical or health passports or cards have thus come a long way during the past 40 years. However, do they present any problems?

The field is becoming increasingly complicated, evolving seemingly without coordination [5]. There is definitely a need for a thorough review and cataloging of the numerous varieties of personal health documents. They also need to be evaluated in the field for practicality and impact on medical or health care. In a subsequent stage, these potentially useful instruments, of particular importance in travel medicine, should be optimized for design and techniques with respect to their given purpose. A forum, concerned with this task and willing to undertake it, still has to be identified.

## References

1. World Health Organization (1951) International sanitary regulations (WHO Regulations no 2). WHO Tech Rep Ser 41
2. Fenner F, Henderson DA, Arita I, Jezek Z, Ladnyi ID (1988) Smallpox and its eradication. World Health Organization, Geneva

3. World Health Organization (1988) Vaccination certificate requirements and health advice for international travel. Situation as on 1 January 1988. World Health Organization, Geneva
4. European Communities (1986) Resolution of the Council and representatives of the Fovernments of the Member States, meeting within the Council, of 29 May 1986 concerning the adoption of a European emergency health card. Official Journal of the European Communities C184:4–15
5. McGuire R (1987) Optical memory cards – the emergency answer? Med Tribune 28:3,18–19

# Computerized Registration and Administration of a Vaccination Outpatient Department

H. J. van der Kaay, L. de Klerk, J. W. M. van der Meer, and D. Overbosch

## Introduction

In 1981 the vaccination outpatient department (OPD) of the Leiden University Hospital initiated computerized registration and administration. The main objectives for computerization were improvement of the quality of the standardized and objective advice on the required and internationally obligatory vaccinations in addition to prophylaxis for malaria and other diseases. The vaccination OPD is run by the Institute of Tropical Medicine together with the Department of Infectious Diseases of the University Hospital.

The computerized system has been developed in Leiden University Hospital and is part of a still-expanding integrated Hospital Information System (HIS), which has been in development since 1972 and in use by 30 hospitals in the Netherlands (Bakker 1984). The system is an on-line terminal system and is used for, but not limited to, approximately 3000 annual consultations to the vaccination OPD. All registration items are coded by the user of the system and provide for appointment and financial administration. Because of the computerized registration, it is very easy to obtain information on the number of visits, the number of travelers to a certain destination, and the amount of vaccine used, all on a monthly, quarterly or annual basis.

## Recording of Health Status of Clients

The medical officer on duty starts his OPD by activating the programme by typing the name of the programme TROVAC. The developed programme flow is shown in Fig. 1. After giving the traveler's identification, i.e. either the registration number and date of birth; or the date of birth, full name and sex, the visual display unit (VDU) presents the first page of the programme showing questions on the health status of the traveler and subjects that may be of importance for the advice to be given.

## Registration of Vaccination and Prophylaxis Plan

After the registration of the health status has been completed, the physician turns to the second page on the VDU, which deals with the vaccination status. This page shows the number of visits, date of consultation, destination, doses of vaccination and drugs advised for malaria prophylaxis.

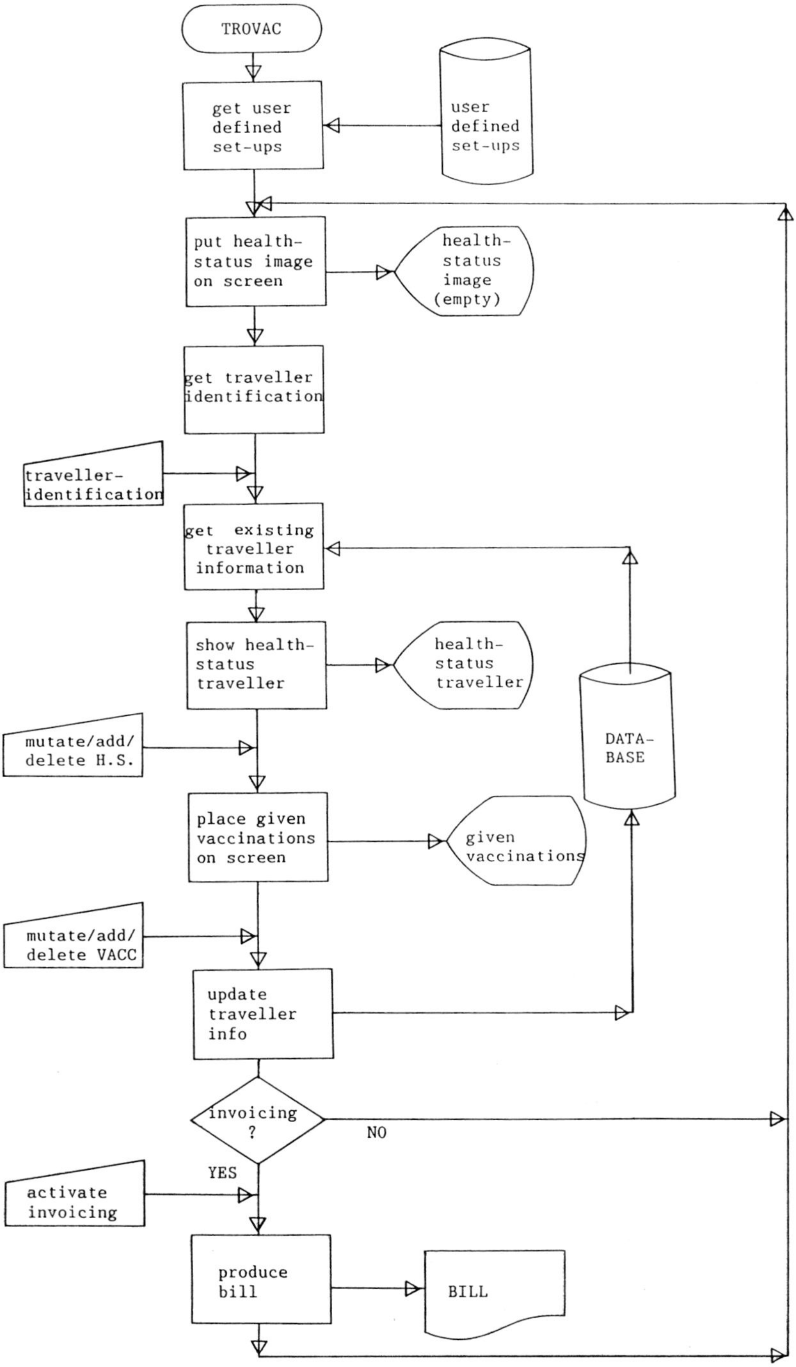


**Fig. 1.** Vaccination record programme flowchart

## Execution of Vaccination Programme and Administrative Settlement

When all advice as well as the subsequent appointments have been registered, the results are passed for a printout in the vaccination room. The nurse in her vaccination room receives a printout of the vaccination plan and bill in triplicate: one for the client, the second for the administration of the OPD and the third for financial and administrative purposes.

## Reference

1. Bakker AR (1984) The development of an integrated and co-operative hospital information system. Med Inf (Land) 9:135–142

# Computerized-Assisted Travel Information System (CATIS)

D. Lawee and F. P. Scappatura

The Computerized-Assisted Travel Information System is designed to provide comprehensive information regarding travel risks, required immunization and pre-travel advice.

The system supports expert problem-solving capability presently only available in specialized travel clinics. An interviewer reads questions to the traveler from a computer screen and types "yes" or "no" responses from the traveler; these are entered into the computer terminal. The system gathers, stores, and analyses the responses. Additional information is requested only if the responses suggest a "developing suspicion of greater risk". The system would then direct the interviewer to obtain additional focused responses so as to "rule in" or "rule out" the "risk". Based on a combination of predefined hierarchical criteria and a heuristic problem-solving approach algorithms are developed in our travel clinic. System decisions are constantly evaluated by the clinic personnel and in the light of newer information.

The basic information required to produce a personalized printout can also be prepared by completing a self-administered questionnaire and mailed to the travel clinic for processing and forwarding by mail. The customized printout could be duplicated and kept in the medical file or be given to the traveler for future reference.

The printout generated by the system has the following features:

1. The pre-travel recommendation takes into account age, geographical, occupational risks, length of stay and health status of the traveler (pregnancy, immune suppression, chronic obstructive pulmonary disease, diabetes). Other protocols are being developed to include high-altitude travel and isolated travel.
2. The prescription of malaria prophylaxis, which includes calculation of the dosage, the number of tablets required and a schedule of administration. The system gives the interviewer a number of drug options, the choice of which depends on local availability or preference.
3. A summary of chronic and acute geographical risks (e.g. malaria, yellow fever, hepatitis, rabies, meningococcal, dengue).

The system is designed to function as a stand-alone expert system. The inexpensive hardware (IBM PC with hard disk drive) eliminates the need for long-distance communication with specialized information sources.

The customized printout could be duplicated and kept in the medical file or be given to the traveler for future reference. Since the printout contains all the relevant travel advice, it frees the health worker to interact creatively with the traveler.

# Development of a Computerized Expert System for Itinerary – Specific Recommendations for Immunizations and Chemoprophylaxis

W. P. McKinney and G. P. Barnas

The widespread availability of microcomputer systems has made it possible to maintain current information on health risks and immunization requirements throughout the world. We have designed a rapidly updatable software system capable of analyzing specific itineraries to determine the requirement or recommendation for cholera and yellow fever vaccines, risks of exposure to chloroquine-sensitive and -resistant strains of malaria, countries with special immunization considerations, and specific reminders for otherwise routine immunizations. This system allows physicians, who are infrequently able to give accurate information on malaria prophylaxis and recommended vaccinations for travelers [1], and nonphysician health care providers to respond rapidly, after minimal training, to inquiries and determine optimal strategies for maintaining health of citizens while abroad.

## Methods

The software system Travax (contraction of travelers' vaccinations) is a microcomputer-based software package which utilizes an expert system approach of integrating a set of specific rules for determination of need for immunizations with a comprehensive data base of country information. Written in the BASIC computer language, it is designed to run on IBM or IBM-compatible microcomputers with a minimum of 128K memory. Two data bases are utilized in the analysis of requirements for cholera and yellow fever vaccines: (1) the list of vaccine entry requirement codes reported to the World Health Organization (WHO) and (2) the list of currently infected countries as reported in the biweekly *Summary of Health Information for International Travel* [2]. For nations requiring yellow fever vaccine for persons transiting countries in the so-called endemic zones or any other specified grouping, these lists are used instead. Country vaccine requirements are coded as follows: I, required for all entrants; II, required only for travelers arriving from currently infected areas of countries, as reported by WHO; III, required for travelers arriving from a country any part of which is infected.

The program is accessed by entering a list of all countries to be visited in the correct sequence of entry (the itinerary). Entries are compared with a built-in atlas of 210 country names to insure proper nomenclature. The logic module is constructed such that all countries transited prior to entry of a given country are considered in light of that country's requirement. This cycle is repeated for each nation on the itinerary and, if no requirement is determined, "not necessary" is the generated response. If any of the countries visited has an infected area, but vaccination is not required, an "optional" response is generated in the case of cholera or "recommended" in the case of yellow fever. In these cases, the specific area of travel within the country must be carefully reviewed with the traveler before a definitive recommendation can be given.

Next, a printout is given of all listed countries having a reported risk of malaria infection, specifying the provinces, districts or regions of the country posing a risk for transmission together with a statement of whether or not chloroquine-reistant strains of *P. falciparum* occur there. This list is generated from *Health Information for International Travel* [3].

The next level of information contains supplementary data on cholera and yellow fever vaccines, if applicable, followed by all nonstandard vaccine considerations for countries to be visited. These include meningococcal vaccination for travel to Nepal or New Delhi, India and Japanese encephalitis vaccine for travel to endemic areas of Asia. Finally, a prompt is given to review the routine immunizations usually given in childhood: tetanus/diphtheria toxoid; poliomyelitis vaccine; and measles/mumps/rubella vaccines. The statement also prompts a review of the need for typhoid vaccine or immune globulin,

**Table 1.** Sample of a Travax printout for a four-country itinerary[a]

| Country | Cholera | | Yellow fever | |
|---|---|---|---|---|
| | Infected | Requirement | Infected | Requirement |
| Nigeria | Yes | None | Yes | II |
| Ghana | Yes | None | Yes | I |
| Lesotho | No | II | No | II |
| Nepal | No | None | No | II |
| Immunization is: | Required | | Required | |

Malaria risk information

| Country | Resistant strains | Areas of risk within country |
|---|---|---|
| Nigeria | Yes | All |
| Ghana | Yes | All |
| Nepal | Yes | Rural areas in Terai District and Hill districts below 1200 m (Dhanukha, Mahotari, Sarlahi, Rautahat, Bara, Parsa, Rupendehi, Kapilvastu). No risk in Katmandu |

Additional recommendations

Nepal – Meningococcal vaccine is also recommended, especially for trekkers
Nepal – Consider need for Japanese encephalitis vaccine

[a] Reminder of routine immunizations not shown

based on details of the visit such as type of accommodation, contact with the indigenous population, or other similar risk factors. This microcomputer system may be readily updated as often as required when changes in country vaccination requirements, changes of infected status for cholera or yellow fever, or bulletins on disease outbreaks occur.

## Results

An example of a printout based on a specific itinerary can be found in Table 1.

## Discussion

The Travax system was designed to relieve health care providers of the burden of time estimated at from 10 to 20 min [4] required to research current publications and coordinate information about multiple countries in order to obtain the necessary data to formulate recommendations. Considering that some 5 million trips are made annually from the United States alone to tropical countries [5], appreciable time savings may be realized. Use of Travax, however, is no substitute for an informed health care provider with a sufficient knowledge base about emporiatric medicine, but can provide the essential framework for an expanded discussion on the full spectrum of health promotion for the international traveler.

## References

1. Raeber PA, Scheidegger C, Vodoz A et al. (1982) Enquete sur les recommendations prodiguées aux voyageurs en zone tropicale. Med Soc Prev 27:266–267
2. Centers for Disease Control (1988) Summary of health information for international travel. United States Department of Health and Human Services, Atlanta
3. Centers for Disease Control (1987) Health information for international travel. United States Government Printing Office, Washington
4. Dardick KR (1985) A computer program for international travel advice. J Fam Pract 20:85–87
5. Cahill KM, Gorbach SL, Mitler MM, Salata RA (1987) Preparing patients for travel. Patient Care 21:217–241

# A Computerized Data Base of Travel Information for Doctors Advising the General Public on Immunization and Malaria Precautions

E. Walker, R. Dewar, and D. Reid

The long-standing involvement of the Communicable Diseases (Scotland) Unit, Ruchill Hospital, Glasgow, with the providing of advice to travellers on avoiding infections while abroad has been developed into an "on-line" data base which can be accessed by interested medical parties. This development has been made possible by the amalgamation of the resources of the CD(S)U with the facilities of the Scottish Poisons Bureau and its established connections to hospitals and health centres.

The advice is directed mainly at the short-term holidaymaker or business traveller. It is recognized that the longer-term overseas worker, especially if children are involved, usually needs personal counselling in addition to factual advice about the availability of different vaccines and tablets used for malaria prophylaxis.

With this proviso, advice is offered country-by-country on recommended vaccinations and those which might need to be considered. If there is a malaria risk this is tated with an assessment of the degree of risk and precautions necessary.

The sources of advice for continuous updating include the World Health Organization, the annual publication for travellers produced by the British Department of Health and Social Security, embassies and informed persons or publications.

The Communicable Diseases (Scotland) Unit provides a surveillance service for Scotland of infections and infection-related problems and acts as a resource centre for advice on management and prevention with a two-way flow of infection being actively encouraged. The advisory service for travellers is a part of this overall function.

# Traveler Service of the Italian Society of Tropical Medicine: Analysis of Its Impact After 1 Year

E. Missoni, G. Bertolaso, M. di Gennaro, F. Vichi, C. Djeddah, and R. Guerra

## Introduction

In the next paper the characteristics and activities of the Traveler Service of the Italian Society for Tropical Medicine (SIMET) are described. Here, results and possible impact are analysed in more detail.

## Analysis

As expected, the trend of the Traveler Service's activities corresponded to the period of most intensive touristic flow to the tropics (Fig. 1) (December–January; July–September). The Centre was consulted by 780 people between February 1987 and March 1988; 70% knew about it through the information contained in the ALITALIA timetable, published March 1987. The remaining 30% became aware of our service through former users. The travelers consult-

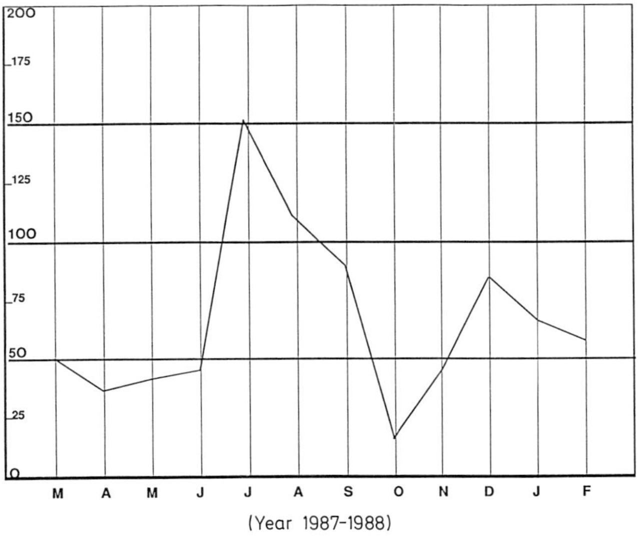


**Fig. 1.** Number of enquiries by month. The increase of enquires before and during summertime and Christmas time is clearly shown

ing SIMET's service were further analysed by category, age, sex, reason of travel and average period of stay.

Out of 780 consulting travelers (family members traveling together are not included), 38% were non-professionals, 27% were non-medical professionals, 20% were doctors and 15% were tourist operators.

The age structure of our traveler's population (including family members traveling together) was as follows: 5% were children under 5 years of age, 10% were aged 5–19, 23% were aged 20–29, 47% were aged 30–59 and 15% were over 60 years of age.

Sixty-four percent of travelers were males and 36% females.

Sixty percent of people seeking advice from our centre were traveling for business and only 40% declared that they were on a tourist trip.

Fifteen percent of the travelers went abroad for less than 1 week; 54% left for periods between 8 and 21 days; 27% left for periods between 22 and 50 days; finally, 4% prolonged their stay for more than 60 days.

In order to evaluate the usefulness of the service, 70 randomly chosen travelers were interviewed. Of these, 84% declared themselves very satisfied with the advice obtained; 13% were satisfied, and 3% were only moderately satisfied because:

- They had not received the information booklet.
- They became ill during the trip, or the information they received was in contrast with that given by other institutions, or by their doctors.

No one considered himself not satisfied.

Among the illnesses acquired abroad and considered as serious by the interviewed traveler we found in one case a scorpion bite and in two cases, amoebic and shigella dysentery.

## Future Perspectives

Future aims must be to increase awareness of preventive measures against tropical diseases and promote the SIMET's Traveler Service as a national centre of reference which will allow Italian health institutions to disseminate correct and non contradictory information regarding preventive measures to be taken while visiting tropical countries.

# Traveler Service of the Italian Society of Tropical Medicine: Activities, Methodology and Results

F. Vichi, E. Missoni, G. Bertolaso, M. di Gennaro, C. Djeddah, and R. Guerra

The Traveler Service is part of a more comprehensive programme of the Italian Society of Tropical Medicine (SIMET). All the services including the Traveler Service are public and free of charge.

What is SIMET? The Italian Society of Tropical Medicine (SIMET), a non-profit-making organization, is a scientific society founded in 1983 under the patronage of the Ministry of Foreign Affairs (more precisely the *Direzione Generale per la Cooperazione allo Sviluppo*) to promote on a national level a better knowledge and more information about social problems and public health in developing countries.

The Italian Society of Tropical Medicine runs a Documentation Centre where scientific, informative and educative materials, such as journals, books, scientific papers, slides, films and others, are made available to the public, and an information service for doctors, general practitioners or specialists in other disciplines, regarding prophylaxis and health precautions for patients traveling to the tropics. Congresses, round tables, symposiums, and conferences on specific subjects are organized as frequently as possible to promote knowledge of tropical medicine in development cooperation on a wide basis. A journal, *La Medicina Tropicale nella Cooperazione allo Sviluppo*, dealing with topics related to technical cooperation and tropical medicine is edited and regularly sent to members of the society.

The objective of the Traveler Service is to inform and advise people traveling to tropical countries, as well as health offices, travel agencies, medical doctors, and others about the risks to which one may be exposed in the tropics, the prophylactic measures to be followed and the institutions which provide provide specialized medical care in Italy.

The Traveler Service has three activities: data collection, organization and dissemination of the information.

Data collection is carried out by the Documentation Centre of SIMET, which regularly receives up-to-date scientific information on tropical diseases (WHO publications, scientific journals, news letters, news bulletins, etc.). In addition, health experts of the Italian Ministry of Foreign Affairs, General Direction of Cooperation Development, and physicians of non-governmental organizations provide the latest information about health problems in the areas where they are on duty. After data are collected, the information is selected, specifically systemized, organized and made available upon request.

Information is given through different channels:

- Personal advice. A medical doctor specialized in tropical medicine is available 8 h/day to answer specific questions. People make enquires at our service by phone, letter, or personally.
- A booklet "Health advice for travelers to developing countries" is edited annually and is sent to all those who request it at our office.
- The national airline (Alitalia): essential information is included in the national timetable.

Similarly information will be included on the on board "magazine" (*Ulisse 2000*) and possibly an on board video film will be produced.

- Mass media.

Between 18 February 1987 and 11 March 1988, 780 people made enquires: 265 by phone, 310 by personally visiting SIMET and 205 by letter. With regard to destination, of these 780, 395 were going to Africa, 121 to Asia, 124 to South America, 7 to the Caribbean, 11 to the Middle East, 105 to the Far East, 8 to Polynesia and 6 to Malta.

# Practical Aids in Disease Prevention and Post-Travel Diagnoses: "The Global Disease Guide", "The Pocket Doc", and "The Diagnostic Digest"

M. E. Gordon

Unlike other standard references, the "Global Disease Guide" has been created as a desk-top, record-sized informational disk that permits instant fingertip dialing of diseases prevalent in each of 170 countries. Color codes direct the physician to the prevalence of viruses, helminths, protozoa, bacteria and rickettsia. Hazardous arboviruses are code classified and readily distinguishable, e.g., lassa fever in Sierra Leone, Japanese encephalitis in mainland China, Rift Valley fever in the Sudan or schistomiasis japonicum in Indonesia and toxoplasmosis in France. Thus the clinician is further alerted to the subtleties of various travel-related diseases. Guidelines for prevention are also itemized on side two of this physician's desk reference.

The "Pocket Doc" is a practical sliderule device designed for the pocket of the millions of travelers who, once alerted to the potential health hazards inherent in their destinations, would be able to carry out preventative measures both conjointly with their physician and, when needed, by themselves. Pre-travel planning and packing information, flight notes, land and sea precautions, some food and water hazards and a glossary of world disease clues all guide the traveler during any trip. Together, the "Global Disease Guide," the physician's world scanner and the "Pocket Doc," the traveler's medical guide, may foster better health prevention, earlier diagnosis and treatment of the many puzzling and other ubiquitous emporiatric diseases.

The evaluation of the many signs and symptoms that occur during and subsequent to travel can be assessed by a diagnostic outline displayed with this poster (soon to be made available as a hand-sized "Diagnostic Digest"). It contains laboratory clues such as eosinophilic leukocytosis occurs most commonly with nematode infections; the erythrocyte sedimentation rate often remains normal despite the leukemoid reaction in trichinosis; hypergammaglobinemia is often a hallmark of toxocariasis, kala azar, African trypanosomiasis and viral hepatitis. The leukopenia of brucellosis is readily recognized but its association with hydatidosis may be overlooked. Other illustrated signals aiding emporiatric diagnoses include the pig-pen fetid odor of balantidiasis, the taste aberrations of ciguatera poisoning and dengue, the ascites of anthrax, the salt craving of diphyllbothriasis, the cardiomyopathy seen in Chagas' disease, toxoplasmosis, Lyme disease and trichinosis and many other correlates are displayed. These three educational devices may further aid disease prevention and facilitate the resolution of the frequently deceptive diagnostic problems of the traveler.

# Inadequate Pre-Travel Health Advice – An Answer?

J. H. Cossar

There has been a spectacular growth in the number of travelers worldwide between 1949 and 1986. During this time the numbers of international tourist arrivals have increased 13-fold to 341.5 million [1], the number of passengers carried on scheduled air services have reached 955 million [2] (a 31-fold increase), and the number of United Kingdom residents traveling abroad has risen 15-fold to 25.2 million [3], with the proportion traveling beyond Europe increasing 23-fold (now 3.1 million).

Studies of illness in travelers show attack rates of 30% to over 50%, varying with age, life style, season and country visited [4–6]. Attacks usually comprise a mild diarrhoeal upset, which rarely results in more than a minor self-limiting inconvenience, but more serious illnesses acquired abroad – for example, malaria [7] – continue to be recorded. Surveys were conducted to assess the measures taken by the travel trade to address this problem [8], to enquire into the numbers of holidaymakers seeking pre-travel health advice and the source consulted (the methodology used was identical to other questionnaire studies [9]), with a view to improving the advice available for travelers.

## Findings of Travel Brochure Survey

Examination of a representative sample of 64 travel brochures for 1985 revealed that 33% carried no health information for United Kingdom travelers. Winter travelers and travelers to Europe were likely to have even less guidance (47% and 62% of brochures respectively, without health advice). Fifty-six percent carried "general" and 11% "specific" advice; the latter health advice was inconsistent. Some brochures carried general recommendations on immunizations, dietary caution, and the use of antimalarial tablets; others were both more and less specific for the same destination country. Reciprocal health arrangements with the National Health Service were mentioned occasionally.

## Findings of Questionnaire Survey

Almost 90% of the 726 travelers who returned questionnaires in 1985 completed the enquiry section on pre-travel health advice taken. Only 32% of these respondents had sought advice, of whom 37% reported illness compared with 26% of the rest. This suggests that there is scope for improvement in the quality of advice provided, or that those not seeking advice were more experienced travelers knowledgeable about avoiding illness whilst abroad.

It is of note in this sample that the family doctor was least consulted for advice compared with travel agents or other sources and this has obvious implications in terms of choice of location to provide advice for travelers. It is surprising that the minority who consulted their family doctor for advice reported the highest attack rate, but perhaps this group were the least fit of the travelers and therefore the most at risk of illness.

## A Pre-Travel Health Advice Booklet

Following market research conducted by the University of Strathclyde Business School a pre-travel health advice booklet [10] was designed, produced and test-marketed by the Communicable Diseases (Scotland) Unit (CDSU) in association with the Scottish Health Education Group (SHEG). It is airline ticket sized such that it can be carried in existing ticket wallets, is attractively designed to compete with the existing "glossy" travel trade literature, and has been accepted by representatives of the travel trade in Scotland as being informative without being inhibitory to holiday enjoyment or the commercial interests of the trade. It is a general pre-travel health advice booklet which directs the traveler to sources of expertise on such subjects as immunizations and antimalarial tablets. There are advice sections directed towards pre-travel, whilst in transit, whilst abroad and on return, as well as sections for personal use about health and other subjects, thereby encouraging the traveler to use and carry the booklet.

## Conclusions

In view of the obvious inadequacies and inconsistences in both the quality and presentation of advice to travelers, there seems to be common ground where health educators and the medical profession could collaborate with the travel trade for the benefit of all concerned.

*Acknowledgements.* I would like to thank Dr. D. Reid, Mr. R. D. Dewar, Mr. M. Raymond, Mr. S. Mitchell, SHEG and CDSU secretarial staff, Messrs. Donald Mackenzie (Travel) Ltd., and the travelers who gave their time to complete the questionnaire.

## References

1. World Tourism Organisation (1987) Tourism compendium. World total, Madrid
2. International Civil Aviation Organisation (1987) Development of world scheduled revenue traffic 1945–1986. Statistics. ICAO, Montreal
3. Business Statistics Office (1986) Business monitor annual statistics. Overseas travel and tourism. HMSO, London, p 13 (MQ 6, Table 8A)
4. Steffen R, van der Linde F, Syr K, Schär M (1983) Epidemiology of diarrhoea in travelers. JAMA 249:1176–1180
5. Peltola H, Kyronseppa H, Holsa P (1983) Trips to the south – a health hazard. Scand J Infect Dis 15:375–381

6. Cossar JH, Reid D, Grist NR, Dewar RD, Fallon RJ, Riding MR, Bell EJ (1985) Illness associated with international travel: a ten year review. Travel Med Int 3:1,13–18
7. Phillips-Howard PA, Bradley DJ, Blaze M, Hurn M (1988) Malaria in Britain: 1977–1986. Br Med J 296:245–248
8. Reid D, Cossar JH, Ako TI, Dewar RD (1986) Do travel brochures give adequate advice on avoiding illness? Br Med J 293:1472
9. Cossar JH, Dewar RD, Fallon RJ, Grist NR, Reid D (1982) *Legionella pneumophila* in tourists. Practitioner 226:1543–1548
10. The Scottish Health Education Group (1986) Holiday information and checklist (a guide to good health on holiday for travelers). SHEG, Edinburgh

# Providing Health Advice to Travelers by a Tour Operator

K. Plentz

Public health authorities are historically sources of information regarding vaccination requirements and other health advice to travelers.

In 1977 2207 tourists to five different destinations were interviewed [1]. It was found that 28.9% of those questioned used the services of the public health authorities and only 16.5% those of a family doctor. This same study showed that 60.7% of the tourists were not advised regarding hygiene and preventive measures in, for example, subtropical and tropical areas (Table 1).

With the support of the Touristik Union International (TUI) – the largest tour operator in Europe, with 2.7 million clients per year – the following activities were developed:

**Table 1.** Numbers of tourists receiving advice about hygiene ($n = 1\,735$)

| | Total | Family doctor | Public Health Office | Government Medical Department | Other institutions and doctors |
|---|---|---|---|---|---|
| No reply | 79 | 19 | 24 | 7 | 21 |
| Yes | 611 (35.2%) | 204 (43.6%) | 275 (31.2%) | 34 (36.2%) | 98 (33.6%) |
| No | 1053 (60.7%) | 245 (52.4%) | 582 (66.1%) | 53 (56.4%) | 173 (59.2%) |

## Medical Travel Adviser

In 1978 a 16-page pamphlet was published, which was automatically included in the travel documents given to all tourists to distant destinations. The contents of this pamphlet with the title "Our medical service makes traveling easier with less complications" were based on communications with TUI personnel and on current medical criteria. The pamphlet explains facts and details in simple, everyday language. The introduction explains to the lay reader that carelessness and thoughtlessness can seriously endanger his vacation. The reader is also cautioned that explanations, advice, and comments are there to help him enjoy his vacation in distant countries without the complications of illness and disease, and to return home healthy and fit. The traveler is urged to relate his experiences and criticisms and the travelers have themselves contributed greatly to this pamphlet. The pamphlet has also been issued by the TUI affiliate "Airtours International" and has been organized in the following format:

1. Prevention at home
   a) Required vaccinations: yellow fever – vaccination intervals, vaccination procedures (time periods, validity, etc.)
   b) Recommended vaccinations: typhoid fever, tetanus, poliomyelitis, hepatitis A
   c) Vaccinations for children
   d) Malaria protection: malaria regions, malaria prophylaxis, other important protection measures
   e) Dentists
   f) Medical insurance
   g) Traveler's medical kit
   h) Glasses/contact lenses/hearing aids
2. Behavior during air travel
3. Behavior on vacation: Eating and drinking, clothing, personal hygiene and body care, air conditioning, healthy tanning, traffic, sexually transmitted diseases and AIDS
4. Behavior during sea cruises
5. At home after the journey

About 300000 pamphlets have been printed. Limited editions offer the possibility of a rapid and continual updating. The seventh edition appeared in May 1987. The next one will be published shortly.

If regional or local changes in the epidemic situation warrant, a page is inserted to indicate the preventive measures.

The TUI has approximately 800 employees abroad. Through contacts with medical and health authorites, it has often been possible for TUI to use the internal information system (Central Operations and a regular weekly report system) to acquire information about health problems. For example, epidemics may be reported sooner than through the WHO. The regular weekly reporting system also requires that employees indicate health problems in their areas.

## Catalogues

Catalogues are published by the tour operator in large numbers twice a year. Normally, they contain little or no health information regarding required vaccinations, recommended vaccinations, or preventive measures against malaria. For several years, however, TUI has included tables in their catalogues which clearly indicate the latest prophylactic requirements and measures for particular destinations.

## Special pamphlets for the Traveler

The TUI has published special pamphlets for several destinations, known as "The little geography book". These also include short health recommendations and tips. At the destination itself, the tourist receives local information at briefings upon arrival, as well as a specific pamphlet, which include the latest updates regarding health problems, including, for example, potable water; the possibility of infections resulting from the consumption of ice cream, fruits and vegetables; clothing; bathing; and protection from the sun.

## Training of Travel Agents and Their Employees

The TUI has over 2600 travel agencies selling its product. Several hundred employees of these travel agencies are invited each year to participate in 3-day seminars. Besides presentation of the new programs and schooling in sales techniques, these seminars usually include the theme "Health and Traveling". The travel agents and their employees are trained so that they can inform the customer regarding health and medical facts in a positive light. New employees of the TUI guide and representative department are trained in seminars which now include all aspects of dealing with healthy and sick tourists. These aspects include health and medical information, including medical crisis management.

## Touristik Union International Magazine "The Journey" (*Die Reise*)

Since 1979, TUI publishes its own newspaper four times a year, with a total of 10 000 copies. From the very first issue, there has been a column "Medicine Abroad". This column includes, in layman's language, current or other important subjects of health and medicine. Subjects include protective and preventive measures, medical travel kits, malaria, and AIDS. It is distributed to all employees worldwide, and to all TUI travel agencies.

The most important commodity on vacation is good health. This outline demonstrates how a tour operator has, step by step, over the years adapted to the preventive and protective health needs of the traveler.

## Reference

1. Plentz K (1978) Impfschutz im Ferntourismus als Problem des öffentlichen Gesundheitsdienstes. Off Gesundheitswes 40:497–506

# Epidemiology of Travel to the Developing World from Connecticut, USA

D. R. Hill

International travel has become a major pursuit of modern Americans, with visits to the developing world frequently included on their itineraries. It is estimated that more than 8 million Americans travel to the developing world each year for business, vacation, study or missionary activities. There is little epidemiologic information, however, about these persons.

The goal of this study was to obtain information on a broad spectrum of travelers. This basic information is important as strategies are developed for preventive medicine for the traveler to the developing world.

## Methods

All patients visiting the International Travelers Medical Service at the University of Connecticut Health Center were interviewed as part of their pre-travel medical care, prior to receiving immunizations or preventive advice. Patients were asked about basic demographic data, their itinerary, reason for travel, and if they had any concomitant medical problems. The information was entered into a data base (File Maker Plus, Nashoba Systems, Inc., Concord, Mass.) and then analyzed. In general, these individuals represent travelers to the developing world and are exclusive of travelers to North America, the Caribbean, Europe, Japan, Australia and New Zealand.

The International Travelers Medical Service draws patients primarily from Hartford County, Connecticut. This county of approximately 1 million people includes both the city of Hartford and many surrounding towns. Within this area there is a large corporate and university community.

## Results

From 1 January 1984 to 29 February 1988, 1238 travelers were seen. Their mean age was 43.3 years, with 3.7% of persons 12 years old and younger and 4.5% greater than 70 years old. Fifty-four percent were female. A chronic medical condition, most often hypertension, diabetes, acid peptic disease and arthritis was present in 29.8%. Sulfonamide intolerance was reported by 3.6%.

Seventy percent of travelers were going for vacations, which included African safaris, mountain treks, sightseeing, cruises and visits to family members in foreign countries. Fourteen percent were going for business, 12% for teach-

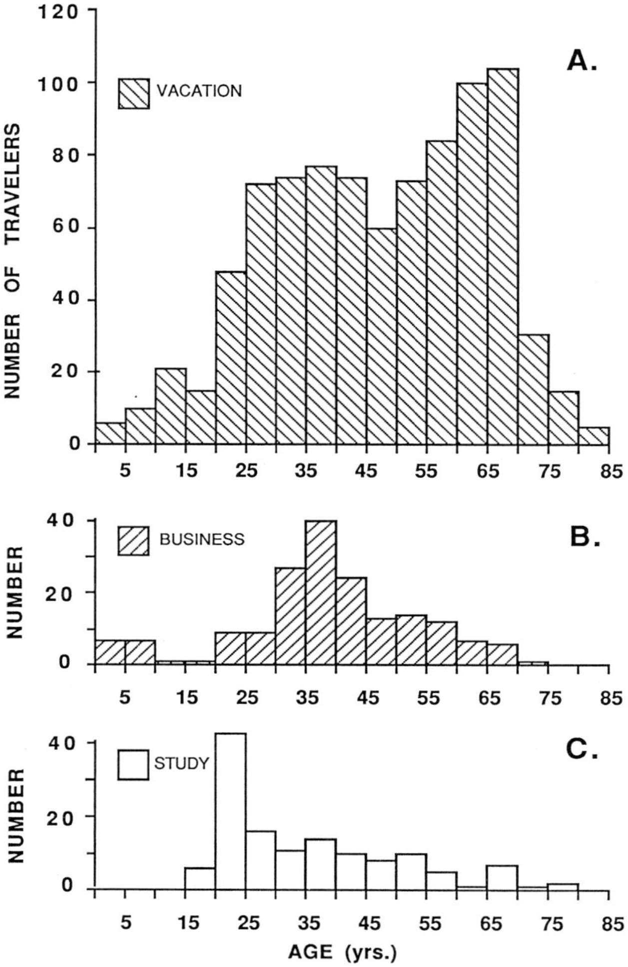


**Fig. 1.** Age of travelers to the developing world for those who are going for vacations (**A**) (mean age 46.5 years, $n=870$), for business (**B**) (mean age 38.5 years, $n=178$), and for teaching or study (**C**) (mean age 34.8 years, $n=134$). Those business travelers who were <20 years old were dependants. The mean age for persons traveling for all reasons was 43.3 years

ing or study, and 4% for missionary activities. The median duration of travel was 21 days; 5% traveled for longer than 1 year.

The most frequently visited countries are listed in Table 1. Countries in East Africa, the Indian subcontinent, the Far East and South America were most popular.

Business travelers (excluding dependants <20 years of age) were more often male (68.9% vs. 41.4%) and younger (41.9 vs. 46.5 years, $P=0.001$) than

**Table 1.** Most frequently visited countries[a]

| Name of country | % of travelers |
|---|---|
| Kenya | 26.4 |
| India | 19.3 |
| Nepal | 11.4 |
| Thailand | 9.1 |
| Tanzania | 8.9 |
| Peru | 8.5 |
| Hong Kong | 8.4 |
| Peoples' Republic of China | 7.1 |
| Singapore | 6.1 |
| Brazil | 4.8 |

[a] Travel to these ten countries (7.9% of the 126 countries visited) represented 54% of all travel

those traveling for vacations. The age profile for vacationers, business travelers, and those going for teaching or study is illustrated in Fig. 1.

Business travelers tended to be seen evenly throughout the year, whereas vacationers were seen most frequently during the months of May, and September through January. For the years 1985–1987, $28 \pm 4$ vacation travelers were seen during each of these months compared with $13 \pm 2$ per month during the rest of the year ($P = 0.001$). Many of the months with an increased number of vacation travelers were associated with visits by persons going to Kenya. The median interval between the clinic visit and travel was 29 days, with 11% of travelers seen 1 week or less before departure.

## Discussion

This prospective study demonstrates that there is a wide range in age of American travelers, most of whom travel to the developing world for vacations. Many of these persons have associated medical problems. For the majority of travelers their trip is of short duration (<1 month) and is concentrated in a small number of geographic areas. The popularity of areas of the world where chloroquine-resistant *Plasmodium falciparum* malaria occurs, especially East Africa, to where 26% of all travelers went, emphasizes the importance of pre-travel advice in malaria prevention.

Most studies of American travelers describe small groups or are retrospective. Further prospective study of travelers will allow the physician and travel medical services to target the areas of emphasis in the prevention of illness in travelers.

# Round Table Discussion

# Providing Health Information for Travelers, in Search of an Optimal Solution

B. Federspiel

With the change of the travel pattern after the Second World War charter travel has developed at a pace which was not considered possible from the start. Not only business people travel, ordinary consumers travel and the urge has come to travel still further – also to strange, remote places. At the same time consumers are demanding more protection and information when buying goods and services, and this also includes services from doctors and from society in general. As a traveler the consumer also wants to be well informed and well treated.

Information about travel medicine and treatment of travelers is very different in different countries. It is clear from the discussion that information is neither at the same level nor distributed in the same way. The various representatives on the panel, speaking from the experience of travel agencies, holiday resorts and professional distributors of travel information, all explained how they advised travelers orally, in writing, etc. There was some disagreement as to what kind of information was most important: vaccinations or general advice about food hygiene, proper clothing, etc. Canadian research had shown that the majority of travelers were quite knowledgeable in the latter field.

It followed from the discussion both between participants in the panel and from the audience that there was a world of difference between the various ways of getting information about health advice, vaccinations and other precautions which you got from various travel agencies, air transport companies, package-tour companies, and professional medical travel information based on data bases in close connection with health authorities. It was also explained that ordinary health authorities sometimes got information very late, and it was at times difficult to obtain reliable information from the respective countries, who were not necessarily interested in giving too precise information which might hamper the tourist interest of the country. Pilots and other flight personnel were mentioned as information sources together with local newspapers, etc. Larger tour operators represented were making a substantial effort to provide reliable and up-to-date information for travelers, but these individual examples did not cover more than the companies themselves, and doubt was therefore expressed as to which information consumers in general would expect to get, no matter which travel agency or authority he approached.

Hope was expressed that new technology and use of data bases in future would provide more secure, immediate and up-to-date information which could also be controlled by outside authorities and used not only by travel professionals, but also by general practitioners, who in most cases would not be expected to be up to date about the newest information on vaccinations in remote countries. Much could probably be learnt from the professional travel information, magazines and booklets, which would normally include not only information about required vaccinations, but also good advice based on information from all kinds of sources. The good examples, however, do not solve the global problem that consumers have. It is not any help for a traveler from one country that travelers from another country are well informed, if he is not.

Severe doubt was raised about a system where companies and many different people including doctors are giving often insufficient, sometimes even wrong, information due to lack of centralized, reliable and speedy information. The general attitude was that official information, for instance from WHO, came too late and was not sufficiently extensive.

There was a general demand for improvement and for reliable, uniform and up-to-date information, which might in future be based on a reliable network in each country combined with a central international data base. There was thus hope that new technology would bring progress also in this area.

# Medical Care Abroad

# Emergency Abroad: What Are the Options?

J. P. McCann

## Summary

An overview of the factors to be considered in the handling of medical emergencies abroad is provided. This includes a discussion of medical and health matters to be considered by the traveler prior to departure from home and options available when an emergency occurs. Separate attention is given to those problems that may be encountered by the short-term holiday or business traveler and those concerned with extended assignments of the expatriate. Emphasis is placed on the accessing of health care systems in selected countries for both emergency and health maintenance needs. Also a review of services available via international health care providers is presented. The latter review includes a presentation of aeromedical evacuation services that are available.

## Introduction

In general, if you are ill postpone the trip until you are well. If you have a medical or physical handicap, build your needs into your overall plans.

The most frequent traveler's destinations seldom present major problems. Enough people, trade and commerce have gone before you to ensure the availability of health care services and medical supplies. Communication systems, including telephone, teletype and facsimile transmissions, are almost global in nature. Language differences, however, can continue to be a problem. English, French and Spanish-speaking people have advantages over most others in this respect. Non-English or French-speaking elderly may find communications in such countries as the United States quite difficult; thus pre-trip planning should include a knowledge of where and how translation assistance can be obtained. Usually friends, relatives, business contacts or home country embassies and consulates are the most frequent sources of assistance. In large cities the better hotels and ethnic civil organizations can also be of great help.

## Planning the Trip

In the planning phase, review the special health problems peculiar to the area to be visited, taking into consideration your own special health care needs. Information can be found from a variety of sources. Travel agents and commercial land, sea and air carriers are good practical places to start. Public libraries usually carry general reference material concerning health and sanitation subjects on a country-to-country basis. World Health Organization publications and material available through one's own state department are usually excellent. Many countries also have schools of public health and tropical medicine or government agencies who provide even more definitive guidelines on local or world health concerns.

An excellent example of the type of material available is the booklet entitled "Medizinischer Reiseratgeber" from Switzerland [1]. In the United States the Center for Disease Control annual publication "Health Information for International Travel" is also of value [2].

Some basics in regard to personal health needs: take along enough required maintenance medication to last until resupply can be established; know what your eyeglasses prescription is and, if corrective lenses are critical to your functioning, take an extra pair; share your travel plans with your physician and dentist so that you can avoid the need for care while abroad to the greatest extent possible. This is the time for an update of required and recommended immunizations. Be sure to match your itinerary with immunization requirements, since they are often difficult to acquire when en route. If travel is taking you into malarial environments, even as a transient, be sure to follow recommended prophylactic measures.

Review the simple, but effective, do's and don'ts regarding the intake of food and drink. If your activities will include potentially hazardous exposure, know them well and the required safety procedures to be observed. These can range from avoiding potential animal and insect bites to knowing in detail the medical concerns of mountain climbers or deep-sea divers. Despite all the preplanning one can do, accidents and illnesses will occur. The ongoing chances of illness and death cannot be expected to take a holiday, even if the trip is for that purpose. Most of the health problems encountered will be a function of your own risk profiles.

Requirements for care when abroad are made up of those basic to your existence plus those peculiar to the plan of travel. Time away from home, itinerary involved and activities to be engaged in are key points to estimating what one's chances are that a medical emergency requiring immediate attention will occur. Taking into consideration the ability to postpone certain types of medical care requirements until one returns home, the need to seek the attention of a physician when away is most likely considerably less than one might expect. As an estimate, fewer than 10% of travelers will require care when away. Despite the relatively low probability of a medical emergency, it is worthwhile to consider just how and where assistance can be obtained should the situation arise. This brings up the question of what services are available during the en route phase of your travel. Since the majority of transit is now by air, remarks are limited to this mode of transport. In the early days of commercial aviation, rather extensive medical kits were commonly carried on board. At one time a number of carriers even required all cabin personnel to be professional nurses. Shortening of in-flight time and the increase in number of alternative landing sites now largely replaces this approach with a concept that relies on first aid and aircraft diversion if the medical emergency is serious.

## Aircraft First Aid Facilities

In general, all the major air carriers provide training in first aid to their air crews. They are also provided in-flilght manuals with instructions on how to handle common medical emergencies. Furthermore, a number of health-care professionals continue to be attracted to flying as a career and bring with them medical expertise as an avocational skill. To augment the above, it is rather typical to ask assistance from fellow travelers who are on board and are physicians or allied medical professionals. In one airline, which carries some 14 million passengers a year, the request for this type of good samaritan assistance occurs approximately once a day somewhere in the carrier's entire route structure. In over 70% of the calls for assistance, a physician is on board and responds. In nearly 100% of such requests there is some category of health care professional on board who is willing to help. As might be expected, the qualifications of these volunteers vary widely. In fact many anecdotal stories relating to the kind of care rendered have become part of aviation folklore. All in all, however, the response on the part of the medical profession is a real tribute to its universality and adherence to the principles of Hypocrites.

There are usually three kinds of medical kits on board. The first is one made up of common over-the-counter preparations. Most often it contains a mild analgesic plus some type of antacid for gastrointestinal upset. It is carried by cabin crew and is available on request. The second type kit contains first aid materials, including simple instructions and bandaging supplies. The third type of kit is one for use by doctors only. The contents of such kits and the flights on which they are carried are highly variable. As a rule of thumb, United States carriers are the least comprehensive in content. In several countries, major carriers may provide a rather extensive array of both medications and instruments. A number of these airlines, however, limit these kits to certain type aircraft and routes, for example, those involving extended overwater flights. At least one carrier has a cardiac defibrillator on board; however, to date its use has not been required. Over and above this variety of kits, special provisions can be made to meet the needs of the handicapped, including stretcher-bound aeromedical evacuation cases.

## The Handicapped passenger

In this regard, the International Air Transport Association (IATA) has developed a guide for standardization of certain aspects of travel that relate to individuals with major medical problems or handicaps [3]. First is the acquisition of medical information pertaining to the incapacitated passenger. The process begins by a call to the airline reservations agent. Although not all airlines will accommodate such passengers, most do. If time permits, airlines will supply a medical information sheet to be completed by the attending physician. This is a standardized "MEDIF" form (Fig. 1 a, b) for documentation of basic demographic data on the traveler and attending physician. Diagnosis, degree of incapacitation and need for special assistance are key in arriving at a decision

| PART 1<br>To be completed by SALES OFFICE/AGENT | M E D I F<br>STANDARD MEDICAL INFORMATION FORM FOR AIR TRAVEL<br>Answer ALL questions - Put a cross (x) in "YES" or "NO" boxes<br>Use BLOCK LETTERS or TYPEWRITER when completing this form |
|---|---|

**A** NAME / INITIALS / TITLE:

**B** PROPOSED ITINERARY (airline(s), flight number(s), class(es), date(s), segments(s), reservation status of continuous air journey) — Transfer from one flight to another often requires LONGER connecting time

**C** NATURE OF INCAPACITATION: — MEDICAL CLEARANCE REQUIRED? No ☐ Yes ☐

**D** IS STRETCHER NEEDED ON BOARD? (all stretcher cases MUST be escorted) No ☐ Yes ☐ — Request rate if unknown

**E** INTENDED ESCORT (Name, sex, age, professional qualification, segments if different from passenger) If untrained, state "TRAVEL COMPANION" — For blind and or deaf, state if escorted by trained dog.

**F** WHEELCHAIR NEEDED? No ☐ Yes ☐
Categories are: WCHR WCHS WCHC
Wheelchair Category ☐

| OWN wheelchair | Collapsible | Power driven? | Battery Type (spillable?) |
|---|---|---|---|
| No ☐ | No ☐ | No ☐ | No ☐ |
| Yes ☐ | Yes ☐ | Yes ☐ | Yes ☐ |

Wheelchairs with spillable batteries are "restricted articles" and are permitted on passenger aircraft only under certain conditions, which can be obtained from the airline(s). In addition, certain countries may impose specific restrictions

**G** AMBULANCE NEEDED? No ☐ Yes ☐
To be arranged by AIRLINE
No ☐ → specify Ambul. Company contact
Yes ☐ → specify destination address
Request rate(s) if unknown

**H** OTHER GROUND ARRANGEMENTS NEEDED No ☐ Yes ☐ — If yes, SPECIFY below and indicate for each item: (a) the ARRANGING airline or other organisation, (b) at whose EXPENSE and (c) CONTACT addresses/phones where appropriate, or whenever specific persons are designated to meet/assist the passenger

1 Arrangements for delivery at air port of DEPARTURE — No ☐ Yes ☐ specify

2 Arrangements for assistance at CONNECTING POINTS — No ☐ Yes ☐ specify

3 Arrangements for meeting at air port of ARRIVAL — No ☐ Yes ☐ specify

4 Other requirements or relevant information — No ☐ Yes ☐ specify

**K** SPECIAL IN-FLIGHT ARRANGEMENTS NEEDED, such as: special meals, special seating, leg-rest, extra seat(s), special equipment, etc. (See "Note *" at the end of PART 2 overleaf) — No ☐ Yes ☐ → If yes, DESCRIBE and indicate for each item: (a) SEGMENT(s) on which required, (b) airline ARRANGED or arranging third party, and (c) at whose expense. Provision of SPECIAL EQUIPMENT such as oxygen etc. always requires completion of PART 2 overleaf.

**L** DOES PASSENGER HOLD A "FREQUENT TRAVELLER'S MEDICAL CARD" VALID FOR THIS TRIP? (FREMEC) — No ☐ Yes ☐ — If yes, add below FREMEC data to your reservation requests. If no (or if additional data needed by carrying airline(s)) have physician in attendance complete PART 2 hereof

FREMEC (FREMEC Number) | (issued by) | (valid until) | (sex) | (age) | (Incapacitation)
(Incapacit. cont.) | (Limitations)

PASSENGER'S DECLARATION

"I HEREBY AUTHORIZE

(name of nominated physician)

to provide the airlines with the information required by those airlines' medical departments for the purpose of determining my fitness for carriage by air and in consideration thereof I hereby relieve that physician of his/her professional duty of confidentiality in respect of such information, and agree to meet such physician's fees in connection therewith.

I take note that, if accepted for carriage, my journey will be subject to the general conditions of carriage/tariffs of the carrier concerned and that the carrier does not assume any special liability exceeding those conditions/tariffs.

I am prepared, at my own risk, to bear any consequences which carriage by air may have for my state of health and I release the carrier, its employees, servants and agents from any liability for such consequences.

I agree to reimburse the carrier upon demand for any special expenditures or costs in connection with my carriage."

*(Where needed, to be read by/to the passenger, dated and signed by him/her, or on his/her behalf)*

| Place: | Date: | Passenger's Signature |
|---|---|---|

a

**Fig. 1 a, b.** MEDIF-IATA standard medical information form

| PART 2 | MEDIF MEDICAL INFORMATION SHEET | (for official use only) |
|---|---|---|
| To be completed by ATTENDING PHYSICIAN | This form is intended to provide CONFIDENTIAL information, to enable the airlines MEDICAL Departments to assess the fitness of the passenger to travel as indicated in PART 1 hereof. If the passenger is acceptable, this information will permit the issuance of the necessary directives designed to provide for the passenger's welfare and comfort.<br>The PHYSICIAN ATTENDING the incapacitated passenger is requested to ANSWER ALL QUESTIONS. (Enter a cross "×" in the appropriate "yes" or "no" boxes, and/or give precise concise answers).<br>COMPLETING OF THE FORM IN BLOCK LETTERS OR BY TYPEWRITER WILL BE APPRECIATED. | The form must be returned to:<br>(Carrier's Designated Office) |

| Airlines' Ref. Code | | |
|---|---|---|
| MEDA01 | PATIENT'S NAME, INITIAL(S), SEX, AGE: | |
| MEDA02 | ATTENDING PHYSICIAN Name & Address<br>Telephone Contact | Business: Home: |
| MEDA03 | MEDICAL DATA:<br>- DIAGNOSIS in details (including vital signs)<br>- Day/month/year of first symptoms: | Date of diagnosis: |
| MEDA04 | - PROGNOSIS for the trip: | |
| MEDA05 | - Contagious AND communicable disease? | No ☐ Yes ☐ Specify: |
| MEDA06 | - Is patient in any way OFFENSIVE to other passengers? (smell, appearance, conduct) | No ☐ Yes ☐ Specify: |
| MEDA07 | - Can patient use normal aircraft seat with seatback placed in the UPRIGHT position when so required? | Yes ☐ No ☐ |
| MEDA08 | - Can patient take care of his own needs on board UNASSISTED * (including meals, visit to toilet, etc.)? | Yes ☐ No ☐<br>If not, type of help needed: |
| MEDA09 | - If to be ESCORTED, is the arrangement proposed in PART 1/E hereof satisfactory for you? | Yes ☐ No ☐<br>If not, type of escort proposed by YOU: |
| MEDA10 | - Does patient need OXYGEN ** equipment in flight? (If yes, state rate of flow) | No ☐ Yes ☐ Litres per Minute ☐ Continuous? Yes ☐ No ☐ |
| MEDA11 | - Does patient need any MEDICATION *, other than self-administered, and/or the use of special apparatus such as respirator, incubator, etc. **? | (a) on the GROUND while at the airport(s): No ☐ Yes ☐ Specify |
| MEDA12 | | (b) on board of the AIRCRAFT: No ☐ Yes ☐ Specify |
| MEDA13 | - Does patient need HOSPITALISATION? (If yes, indicate arrangements made or, if none were made, indicate "NO ACTION TAKEN") | (a) during long layover or nightstop at CONNECTING POINTS en route: No ☐ Yes ☐ Action |
| MEDA14 | | (b) upon arrival at DESTINATION: No ☐ Yes ☐ Action |
| MEDA15 | Other remarks or information in the interest of your patient's smooth and comfortable transportation: | None ☐ Specify if any** |
| MEDA16 | - Other arrangements made by the attending physician: | |

NOTE (*): Cabin attendants are NOT authorized to give special assistance to particular passengers, to the detriment of their service to other passengers - Additionally, they are trained only in FIRST AID and are NOT PERMITTED to administer any injection, or to give medication.

IMPORTANT: FEES IF ANY RELEVANT TO THE PROVISION OF THE ABOVE INFORMATION AND FOR CARRIER-PROVIDED SPECIAL EQUIPMENT (**) ARE TO BE PAID BY THE PASSENGER CONCERNED.

| Date: | Place: | Attending Physician's Signature |
|---|---|---|

b

**Table 1.** Advice to physicians and passengers

1. Conditions usually considered unacceptable for air travel:
   a) Severe cardiac decompensation. Myocardial infarction within 4–6 weeks depending on severity, progress and complications. Severe immobilizing chronic obstructive airway disease (COAD)
   b) Recent pneumothorax if air is still entrapped. Residual air in the CNS, e.g., after radiology
   c) Psychoses not adequately controlled. An escort may be required by the airline for any psychiatric patient
   d) Otitis media with eustachian block
   e) Communicable diseases if possibility of spread exists
   f) Pregnancy beyond the 35th week
   g) Disorders with increased intracranial pressure, intestinal obstruction, large unsupported hernias, recent skull fractures, large mediastinal tumors
   h) Postoperative cases before wound is sufficiently healed (usually about 10 days following major abdominal surgery)
2. Any attendant or escort must be approved by the airline and must accept full responsibility for the care of the patient and supply and administration of drugs and dressings. All costs including attendant's fares and expenses are the patient's responsibility. Stretcher cases must always be escorted. Aircraft crews are not permitted to give injections nor assist with passengers' toilet requirements
3. Given notice at most airports, ambulances and wheelchairs can be provided. The patient must pay any charges
4. Safety regulations forbid the use of passengers' own oxygen equipment in flight. The company will provide such equipment; a charge will be made
5. Cases will not be accepted which the Company considers may prejudice the normal operation of the aircraft
6. Use of this form does not guarantee specific seats
7. Patients with COAD cause many problems of assessment. Please give latest levels of Hb, $pO^2$, $pCO^2$, date of tests and present need for supplemental oxygen
8. If psychiatric conditions exist please state if suicidal tendencies are present, or if the passenger has been violent, noisy or required restraint and the date of such an incident

as to whether the individual can be safely carried. Along with the questionnaire, the passenger and physician are provided a brief description of conditions usually not acceptable for travel (Table 1). Once it is in the hands of the airline it is transmitted to the medical department for review and final decision. In a number of carriers this is handed off to one of the various medical assistance companies, who will make all the arrangements and coordinate final approvals with the carrier. This is done on a fee-for-service basis. A significant advantage found in the use of medical assistance companies is their ability to provide in-flight attendants and equipment on an as-needed basis. Airlines, on the other hand, most often limit their services to on-board stretchers and supplemental oxygen supplies.

A very important additional feature of the IATA system is its ability to recognize the frequent medical traveler who has a significant, but static, handicap. If these individuals have demonstrated their ability to travel alone, many airline medical departments will issue them a frequent traveler medical card.

FREQUENT TRAVELLER'S MEDICAL CARD (FREMEC)

Honouring instructions: The data contained in the shaded fields MUST always be transmitted with any reservation request. - Journeys requested but not authorised by this Card, require completion of the Standard Medical Information Form (MEDIF).

FREMEC Number: ______ / ______ (Airline's Code Number) (Serial Number) Issued by: ______ (Airline's Medical Dept.'s Telex Code) Valid until: ______ (day/month/year)

The holder of this Card, ______ (Surname) ______ (Init.) ______ (Title) ______ (Sex) ______ (Age)

______ (Permanent Address) ______ (Phone)

has the following permanent/chronic incapacitation ______

______ ______ (Code, if any example: BLND, DEAF, WCHC, etc.)

The holder is authorized by the Medical Department issuing this Card, to travel by air within the validity of this Card, subject to: (a) the Conditions stated on the reverse, (b) no worsening of the Holder's present health conditions, and (c) full observance of all carrier rules, regulations and instructions, and with the following LIMITATIONS:

______

(Insert limitations, including any permanent dietary requirements)

(2)

CONDITIONS OF ISSUE

1. Cardholders are responsible to REPORT ALL CHANGES in their present handicap or incapacitation, and/or the deterioration in their physical or medical condition, to the airline representative or agent with whom they are in contact.
2. Subject to all terms and conditions stated on this Card, the authorisation for air travel is valid only up to the date stated on the front.
3. This Card is not transferable and must be produced, together with proof of the cardholder's identity, on every occasion whenever airline reservations are made for the cardholder, at time of ticket issuance, and when so requested by the airlines or their agents or representatives.
4. Cardholders are reminded that arrangements for travel should be made as much in advance as possible. They should also allow sufficient time for check-in formalities.

Date and Place of Issue ______

Passenger's Signature ______

(Legal guardian or Passenger's witness may sign if passenger is physically unable to do so).



**Fig. 2.** Frequent traveler's medical card (FREMEC)

This card is recognized by the name "FREMEC" within the industry (Fig. 2). A handicapped person in possession of such a card would have his travel facilitated with little or no requirement to undergo further approval. Travelers most affected by this agreement are paraplegics who have become, for the most part, self-sufficient. In this same light it is worthwhile to know that there is a growing trend to design aircraft and air terminals in a manner that facilitates the travel of the handicapped. This includes changes in aircraft lavatories, fold down arm rest on aisle seats, the provision of on-board wheelchairs and a wide selection of special diets.

## Airport Medical Facilities

On arrival a significant number of airports have medical facilities either on site or nearby. These facilities usually have a dual role, first to provide occupational and aviation medical support to the airport workers and second to respond to the emergency needs of the traveler. Of great value is their ability to provide a point of entry into local health care systems if more extensive care is required. On the negative side, services can be expensive and have even been known to be withheld if one cannot pay. Another option is the airline itself; as a rule, airlines have arrangements with health care providers in each of the stations they serve. Several even publish booklets for the travelers that contain names and addresses of available medical facilities and doctors. Although their primary purpose is to serve company personnel, many welcome the opportunity to provide this added service to the traveler. The point of contact is the station manager. There is no question that individuals and lay people do a reasonable job of triage. Thus a number of emergencies may completely bypass the airport medical facility and be transported directly to a hospital. Transport may be of the private or public type ambulance. Again, fees will most likely be encountered. Many localities have a single telephone number to handle calls for help, for example 911 in the United States and 144 in Zurich, Switzerland.

## Country Health Services

Once the traveler is away from the airport environment, the options remain pretty much the same; however, the point of contact usually becomes the hotel doctor or one recommended by the hotel staff. If time permits, consulates, friends and business contacts will substantially improve the range of choices. Another possibility is to belong to one of the many service companies who, as part of either a traveler's insurance plan or as a feature of other services they offer, include names and addresses of health care facilities who have agreed to care for their members. These include many credit card companies, specialized medical assistance organizations, travel associations and insurance companies. Access to care may also be found in telephone directories that have special listings in the yellow pages for health care facilities and doctors. These may be categorized by medical specialty. The most frustrating aspect of this source of information is usually the language limitation of travelers when in a foreign land.

**Table 2.** Guidelines for acceptance of newborn babies and pregnant women

| Category | Age of baby/time of expected birth | Acceptance | Equipment |
|---|---|---|---|
| 1. Babies (normal or prematurely born) | Within first 7 days | Not accepted | – |
| 2. Babies, healthy (normal birth) | At least 7 days and up to age specified in airline's rules | Accepted if accompanied by mother or other suitable escort (nurse, etc.) medical clearance not required | Normal |
| 3. Babies, not healthy (normal birth) or prematurely born (including incubator cases | At least 7 days and up to period established by doctor, not exceeding 2 years old | Accepted only after positive medical clearance. Must be escorted by qualified escort (doctor, specialized medical nurse/attendant) IATA Resolution 401/RP 1401 applies | As specified by medical department/advisor. See sections on incubators and oxygen |
| 4. Expectant mothers in normal health, no previous multiple birth, no complication in delivery expected, progress of pregnancy certain | Four weeks or more after date of travel | Accepted without restrictions. Medical clearance not required | If needed, supply WCHR or WCHS |
| 5. Expectant mothers otherwise "incapacitated," or with complications in delivery expected, or with progress of pregnancy uncertain | Four weeks or more after date of travel | Accepted only after positive medical clearance. Medical Information Form (MEDIF) to be issued within 7 days before commencement of travel. Escort if/as required by Medical Clearance. IATA Resolution 401/RP 1401 applies | As specified by medical department/advisor |
| 6. Expectant mothers, any condition/case history | Within 4 weeks after date of travel | | |
| 7. Expectant mothers, any condition/case history | Within 7 days after date of travel | Not recommended. Medical clearance required | |
| 8. New mothers, normal, premature, or with complications | Within 7 days after birth | Not recommended. Medical clearance required | |

*Note:* Infant's bassinet/carrycot/baby basket (with infant's food for consumption in flight, wrap or blanket) carried free of charge. However, this requirement must be notified at time reservations are requested

As one travels further away from population centers the choice of what to do most often becomes simple because the range of alternatives eventually reduces itself to zero. When Dr. Smith is the only doctor in town there is no other one to go to. If Dr. Smith cannot help, then medical evacuation may be in order.

In this regard there are now very specialized services to be found in air ambulance rescue organizations. The helicopter is becoming the most prominent carrier used for emergency response in the nonurban areas. They may be public or private, but both usually provide service with a well-equipped and well-trained staff. One of the most advanced systems can be found in Switzerland, and an excellent service even exists in the remoteness of Nepal. Almost all countries have some ability for aeromedical evacuation. Transportation is usually to a definitive treatment facility or at least to a point where the patient can be stabilized and then be further evacuated to selected specialty centers. This second echelon of evacuation may be by special air ambulance of the fixed wing variety or in a partitioned off portion of a larger airliner. Again medical assistance companies can play a very valuable role in coordinating such moves and in providing for special en route medical attention.

We have now completed the circle with the traveler either recovering to a degree that travel can be continued or that repatriation home as a patient can be accomplished.

Considering the more than 350 million annual travelers worldwide, the fact that fewer than 10,000 come home by stretcher as patients is further evidence of the low probability of serious medical problems occurring when away from home.

Although there are many stories concerning inadequate medical treatment provided travelers, all in all, the worldwide system of health care providers actually responds remarkably well. Really true emergencies receive international attention. Help pours in from everywhere. The international response that occurred after the recent earthquake in Mexico City and that which followed the terrorist hijacking at Karachi, Pakistan, in 1986 was truly remarkable. Local hospitals, doctors and nurses immediately turned out in force to render care to the many badly injured persons and to attend to those who were killed. In hours, similar international help followed. In the terrorist incident, India and the United States brought in special aeromedical evacuation and treatment teams. Sister airlines further augmented evacuation capabilities. Within 24 h a number of casualties were already hospitalized in specialty treatment centers as far away as London, Frankfurt, Delhi and Bombay. Within 2 weeks almost all casualties were back to their country of origin or original destination despite the severity of their wound. Although improved triaging may have provided for better utilization of available medical resources, there were few primary treatment problems and only a limited number of secondary complications. Examples such as these again speak well of the capability of the international medical community.

## Conclusions

In summary, the fear of being unable to cope with medical emergencies when away from home is not as formidable as it may seem. Proper planning will reduce the possibility of medical problems. Although medical assistance when airborne is limited, experience indicates a low incidence of in-flight medical emergencies. On-board first aid and diversion to the nearest airport are the preferred courses of action if major problems occur. Most airlines will carry handicapped and ill passengers if given adequate notice, provided safety is not compromised. Individuals with static physical limitations may be eligible for a frequent traveler's medical card that is issued by a number of international carriers. Possession of such a card facilitates travel for these persons. A number of airports now have on-site medical facilities available to the traveler. In addition, many medical assistance companies, travel organizations, insurance and credit card companies are able to recommend available medical care facilities on a worldwide basis. For major illnesses and injuries the availability of air ambulances and medical assitance companies provide a means for aeromedical evacuation when local facilities are inadequate. The sum total of these options is such that even individuals with significant health concerns can now be optimistic in their ability to undertake safe worldwide travel.

## References


1. Medizinischer Reiseratgeber (1988) Schweizerische Stiftung für Gesundheitserziehung, Zürich
2. Centers for Disease Control (1988) Health information for international travel. US Department of Health and Human Services, Public Health Service, Center for Prevention Services, Division of Quarantine, Atlanta (HHS publ no (CDC) 85-8280)
3. Traffic Services Administrator (1981) Incapacitated passengers air travel guide. International Air Transport Association, Montreal; IATA, Geneva

# A Rational Model for Access to Medical Care for Travelers

L. van der Reis

During the past few decades the annual increase in the number of air travelers has been in the millions. Current predictions do not suggest a diminution in that rate of increase. In the Pacific rim an annual increase of 9% may well be exceeded. The annual increments in the number of passengers worldwide will remain in the millions.

The characteristics of these vast numbers of passengers include all varieties and ranges of age, physical condition and ability to communicate. It is self-evident that the incidence of illness among these passengers will keep pace with the increased numbers of travelers.

Most of those who venture into foreign countries do not have the contacts in those countries which provide for immediate access to medical services. Rather, in most instances it is a hit-and-miss proposition to gain access to medical care.

A number of organizations exist which in one manner or another make an attempt to provide some type of service, but in general these programs do not meet the requirements of most travelers – nor do they comply with a number of conditions which assure quality and scrutinize costs.

In response to a definite demand, we have undertaken the design and development of a system which in our opinion satisfies the conditions needed to provide immediate access to high-quality medical services at controlled costs.

The features/subsystems of the model include:

1. Twenty-four-hour access
2. Physician orientation
3. Quality assurance
4. Cost containment

## Access

Access must be continuous. Thus, the physicians and communications support system must be accessible 24 h/day, 365 days/year. Determination of a substitute physician acceptable to the network's supervisory board is part and parcel of the physician selection protocol.

## Physician Orientation

When one looks at the manner in which medical services are delivered and how decisions are made, it becomes obvious that physicians constitute the axis around which the processes revolve and evolve.

Physicians are indeed the focus of the decision-making processes in medicine – in contrast to "hospitals," "service bureaus" and other institutional agencies which at times are depersonalized and dehumanized. Physicians can and do respond in a personalized, professional manner, can make referrals and perform other aspects of therapeutic and diagnostic triage.

## Quality Assurance

Quality assurance plays a very crucial role if one wants to provide first-class care. Thus, the selection of physicians must be very deliberately planned and executed based on a finely tuned selection protocol. Maintenance of quality must be exercised through frequent monitoring and follow-up. Participating physicians should be able to provide care themselves. Thus, whenever possible internists or general practitioners are selected for inclusion in the network.

## Cost Containment

Cost containment is accomplished in a number of ways. A "usual and customary fee" schedule is on file for each physician participant. Follow-up allows for confirmation of adherence to the fee schedule. Furthermore, the careful selection of the physician and the likelihood of being dropped as a participating physician without a chance for appeal constitutes a deterrent against abuse.

## Communications Network

Reliable telecommunications on a worldwide scale are a reality. In our model, a central office is the core for 24-h access. This office can be situated in any location in the world which has a well-functioning, up-to-date communications system.

Communications with and between participating physicians, field offices and other agencies via telephone, telex, telegraph or telefax are the channels which keep the system on "real time," responsive to the customers' needs and demands.

A properly planned, dedicated communications system together with a network of quality physicians make for an efficient, medically reliable and economically sound system. From a financial point of view, the model allows for a number of options. Thus, the system can be operated as a "for profit" network or a charitable, "non-profit" organization.

Our experience with this type of system has been most satisfactory. We anticipate expansion and widespread adoption and adaptation of our model and its subsystems.

# Investigation, Control and Surveillance of an Outbreak of Gastroenteritis in a Portuguese Holiday Resort

R. Y. Cartwright and J. Albuquerque

Albufeira is a coastal holiday resort in the Algarve of Portugal. It has a municipality potable water supply and sewage disposal system. The public health surveillance is under the jurisdiction of the Algarve Health Department. It is a popular holiday both with Portuguese tourists and tourists from Britain and Scandinavia. Holiday accommodation is mainly in hotels and time share apartments. Most of the British tourists travel with a package tour operator. In the latter part of the summer season 1983, tour operators reported an increased number of clients with diarrhoea. Concern was expressed about the quality and availability of potable water. The incidence of travellers' diarrhoea returned to the norm for the resort at the end of 1983 and was not raised in the early part of the summer season 1984. An explosive outbreak of gastroenteritis occurred in August 1984 and the outbreak was investigated by the Algarve Health Department with the assistance of a British microbiologist and epidemiologist.

## Outbreak Onset

In mid-August, tour operator representatives were reporting a sudden increase in the incidence of diarrhoea among clients. In some units attack rates of 100% were reported. The possibility of overreaction by the representatives was considered and local officials were of the opinion that the cause was excessive alcohol intake, too much sun, differences in food and/or chemicals used to spray fruit. Preliminary bacteriological examination of potable water from some holiday units revealed the presence of coliforms and thermotolerant coliforms. Laboratory reports of enteropathogens isolated from visitors to Albufeira showed a range of *Salmonella* spp., *Campylobacter* spp., *Giardia lamblia* and *Shigella sonnei*. Other resorts in the Algarve and other parts of Portugal were not affected (Fig. 1). This suggested a local cause and not alcohol consumption, food or excessive sun!

Examination of the records from the Albufeira hospital clinic revealed a sudden rise in the number of patients complaining of diarrhoea. The rise occurred over 3 days and involved the indigenous population, Portuguese tourists and foreign tourists (Fig. 2). An in resort questionnaire study among British tourists gave an incidence rate of over 80%. A working hypothesis was proposed – that the source of infection was most likely human sewage contaminating both the potable water supplies and recreational waters.

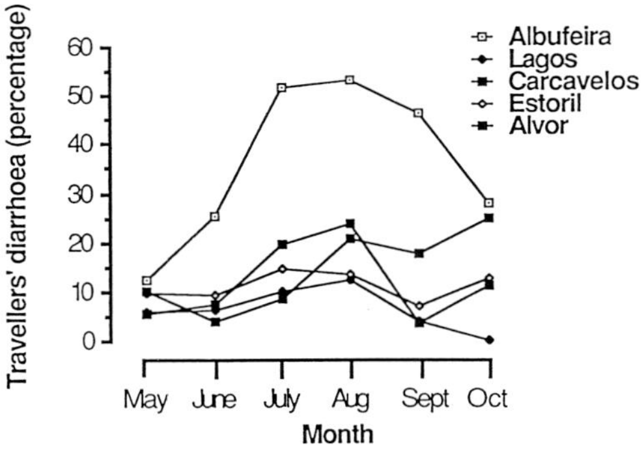


**Fig. 1.** Incidence of travellers' diarrhoea in Portuguese resorts 1984

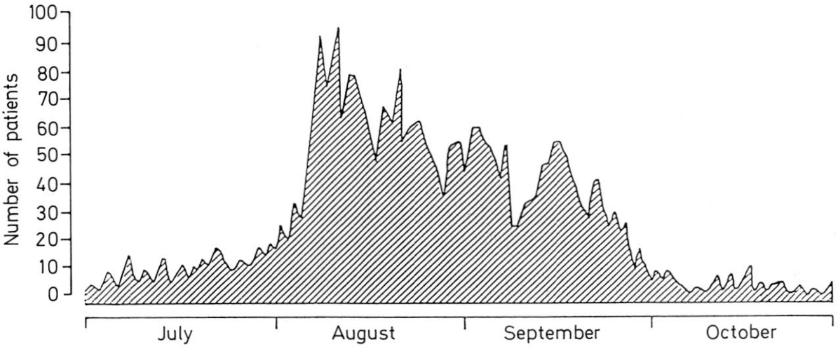


**Fig. 2.** Patients with diarrhoea presenting to the Albufeira Hospital Clinic, August–October 1984

## Potable Water

The municipality water supply was obtained from 21 bore holes all of which were said to have chlorinators. Water storage depots were situated at various parts of the distribution network. Every bore hole was inspected and samples taken for bacteriological examination. Seventeen bore holes were supplying water to the network, but the chlorinator was working properly at only one. Failure of chlorination was due to broken chlorine infection pumps, lack of chlorine cylinders or the absence of a pump. No free available chlorine could be detected at the periphery of the water distribution network. The majority of water samples contained coliforms and many also contained thermotolerant coliforms. It was concluded that the municipality water was bacteriologically unsafe.

## Sewage Systems

The municipality was served by four treatment works, three discharging their effluent into the sea and the other into the river Quateria. One of the treatment works was not being operated correctly, due to operator error. The sea outfall pipes were either just below the water line or onto rocks producing an effluent stream onto the beach. In the course of the inspections raw sewage was found to be discharged from some hotels into a river bed providing a sewage stream which ran across a popular beach. A large apartment block was not connected to the main drainage, discharging raw sewage into a river bed near to a bore hole. Another discharge of raw sewage from a holiday village onto ground adjacent to a bore hole was observed. At the end of the popular Fishermans' Beach, the concrete structure was the old town sewer still discharging raw sewage into the sea frequented by many tourists. Bacteriological testing of sea water from all main beaches showed bacterial levels exceeding the EEC recommendations. It was concluded that recreational water was contaminated with sewage and that sewage contamination of potable water sources was probable.

## Action

Immediate action was taken to chlorinate the municipality water supply by adding sodium hypochlorite to strategic water storage depots. Chlorination was achieved within a day. Recommendations were made to ensure adequate and continued chlorination of the water. It was not possible to take immediate action to improve the sewage systems but fortunately the number of tourists diminished, as it was the end of the season, thus reducing the load on the system. Plans which had been made to improve the sewage system were urgently reviewed and work commenced so that by summer 1985 raw sewage was no longer contaminating recreational or potable water. The effluent from treatment plans was chlorinated until long sea outfalls were operational.

## Surveillance

The incidence of travellers' diarrhoea was monitored by Thomson Holidays using their client satisfaction questionnaire. The results (Fig. 3) show that the

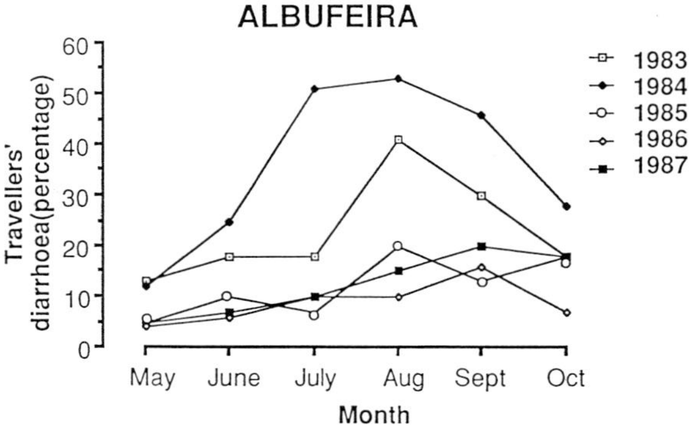


**Fig. 3.** Incidence of travellers' diarrhoea, Albufeira, 1983–1987

actions taken were effective. The hospital clinic attendance figure also indicated a return to expected numbers of diarrhoea cases. Bacteriological monitoring of potable and recreational water ensured that required standards were being maintained.

## Discussion

The international team approach used in the investigation, control and monitoring of this outbreak was successful. Data obtained from returning tourists both from questionnaires and on faecal isolates were made available to the Algarve health department. Five outbreaks of *Shigella sonnei* dysentery in England and Wales were associated with visitors to Albufeira during this period. The British tour operators supported this investigation, expressing their concern through the Portuguese Toruist Office. British tourists continued to use the resort in contrast to the Scandinavians, who pulled out of Albufeira. Although help and assistance from the home country of tourists can be of value, it is important that the investigation is led by the medical officer from the affected country responsible for public health.

## Conclusion

An outbreak of gastroenteritis in the Portuguese resort of Albufeira in August 1984 was investigated by a joint Portuguese-British team led by a medical officer from the Algarve Health Department. Data from Portugal and Britain were of value in both the investigation and subsequent monitoring. The health of tourists involves the holiday country, the home country and the tour operators. Combining their resources has shown to facilitate the investigation and control of an outbreak of gastroenteritis.

# Diagnoses and Related Medical Costs Among Swedish Citizens Working and Living Abroad: A 2-Year Follow-up of Insurance Statistics

R. Sinclair

To live and work abroad is to many Swedish employees, and their families, a natural part of their career within companies and organizations with international interests. Most of these people are relatively young and often take their children. The majority undergo a medical examination before their foreign assignment.

To get an idea of what kind of medical problems these people will run into during their stay abroad, an investigation of insurance company (Trygg-Hansa) statistics from 1986 and 1987 was made. All the registered cases with medical costs, including necessary transportation, exceeding about US$ 325 are included in the survey – except certain cases with accidents at, on the way to or from their place of work.

## Results

In 1986 there were 1989 and in 1987 1628 persons covered by medical insurance. Thirty percent of these were children under the age of about 18 years. From this population there were 91 registered cases meeting the above-men-

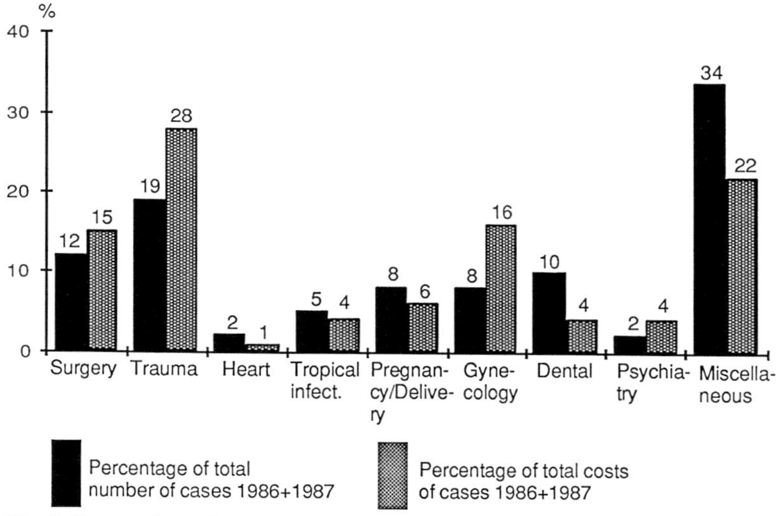


**Fig. 1.** Proportion of cases and of costs attributed to various diagnostic groups

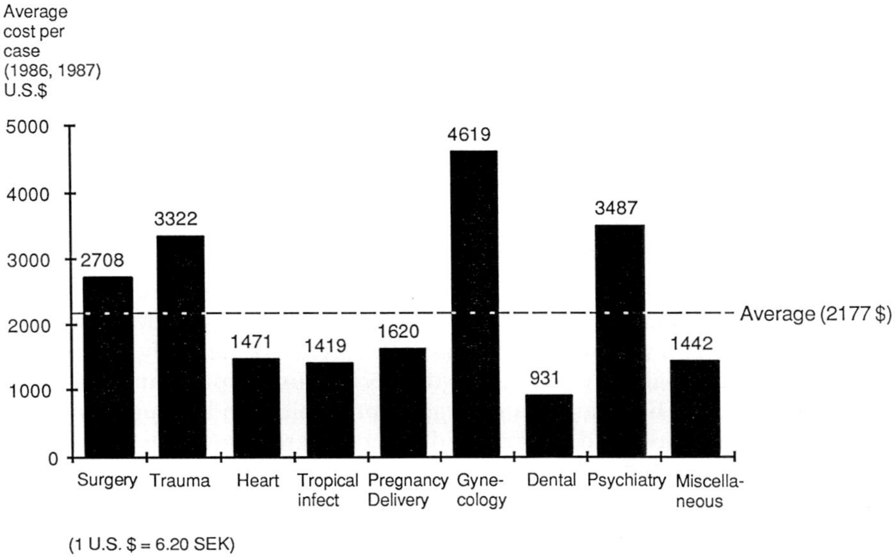


**Fig. 2.** Average cost per case in various diagnostic groups

tioned criteria during the 2 years of study, giving an annual average incidence of 2.5% of the people insured that used the insurance. The incidence among the employees (almost all males) was slightly above that among their spouses, but was lower among the children (about 1%).

When separating the 91 cases into nine diagnostic groups (Fig. 1) in this specific population it was found that – apart from a big group of "miscellaneous" diagnoses which included, e.g., lower back pain, middle ear infection and muscle pains – trauma, surgical, dental, gynecological and pregnancy/delivery cases were the most common. The costs of the cases in the different groups were calculated, both as a percentage of the total costs (Fig. 1) and as an average cost per case (Fig. 2).

## Discussion

This survey indicates that in this specific population the gynecological, traumatic and surgical cases were not only among the most frequent but also the most expensive. Heart and chest pain problems were, as expected, infrequent in this relatively young and well-controlled population. Tropical medical diseases were also infrequent, partly probably because these people have favorable living conditions they are not highly exposed, partly because of information, vaccination and prescription of malaria chemoprophylaxis and other preventive steps. The psychiatric cases were few, but costly, mainly because the patients had to interrupt their stay abroad and be sent home to Sweden. The dental cases were not as expensive but made up as many as 10% of the total number of cases. About half of these were caused by acute damage, and the rest had diagnoses like parodontitis complications and apical infection. To a certain extent these latter problems might have been prevented if a better dental check-up with a teeth X-ray and peridental areas had been made before the expatriation.

## Conclusions

To identify people at risk of suffering from medical problems and for an opportunity to give advice and information about general and local health risks, a medical checkup of the whole family is probably of value before they set out on a foreign assignment. The information given can include a description of trauma risks, e.g., by pointing out that traffic accidents are fairly common in many places, especially in connection with alcohol consumption and when motorcycles are used. Food and water hygiene principles can be taught and also principles of how to avoid malaria and other diseases transmitted by insects as well as how to avoid HIV infection and other sexually transmitted diseases. A thorough history, and if needed a further investigation, of gynecological symptoms and problems will probably be well worthwhile, and the same seems to be applicable to psychiatric and dental problems.

# Company Medical Policy for Expatriates in Third World Countries

D. G. Dawson

It is the responsibility of the company medical director to develop a medical policy to cover all aspects of health when employees and families are transferred to a Third World Country. Failure to do so may result in unnecessary suffering with possible tragic consequences. Prior consultation with professional colleagues knowledgeable of the particular area is useful. Policy should be focused on the best available facility in the area, which will usually be located in the capital city of that particular country. When visiting the country, the medical director should assess six key factors – profession, equipment, construction, administration, logistics and epidemiology – "PECALE".

## Profession

The most important single factor concerning the health of the expatriate is the physician with whom he or she will deal.

*Training.* Enquiries should be made concerning the training of available specialists. Key physicians covering internal medicine, surgery, obstetrics, gynaecology and paediatrics should be identified. It is important to assess any dental facilities that are available, and to note the experience and training of the dental surgeon. Many hospitals visited will have their own training school for nurses. This is usually an added bonus, as the standards of nursing will probably be more closely supervised.

*Postgraduate Experience.* Enquiries should be made of any medical staff who have had overseas postgraduate experience. They will usually have a better understanding of western culture and be able to relate more easily to the expatriate.

*Language.* Locating medical staff who are fluent in the language of the expatriate is most helpful. Usually this will be more easily found among the physicians than in the nursing staff.

*Dress Code.* It is important to notice the dress code, which should be compatible with persons of professional standing. The nurses' uniform should be neat and clean, portraying a feeling of trust and confidence.

## Equipment

Second only in importance to the skills of the professional are the tools with which he or she has to work.

*Invasive Procedures.* All equipment used to penetrate the skin, especially that which enters directly into the bloodstream, *must* be disposable. Sterilizing procedures for needles cannot be relied upon. If disposable syringes and needles, fluid administration sets and suture needles are not available, and the Company Medical Director wishes to utilize that particular medical facility, then he must supply the necessary equipment for use in the hospital. Anything less places the expatriates at risk of contracting AIDS, hepatitis B or other infections from inadequately sterilized equipment.

*Resuscitation.* Check the equipment available for resuscitation. This gives an opportunity to visit the 24-h emergency receiving room. Simple equipment can be very effective when used in the right hands.

*Diagnosis.* Diagnostic equipment need not be sophisticated, but facilities for X-ray, electrocardiograph, haematology, blood chemistry, bacteriology and parasitology are essential. Enquiries should be made regarding the ability to check blood groups and to test for human immunodeficiency virus (HIV) antibody and hepatitis B surface antigen (HBsAG). Should very sophisticated equipment be available, such as a scanner, then it is worth enquiring what operational training has taken place, and by how many staff. It is important to ascertain whether blood gases can be estimated, although in most cases this analysis will probably not be available.

*Surgery and Obstetrics.* The operating theatres should be visited and note made of the standard of sophistication. Enquiries should be made about anaesthetists and their availability; sometimes this is undertaken by nurses who have undergone training in this field. Enquire about blood availability and whether checked for HIV antibody, HBsAG and malaria parasites. Reliability may need to be placed on the expatriate community to act as a walking blood bank. The method of sterilization of all surgical equipment should be checked.

*Cardiac Monitoring.* A visit should be paid to the intensive care unit, if one exists, and checks made on the ability to monitor cardiac disease, and to stabilize prior to evacuation.

*Renal Dialysis.* It is of interest to note whether renal dialysis is performed. While it is unlikely this facility would need to be utilized by an expatriate, it does indicate the degree of sophistication which the hospital has reached.

*Chemotherapy.* A visit to the hospital pharmacy helps determine the range of treatments available. Checks particularly should be made for drugs used in the treatment of tropical parasitology. If supplies are short (e.g. i.v. quinine), offer to import selected items.

*Inpatient Care.* Check how well the inpatient rooms are equipped, and note whether rooms are provided with central oxygen and suction. It may be necessary to provide anything from essentials such as sheets and blankets to a luxury television set. Enquire about the diet provided (may be vegetarian or non-western) and check whether meals need to be supplemented from outside.

## Construction

*Cleanliness.* Cleanliness throughout the entire hospital is an indicator of good housekeeping. Complications can be expected from infection in dirty premises.

*Space.* Overcrowding or lack of space encourages cross-infection. There will be little privacy in cramped quarters.

*Maintenance.* Lack of maintenance indicates poor financial resources. This situation occurs worldwide, not only in Third World countries.

*Temperature and Humidity Control.* Hospital rooms with overhead fans and a through air draught are usually very comfortable and cool. Air conditioning, while often installed, can be noisy and may keep the humidity at a level too low for comfort.

*Private Rooms.* Check the private rooms and any extra facilities available, such as adjacent bath/shower room, telephone and general comfort.

*Kitchen.* It is not always possible to visit the kitchen, but if an invitation is extended, it is useful to make a quick survey.

## Administration

*Outpatient.* It is important to check the appointment system for choice of doctor and likely waiting time. A list of specialists and general practitioners should be obtained. It will be useful to ascertain the fluency of language of the appointment clerks. Ensure there is a 24-h emergency receiving capability.

A list of specialists and general practitioners should be obtained from the outpatient department, and the consultation facilities for privacy, or lack of it, observed. Enquire whether home visits can be arranged and, if so, which physicians are prepared to undertake them.

*Inpatients.* Many hospitals will require a retainer from the company. This will generally guarantee a bed at any time and, in some instances, special private rooms are permanently reserved. Generally a letter guaranteeing payment of an employee's account is required for each admission. Some hospitals require a list of expatriates resident in the country who may wish to utilize the hospital's facilities. It is vitally important that there is good understanding between the hospital and the company concerning willingness to repatriate a patient providing the patient is deemed fit to fly. The hospital administrator or one of the senior physicians should be used for liaison between the company medical director and the hospital. Mutual respect and confidence should be estblished in order to smooth over any problems that may arise in the future.

## Logistics

*Transportation to Hospital.* Enquire about ambulance services, but also ensure the company has adequate transportation available to bring personnel to the hospital. Air transport may be required from outlying districts. Check charter flight availability. If personnel are in remote areas (e. g. offshore) confirm helicopter availability, permit to fly over land, and location of nearest heliport to the hospital.

*Repatriation.* An arrangement or contract should be made with an international air evacuation company to repatriate ill or injured personnel. Check on availability of exit visas, if these are required. Note the schedule of regular commercial flights out of the country, and identify local airline offices for future reference, in case repatriation is required by a commercial line.

*Telephone Communications.* Ensure that overseas telephone communication can be made with the hospital. List all relevant numbers, including home and hospital numbers of the hospital liaison administrator.

*Hospital Location.* If possible, it is helpful to identify a hospital close to the general expatriate living area, particularly if operating in a crowded traffic-congested city. However, quality of service is far more important than location.

## Epidemiology

It is most important to talk to the local physicians regarding disease trends, particularly infectious, in the particular area. It is surprising how much variation there can be, both geographically and seasonally. Look for the unexpected; in certain areas in a Third World country, for example, if the rains fail, cholera can be contracted from eating water melons. The reason – the local farmers inject the water melons with river water in order to increase the weight prior to marketing.

It cannot be overemphasized how important it is for the medical director to follow a definitive plan such as "PECALE," when formulating a medical policy for company expatriates residing in a Third World country.

# Health Protection Measures in Remote Locations of Club Méditerranée

M. Binder


## Summary

The health concerns of Club Méditerranée comprise two major components. First, to meet the needs of the members who come mostly from industrialized countries and may find it difficult to adapt to a different environment, especially when they become ill or have an accident. Also, vacationers may be tempted to relax their normal standards of behavior. Second, the geographical, environmental, and medical conditions which prevail in developing countries have to be dealt with so that safe conditions can be maintained.


The purpose of resort operators is to provide a pleasant and relaxing environment of their guest. This includes providing environmental conditions of high hygienic and safety standards and the availability of medical attention. The French village resort operator Club Méditerranée is the world's ninth largest tour operator which offers all-inclusive travel packages: travel, accomodation, catering, entertainment, sports and excursions. The Club Med operates 98 villages in 26 countries with a total of 64 500 beds. Each year some 20 million meals are served. The Club Med has 1 million members, 39% of whom are from France, 23% from other European countries, 23% from North America, 8% from sia and 3% from South America. The average length of stay is 8.2 days and the average age of the guests is 42 years.

Club Med employs 6700 staff from 52 different nationalities. In 1987 a total of 18 000 h training was provided to more than 2000 staff members. In addition, there are about 12 000 service personnel, two-thirds of which are locally hired.

Health advice is provided in a brochure sent to all travelers in their own language before their departure. Topics include vaccinations, climatic and environmental adjustment, food, malaria, sexually transmitted diseases (STDS), and diarrhea.

Medical supervision of the staff and sanitary inspections of the facilities are conducted twice a year by physicians. These visits include medical examination and immunizations for the entire staff with special attention to food handlers (including stool examinations) and scuba diving instructors. The inspections regularly check the hygienic conditions of the food preparations and the environment. Bacteriological examinations are carried out of foods, drinking water and swimming pool water in accordance with a detailed protocol. Educational programs are presented to the entire staff which review the basic rules of food hygiene, the dangers of food poisoning, the need for handwashing and the use of chlorinated water, and general aspects of hygiene such as vector control and water conditions.

Information is provided to the guests on STDs and AIDS with oral, written, and video presentations. Condoms are available in each village.

The Club Med has established an infirmary in each of its villages under the guidelines of its International Epidemiological Medical Committee. Each infirmary is staffed by two nurses and sometimes a physician. Most medical care is limited to dealing with emergencies and providing for medical evacuation. The infirmaries are provided with nonprescription and emergency drugs and equipment includes resuscitation kits, oxygen, and first aid kits. All members are insured for medical evacuation.

Weekly statistics on the occurrence of diarrhea are reported to the Medical Office in Paris. All unusual events are reported immediately so that the Medical Office can conduct an investigation and take control measures.

# Medical Care of Tourists in the Maldives

K. Plentz

With the support of the Touristik Union International (TUI) – the largest tour operator in Europe, with 2.7 million clients a year – the weekly reports were analyzed of health impairments among tourists to five destinations in 1982/1983. These included unusual events, such as in- and outpatient cases as well as fatalities.

The rate of complications of 0.32% (Table 1) was very small, but the occurrence of 6 deaths and 27 hospital admissions led to the establishment by the TUI of medical services and support in a remote destination without medical facilities on an island of the Republic of the Maldives.

The Maldives, located in the Indian Ocean, have about 150000 inhabitants. They consist of 19 atolls with 1302 islands spread out over hundreds of kilometers. Only 202 islands are inhabited and 55 are tourist resorts. In 1986/1987 almost 29000 German tourists went there, of whom 8000 were TUI clients. These tourists are dispersed over many islands, with varying distances from Male, the capital.

The 120-bed hospital in Male has, for example, internal medicine, surgical, and obstetrics departments with about 11 physicians on duty in the mornings. The rest of the time there is an emergency service. Male Hospital takes care of about 80000 in- and outpatients/year.

**Table 1.** Rates of health impairment among travelers (1982/1983)

| Destination | Number of tourists | Incidence (%) |
|---|---|---|
| South America (including Brazil, Andes, Amazon) | 3381 | 0.35 |
| Africa (including Kenya, Seychelles, Tanzania, Mauritius) | 13796 | 0.11 |
| South India (including Sri Lanka, Maldives, southern India) | 12343 | 0.11 |
| Southeast Asia (including Thailand, Burma, Hongkong, Indonesia, Singapore, Malaysia, Nepal, Philippines) | 8126 | 0.69 |
| | 37646 | 0.32 |

The number of practicing physicians/10000 inhabitants is 0.72. (In comparison, the Federal Republic of Germany has 237.) The urban and rural infant mortality rate in total is about 70.0 [1].

With the approval of the Ministry of Health, TUI started a pilot project in the winter season of 1983/1984. This project consisted of stationing of German doctors on one island to take care of the TUI clients. In October 1985, this became a permanent arrangement with the support of the local tour operator. Universal Enterprises, as well as TUI, who carry the costs of transportation, lodging and board jointly. The selection of physicians is based on knowledge of general and intensive care medicine and of diving medicine. The tour of duty is normally 2–4 weeks. The physicians receive free transport, room and board, and an accompanying person pays a special reduced rate.

The physicians are stationed at Kuramathi, about 3 h by boat from Male. This island has a capacity for 210 TUI clients and 130 clients from other tour operators. In addition, about 60 natives make up staff and personnel. Nearby is the island Rasdu, on which about 500 Maledivians live. There is a windsurfing school and a diving school on Kuramathi.

The physician has his own bungalow. It is equipped for primary treatment. It has a refrigerator, and an assortment of medicines. If these run low, replacements can be ordered from Germany. In special cases, medicine is available from the hospital on Male.

The physician on duty on the island can be reached at any time. It has become the custom that this doctor holds a consultation period 1 h before sundown on a daily basis. All medical services are free. TUI and other tourists, staff and personnel of Kuramathi Island, as well as sick natives of the Island of Rasdu, all are treated by this physician. This has become a sort of development aid, which is welcomed by both the visiting doctors and the natives.

**Table 2.** Diagnosis and frequency of health impairments[a] in the Maldives 3 January 1986–15 January 1987

| ICD · 9 code | Condition | | Number | (%) |
|---|---|---|---|---|
| 380–389 | Ear disease | | 164 | 24.6 |
| 910–919 | Superficial injuries | | 93 | 13.9 |
| 990–995 | Sun allergies | | 84 | 12.6 |
| 460–496 | Respiratory diseases | | 65 | 9.8 |
| 680–698 | Dermal diseases, | 21 | 51 | 7.7 |
| | sunburn | 30 | | |
| 530–579 | Digestive system | 30 | 47 | 7.1 |
| | diarrheas | 17 | | |
| 920–949 | Sprains, contusions | | 27 | 4.1 |
| 700–724 | Arthropathies, dorsopathies | | 23 | 3.5 |
| 820–854 | Fractures, dislocations | | 22 | 3.3 |
| 401–459 | Circulatory system | | 18 | 2.7 |
| | Other diseases | | 72 | 10.7 |
| | Total | | 666 | 100.0 |

[a] Classified in accordance with the ICD · 9 code

Every physician stationed on Kuramathi is obliged to keep careful statistics of his diagnosis and therapies in accordance with a given format. This is to keep an objective record of the occurrence of illness in the destination. I hereby return to the initially mentioned lack of hard statistics and data.

There have been no diving accidents in the last few years but the medical diving specialist from the neighboring island occupied by the Club Méditerranée is available. This island also has a two-man decompression chamber. The department for medical technical emergency service of the Naval medical Institute of the German Navy in Kiel can be consulted via telex.

Table 2 shows the diagnostic ICD.9 categories [2] between 3 January 1986 and 15 January 1987 for 666 treated tourists.

Ear diseases (all forms of otitis) were the most frequent complaint. This demonstrates that in a tropical paradise for bathing and diving, in warm water, the tourist does not know how to take care of himself, and thereby encourages laceration of the outer ear. The great number of superficial injuries is largely caused by walking around barefoot. The superinfections caused by the tropical climate often cause minor cuts to become major wounds. Only 2.5% of the tourists consulted the physician because of diarrhea. Of interest were injuries on the upper extremities, resulting from contact with moray eels and stingrays.

The "medical care for tourists" project has proven to be useful. Early treatment of illness and injury made it posible to avoid or at least lessen the typical tropical superinfections. It also avoided burdening the Male Hospital with additional outpatients and language was not a problem.

## References

1. Statistical Year Book of the Maldives 1983
2. Internatinal Classification of Diseases (ICD) 1979, 9th Revision

# First Aid Kits of International Air Companies: Are They Really Appropriate?

E. Missoni, G. Bertolaso, M. diGennaro, F. Vichi,
C. Djeddah, and R. Guerra

During long flights it is not unusual to hear a passenger asking the steward(ess) for treatment of minor ailments; less often, however, it happens that a physician is paged to assist a real medical emergency. In both cases appropriate intervention needs to rely on the availability of a set of basic instruments and drugs. The preparedness of flying staff members is equallly important.

The idea of this work originated from a few experiences that some of us had on board aircraft on intercontinental flights. Three episodes, which we consider significant for the present discussion, are described below.

The first case refers to an infant 6 months of age traveling with his mother from Europe to Latin America. After a few hours' flight the child experienced worsening of acute diarrhea he had been suffering since the day before. Worried by the frequent watery stools and by the fact that her child looked unwell, the mother sought help from the flight attendant. Purely by chance, a physician realized that somebody was ill on board and offered his help, which was gratefully accepted. When the physician took over, the child had already suffered one episode of vomiting, had repeated liquid stools and presented signs of moderate dehydration. By that time he had already received a diphenoxylate-based antidiarrheal drug and intake of food had been suspended as well as intake of fluids after the child vomited. Surprisingly enough, 1 liter oral rehydration salts packets of WHO-recommended composition were included in the first aid kit and oral rehydration could immediately be started with an adequate solution. The general condition of the child improved soon and his mother was reassured that there was no need to interrupt the journey at the first stopover after having crossed the ocean; she happily reached her final destination.

The second case refers to a man in his forties who fainted, knocked his head and remained unconscious for about 1 min. A physician was immediately paged and on examination he found the injured passenger still cyanotic and with a feeble pulse. Oxygen was immediately administered, but neither a sphygmomanometer nor a stethoscope was available. A diagnosis of seizure was finally made, but no antiepileptic drugs were on board. The patient slowly recovered and an emergency landing at the nearest airport was not considered essential.

The last case refers to a young European woman returning from a prolonged stay in a western African country presenting with chills and fever. On board there was not even a thermometer; a malaria attack was strongly suspected; however, only salicylic acid could be administered, because no antimalarial drugs were available.

These and other experiences led us to review the contents of first aid kits of international airlines. Information was not easy to obtain, mainly because of bureaucratic obstacles and/or inadequate answers from the airlines contacted.

Only one study on the subject has been found in the literature of the last 5 years [1]. A basic cabin attendant medical kit and a more complete first aid kit is present in all aircraft of the main airlines on international flights. Recently a more comprehensive "doctor's kit" has been introduced both by European and North American commercial airlines; an initial evaluation of it has been traced in the above-mentioned study [1]. The "doctor's kit" adopted by certain companies is a rather sophisticated resuscitation kit complete with airways, ambu, aspirator, endotracheal tubes, scalpels, scissors, forceps and other instruments. Drugs include epinephrine, atrophine, diuretics, digoxin, cortisone and others; surprisingly intravenous fluids seem not to be always included. This type of professional emergency kit is obviously only for use by qulified medical personnel.

Both the "first aid kit" and the "cabin attendant medical kit" contain basic tools for dressing of minor injuries and drugs for common ailments, use of which is not restricted to professionally trained personnel. While antimalarial drugs seem to be included in most airline's emergency equipment, unfortunately oral rehydration solutions are not. In most cases drugs contained in the emergency kits are labeled with proprietary names, which may cause some difficulty for a foreign doctor on board wanting to act rapidly, especially when further description on the packing is not in English or another widely used language. Examining the instructions for the flight attendant included in first aid kits, we found in some cases the indicated use of drugs inadequate if not potentially harmful, such as the use of *salicylic acid* for vomitus, *hyoscine butylbromide* for "excitment or psychic tension" and combination of *bacitracin, neomycin, phtalylsulfathiazol* and *pectin* for diarrhea, including in children. Finally, we were surprised to know that refill of used kits is generally made only at the airline's home base, with the possible risk of inadequate intervention in subsequent emergencies on the same aircraft.

## Conclusions and Recommendations

Experience shows that an appropriate emergency kit is needed on board aircraft on long flights. The level of sophistication of equipment needed needs to be evaluated further on the basis of extensive studies on the incidence of medical emergencies on board. Standardization must then be advocated and reduced specific lists of WHO essential drugs must be adopted with international nonproprietary names and instructions for use in English and possibly other official languages. Flight attendants should receive specific periodic training and simple but comprehensive instructions should be included in every first aid kit. Standardization must be advocated for drugs and instructions contained in every first aid kit.

## Reference

1. Rodenberg H (1987) Medical emergencies aboard commercial aircraft. Ann Emerg Med 16:1373–1374

# Conclusions

# The Present and Future of Travel Medicine: Summary of and Outlook from the Conference

D.J. Bradley

This meeting has provided all those attending with a feast, both educationally and intellectually, and also culinarily at the banquet! Indeed some may now have some degree of indigestion – intellectual or physical. To summarize such an array of papers and other material is scarcely feasible, even if it were desirable. The principle once recommended by a preacher may apply in educating travellers, but is not really applicable to summarizing a conference: "Tell them what your are going to say, then say it, then tell them what you have said."

Some at the conference would wish to know in full what took place at the simultaneous sessions they could not attend, but this can be gained from the Proceedings rather than from a summary, though the very high attendance at all sessions has been a striking feature of the conference.

At the opening of the conference I made three main general points, which were to draw attention, firstly, to the greatly increased range and possibilities for travel at present and secondly to the diversity of types of migrant or traveller.

Parenthetically, one might note the very different mental picture produced by the words "migrant" and "traveller". My first doctoral student was an Iranian epidemiologist of immense dedication who studied the migrating Kashgai tribe in Iran with enormous diligence, dragging many thousands from their camels in order to administer a detailed questionnaire to each one. Yet somehow, though all three terms fit, it gives a differing impression if we consider them as "nomads" or "seasonal migrants" or "overland travellers". The third general point made at the start of the conference was to let the subject of travel medicine define itself in the papers given.

The conference has indeed shown the range of travel now available. The scale of many travel activities has been shown to be very great. Not only are there hundreds of millions of air passengers each year but we are told of some 50000 trekkers in Nepal annually and several million visitors to China. The diversity of travellers and their needs have also been made abundantly clear and is a topic to which I shall revert later.

The subject of travel medicine has to some extent defined itself, and it is instructive, with hindsight "to count the trees in order to describe the wood." In Table 1 are listed the broad subject categories dealt with in the conference. The activity in each category is measured in three ways: by the number of papers (excluding posters), which happen to total 100; by the number of contributions weighted as follows: 4 points for a longer paper, 2 points for a short

**Table 1.** Travel medicine as defined by papers at the conference

| | Papers | Weighted[a] contributions | |
|---|---|---|---|
| | | Units | % |
| General | | | |
| General papers | 6 | 24 | 7 |
| Disease patterns | 9 | 22 | 7 |
| Infections | | | |
| Diarrhoea | 11 | 35 | 11 |
| Malaria | 12 | 48 | 15 |
| STD/HIV infection | 3 | 16 | 5 |
| Other infections | 9 | 29 | 9 |
| Non-infective disease | | | |
| Miscellaneous non-infective disease | 3 | 10 | 3 |
| Advice | | | |
| Immunization | 16 | 42 | 13 |
| Advice | 11 | 38 | 12 |
| Care | | | |
| Care of travellers | 6 | 11 | 3 |
| Specific groups of travellers | 4 | 18 | 6 |
| Transport | | | |
| Ships | 2 | 4 | 1 |
| Flight | 3 | 11 | 3 |
| Locations | | | |
| Altitude | 5 | 14 | 4 |
| Total | 100 | 322 | |

[a] See text

paper and 1 point for a poster. The total comprised 322 points, expressed in percentage terms in the last column. The table thus illustrates both the range of topics covered by the conference and also those of greatest present interest and activity. In Fig. 1 these topics are rearranged along the course of the "simple journey" or the "travel cycle," where travel is viewed as beginning with advice and immunization, passing through various potential hazards whilst away and on the journey and returning to the point of origin, possibly with needs for diagnosis and therapy. In general, specific diseases are placed on the convex side of the journey curve in the figure and traveller concerns on the concave aspect. A simple diagram has to omit much, and cannot make clear the distinction, that affects much leisure travel, between the journey itself as simply a means – as when the package tourist flies to Kenya – and the journey as an end in itself, for the person cruising in the Greek islands, trekking in the Himalaya, or on a safari. It also cannot reflect the diverse forms of travel discussed in my opening talk nor the "mirror-image" traveller from a tropical or third world country to Europe and his or her return.

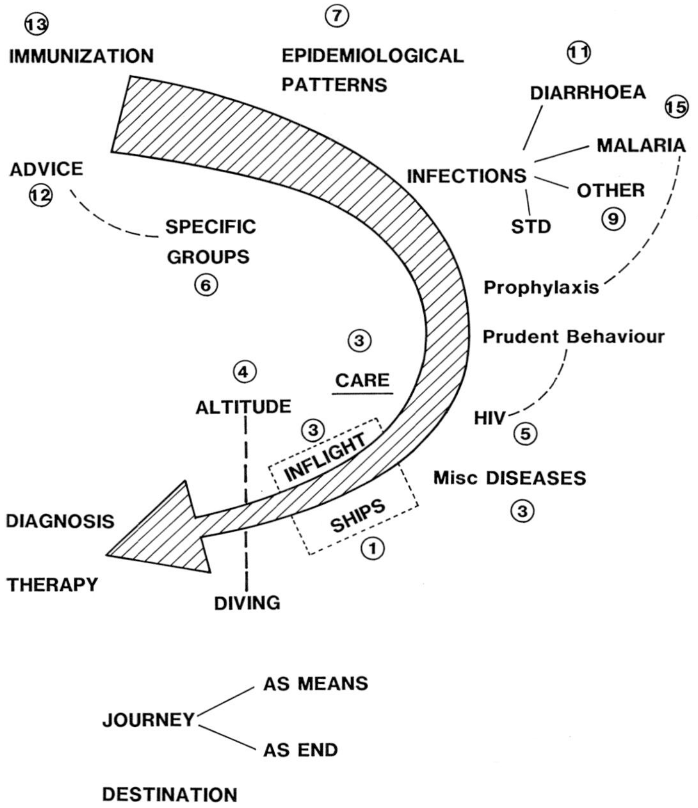


**Fig. 1.** Distribution of the conference papers by subject (percentage of total *in circles*) arranged along a schematic journey

Certain emphases emerge clearly from Fig. 1, and they provoke questions for a future conference on travel medicine. In particular, there is an emphasis on specific diseases, their problems and prevention or management. This partly reflects the way in which science advances by considering one particular issue at a time and partly the work of those presenting papers. There is a relative scarcity, by comparison, of papers addressing the needs of particular groups of travellers. The needs of pregnant travellers and of small children were considered, but it may be that at a subsequent conference these needs, and those of other particular groups – overlanders in Asia, those who dive near coral reefs, small babies being taken to the tropics for a prolonged period – may receive detailed attention. The other area where several speakers pointed to our limited organized solutions concerned access to effective care whilst abroad. If one has the misfortune to get ill or injured as a visitor, where can one seek competent and reliable medical care? Often there is little information quickly available, unless the traveller is part of a business enterprise or organized party, and such information is usually needed at short notice.

Three groups of infections understandably dominated the discussions: the diarrhoeal diseases because of their extremely high incidence in travellers, malaria because it is potentially lethal but is treatable, and HIV-AIDS because there is no vaccine, no chemoprophylaxis, and it is not curable. On the positive side are both the emphasis given to advisory services and the progress achieved in improving vaccines and immunization schedules.

These are the topics covered in our conference. To turn to the *outlook* for travel medicine involves becoming frankly subjective, but some guidance is obtained from considering which papers have been especially memorable.

Two particular types of study stand out – those based on long experience, and careful population-based studies.

Papers in which the authors have shared their long and special experience of particular problems have been the most readily appreciated as being both helpful and applicable. This has been especially the case where workers have moved from a description of their own experience to an analysis of it so as to present a more generally applicable structured system for approaching a problem. It seems invidious to mention only a few contributions when so many of the papers at the meeting were outstanding, but illustrations of my main points may make them clearer. The very clear account of the psychiatric problems of travel (E. F. Rigamer, this volume) took what needs to be viewed as a very confused area and applied the fruits of long and deep experience to produce a structured approach to this area which all will find helpful.

In many ways the less-studied subjects have proved to provide the most satisfying papers. Some have covered topics of which we were previously unaware and so we are conscious of having learned a great deal. Where there has been a single good paper on a topic the subject has perhaps acquired a spurious clarity, which disappears as more people study the area and come up with differing conclusions.

In the key areas for travel medicine many have shared their experience and studies so that the subjects re-acquire their complexity. This applies especially to diarrhoea prevention and to malaria prophylaxis where the vast amount of information is still inadequate for rational choice and where the clarity which comes from restricted information has certainly been dispersed. One is reminded of the lines of Alexander Pope on that tidier subject, physics, modified:

Natute and nature's laws lay sunk in night
God said "let Newton be", and all was light.

To which a more cynical poet, mindful of a great man who worked in Zurich, added:

It could not last; the devil shouting "Ho,
Let Einstein be", restored the status quo.

Once we reach that ampler disorder that comes from fuller knowledge, how can we reach through to wise practice? There are at least two main approaches. First is the need to understand processes, to get beyond the anecdotes and clinical experience to the underlying physiology, epidemiology or pathogenesis, as was illustrated in the papers on jet lag. The second approach is by way of the controlled trial – the work of Dr. Fogh, reported to the conference, on a controlled comparison of two antimalarial regimes is an example of how clear data may be obtained.

It was good to see the number of population-based studies of an epidemiological type presented to the conference. These included Dr. Steffen's remarkable large studies of airline passengers on package tours and several others. There is still a long way to go in this area. More such studies are needed. Dropout rates are still higher than is desirable, especially when one is seeking rare events such as deaths, severe side effects of prophylactics, uncommon diseases. They can be too easily missed if losses from follow-up are at all numerous. Nor are issues of bias – more in the selection of the study population than in sampling – yet faced up to fully. But a great step forward is marked by these population-based studies. There is an increasing need for travel physicians to think epidemiologically and to plan any studies they do accordingly.

Although there is much inevitable diversity in the recommendations for malaria prophylaxis, there is also great uneveness in the way advice on the prevention of malaria is given. The same applies to other travellers' health problems. I was much impressed that among the many examples of different aspects of the provision of advice there were examples of very good practice in each area of work at the conference, as well as poor examples in many areas. Examples of education and advice of a very high standard included the Club Med simple colourful health brochures for package tourists, several clinics for individual advice, the Danish video film for HIV/AIDS prevention, Masta for computer-based personal written advice to fit individual journeys, British Airways for announcements of malaria risk prior to landing, Swiss and German airlines for collaboration with surveys, and so on. If all advice and health education reached the standards of the best in each area we should have much of which to be proud. Perhaps the conference, or a successor, could promote and disseminate examples of good practice. The manuals by Maurice King on third world health care come to mind. They are immensely comprehensive and detailed and each country tends to plagiarize selected parts of the manuals to meet national needs.

It is certainly important to make the advice appropriate to the person. The package tourist does not want to read a monograph on health. The leader of a Himalayan expedition may be glad of and need a full account of how to deal with the health problems he may encounter. The long-term expatriate tropical resident has yet other needs and a future conference could specifically aim to focus on good material to advise each group of travellers.

There are other areas where standardization rather than personally appropriate diversity is needed. This especially applies to reporting of data on imported disease and collection of travel statistics for the comparative assessment of health risks. There is also a need for reliable lists of good health care facilities for travellers taken ill in each country and the conference highlighted the need for information of this sort.

This confernce, and that held earlier in the year at Rimini, which addressed problems of the Mediterranean aera in particular, have served to bring travel

**Table 2.** Features of this conference and for the future of travel medicine

| |
|---|
| Strengths of the present |
| Experiences of particular travel situations |
| Studies of diarrhoea and of antimalarials |
| Good examples of the provision of different types of advice |
| Shared experience |
| Issues for future emphasis |
| Analysis of experience to give a structured view |
| Population-based studies |
| Controlled trials of interventions |
| Understanding processes |
| Provision of advice to specific groups |

medicine as a subject to the crossroads. It needs to gain a philosophy and a coherent way of viewing its subject. One approach is a restrictive and solely practical one. It would be pragmatic and confine its interest to tourists, dealing with prevention and with care on returning to the United Kingdom. This is in part very sound, but also is a narrow view. The physician views the visited country nationals simply as environment, he thinks only as a clinician and does not worry about sources of bias in any data. Such a narrow approach also omits the interests of many here – the long-term tropical residents, visitors to the United Kingdom from developing countries and long-term students from the tropics in Europe.

To cope with all these needs of travellers and concerns of physicians requires broad bases of understanding. Migration is the key issue or feature, including multilocal residence and transfer between different places or habitats. The traveller is characterized by changes in his or her environment and also behavioural changes. For the future we need much more careful population-based information on health, better understanding of the processes leading to illness in travellers, and clearly formulated advice, usually on a group-specific base (e.g. for babies being taken to live in the tropics, alpine climbers, or other defined groups). We need to give more attention to access to health care overseas, and especially dissemination of the best practice in each aspect of travel medicine.

There is thus a substantial travel medicine agenda, and it would be very desirable to meet again in 2–3 years' time to review progress (see Table 2).

In conclusion, the arrangements made for this Conference on International Travel Medicine by Dr. Steffen and his organizing committee were an outstanding example of healthy and well-planned travel. If all travellers' journeys were as well looked after and our stays abroad so perfectly managed, we would indeed be fortunate. The conference was indeed grateful to the Committee.